Lecture Notes in Networks and Systems

Volume 519

AF892971

Series Editor

Janusz Kacprzyk, Systems Research Institute, Polish Academy of Sciences, Warsaw, Poland

Advisory Editors

Fernando Gomide, Department of Computer Engineering and Automation—DCA, School of Electrical and Computer Engineering—FEEC, University of Campinas—UNICAMP, São Paulo, Brazil

Okyay Kaynak, Department of Electrical and Electronic Engineering, Bogazici University, Istanbul, Turkey

Derong Liu, Department of Electrical and Computer Engineering, University of Illinois at Chicago, Chicago, USA
Institute of Automation, Chinese Academy of Sciences, Beijing, China

Witold Pedrycz, Department of Electrical and Computer Engineering, University of Alberta, Alberta, Canada
Systems Research Institute, Polish Academy of Sciences, Warsaw, Poland

Marios M. Polycarpou, Department of Electrical and Computer Engineering, KIOS Research Center for Intelligent Systems and Networks, University of Cyprus, Nicosia, Cyprus

Imre J. Rudas, Óbuda University, Budapest, Hungary

Jun Wang, Department of Computer Science, City University of Hong Kong, Kowloon, Hong Kong

The series "Lecture Notes in Networks and Systems" publishes the latest developments in Networks and Systems—quickly, informally and with high quality. Original research reported in proceedings and post-proceedings represents the core of LNNS.

Volumes published in LNNS embrace all aspects and subfields of, as well as new challenges in, Networks and Systems.

The series contains proceedings and edited volumes in systems and networks, spanning the areas of Cyber-Physical Systems, Autonomous Systems, Sensor Networks, Control Systems, Energy Systems, Automotive Systems, Biological Systems, Vehicular Networking and Connected Vehicles, Aerospace Systems, Automation, Manufacturing, Smart Grids, Nonlinear Systems, Power Systems, Robotics, Social Systems, Economic Systems and other. Of particular value to both the contributors and the readership are the short publication timeframe and the world-wide distribution and exposure which enable both a wide and rapid dissemination of research output.

The series covers the theory, applications, and perspectives on the state of the art and future developments relevant to systems and networks, decision making, control, complex processes and related areas, as embedded in the fields of interdisciplinary and applied sciences, engineering, computer science, physics, economics, social, and life sciences, as well as the paradigms and methodologies behind them.

Indexed by SCOPUS, INSPEC, WTI Frankfurt eG, zbMATH, SCImago.

All books published in the series are submitted for consideration in Web of Science.

For proposals from Asia please contact Aninda Bose (aninda.bose@springer.com).

Jyotsna Kumar Mandal · Debashis De
Editors

Frontiers of ICT in Healthcare

Proceedings of EAIT 2022

Springer

Editors
Jyotsna Kumar Mandal
Department of Computer Science
and Engineering
University of Kalyani
Kalyani, West Bengal, India

Debashis De
Department of Computer Science
and Engineering
School of Computational Science
Maulana Abul Kalam Azad University
of Technology
Kolkata, West Bengal, India

ISSN 2367-3370 ISSN 2367-3389 (electronic)
Lecture Notes in Networks and Systems
ISBN 978-981-19-5190-9 ISBN 978-981-19-5191-6 (eBook)
https://doi.org/10.1007/978-981-19-5191-6

© The Editor(s) (if applicable) and The Author(s), under exclusive license to Springer Nature Singapore Pte Ltd. 2023
This work is subject to copyright. All rights are solely and exclusively licensed by the Publisher, whether the whole or part of the material is concerned, specifically the rights of translation, reprinting, reuse of illustrations, recitation, broadcasting, reproduction on microfilms or in any other physical way, and transmission or information storage and retrieval, electronic adaptation, computer software, or by similar or dissimilar methodology now known or hereafter developed.
The use of general descriptive names, registered names, trademarks, service marks, etc. in this publication does not imply, even in the absence of a specific statement, that such names are exempt from the relevant protective laws and regulations and therefore free for general use.
The publisher, the authors, and the editors are safe to assume that the advice and information in this book are believed to be true and accurate at the date of publication. Neither the publisher nor the authors or the editors give a warranty, expressed or implied, with respect to the material contained herein or for any errors or omissions that may have been made. The publisher remains neutral with regard to jurisdictional claims in published maps and institutional affiliations.

This Springer imprint is published by the registered company Springer Nature Singapore Pte Ltd.
The registered company address is: 152 Beach Road, #21-01/04 Gateway East, Singapore 189721, Singapore

Preface

With the explosive growth of e-business, artificial intelligence, intelligent systems, and computer visions in the healthcare systems, the researchers in academics and industry face more and more technological challenges. Computational intelligence requires of catering intelligent healthcare applications with the significant associations with high-speed wireless networks, autonomous systems, and the Internet of Things with enhanced quality of healthcare services. The IoT empowers the healthcare professionals and researchers to be more observant and associate with the patients prognostically. Healthcare information gathered from the essential IoT devices can assist medical practitioners recognise the finest treatment procedure for patients and influence the anticipated consequences.

The Seventh Edition of the International Conference on Emerging Applications of Information Technology (EAIT 2022) organised by the Computer Society of India (CSI) Kolkata Chapter emphasises Frontiers of ICT in Healthcare organised during 27–28 March 2022 in hybrid mode. The 1st day of the conference was organised at Sister Nivedita University, Kolkata. The 2nd day was organised at MAKAUT, West Bengal, Salt Lake City, Kolkata, and the last day of the conference was held at the University of Kalyani, West Bengal. The previously organised EAIT conference series with the accepted and peer-reviewed papers had been published by Springer.

The conference is planned to host in every year to access the new development/advances in computing. Nowadays, specifically in the COVID-19 pandemic, the healthcare analytics have gained the momentum towards the critical healthcare services, diagnosis, treatment, and entire management.

The essential utilities of information and communication technologies (ICT) in the hospitals and medical care units are for digital storage of medical information that assistances to reclaim the medical information straightforwardly. Through the ICT, the information can be transmitted to the patients as well as to the doctors and medical care units for consultation. The patient can have medical repository that can be used anywhere and/or anytime. Additionally, the 5G and 6G heterogeneous networks are developed based on quantum computers. Post-quantum cryptography, IoT connecting edge devices need security using blockchain and real-time computations in ICT-induced health care. AI-enabled intelligent mobile connectivity is the future arena of communication. The integrated theme of this seventh edition of the conference EAIT 2022 is the "Frontiers of ICT in Healthcare". The domain experts on ICT-based health care, Internet of Health Things, medical things, cloud-dew-edge-fog computing in ICT-health care, blockchain technology, medical image processing, have participated in this event as the keynote speakers, contributors, and resource persons to elaborate their significant thoughts and contributed with their original research manuscripts. More than 400 participants joined both in the online and offline modes in the event across the globe.

The conference's main objective was to bring together academic and industrial experts of the research community and to highlight critical issues, identify trends, and develop a vision of the intelligence systems for future applications from a design, deployment, and operational standpoint. Total 272 original research manuscripts have been received. Out of 272 articles from 11 countries, only 57 articles have been selected for publications into the proceedings by Springer Nature. The entire conference proceeding is published within a single volume.

This volume contains the chapters authored by various researchers worldwide. This volume contains the research articles which are classified into six parts, such as (a) Healthcare Informatics, (b) Machine Learning in Health care, (c) Healthcare Security and Blockchain, (d) Health care in COVID-19 Scenario, (e) IoT in Health care, and (f) Image Processing in Health care.

Part One consists of the ten research articles, contributed by the allied researchers, and principally illustrates the healthcare informatics, such as AI- and ML-inspired speech recognition and sentiment analytics in health care, malaria diagnosis, fake news identifications during pandemic, melanoma detection, and stress prediction.

Part Two consists of thirteen articles mainly focused on the performance evaluations of the healthcare parameters through the advanced strategies of representation learning and explainable artificial intelligence mechanisms. The healthcare diagnosis and identification contexts of medical features consist of visualisations of genome sequences, prediction of heart diseases, emotion recognition, e-healthcare management, cerebral attacks, breast cancer, lung cancer, faetal and mental health, thyroid identification.

Eight research articles are included in Part Three. The significant contributions by the researchers include in this part, viz. healthcare security and blockchain. The authors have depicted their significant contributions on the development of healthcare ecosystems, clinical data communication, medical image authentication, secured and authenticated e-Health record storage paradigms.

Furthermore, eight original research articles are included in Part Four. This part categorically illustrated the researches on health care in the COVID-19 scenarios. Studies on Spike Protein of coronavirus, data analytics on COVID epidemic data, coronavirus detection models, and identifications of diverge variants of COVID-19 have been illustrated in this part.

Part Five consists of six original research articles, typically focussed on the healthcare analytics in the context of Internet of Things (IoT). The researchers have illustrated IoT-based health monitoring devices, smart safety applications, medical or health resource sharing applications, privacy preservation on the biometric data in

Internet of Medical Things, IoT-enabled sleep monitoring framework, and encryption mechanism in the domains of Internet of Medical Things.

The last part, Part Six, consists of twelve research contributions that have been titled as the image processing in health care. In this part, cardiovascular disease prediction models, medical image security strategies, vessel segregation model, medical image segmentation and formalisations methodologies, breast cancer diagnosis framework, brain tumour segmentation algorithm, online patient monitoring mechanism, multi-lingual textual pattern recognition paradigms, and so forth are well illustrated.

Eventually, on behalf of the organization committee, we would like to express our sincere gratitude to all keynote speakers, esteemed reviewers, authors, and participants making our conference programme a grand success. This proceeding will be a valuable document to the researchers, budding engineers, graduate, postgraduate students, and the entire healthcare professionals.

Kalyani, India — Jyotsna Kumar Mandal
Kolkata, India — Debashis De

Contents

Editors and Contributors

About the Editors

Jyotsna Kumar Mandal, M. Tech. (Computer Science, University of Calcutta), Ph.D. (Engineering, Jadavpur University) in the field of Data Compression and Error Correction Techniques and Professor in Computer Science and Engineering, University of Kalyani, India. Former Dean Faculty of Engineering, Technology and Management 2008–2012 (two consecutive terms), 32 years of teaching and research experiences. Served as Professor, Computer Applications, Kalyani Government Engineering College for two years. Served as Associate and Assistant Professor at University of North Bengal for sixteen years. Life Member of Computer Society of India since 1992 and Life Member of Cryptology Research Society of India. Member of AIRCC. Honorary Chairman of CSI Kolkata Chapter 2016–17. Working in the field of Network Security, Steganography, Remote Sensing and GIS Application, Image Processing, Wireless and Sensor Networks. Domain Expert of Uttarbanga Krishi Viswavidyalaya, Bidhan Chandra Krishi Viswavidyalaya for planning and integration of Public domain networks. Chief Editor, *Advanced Computing: An International Journal*, Associate Editor (Guest), *Microsystem Technologies*, Springer, Chief Editor, *CSI Journal of Computing*, Editor of Proceedings of ETCS 2012, NIDS-98 and ERC-95 of CSI. Twenty-four scholars awarded Ph.D., four submitted till January 2017, and 8 scholars are pursuing for their Ph.D. degree. Published five books from LAP-Lambert Academic Publishing, Germany, and one book from IGI Global publishers, Indexed by Thomson Reuters. Total number of publications is more than 400 including 180 publications in various International Journals. Edited fifteen volumes as volume editor from Science Direct, Springer, CSI, etc., Organizing various international Conferences of Springer and Science Direct. Director, IQAC, University of Kalyani, Chairman, Center for Information Resource Management (CIRM), Kalyani University. He has successfully executed five Research Projects funded by AICTE, Ministry of IT Government of West Bengal. Department of Higher Education, Government of West Bengal conferred him the "Siksha Ratna" award in 2018.

Prof. Debashis De earned his M.Tech. from the University of Calcutta in 2002 and his Ph.D. (Engineering) from Jadavpur University in 2005. He is the Professor and Director in the Department of Computer Science and Engineering of the West Bengal University of Technology, India, and Adjunct Research Fellow at the University of Western Australia, Australia. He is a Senior Member of the IEEE. Life Member of CSI and Member of the International Union of Radio science. He worked as R&D Engineer for Telektronics and Programmer at Cognizant Technology Solutions. He was awarded the prestigious Boyscast Fellowship by the Department of Science and Technology, Government of India, to work at the Herriot-Watt University, Scotland, UK. He received the Endeavour Fellowship Award during 2008–2009 by DEST Australia to work at the University of Western Australia. He received the Young Scientist award both in 2005 at New Delhi and in 2011 at Istanbul, Turkey, from the International Union of Radio Science, Head Quarter, Belgium. His research interests include mobile cloud computing, green mobile networks. He has published in more than 250 peer-reviewed international journals in IEEE, IET, Elsevier, Springer, World Scientific, Wiley, IETE, Taylor Francis and ASP, 100 International conference papers, six researches monographs in springer, CRC, NOVA and ten text books published by Person education. He is Associate Editor of journal IEEE ACCESS, Editor Hybrid computational intelligence, Journal Array, Elsevier.

Contributors

Isha Agarwal Sardar Vallabhbhai National Institute of Technology, Surat, Gujarat, India

Akshat Agrawal Amity University, Gurgaon, Hariyana, India

Ravin Ahuja Center of ICT/ICE, Covenant University, Ota, Nigeria

Ankit Anand Department of Computer Science and Engineering, Meghnad Saha Institute of Technology, Kolkata, India

Adithya Sreemandiram Anil School of Computer Science and Engineering, Vellore Institute of Technology, Vellore, Tamil Nadu, India

Sameer Antani National Library of Medicine, National Institutes of Health, Bethesda, MD, USA

Md. Safkat Azad Arnab Department of Information and Communication Technology, Bangladesh University of Professionals, Dhaka, Bangladesh, India

Chinmay Ashtikar School of Computer Science and Engineering, Vellore Institute of Technology, Vellore, Tamil Nadu, India

Joseph Bamidele Awotunde Department of Computer Science, University of Ilorin, Ilorin, Nigeria

Femi Emmanuel Ayo Department of Computer Science, McPherson University, Seriki-Sotayo, Abeokuta, Nigeria

Tina Babu Department of Computer Science and Engineering, School of Engineering, Dayananda Sagar University, Bengaluru, Karnataka, India

Aritra Bandyopadhyay Department of CSE, Supreme Knowledge Foundation Group of Institutions, Mankundu, India

Rathit Bandyopadhyay Siliguri Government Polytechnic, Siliguri, India

Sakhi Bandyopadhyay Department of Computer Science and Engineering, Assam University, Silchar, Assam, India

Saradwata Bandyopadhyay University of Engineering and Management, Kolkata, India

Aniket Banerjee IIEST Shibpur, Howrah, West Bengal, India

Shubhendu Banerjee Department of CSE, Narula Institute of Technology, Kolkata, India

Sinjini Banerjee Department of CSE, Hooghly Engineering & Technology College, Pipulpati, Hooghly, West Bengal, India

Md. Hasan Al Banna Bangladesh University of Professionals, Dhaka, Bangladesh

Subhas Barman Jalpaiguri Government Engineering College, Jalpaiguri, India

Arghya Basu St. Xavier's College (Autonomous), Kolkata, India

Dougani Bentabet Lab Smart Grids Renewable Energies, Tahri Mohammad University of Bechar, Béchar, Algeria

Dhritesh Bhagat Department of Computer Science and Engineering, Institute of Engineering and Management, Kolkata, India

Vandana Bhattacharjee Department of Computer Science and Engineering, Birla Institute of Technology, Jharkhand, India;
Birla Institute of Technology, Mesra, Ranchi, India

Dilip Kumar Bhattacharya University of Calcutta, Kolkata, India

Tanmay Bhattacharya Department of IT, Techno Main, Kolkata, India

Soumen Bhowmick Indian Institute of Engineering Science and Technology (IIEST), Shibpur, India

Suparna Biswas Department of Computer Science & Engineering, Maulana Abul Kalam Azad University of Technology, Kolkata, West Bengal, India

Sima Boro Central Institute of Technology, Kokrajhar, India

Sumit Chahar Amity School of Engineering and Technology, Amity University Maharashtra, Mumbai, India

Avishek Chakraborty Department of Engineering Science, Academy of Technology, Adisaptagram, West Bengal, India

Debasish Chakraborty RRSC-East, Indian Space Research Organization, Kolkata, India

Rajdeep Chakraborty Department of CSE, Chandigarh University, Chandigarh, India;
Department of CSE, Netaji Subhash Engineering College, Kolkata, India

Somenath Chakraborty Department of Computer Science and Information Systems, West Virginia University Institute of Technology, Beckley, United States

Bibhas Chandra Dhara Jadavpur University, Kolkata, India

Ayan Chatterjee Department of Information Technology, Center for eHealth, University of Agder, Kristiansand, Norway

Runa Chatterjee Department of CSE, Netaji Subhash Engineering College, Kolkata, India

Partha Chowdhuri Department of Computer Science, Vidyasagar University, Midnapore, West Bengal, India

Aditi Roy Chowdhury Women's Polytechnic, Kolkata, India

Debkumar Chowdhury University of Engineering and Management, Kolkata, India

Sasank Chunduri School of Computer Science and Engineering, Vellore Institute of Technology, Vellore, Tamil Nadu, India

Dhrupadi Das IIEST Shibpur, Howrah, West Bengal, India

Jishnu Das Department of Library and Information Science, University of Calcutta, Calcutta, India

Malabika Das Department of Mathematics, Heramba Chandra College, Kolkata, India

Nibaran Das CMATER Department of CSE, Jadavpur University, Kolkata, India

Priya Das Department of Computer Science, Chakdaha College, Chakdaha, West Bengal, India

Rajrupa Das University of Engineering and Management, Kolkata, India

Kousik Dasgupta Kalyani Government Engineering College, Kalyani, India

Shuvayan Ghosh Dastidar CMATER Department of CSE, Jadavpur University, Kolkata, India

Kakali Datta Department of Computer and System Sciences, Visva-Bharati University, Santiniketan, West Bengal, India

Debashis De Department of Computer Science and Engineering, Maulana Abul Kalam Azad University of Technology (MAKAUT), Kolkata, West Bengal, India

Susmit De University of Engineering and Management, Kolkata, India

Asish Debnath Department of Computer Science, Vidyasagar University, Midnapore, West Bengal, India

Shirsendu Dhar Fractal Analytics, Bengaluru, India

Trishita Dhara Department of Information Technology, Jadavpur University, Kolkata, West Bengal, India

Jhuma Dutta Jalpaiguri Government Engineering College, Jalpaiguri, India

Kalpita Dutta CMATER Department of CSE, Jadavpur University, Kolkata, India

Paramartha Dutta Visvabharati University, Santiniketan, India

Nilanjana Dutta Roy Department of Computer Science and Engineering, Institute of Engineering and Management, Kolkata, India

Raghav Gaur Symbiosis University, Symbiosis Institute of Technology, Pune, India

Mithlesh Gautam Truba College of Science and Technology, Bhopal, India

Arnobrata Ghosh University of Engineering and Management, Kolkata, India

Moumita Ghosh Siliguri Institute of Technology, Siliguri, India

Soumen Ghosh Narula Institute of Technology, Kolkata, India;
National Institute of Technology, Durgapur, India

Sudip Ghosh Indian Institute of Engineering Science and Technology (IIEST), Shibpur, Howrah, West Bengal, India

Supratim Ghosh Techno India University, Kolkata, West Bengal, India

Jayati Ghosh Dastidar St. Xavier's College (Autonomous), Kolkata, India

Ranjit Ghoshal St. Thomas' College of Engineering and Technology, Kolkata, India

Aman Gupta Department of CSE, National Institute of Technology Raipur, Raipur, Chhattisgarh, India

Pritish Gupta School of Information Technology and Engineering, Vellore Institute Technology, Vellore, Tamil Nadu, India

Angira Halder University of Engineering and Management, Kolkata, India

Md. Yeaminul Haque Bangladesh University of Professionals, Dhaka, Bangladesh

Joydev Hazra Heritage Institute of Technology, Kolkata, India

Savitha Hiremath Department of Computer Science Engineering, Dayananda Sagar University, Bengaluru, India

Sirshendu Hore Department of CSE, Hooghly Engineering & Technology College, Pipulpati, Hooghly, West Bengal, India

Sadaf Hussaini Truba College of Science and Technology, Bhopal, India

Sumaiya Thaseen Ikram School of Information Technology and Engineering, Vellore Institute Technology, Vellore, Tamil Nadu, India

Varun Iyengar Amity School of Engineering and Technology, Amity University Maharashtra, Mumbai, India

Ashika Jain Department of Information Technology, Amity University, Kolkata, India

Garima Jain Department of Computer Science and Engineering, Noida Institute of Engineering and Technology, Gr. Noida, India

K. Jairam Naik Department of CSE, National Institute of Technology Raipur, Raipur, Chhattisgarh, India

Biswapati Jana Department of Computer Science, Vidyasagar University, Midnapore, West Bengal, India

M. Shamim Kaiser IIT, Jahangirnagar University, Savar, Dhaka, Bangladesh

Gadisa Kana Department of Information Technology, Dambi Dollo University, Dembi Dolo, Welega, Ethiopia

Naveen Kanuri Department of Electronics and Communication, MLR Institute of Technology, Hyderabad, India

Mithun Karmakar Department of Computer Science and Engineering, CITK, Kokrajhar, Assam, India

Munia Sarwat Khan Department of Information and Communication Technology, Bangladesh University of Professionals, Dhaka, Bangladesh, India

Radha Krishna Bar Department of Computer Science and Engineering, Assam University, Silchar, India

Chandan Kumar SAGE University, Bhopal, India

Arju Kumari University of Engineering and Management, Kolkata, India

Mahantapas Kundu CMATER Department of CSE, Jadavpur University, Kolkata, West Bengal, India

Anto Rahul Mahiban School of Information Technology and Engineering, Vellore Institute Technology, Vellore, Tamil Nadu, India

Mufti Mahmud Department of Computer Science, Nottingham Trent University, Clifton, Nottingham, UK;
Medical Technologies Innovation Facility, Nottingham Trent University, Clifton, Nottingham, UK;
Computing and Informatics Research Centre, Nottingham Trent University, Clifton, Nottingham, UK

Bansibadan Maji National Institute of Technology, Durgapur, India

J. K. Mandal Department of CSE, Kalyani University, Kalyani, West Bengal, India

Sandip Mandal University of Engineering and Management, Kolkata, India

Kamta Nath Mishra Department of Computer Science and Engineering, Birla Institute of Technology, Jharkhand, India

Sanjukta Mishra University of Engineering and Management, Kolkata, India

Shashank Mishra Department of CSE, National Institute of Technology Raipur, Raipur, Chhattisgarh, India

Shivam P. Mishra Department of Computer Science and Engineering, Birla Institute of Technology, Jharkhand, India

Sanjay Misra Department of Computer Science and Comunication, Ostfold University, Halden, Norway

Sujoy Mistry Department of Computer Science and Engineering, Maulana Abul Kalam Azad University of Technology, Kolkata, India

Soma Mitra Department of Computational Science, Brainware University, Barasat, India

Rohan Molia Central Institute of Technology, Kokrajhar, India

Subhash Mondal Department of Computer Science and Engineering, Meghnad Saha Institute of Technology, Kolkata, India

Uttam Kr. Mondal Department of Computer Science, Vidyasagar University, Midnapore, West Bengal, India

Akash Mourya Truba College of Science and Technology, Bhopal, India

Subhadip Mukherjee Department of Computer Science and Engineering, Assam University, Silchar, Assam, India

Sumit Mukherjee Tata Consultancy Services, Kolkata, India

Tamoghna Mukherjee Department of CSE, Amity University, Kolkata, India

Somnath Mukhopadhyay Department of Computer Science and Engineering, Assam University, Silchar, Assam, India

Beddhu Murali Department of Computer Science and Information Systems, West Virginia University Institute of Technology, Beckley, United States

Amitava Nag Department of Computer Science and Engineering, Central Institute of Technology, Kokrajhar, Assam, India

Rekha R. Nair Department of Computer Applications, School of Engineering, Dayananda Sagar University, Bengaluru, Karnataka, India

Mauparna Nandan Department of Computer Applications, Haldia Institute of Technology, Haldia, India

Swathi Jamjala Narayanan School of Computer Science and Engineering, Vellore Institute of Technology, Vellore, Tamil Nadu, India

Mita Nasipuri CMATER Department of CSE, Jadavpur University, Kolkata, West Bengal, India

Nibedita Pahari Department of Software Engineering, Knowit AS, Oslo, Norway

Akash Pal Department of Computer Science and Engineering, Noida Institute of Engineering and Technology, Gr. Noida, India

Anabik Pal SRM University, Amaravati, Guntur District, Andhra Pradesh, India; National Library of Medicine, National Institutes of Health, Bethesda, MD, USA

Jayanta Pal Narula Institute of Technology, Kolkata, India;
National Institute of Technology, Durgapur, India

Mahua Pal Department of Sciences and Commerce, J. D. Birla Institute, Kolkata, India

Pabitra Pal BSTTM, IIT Delhi, New Delhi, India

Amartya Pandey Department of Computer Science and Engineering, Meghnad Saha Institute of Technology, Kolkata, India

Deepa Parasar Amity School of Engineering and Technology, Amity University Maharashtra, Mumbai, India

Lopamudra Pathak Central Institute of Technology, Kokrajhar, India

Isha Patil Symbiosis University, Symbiosis Institute of Technology, Pune, India

Seema Patil Symbiosis University, Symbiosis Institute of Technology, Pune, India

Abhijit Paul Department of Information Technology, Amity University, Kolkata, India

Shubhojeet Paul Birla Institute of Technology, Mesra, Ranchi, India

Rishabh Pipalwa Department of Information Technology, Amity University, Kolkata, India

Aishi Pramanik IIEST Shibpur, Howrah, West Bengal, India

Vivek Prasad Amity School of Engineering and Technology, Amity University Maharashtra, Mumbai, India

Andreas Prinz Department of Information Technology, Center for eHealth, University of Agder, Kristiansand, Norway

R. Priya Vels Institute of Science, Technology and Advanced Sciences (VISTAS), Chennai, Tamilnadu, India

Santanu Purkait National Institute of Technology, Raipur, India

Safwon Sadif Rahman Department of Information and Communication Technology, Bangladesh University of Professionals, Dhaka, Bangladesh, India

Aditya Raj School of Information Technology and Engineering, Vellore Institute Technology, Vellore, Tamil Nadu, India

Aman Raj Department of Computer Science and Engineering, Meghnad Saha Institute of Technology, Kolkata, India

Dipti Rana Sardar Vallabhbhai National Institute of Technology, Surat, Gujarat, India

Dipti P. Rana Sardar Vallabhbhai National Institute of Technology, Surat, Gujarat, India

R. Ranjani Vels Institute of Science, Technology and Advanced Sciences (VISTAS), Chennai, Tamilnadu, India

Aritra Ray Department of Computer Science and Engineering, Institute of Engineering and Management, Kolkata, India

Michael Alexander Riegler Department of Holistic Systems, Simula Research Laboratory, Oslo, Norway

Chowdhury Saleh Ahmed Rony Bangladesh University of Professionals, Dhaka, Bangladesh

Abhijit Roy Dr. Bhupendra Nath Dutta Smriti Mahavidyalaya, Purba Barddhaman, West Bengal, India

Ishita Roy Department of Computer Science and Engineering, Noida Institute of Engineering and Technology, Gr. Noida, India

Sujan Kumar Saha Birla Institute of Technology, Mesra, Ranchi, India

Nunna Naga Surya Sai Daivik Sardar Vallabhbhai National Institute of Technology, Surat, Gujarat, India

Sohail Saif Department of Computer Applications, Maulana Abul Kalam Azad University of Technology, Kolkata, West Bengal, India

Shashwat Saket Department of Computer Science and Engineering, Birla Institute of Technology, Jharkhand, India

Sangeetha Saman School of Computer Science and Engineering, Vellore Institute of Technology, Vellore, Tamil Nadu, India

Souvik Samanta Deloitte US-India, Kolkata, India

F. Sammy Department of Information Technology, Dambi Dollo University, Dembi Dolo, Welega, Ethiopia

Adarsh Sarda Department of Computer Science and Engineering, Institute of Engineering and Management, Kolkata, India

Arun Sarkar Department of Mathematics, Heramba Chandra College, Kolkata, India

Puja Sarkar Central Institute of Technology, Kokrajhar, India

Randrita Sarkar Department of Information Technology, B. P. Poddar Institute of Management and Technology, Kolkata, India

Sunita Sarkar Department of Computer Science and Engineering, Assam University, Silchar, Assam, India

Kartik Sau University of Engineering and Management, Kolkata, India

Diganta Sengupta Department of Computer Science and Engineering, Meghnad Saha Institute of Technology, Kolkata, India;
Department of Computer Science and Business Systems, Meghnad Saha Institute of Technology, Kolkata, India

M. Shahina Parveen Computer Science Technology Department, Dayananda Sagar University, Bengaluru, India

Md. Faiyaz Shahriar Department of Information and Communication Technology, Bangladesh University of Professionals, Dhaka, Bangladesh, India

Sumit Sharma Department of Computer Science and Engineering, Noida Institute of Engineering and Technology, Gr. Noida, India

Sunil Kumar Sharma University of Engineering and Management, Kolkata, India

Akash Kumar Singh University of Engineering and Management, Kolkata, India

Aryaa Singh Amity School of Engineering and Technology, Amity University Maharashtra, Mumbai, India

Avtar Singh Department of Computer Science and Engineering, Dr B R Ambedkar National Institute of Technology, Jalandhar, India

Pawan Kumar Singh Department of Information Technology, Jadavpur University, Kolkata, West Bengal, India

Prabhash Kumar Singh Department of Computer Science, Vidyasagar University, Midnapore, West Bengal, India;
Department of Computer and System Sciences, Visva-Bharati University, Santiniketan, West Bengal, India

Ravneesh Singh Symbiosis University, Symbiosis Institute of Technology, Pune, India

Sumit Kumar Singh Department of CSE, University of Essex, Colchester, UK

Yash Raj Singh Department of Computer Science and Engineering, Meghnad Saha Institute of Technology, Kolkata, India

Tirtharaj Sinha University of Engineering and Management, Kolkata, India

N. Tabassum Department of Computer Science, Vidyasagar University, Midnapore, West Bengal, India

Ch Surya Teja Sardar Vallabhbhai National Institute of Technology, Surat, Gujarat, India

Teegala Tejaswi Department of Electronics and Communication, MLR Institute of Technology, Hyderabad, India

Shweta A. Tikhe Sardar Vallabhbhai National Institute of Technology, Surat, Gujarat, India

Bhaskar K. Uday Department of Electronics and Communication, MLR Institute of Technology, Hyderabad, India

Anurag Unnikannan University of Engineering and Management, Kolkata, India

Hirdesh Varshney Department of Computer Science and Engineering, Dr B R Ambedkar National Institute of Technology, Jalandhar, India;
Department of Computer Science and Engineering, Babu Banarasi Das University, Lucknow, India

Aayushi Verma Symbiosis University, Symbiosis Institute of Technology, Pune, India

Preet Viradiya Amity School of Engineering and Technology, Amity University Maharashtra, Mumbai, India

Zhiyun Xue National Library of Medicine, National Institutes of Health, Bethesda, MD, USA

Ramjeet Singh Yadav Department of Business Management and Entrepreneurship, Dr. Rammanohar Lohia Avadh University, Ayodhya, UP, India

Md. Rahat Shahriar Zawad Bangladesh University of Professionals, Dhaka, Bangladesh

Healthcare Informatics

Continuous Speech Recognition in Hindi for Health Care Using Deep Learning

Shubhojeet Paul, Sujan Kumar Saha, and Vandana Bhattacharjee

Abstract Speech is the most natural, convenient, and effective way of communication among human beings. An automatic speech recognition (ASR) system is an effective way for converting speech signals into text. This paper proposes a continuous speech recognition system for the healthcare domain in the Hindi language. Although ample effort has been taken to develop general-domain ASR systems in Hindi, we could not find any ASR system in the healthcare domain. The system is built using convolutional neural network (CNN), bidirectional gated recurrent units (Bi-GRU) using connectionist temporal classification (CTC). We prepare a healthcare domain speech corpus for the task. However, as the training corpus was insufficient, we employed another openly available general-domain corpus and the domain data. A combined corpus has been used to train and evaluate the system. The system is then evaluated using character error rate (CER) and word error rate (WER), and the performance is promising. We achieved a CER of 0.1285 in the developed system.

Keywords Automatic Speech Recognition · Hindi ASR · Healthcare domain · Deep learning for ASR

1 Introduction

The healthcare industry has witnessed a drastic change over a few decades with the advancement of technologies. With the advancement of speech recognition systems, it is now possible to improve delivery services' productivity and efficient flow. There are a lot of applications of speech recognition systems in health care, including clinical documentation, medical voice assistance, reducing language barriers

S. Paul · S. K. Saha (✉) · V. Bhattacharjee
Birla Institute of Technology, Mesra, Ranchi 835215, India
e-mail: sujan.kr.saha@gmail.com

S. Paul
URL: https://www.overleaf.com

V. Bhattacharjee
e-mail: vbhattacharya@bitmesra.ac.in

© The Author(s), under exclusive license to Springer Nature Singapore Pte Ltd. 2023

J. K. Mandal and D. De (eds.), *Frontiers of ICT in Healthcare*, Lecture Notes in Networks and Systems 519, https://doi.org/10.1007/978-981-19-5191-6_1

between doctors and patients, development for interactive voice response (IVR) systems, and remote monitoring of patients.

In speech recognition systems, the capability to generate text from speech enables the ease of documenting medical records in electronic form by reducing the latency and increasing the correctness of the records by minimizing the potential of errors and reducing redundancy. Successful implementation of a speech recognition system requires a well-planned infrastructure to integrate into the current healthcare systems. The application of the automatic speech recognition system is not only limited to transcription-based systems but also capable of building IVR systems that can be streamlined in many communication-intensive aspects of the healthcare systems.

Despite all the benefits of automatic speech recognition systems, there is much scope to penetrate such technologies in current healthcare systems [1], especially in India. India is among the fast-developing nation, and healthcare is among one of the major challenges, which the nation is facing several problems to provide universal access to all the patients like accessibility, affordability, and quality to cover maximum population. Apart from these challenges, language diversity in India also creates a massive gap in accessibility and communication to avail healthcare services. In India, Hindi is the most common and major spoken language with almost 43.63% speakers throughout the nation.[1] So, the ASR system in health care for the Hindi language can hugely impact the current workflow by improving the healthcare system by enhancing the information systems that currently lack coherent integration.

Recent ASR systems in the Hindi language are built by the use of generic Hindi vocabulary, which lacks the domain-specific vocabulary related to health care. This paper proposes an ASR system for Hindi language for healthcare using deep neural networks (DNN).

The proposed system is built using convolutional neural networks (CNN) followed by bidirectional gated recurrent units (Bi-GRU) as a variant of recurrent neural networks (RNN) layers with a softmax layer for continuous speech recognition. We created a speech dataset consisting of 5 h of Hindi healthcare speech data for the task. We also employed another generic Hindi speech data.[2] Speech data and their transcription are passed in the system as inputs for training and evaluation. The system generates transcription of each sentence corresponding to the speech data as output. The system is evaluated using character error rate (CER) and word error rate (WER) as the standard metric. The experimental results show that the concept of merging domain-specific speech data with general-domain speech data in Hindi is promising.

[1] https://censusindia.gov.in/2011Census/C-16_25062018_NEW.pdf.

[2] http://www.openslr.org/103/.

2 Related Works

In recent years, the growing interest in developing ASR systems for Indian languages led to the exploration of various approaches ranging from the hidden Markov model (HMM) and Gaussian mixture model (GMM)-based models to the use of deep learning-based models. In most Indian languages systems, HMM- and GMM-based models are used with acoustic and language models. MFCC has been the most used method for feature extraction of speech signals.

The most commonly implemented ASR systems for Indian languages are based on HMM and GMM for acoustic and language modeling. MFCC is primarily used for the feature extraction from the speech signals, [2–4] are some of the ASR systems implemented for Hindi language, [5] is implemented in the Bengali language, and [6] is implemented in the Kannada language. There are also some ASR systems based on DNN implementation using CNN and RNN with MFCC for feature extraction which has been explored and experimented with for Indian languages, and [7–9] used DNN method to implement ASR system in the Bengali language.

3 Proposed System

The system is built using three layers of CNN followed by a fully connected linear layer, five layers of Bi-GRU layers, and a fully connected linear layer with a softmax layer and connectionist temporal classification (CTC) loss function to recognize individual characters, thus generating the whole sentences of the speech data. The representation of the system is depicted in Fig. 1, and the individual components are discussed below.

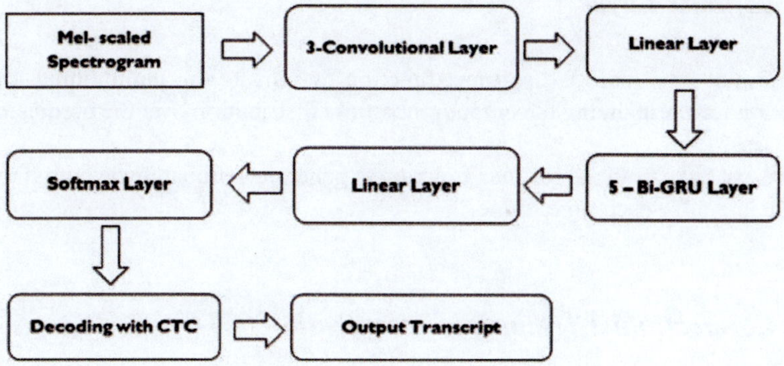

Fig. 1 Proposed system for ASR in Hindi healthcare domain

3.1 Convolutional Layers

Like the response system of a neuron in the visual cortex to a specific stimulus, convolutional layers convolve the given input and pass the result into the next layer. It is commonly applied for analyzing visual imagery.

Here, we have used three layers of CNN layers for the acoustic feature extraction from the mel-scaled spectrograms of the speech data.

3.2 Fully Connected Linear Layer

The fully connected linear layer is the simplest form of neural network. It consists of fixed-sized weights and biases. Here, we have used a fully connected linear layer to map the outputs from the CNN layers to map it with the RNN layers.

3.3 Recurrent Layers

In the recurrent layer, the output is obtained using the last frame's input to determine the current frame's output. This means that the information from the last frame is also considered to calculate the output of the current layer. Hence, it is broadly used for sequential data where each frame is dependent on other frames.

Here, we have used five layers of the Bi-GRU variant of RNN to identify the dependencies between the frames across time and extract the context from the frames.

3.4 Softmax Layer

The softmax layer uses the softmax function to activate the multinomial logistic regression for normalizing the output probability distribution over the predicted output classes.

Here, we have used the softmax function to generate a probabilistic output to map the characters for each time frame.

3.5 Connectionist Temporal Classification (CTC)

CTC is typically used for sequence modeling. Here, the use of CTC function eliminates the need for the pre-segmenting of the training data, and it aligns the audio to the transcript by predicting the probability distribution for all characters for each frame (time-step).

4 Experimental Setup

4.1 Collection of Healthcare Text Corpus

The text corpus is collected from various online healthcare portals of commonly occurring diseases in Hindi language using the Devanagari script. The text corpus contains various symptoms and remedies of the diseases. The text corpus contains a total of 500 sentences containing 10,000 words, with an average of 20 words per sentence having 1900 unique words in which about 800 unique words are related to health care.

4.2 Labeling and Transliteration of the Text Corpus

The originally collected text corpus is in Devanagari script, so a proper transliteration of the corpus is created by labeling the Devanagari characters using the ILSL labeling scheme [10] into English characters for the training and evaluation of the ASR system. Individual transliteration files are created based on the speech data collected from the speakers.

4.3 Preparation of Speech Data

The speech dataset is collected from ten speakers, out of which six are male and are four female. The speaker age group ranges from 25 to 60. The dataset is collected by recording the sentences from the text corpus in an office noise environment. The collected dataset is recorded in .flac format to capture lossless audio data in 16 kHz, monochannel contributing about 8 h duration of the continuous speech data.

Apart from the recorded speech data, OpenSLR [?] generic Hindi train speech dataset is also used in combination with the recorded healthcare speech dataset. OpenSLR Hindi train speech dataset contains about 95 h of speech data recorded from 59 speakers. We have manually analyzed the data and selected a portion containing 15 h based on our requirement. The experiment conducted in this paper used the combination of 15 h of speech data from OpenSLR and 5 h of in-house healthcare speech data.

4.4 Pre-processing of Speech Data and Feature Extraction

We have segmented the raw speech data into a frame size of 25 ms with a 10 ms stride with an overlap of 15 ms and hamming window of 25 ms. Then, it is transformed into mel-Spectrograms with a sample rate of 16 kHz and 128 mel-filterbank and augmented using masking in the frequency domain with the maximum mask length of 30 and masking in the time domain with the maximum mask length of 100. It has been observed that the implementation of the augmentation policies directly to the filterbank significantly reduces the WER of the system [11].

4.5 Hyper-Parameters and Details

The model is trained with ten batch size using one cycle learning rate scheduler coupled with AdamW optimizer [12] with a maximum learning rate of 5e-3. The steps per iteration are calculated by the size of the training data in the batch with a linear anneal strategy. The dropout is taken as 0.1 which randomly drops 10% of the connections in each iteration into each layer of the model for a total of ten epochs.

5 Evaluation Parameters

We used a greedy decoder to process the model output to map it with the characters and then combine it to generate the output transcript. Then, the model is evaluated using word error rate (WER) and character error rate (CER), which is used as a standard metric for the evaluation of ASR systems. Both WER and CER are calculated by measuring the errors using Levenshtein distance for the inserted, substituted, and deleted words and characters for WER and CER, respectively. It compares the output transcription from the model with the original transcription, and hence, error rates are calculated. WER is calculated by:

$$\mathrm{WER} = (\mathrm{Sw} + \mathrm{Dw} + \mathrm{Iw})/\mathrm{Nw} \tag{1}$$

where Sw is the number of words substituted, Dw is the number of words deleted, Iw is the number of words inserted, and Nw is the number of words in the reference. And CER is calculated by:

$$\mathrm{CER} = (\mathrm{Sc} + \mathrm{Dc} + \mathrm{Ic})/\mathrm{Nc} \tag{2}$$

where Sc is the number of characters substituted, Dc is the number of characters deleted, Ic is the number of characters inserted, and Nc is the number of characters in the reference.

6 Results and Discussion

The combined speech dataset of healthcare and generic Hindi speech data has been split into 21 and 2 h for the purpose of training and evaluation of the system. The system is trained and evaluated for ten epochs, and the results are provided in Table 1; in the initial few epochs, there were no significant decrease in WER although the CER was decreasing drastically after which the system showed significant decrease in both CER and WER after each epochs. The decrease in the CER and WER after each epochs is shown in Fig. 2. In this figure, we have shown the values for first ten epochs.

It is observed that the average loss is also decreasing gradually in each epochs as shown in Fig. 3.

Table 1 Results of 10 epochs

Epochs	Loss	CER	WER
1	2.9171	1.0000	1.0000
2	2.7469	0.9878	0.9866
3	1.7292	0.5024	0.9511
4	1.3801	0.4098	0.9140
5	1.0587	0.3234	0.8128
6	0.9631	0.2947	0.7650
7	0.8377	0.2571	0.6922
8	0.7110	0.2197	0.6153
9	0.6681	0.2039	0.5825
10	0.6014	0.1832	0.5372

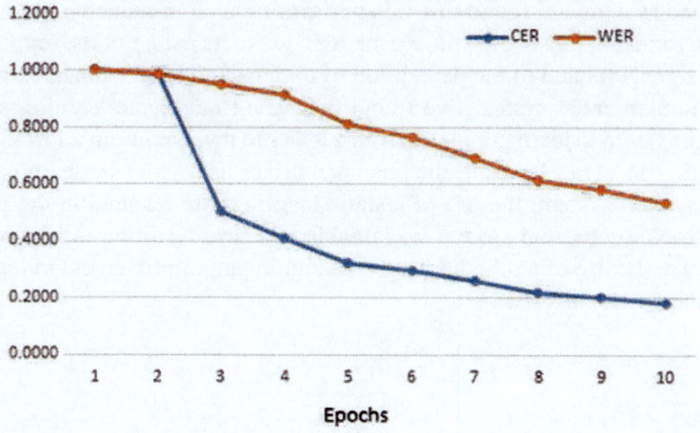

Fig. 2 Decrease in CER and WER after each epochs

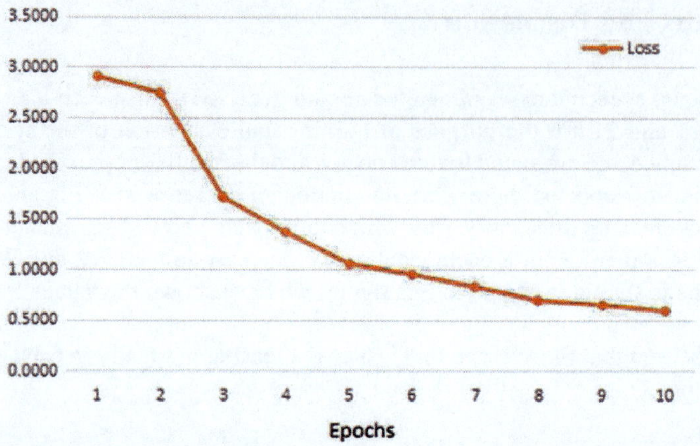

Fig. 3 Decrease in average loss in each epochs

We further continued our experiment for another 15 epochs till it converged. The final CER and WER become 0.1285 and 0.3848, respectively. As our domain-specific recorded data is insufficient, there was no significant decrease in the CER and WER during the last few epochs. Although the final accuracy we achieved is needed further improvement to apply the system in real applications, we feel the approach is quite promising. The system will achieve a reasonable accuracy if the size of the domain data is increased.

Traditional ASR systems were typically based on HMM and GMM, where the use of MFCC was the most popular method and became the standard way for developing most of the ASR systems. In recent years, the implementation of various deep learning methods for speech recognition led to the exploration of other methods to study their implication in improving the system. We have used mel-scaled filter bank in our implemented system and found that it is performing well in reducing the CER. The motivation for using mel-scaled filter bank was due to its nature of the representation of speech signals related to the perception of understanding by human beings.

In the implemented system, we found that using one cycle learning scheduler allowed the system to learn gradually from a lower to the maximum allowed learning rate, resulting in better learning the characters than using a static learning rate. In our implemented system, the use of a static learning rate resulted in the vanishing gradient problem, and the system was unable to learn, resulting in high CER and WER. Hence, the use of a scheduler showed significant improvement in learning by lowering the CER and WER.

7 Future Work

In the implemented system, we used the combination of both Hindi generic and healthcare speech data for training and evaluation because of the limited Hindi healthcare speech data. The performance of the system may increase with larger speech data. However, due to the limited recorded Hindi healthcare speech data, the proposed system can be explored by modifying it by implementing transfer learning to increase the accuracy of the overall system by first training the system with more generic Hindi speech data followed by healthcare speech data. In future experiments, we will implement transfer learning with more generic Hindi speech data to compare the performance with the current implemented system.

References

1. Latif S, Qadir J, Qayyum A, Usama M, Younis S (2021) Speech technology for healthcare: opportunities, challenges, and state of the art. IEEE Rev Biomed Eng 14:342–356. https://doi.org/10.1109/RBME.2020.3006860
2. Kumari P, Shakina Deiv D, Bhattacharya M (2014) Automatic speech recognition of accented Hindi data. In: International Conference on Computation of Power, Energy, Information and Communication (ICCPEIC), pp 68–76. https://doi.org/10.1109/ICCPEIC.2014.6915342
3. Kuamr A, Dua M, Choudhary T (2014) Continuous Hindi speech recognition using Gaussian mixture HMM. IEEE students' conference on electrical, electronics and computer science 2014:1–5. https://doi.org/10.1109/SCEECS.2014.6804519
4. Karra S, Mayuka S, Radhika N, Priya K, Deepa G (2020) Kaldi recipe in Hindi for word level recognition and phoneme level transcription. Proc Comput Sci 171:2476–2485. https://doi.org/10.1016/j.procs.2020.04.268
5. Amin MAA, Islam MT, Kibria S, Rahman MS (2019) Continuous Bengali speech recognition based on deep neural network. In: International conference on Electrical, Computer and Communication Engineering (ECCE), pp 1–6. https://doi.org/10.1109/ECACE.2019.8679341
6. Sajjan SC, Vijaya C (2016) Continuous speech recognition of Kannada language using triphone modeling. In: International conference on Wireless Communications, Signal Processing and Networking (WiSPNET), pp 451–455. https://doi.org/10.1109/WiSPNET.2016.7566174
7. Hosain Sumit S, Al Muntasir T, Arefin Zaman MM, Nath Nandi R, Sourov T (2018) Noise robust end-to-end speech recognition for Bangla language. In: International Conference on Bangla Speech and Language Processing (ICBSLP), pp 1–5. https://doi.org/10.1109/ICBSLP.2018.8554871
8. Islam J, Mubassira M, Islam MR, Das AK (2019) A speech recognition system for Bengali language using recurrent neural network. In: IEEE 4th International Conference on Computer and Communication Systems (ICCCS), pp 73–76. https://doi.org/10.1109/CCOMS.2019.8821629
9. Nahid MMH, Purkaystha B, Islam MS (2017) Bengali speech recognition: a double layered LSTM-RNN approach. In: 20th International Conference of Computer and Information Technology (ICCIT), pp 1–6. https://doi.org/10.1109/ICCITECHN.2017.8281848
10. Samudravijaya K (2021) Indian Language Speech Label (ILSL): a De Facto national standard. In: Biswas A, Wennekes E, Hong TP, Wieczorkowska A (eds) Advances in speech and music technology. Advances in intelligent systems and computing, vol 1320. Springer, Singapore. https://doi.org/10.1007/978-981-33-6881-1_36
11. Park DS, Chan W, Zhang Y, Chiu C-C, Zoph B, Cubuk ED, Le QV (2019) SpecAugment: a simple data augmentation method for automatic speech recognition. Proc. Interspeech 2019:2613–2617. https://doi.org/10.21437/Interspeech.2019-2680
12. Loshchilov I, Hutter F (2019) Decoupled weight decay regularization, ICLR 2019. https://arxiv.org/abs/1711.05101

Improving Mental Health Through Multimodal Emotion Detection from Speech and Text Data Using Long-Short Term Memory

Dhritesh Bhagat, Aritra Ray, Adarsh Sarda, Nilanjana Dutta Roy, Mufti Mahmud, and Debashis De

Abstract In today's world of cut-throat competition, where everyone is running an invisible race, we often find ourselves alone amongst the crowd. The advancements in technology are making our lives easier, yet man being a social animal is losing touch with society. As a result, today a huge part of the population is suffering from psychological disorders. Inferiority complex, inability to fulfil dreams, loneliness, etc., are considered to be the common reasons to disturb mental stability, which may further lead to disorders like depression. In extreme cases, depression causes loss of precious lives when an individual decides to commit suicide. Assessing an individual's mental health in an interactive way with the core help of machine learning is the primary focus of this work. To realize this objective, we have used the most suitable long-short term memory (LSTM) architecture. It is an artificial recurrent neural network (RNN) in the field of deep learning on Ryerson Audio-Visual Database of Emotional Speech and Song (RAVDESS) and FastText datasets to get 86% accuracy when fed with model-patient conversational data. Further, we discussed the scope of enhancing cognitive control capabilities over the psychiatric disorders, which may even lead to severe level of depression and suicidal attacks. Here, the proposed system will help to determine the severity level of depression in a person and will help with the recovery process. The system comprises of a wrist-band to measure some biological parameters, a headband to analyse the mental health and a user-friendly website and mobile application which has an in-built chatbot. AI-based chatbot will talk to the patients and help them reveal their thoughts, which they are otherwise not able to communicate to their peers. A person can chat via text message, which is to be stored in the database for further analysis. The novelty of this work is in the sentiment analysis of voice chat, which therefore creates a comfortable environment for the user.

D. Bhagat · A. Ray · A. Sarda · N. Dutta Roy (✉)
Department of Computer Science and Engineering, Institute of Engineering and Management, Kolkata, India
e-mail: nilanjanaduttaroy@gmail.com

M. Mahmud
Department of Computer Science, Nottingham Trent University, Nottingham, UK

D. De
Department of Computer Science and Engineering, Maulana Abul Kalam Azad University, West Bengal, India

© The Author(s), under exclusive license to Springer Nature Singapore Pte Ltd. 2023
J. K. Mandal and D. De (eds.), *Frontiers of ICT in Healthcare*, Lecture Notes in Networks and Systems 519, https://doi.org/10.1007/978-981-19-5191-6_2

Keywords Mental health · AI-supported chatbot · Sentiment · Emotion analysis · Depression prediction · Neural network

1 Introduction

Mental health of an individual mostly depends on psychological, emotional, and social factors. It determines our ability to handle stress and make choices. It is important to maintain a good mental health at every stage of life. However, instability affects our healthy lifestyle in terms of the way of thinking, mood fluctuation, and change in behaviour. Some biological factors, life experiences and family history may also contribute to mental health issues. It is common but recoverable with proper and timely action. Generally, sufferers of depression tend to internalize their feelings and express hesitation with human interrogation. But with technologies advancing, people have now found a ground of comfort with general chatbots. Considering these to account, our idea is to create an AI implemented model, for better interaction and thus adding a benefit to both ends; detection and proper analysis. A user-friendly chatbot has been built on a cloud-based AI model having detecting capabilities from neural Networking, a close study to tracking a human brain. Further, inclusion of voice support will get this model an extra mile with users. To measure the severity of depression, emotional analysis is essential. We have performed multimodal emotional analysis using AI-bot for necessary remedies. This would be an effective way to reach more people suffering from depression, as the patient will not have to open up about personal troubles to the unknown or have a fear of getting judged. A chatbot can simply lend a helping hand and heed the need. The work is focused on planning to execute the first and foremost thing needed would be the data collection and analysis for understanding human emotions. The most viable option was to get it using any form asking clinically/psychologically relevant questions. AI-based models are then used to analyse the answers. Open-ended answers are preferable here rather than using the MCQ-based versions for more variations (Fig. 1).

The system has been developed for emotion analysis using human interaction. Alongside, an user interface (UI) has also been designed for people to interact with the model. We implemented the LSTM architecture using the w2v method converting each word into a vector. Those vectors can be used to calculate the emotions further. Finally, to achieve the goal for sentiment and emotion analysis, we fed the RAVDESS dataset to our model, which categorized the data into numerous classes along with five basic emotions namely neutral, joy, sad, fear, and anger. It can detect emotion by recognizing voice, text, and social media influenced language. In contrast, advancements in lifestyles and reasons have outnumbered depression reaching heights of statistics. We took the challenge to contribute to the main-field research by incorporating remedies in correspondence with situations. This work also considers specialists' recommendations and active communication with physical help centres.

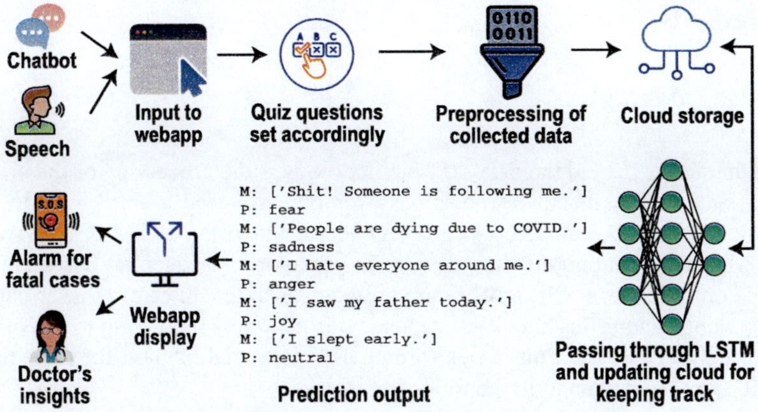

Fig. 1 Block diagram of the multimodal emotion detection system

The main contributions of the work are as follows:

- Multimodal emotion recognition via speech and text.
- Development of a new web application (web app) suitable for all platforms.
- Development of a support system to improve mental health.

Extraction of emotion from different social media is one of the trending works nowadays [16]. There are many state-of-the-art methods which supports emotional detection [5, 6]. The posts given in various social media platforms are being analysed by the researchers to understand the current state of mind. The combination of speech, text, gesture, voice, EEG, and other biomarkers is also being considered as powerful parameters for emotion detection [12]. However, most of the works focuses on a specific content in this case [14]. Voice frequency, modulation of speech, and tone were used in a study to detect emotion [2, 17]. Emotion detection from videos by watching gestures and facial expressions was done in another study [8]. Emotion models can be divided into two categories based on some existing theories. They are categorical and dimensional. Emotions which are discrete in nature, are enlisted into the categorical models. And dimensional category models depend upon some dimensions with parameters. The terms valence, which is the positivity and negativity of emotions, arousal, which is the excitement level of emotion and dominance which is basically the level of control of emotions, are used in dimensional emotional models [13]. Lexicon-based emotion detection is another well-known method against a given input dataset [3, 11].

The organization of the rest of the paper is as follows: The complete methodology has been defined in Sect. 2. Results and discussions are shown in Sects. 3 and 4 draws the final conclusion.

2 Methods

2.1 Methodology

The main motive behind the data flow methodology is the processing of the original data in such a way that it becomes easy for our proposed architecture. In deep learning, long-short term memory recurrent neural networks (LSTM-RNNs) require time-series data, continuous-time data, or in other words sequential data, data that depends on time [1, 4, 15]. LSTMs are quite advanced architecture that is capable of processing time-series data. We proposed this data flow modelling to convert our original dataset into the time-series format. The proposed method for the emotion detection can be explained in the following steps:

- After getting the input, the words have been tokenized first. This segregates each word which would help us embed the sentence properly.
- The length of each sentence being different, becomes difficult if we pass it through the model. The length of each sentence should be equal. So, it is mandatory to convert every sentence to an approximate number of words. For this, we have taken the help of padding.
- Now, each word needs to be embedded in some numeric representation, as the model understands only numeric digits. So for this task, we used FastText []. It is easy to download and import any pre-trained word embedding as it is available. The 300-dimensional w2v pre-trained on Wikipedia articles has been used here.
- The first word of each row is the character that is to be embedded. And from the column to the last column, there is the numeric representation of that character in a 300D vector form.
- Now, the preprocessing part is over, and now, we need to perform the following things:
  - Do one-hot encoding of each emotion.
  - Split the dataset into train and test sets.
  - Train the model on our dataset.
  - Test the model on the test set.

Now, the model is ready to be tried. We observed the emotion we are getting as output, reported in Table 2. The architecture is shown in Fig. 2.

2.2 Datasets for Text and Voice Messages for Emotion Detection

Working on combined models sets would require adequate data for fine analysis and predictions. With two different approaches to design models and detect emotions, we have utilized two datasets namely FastText [10] and RAVDESS [9].

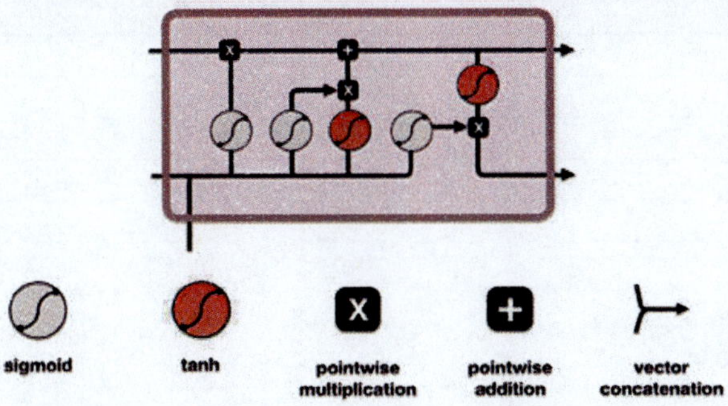

Fig. 2 Architecture of a long-short term memory network model

FastText

FastText is an open-source library, technologically advanced by the Facebook AI Research lab. It focuses its work on achieving scalable solutions exclusively for text classification and illustration while dealing with large datasets in a smaller time frame and accurate results. It enables the processing to be quick, allowing to train models on large corpora. It also permits to compute of word representations for words that did not appear in the training data giving an edge to test data. We came across a table available on FastText blog page comparing with the deep learning classifiers in terms of accuracy, orders of magnitude, and of all, training time. According to the table, it gave better results than most deep learning-based methods tested on various brands like Amazon and Yahoo. Moving with model advancements to implement our idea, we have put our hands on a collection of a million [7] words vectors trained on Wikipedia 2017, UMBC web-based corpus, and statmt.org news dataset (16B tokens). Another million word vectors have been trained on the sub-word information available on Wikipedia 2017 along with other sources like UMBC web-based corpus, etc. It is capable of recognizing modern-day text-style writing, thus providing our end-users with a more comfortable conversation with our models. It is arranged in descending order from the most used words or heavy words to the least likely to be used words. Here, each word is represented as a bag of character n-grams. A vector representation is attached to each character n-gram as the sum of these representations. Basically, incorporating word vectors to preserve some information about the surrounding words and sub-word information appearing near each word. This is very useful for classification applications, as the combination of two string words may echo a different piece of emotion instead of each separately. This improves the prediction of the models with test data.

Table 1 Notations used in implementing LSTM

Notations	Meaning
h_t, C_t	Hidden layer vectors
x_t	Input vector
b_f, b_i, b_c, b_o	Bias vector
W_f, W_i, W_c, W_o	Parameter matrices
$\sigma, tanh$	Activation functions

RAVDESS

According to resources, emotion is a form of high-level paralinguistic information that is intrinsically conveyed by human speech. This dataset is a collection of various recorded emotional states in variable environments and people. The Ryerson Audio-Visual Database of Emotional Speech and Song (RAVDESS) released under the Creative Commons Attribution licence is a validated multimodal database of emotional speech and song. The database is strongly unbiased to gender. It consists of 24 professional actors with neutral North American accents. It was fed with speeches that include a variety of emotions like calm, happy, sad, angry, fearful, surprise, and disgust expressions. Including songs expressing the above list as well. It is calculated with each expression produced at two levels of emotional intensity along with an additional neutral expression. It has a total of 7356 recordings carrying emotional validity, intensity, and genuineness. The mentioned conditions are available in three modality formats: audio-only (16 bit, 48 kHz .wav), audio–video (720p H.264, AAC 48 kHz, .mp4), and video-only (no sound). 247 individuals provided ratings, who were distinctive of untrained research participants from North America. 72-participants further provided test-retest data assuring purity of data. High levels of emotional validity and test-retest inter-rater consistency were reported. Corrected accuracy and composite "goodness" events are offered to assist researchers in the selection of stimuli. There are four distinguishing features of the RAVDESS that build on popular existing sets which will be utilized in our project: (i) scope, (ii) emotional intensity, (iii) two baseline emotions: neutral and calm, and (iv) singing corps (Table 1).

2.3 *Mathematical Formulation of LSTM*

Let us take the LSTM neuron as a reference to understand the mathematical formulation (feed-forward and the backpropagation with time). The feed-forward formulation of the neuron can be represented as

$$f_t = \sigma(W_f * [h_t - 1, x_t] + b_f) \tag{1}$$

$$i_t = \sigma(W_i * [h_t - 1, x_t] + b_i) \tag{2}$$

$$o_t = \sigma(W_o * [h_t - 1, x_t] + b_o) \tag{3}$$

$$C_t = \tanh(W_c * [h_t - 1, x_t] + b_c) \tag{4}$$

$$C_t = f_t \circledast C_t - 1 + i_t \circledast C_t \tag{5}$$

$$h_t = o_t \circledast \tanh(C_t) \tag{6}$$

Now, we will find out the output or the hidden state as a complete mathematical formula.

Combining Eqs. 4, 5, and 6, we get

$$h_t = o_t \circledast \tanh(f_t \circledast C_t - 1 + i_t \circledast \tanh(W_c * [h_t - 1, x_t] + b_c)) \tag{7}$$

Now putting in Eqs. 1, 2 in 7, we get

$$\begin{aligned} h_t = {} & o_t \circledast \tanh(\sigma(W_f * [h_t - 1, x_t] + b_f) \circledast Ct - 1 \\ & + \sigma(W_i * [h_t - 1, x_t] + b_i) \circledast \tanh(W_c * [h_t - 1, x_t] + b_c)) \end{aligned} \tag{8}$$

Now putting in Eqs. 3 in 8

$$\begin{aligned} h_t = {} & \sigma(W_o * [h_t - 1, x_t] + b_o) \\ & \circledast \tanh(\sigma(W_f * [h_t - 1, x_t] + b_f) \circledast C_t - 1 + \sigma(W_i * [h_t - 1, x_t] + b_i)) \\ & \circledast \tanh(W_c * [h_t - 1, x_t] + b_c) \end{aligned} \tag{9}$$

This Eq. 9 that we get is the final equation that the LSTM neuron would give us as an output.

3 Results and Discussion

3.1 *Results*

The goal of the work is to develop a system for emotion analysis using human interaction. To achieve this, the samples have been collected from available datasets. The architecture works initially by tokenizing every word after getting the input. With padding, every sentence has been converted into a number of approximate words. Then, each word has been embedded into numeric representation with the FastText

Table 2 Experimental results based on some random messages

Message	Prediction	Time (in sec)
Oh no, someone is following me	Fear	0.22
People are dying because of COVID-19	Sadness	0.22
Delivery was hour late and my pizza was cold	Sadness	0.06
I hate everyone around me	Anger	0.20
I don't like going to the doctor	Fear	0.21
Why are you not paying attention to me?	Anger	0.22
Bro! I got really good marks	Joy	0.20
I am confused about my life	Sadness	0.21
Life has been too easy	Neutral	0.23
Why do we give exams?	Anger	0.20
This is a fine day	Neutral	0.00
Congratulations thats a big news	Joy	0.00
That room is so creepy	Fear	0.00
That man over there is running fast	Neutral	0.00

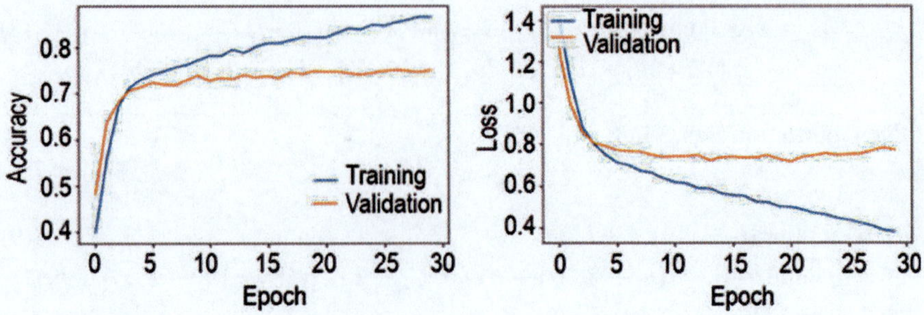

Fig. 3 Model accuracy and loss with 30 epochs

dataset. The performance of the model is around 86%, which is reported in Table 2. The accuracy-loss and confusion matrix of the model are shown in Figs. 3 and 4, respectively. Also, a comparative analysis has been shown in Table 3.

3.2 Comparative Analysis

Here are a few depression detecting applications and a comparative analysis with our proposed model.

We are providing an all round package to our users for accurate measurement of depression level along with educating them with the same.

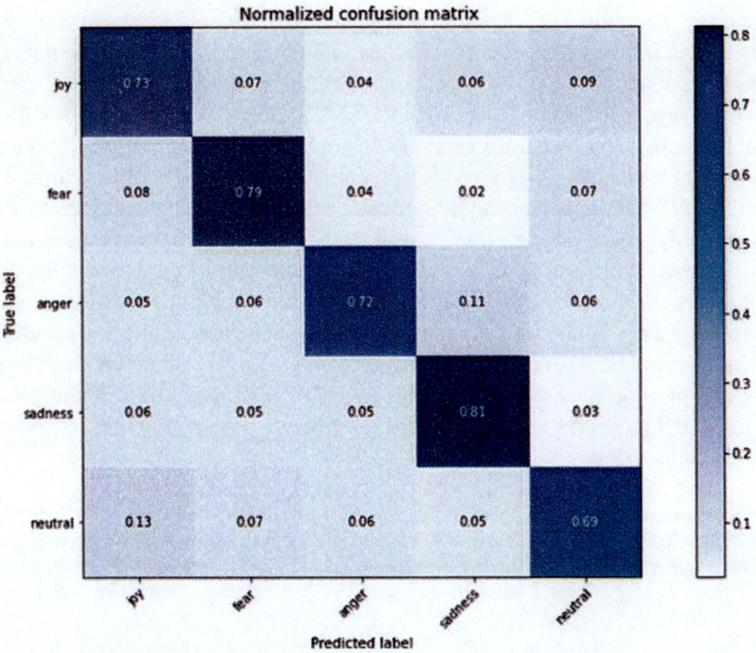

Fig. 4 Confusion matrix with 30 epochs

Table 3 Comparative analysis with some of the existing methods

Name of the apps from Google Play Store	Objective questions	Descriptive	Voice assistant	Interactive games	Awareness or community support	Alerts for emergencies
Moodpath	Yes	No	No	No	Yes	Yes
TalkLife	Yes	No	No	No	Yes	No
Daylio	Yes	No	No	No	No	No
Youper	Yes	No	No	No	No	No
What's Up	Yes	Yes	No	No	Yes	No
Proposed application	No	Yes	Yes	Yes	Yes	Yes

4 Conclusion

Hence, it can be concluded that our elementary research and implementation has strived to provide solutions for emotional analysis, with the implementation of various pathways like AI-bots. The system logically determines the level of emotion and attempting to provide remedial solutions by analysing, with the aid of questions and provided answers. This provides an easily accessible platform that does not require the intervention of actual people, which in most of the cases turn out to be advantageous.

We have primarily implemented RAVDESS and FastText datasets for the prediction and collection of data. FastText illustrates and classifies texts, by comparison with larger datasets and provides precise outcomes, adaptable with the time required. RAVDESS analyses the individual's psychological state and severity of an expression, expressed through a statement. In the LSTM, long-short term memory we applied activation functions namely sigmoid activation function and hyperbolic tangent activation function, for determining whether the input sequences should be stored in long-term or short-term memory. Lastly, we provided the end result of the formative development, to provide an insight to our ultimate objective. In future, the system will be upgraded with the model for depression detection. If the person is found to have depression, our AI-bot will provide necessary remedies, based on the severity of depression.

Acknowledgements MM is supported by the AI-TOP (2020-1-UK01-KA201-079167) and DIVERSASIA (618615-EPP-1-2020-1-UKEPPKA2-CBHEJP) projects funded by the European Commission under the Erasmus+ programme.

References

1. Al Banna MH et al (2021) Attention-based bi-directional long-short term memory network for earthquake prediction. IEEE Access 9:56589–56603
2. Anagnostopoulos CN, Iliou T, Giannoukos I (2015) Features and classifiers for emotion recognition from speech: a survey from 2000 to 2011. Artif Intell Rev 43(2):155–177
3. Dini L, Bittar A (2016) Emotion analysis on Twitter: the hidden challenge. In: Proceedings of LREC'16, pp 3953–3958 (2016)
4. Fabietti M et al (2020) Artifact detection in chronically recorded local field potentials using long-short term memory neural network. In: Proceedings of AICT 2020, pp 1–6 (2020)
5. Ghosh T et al (2021) An attention-based mood controlling framework for social media users. In: Proceedings of brain informatics, pp 245–256 (2021)
6. Ghosh T et al (2021) A hybrid deep learning model to predict the impact of covid-19 on mental health form social media big data. Preprints (2021060654)
7. Humphrey EJ, Bello JP, LeCun Y (2012) Moving beyond feature design: deep architectures and automatic feature learning in music informatics. In: ISMIR, pp 403–408
8. Kahou SE et al (2016) Emonets: multimodal deep learning approaches for emotion recognition in video. J Multimodal User Interfaces 10(2):99–111
9. Livingstone SR, Russo FA (2018) The ryerson audio-visual database of emotional speech and song (ravdess): a dynamic, multimodal set of facial and vocal expressions in North American English. PloS One 13(5):e0196391
10. Mikolov T, Grave E, Puhrsch C, Joulin A (2017) Advances in pre-training distributed word representations. arXiv preprint arXiv:1712.09405, pp 1–4
11. Mohammad SM, Bravo-Marquez F (2017) Emotion intensities in tweets. arXiv preprint arXiv:1708.03696, pp 1–13
12. Poria S, Cambria E, Howard N, Huang GB, Hussain A (2016) Fusing audio, visual and textual clues for sentiment analysis from multimodal content. Neurocomputing 174:50–59

13. Sreeja PS, Mahalakshmi G (2017) Emotion models: a review. Int J Control Theor Appl 10:651–657
14. Sailunaz K, Dhaliwal M, Rokne J, Alhajj R (2018) Emotion detection from text and speech: a survey. Soc Netw Anal Mining 8(1):1–26
15. Satu M et al (2020) Towards improved detection of cognitive performance using bidirectional multilayer long-short term memory neural network. In: Proceedings of brain informatics, pp 297–306
16. Satu MS et al (2021) Tclustvid: a novel machine learning classification model to investigate topics and sentiment in covid-19 tweets. Knowl-Based Syst 226:107126
17. Semwal N, Kumar A, Narayanan S (2017) Automatic speech emotion detection system using multi-domain acoustic feature selection and classification models. In: Proceedings of ISBA, pp 1–6

Hybridized Support Vector Machine and Adaboost Technique for Malaria Diagnosis

Joseph Bamidele Awotunde, Sanjay Misra, Femi Emmanuel Ayo, Akshat Agrawal, and Ravin Ahuja

Abstract One of the most prevalence diseases in developing countries in recent years is still Malaria with global public health concern. Malaria is caused by mosquitoe's parasites which are very common in developing nations. This reason was not far from environmental insanity coupled with inadequate healthcare facilities. Thus, develop a reliable and efficient classification model for early diagnosis and discovery of the malaria symptoms is required. Hence, to reduce malaria endemic globally, the use machine learning models is essentials and paramount. Therefore, this paper proposes malaria diagnosis model using hybrid Support Vector Machines (SVM) and Adaboost. SVM classifiers for malaria classification and eliminating redundant or extraneous features were extracted using Chi-square. The classification accuracy of SVM and Adaboost models gave 97% with the six features removed but from seventh feature the accuracy reduced to 91%. The study revealed that, the developed hybridized model gives optimal solutions by using the most prominent features (symptoms) for malaria classification.

Keywords Malaria · Diagnosis · Support vector machines · Adaboost · Data mining · Malaria fever · Mosquitoes parasites

---

J. B. Awotunde
Department of Computer Science, University of Ilorin, Ilorin, Nigeria
e-mail: awotunde.jb@unilorin.edu.ng

S. Misra
Department of Computer Science and Comunication, Ostfold University, Halden, Norway
e-mail: sanjay.misra@covenantuniversity.edu.ng

F. E. Ayo
Department of Computer Science, McPherson University, Seriki-Sotayo, Abeokuta, Nigeria
e-mail: ayofe@mcu.edu.ng

A. Agrawal (✉)
Amity University, Gurgaon, Hariyana, India
e-mail: akshatag20@gmail.com

R. Ahuja
Center of ICT/ICE, Covenant University, Ota, Nigeria

© The Author(s), under exclusive license to Springer Nature Singapore Pte Ltd. 2023
J. K. Mandal and D. De (eds.), *Frontiers of ICT in Healthcare*, Lecture Notes in Networks and Systems 519, https://doi.org/10.1007/978-981-19-5191-6_3

1 Introduction

Malaria is one of Africa's most dangerous diseases, particularly in Nigeria [1, 2]. A reliable and timely parasite-based identification is always welcome. Further malaria control initiatives, such as the use of insecticide-treated bed nets and indoor continuous spray, are critical to reduce malaria cases in developing countries. Many donors have aided in this effort by providing medicated bed nets to poor countries. In addition to proper laboratory diagnosis, Plasmodium falciparum resistance to commonly used anti-malarial drugs necessitates the use of substantially more cost-effective immunotherapy [3]. The World Health Organization (WHO) emphasizes the presence of malaria in a human body before using or treating malaria treatments to minimize unintentional use of anti-malaria drugs. However, due to a lack of medical personnel, technical expertise, and an adequate laboratory system in numerous underdeveloped countries, the presumption treatment of malaria and other related fevers remains popular. The mentioned facts have resulted in delays in the diagnosis of other serious feverish conditions, and the assumption of treatment has occasionally resulted in anti-malarial drug usage or abuse [4, 5].

Malaria is as old as humanity since it is an ancient disease that causes societal, financial, and health problems for individuals all over the world [6]. Malaria is a disease that is frequent in hot and humid climates, and it has been around for hundreds of years. Malaria has remained a major public health concern in many countries. In 2008, WHO labeled malaria endemic in 109 countries, with 243 million malaria cases recorded and millions of endemic deaths, mostly among children under the age of five (WHO).

Data mining has been proved to be the most relevant and significant approach for classification, prediction or diagnosis of different diseases. Studies have suggested various classifiers to identify falciparum fever, including Neural Network, Support Vector Machine, Adaboost, Decision Tree, Naive Bayes, and KNN. However, determining which of these data mining approaches performs better and more successfully is difficult. It has also been discovered that single data mining strategies do not always produce the intended results. This study analyzed the effectiveness of the top three most prevalent data mining algorithms used in malaria diagnosis to discover a solution to this problem. Hence, this study only applied three data mining techniques to predict malaria fever using the C 4.5 Decision Tree, Kernel Basis Function Support Vector Machine (SVM), and Adaboost.

Therefore, the aim of this study is to conduct a performance analysis of the malaria diagnostic system using a data mining approach and with the following objectives: Use Chi-square to select relevant attributes from malaria fever patients. Implement the data mining classification methods; Support Vector Machine (SVM), and AdaBoost in Weka data mining tool environment. Finally, conduct comparative performance evaluation on the classification algorithms.

2 Related Work

Data mining is referred to as the method of finding new, interesting and informative tendencies from large-scale data along with concise, comprehensible and prognostic prototypes. Fundamental data mining and investigation algorithms formulate the foundation for the developing area of data science, which integrates computerized techniques for analyzing patterns and prototypes for all forms of data, from systematic research to business intelligence and analytics.

In most cases, well-known mathematical techniques and algorithms are computational tools employed in data mining. While data mining is a new technology, in the data analysis phase alone nothing new is included. The reason for the link between these methods and large databases was the low cost of storage space and processing power. To find patterns, identify information, and extract data from enormous datasets, data mining procedures are employed. Knowledge is usually hidden in large datasets, but data mining techniques can be used to expose it and make it useful.

Data mining, also identified as Knowledge Discovery in Databases (KDD), is concerned with the discovery from large amounts of data of new and potentially valuable knowledge [7, 8]. Data mining techniques, unlike conventional statistical methods, scan for motivating evidence exclusive of having previous assumptions, depending on the data mining tasks performed, the pattern type that can be identified. In general, there are two categories of data mining duties: descriptive data mining duties describing the universal characteristics of prevailing data and predictive data mining duties attempting to make prognostications established on obtainable data inferences. Such procedures are frequently stronger, additionally versatile and more effective than the exploratory analysis statistical techniques.

SVM, Adaboost, ID3, and C4.5 are well-known among the various classification algorithms and play an essential role in medical research [9, 10]. Several studies were conducted to explain malaria fever risk prediction and classification using data mining techniques [11–16]. In cultures, this was done to find a lasting solution to malaria fever. The authors in [17] study concentrated on the assessment of data mining methods and algorithms that can be used for implementing the disease risk forecasting model. Assessment of the performance of the algorithms of data mining was accomplished by being centered on its accuracy. It was established that artificial neural network was regularly used for finding the likelihood of heart disease and it was discovered that it attained the highest accuracy for general heart disease prediction. It was also realized that absence of experimentation by means of diverse type of inputs and algorithms were utilized for other diseases, and it was suggested that there should requirement for extra studies to have a further dependable prognostication on those other sicknesses.

In [18], the authors discussed in their research that the prevailing applications and projections of homeopathic data categorization which are centered on data mining methods were considered in this study. Foremost progressive classification methodologies that can be applied to improve classification correctness were being emphasized by authors of the study. Numerous works of literature had been reviewed and it was discovered that for the classification activities the data mining approaches were very effective. The recent development in the classification of medical data was comparatively investigated and the discoveries from the research suggested that the present classification of the medical data could be enhanced the more. The researchers concluded that there should be further studies to establish and reduce the uncertainties for classification to achieve enhanced accuracy.

In a similar word, the authors in [19] discussed in their research that the three mostly used classification procedures which are support vector machine (SVM), K-nearest neighbor (KNN), and lastly artificial neural network (ANN). These three approaches were considered with a mindset of assessing them for heart disease prediction using Cleveland standard heart disease datasets. The experimental findings presented that the classification accuracy using SVM is 85.1852% which makes it outperform that of the using the other two approaches as they had KNN (82.963%) and ANN is 73.3333%.

In [12], the authors examine the ability of the Geographical Information System (GIS) to investigate the non-linear relationship between malaria and socio-physical conditions, remote sensing data, some machine learning classifiers in Vietnam's DakNong province, and ensemble techniques. To test the accuracy of the proposed system, the receiver operating characteristic (ROC) curve and pair t-test were used. The results obtained under ROC were better achieved than the other models based on statistical measurements of the Random Subspace Ensemble model. After comparing pair t-tests with Area Under Curve values, the findings showed a slight difference of about 1%. Therefore, assembly techniques significantly improved the base classifier's efficiency. Performance, however, may vary from location to location. It is concluded that the combination of these methods is promising for mapping malaria vulnerability so that derived maps can be used as a fundamental basis for programs to control spatial diseases.

Reference [20] reported on the analysis and review of current regression and classification models used to forecast disease outbreaks in datasets. The paper found that there are different techniques for both classification and regression prediction models, but many rely on single techniques as well as hybrid techniques, but are still few available, so there is a need for more complex models to improve the accuracy of classification and prediction of disease outbreaks and the inclusion of theoretical knowledge. The critic provided the specifics of the strengths and weaknesses of the various classification and regression models and concluded that a data mining hybrid model is most likely to predict disease outbreaks with optimum accuracy. Many previous models based either on single data mining methods classification or regression. Therefore, efforts should be moved to a hybrid approach for both the detection and prediction of disease outbreaks, resulting in the advantages of the individual model's best features to achieve the best and reliable outcomes.

The authors in [21] proposed geo-tagging predictive mapping demonstrated a significant impact on mosquito-borne disease prevention and monitoring in a specific resource-limited area. Latent Dirichlet allocation (LDA)-based theme modeling techniques are used to filter out relevant symptom, prevention and fear-related topics. Early detection or anxiety of outbreak associated with real-time monitoring of public feelings. The Naive Bayes and Support Vector method were used for the two phases of fine-grained data classification. The proposed model of the smart monitoring mechanism will help government agencies better manage their time and money. The key factors obtained from Twitter and RSS feeds and the use of regular kernel density estimates (KDE) have been used for predictive mapping. The proposed system has been used to predict the incidence of mosquito-borne disease in India.

Reference [11] using Integrated Management of Childhood Illness (IMCI) Guidelines and Rapid Diagnostic Testing of Malaria (RDT) for Integrated Pediatric Fever Control, including antibiotic over-treatment in Malawi's health facilities in 2013–2014, and the association between RDT-negative outcomes for children aged 2–59 with fever complaints. Classification trees using model-based recursive partitioning estimated the correlation between RDT results and antibiotic over-treatment and learned the impact of 38 other input variables at patient, provider and facility level. Despite common compliance with malaria guidelines, comprehensive pediatric fever management for completed assessments and antibiotic targeting was sub-optimal. RDT-negative results were strongly associated with over-treatment or troubled breathing problems with cough-conditioned antibiotics. In line with recent global commitments to counter-resistance, to improve quality fever care and fair use of both anti-malarias' and antibiotics, a move from malaria-focused testing and treatment approaches to 'IMCI with research' is needed.

In [14], the authors used a supervised learning algorithm to predict specific disease outcomes with various types of data including biological and environmental data. Health social determinants tend to be important predictors of public health issues such as malaria and children's anemia, but very little has been investigated in the health care system. Their contribution capacity was considered based on variable importance in Projection (VIP) in malaria and anemia predictions. The research used five machine learning approaches to identify the two diseases using health data's social determinants. The method has the potential advantages of measuring and comparing the effects of independent variables on disease prediction. Of the five machine learning algorithms used, 94.74% and 84.17%, respectively, were the best results of artificial neural networks for malaria and anemia prediction, and the findings are consistent and demonstrate the importance of non-medical factors in disease prediction.

3 Research Methodology

3.1 The Approach

The development framework used and integrates Weka 3.6 platform with data mining techniques. Data was converted into ARFF and then later loaded into the system. The selection of relevant features was done using the chi-square filter selector to rank the features according to their relevance. This study employed three data mining techniques: Adaboost, Support Vector Machine algorithms together with the ensemble methods to predict the probability of a patient having malaria fever. The analysis was performed to find the most suitable one for the prediction of malaria fever. Weka toolkit was used to experiment with the three data mining algorithms. A program is an ensemble tool for data classification, regression, clustering, association rules, and visualization.

Pre-processing of the input dataset for a knowledge discovery goal using a data mining approach usually consumes the biggest portion of the effort in the proposed study. A chi-square filter algorithm will be applied to extract and clean the raw data from the patient record used. After the input data normalization, the classification will be performed using the three machine learning techniques.

3.2 System Architecture

See Fig. 1.

3.3 Support Vector Machines (SVM)

The most frequent and readily available supervised learning algorithm is the support vector machine (SVM). Based on the kernel principle, this separates incoming data linearly into two groups. SVM is the best machine learning technique for binary classification assignment [21]. SVM is a binary classifier that is great for healthcare classification and prediction since the kernel is set to linear and a search algorithm runs a grid to calculate the cost value of the classification [22, 23]. As a result, SVM is one of the most effective machine learning algorithms for determining the best solution to any classification or prediction problem.

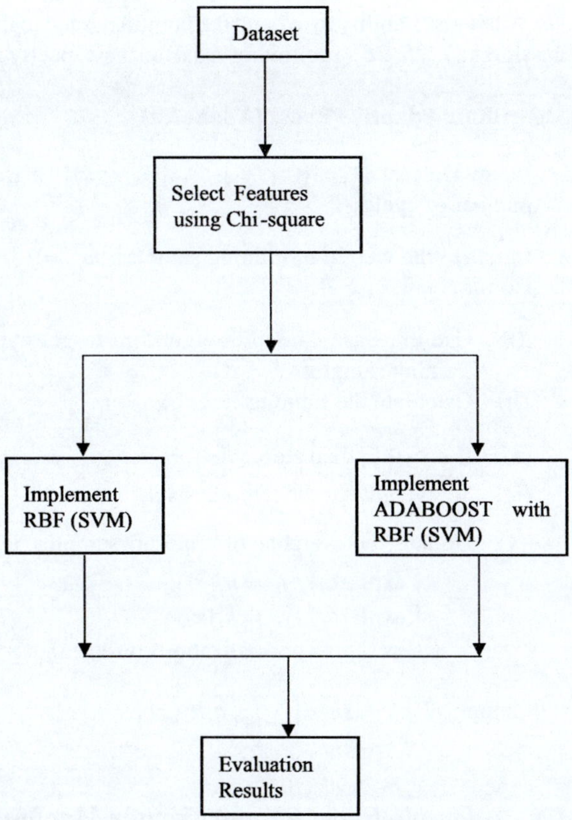

Fig. 1 Block diagram for system architecture

3.4 *AdaBoost Ensemble Classifier*

The ensemble method in recent time is one of the major developments in machine learning that combining more than one accurate component classifiers to finds a highly accurate classifier [24]. Bagging and Boosting are the two commonly used techniques for constructing Ensemble classifiers [25–27]. Boosting performs better when compared with bagging especially when the data do not have much noise [28, 29]. AdaBoost is the most common Boosting method [30, 31] which builds a group of complexity associated by keeping a set of weights across training samples and modifying them after each cycle of boosting. Training samples that were misclassified by the current component classifier will have their weights increased, while training samples that were correctly classified will have their weights increased. Several theories have been proposed to explain Adaboost's weight fluctuation [31,

32]. Adaboost's ability to expand the margin has led to its popularity among ensemble classifiers [7, 25, 26], improving AdaBoost's capacity for generalization.

Algorithm: Adaptive Boost (Adaboost)

1. Input: Dataset D $= \{(x_1, y_1), \ldots, (x_m, y_m)\}$, a Base Classifier algorithm, the number of cycles T.

2. Initialize the weight of training samples: $w_i^1 = 1/m$, for all $i = 1, 2, \ldots, m$.
3. Do for $t = 1, \ldots, T$.

   (i) Use the Base Classifier algorithm to get hypothesis h_t, on the weighted training samples.
   (ii) Calculate the training error of $h_t : \varepsilon_{t=\sum_{i=1}^{m} w_i^t, y_i \neq h_t(x_i)}$.
   (iii) If $\varepsilon_t > 0.5$; then stop.
   (iv) Set weight for the hypothesis $h_t : a_t = \frac{1}{2} ln\left(\frac{1-\varepsilon_t}{\varepsilon_t}\right)$.
   (v) Update the weights of training samples $w_i^{t-1} = \frac{w_i^{t-1} exp(-a_t y_i h_t(x_i))}{Z_t} = \frac{w_i^t}{Z_t} \text{x} \begin{cases} \exp\{-a_t\}, y_i = h_t(x_i) \\ \exp\{-a_t\}, y_i \neq h_t(x_i) \end{cases}$,
   where Z_t is a normalization consant and $\sum_{i=1}^{m} w_i^{t+1} = 1$.

4. Output: $H(x) = sign\left(\sum_{t=1}^{T} a_t h_t(x)\right)$.

3.5 *Adaptive Boost Support Vector Machine (AdaBoost SVM)*

The combination of AdaBoost and SVM as the foundation classifier is called AdaBoost SVM. The algorithm is very similar to the AdaBoost algorithm only because it achieved the SVM method's hypothesis weighting to achieve a better precision. At each cycle, the weight in misclassification error has been increased, while the weight on the already well = classified has been reduced to reduce the weighted potential back in the next cycle, thus predicting the htclass (label) hypothesis.

Algorithm: Adaptive Boost Support Vector Machine (AdaBoost SVM)

1. Input: Dataset D $= \{(x_1, y_1), \ldots, (x_m, y_m)\}$, a Base Classifier algorithm, the number of cycles T.
2. Initialize the weight of training samples: $w_i^1 = 1/m$, for all $i = 1, 2, \ldots, m$.
3. Do for $t = 1, \ldots, T$.

   (1) Use SVM algorithm to get hypothesis h_t, on the weighted training samples.
   (2) Calculate the training error of $h_t : \varepsilon_{t=\sum_{i=1}^{m} w_i^t, y_i \neq h_t(x_i)}$.
   (3) If $\varepsilon_t > 0.5$; then stop.

(4) Set weight for the hypothesis $h_t : a_t = \frac{1}{2}\ln\left(\frac{1-\varepsilon_t}{\varepsilon_t}\right)$.

(5) Update the weights of training samples $w_i^{t-1} = \frac{w_i^{t-1} exp(-a_t y_i h_t(x_i))}{Z_t} = \frac{w_i^t}{Z_t} \text{x} \begin{cases} \exp\{-a_t\}, y_i = h_t(x_i) \\ \exp\{-a_t\}, y_i \neq h_t(x_i) \end{cases}$,where Z_t is a normalization consant and $\sum_{i=1}^{m} w_i^{t+1} = 1$.

4. Output: $H(x) = \text{sign}\left(\sum_{t=1}^{T} a_t h_t(x)\right)$.

3.6 *Instrument for Data Collection and Preparation*

Monthly malaria incidence surveys were obtained from three (3) randomly sampled health centers in Kwara State. That patient has a set of symptoms and the number of MPs identified as the symptoms of malaria data and the results of the laboratory test. The input variables consist of monthly incidences of malaria and were trained and simulated using Microsoft Excel and integrated Weka 3.6 platform Giemsa staining was used for laboratory testing in the sampled hospital laboratories. Red blood cells (RBCs), plasmodium spp, platelets, and other structures have been described. This Plasmodium spp is counted in Malaria Parasite Count (MPcount). Each patient has a set of symptoms and the number of MPs. This malaria dataset is used to train and check the selected algorithm's performance. The report reports 1200 cases of malaria from January 2015 to December 2018. Such main characteristics of the dataset are: Headache (Hd), Fever(F), Dizziness(D), Muscle Weakness (BW), Vomiting(V), Appetite Loss (LA), and Joint Pain (JP).

4 Results and Discussion

4.1 *Performance Measurement Terms*

Accuracy: This is the percentage of the instances which are classified correctly by the classifier.

Time taken to build model: This is the classifier's time to build the model to be used for classification.

4.2 *10-Fold Cross Validations*

In the field of machine learning, ten-fold cross-validation is used to evaluate how effectively a learning algorithm can predict the data on which it is not equipped. The training dataset is split into 10 classes randomly, the first 9 groups are used to train the classifier, and the other group is often used as the test dataset. The process is repeated until all the groups are used as the test dataset, then the performance of the classifier is measured as an aggregate of all the 10-folds.

4.3 *Performance Evaluation*

The first feature removed is vomiting, the second feature removed is Jaundice, the third feature removed is enlarge liver, the fourth feature removed is the loss of appetite, the fifth feature removed is fever, the sixth feature removed is headache, the seventh feature removed is joint pain, the eighth feature removed is body weakness, the ninth feature removed is dizziness, and the tenth feature removed is nausea (Fig. 2 and Table 1).

After ten (10) features were removed, it was observed that none of the classifiers had less than 91% classification accuracy; this shows that the "fever" attribute is the most important feature in determining whether a parasite in the body is mild or severe. But being a medical condition where increased accuracy in classification means the difference between life and death, other features need to be considered.

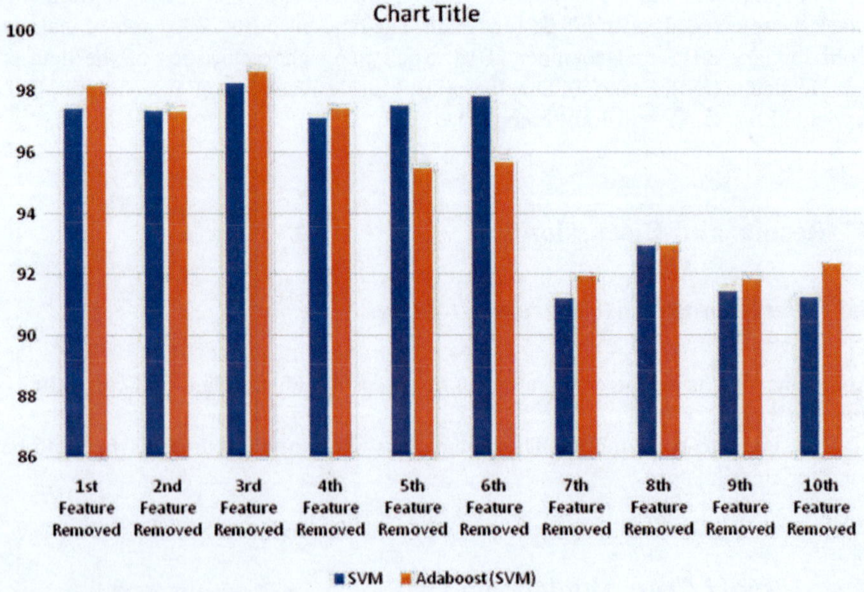

Fig. 2 Classification accuracy

Table 1 The classification accuracy of the algorithms when the feature is removed

	SVM	Adaboost (SVM)
1st Feature removed	97.4213	98.1741
2nd Feature removed	97.3499	97.3473
3rd Feature removed	98.2733	98.6654
4th Feature removed	97.1147	97.4399
5th Feature removed	97.5165	95.4848
6th Feature removed	97.8267	95.6614
7th Feature removed	91.2245	91.9232
8th Feature removed	92.9493	92.9493
9th Feature removed	91.4312	91.7985
10th Feature removed	91.2341	92.3431

Table 2 The time taken to build a classification model of the algorithms when the features are removed

	SVM	Adaboost (SVM)
1st Feature removed	0.95	3.98
2nd Feature removed	0.95	3.98
3rd Feature removed	0.47	3.78
4th Feature removed	0.95	3.98
5th Feature removed	0.44	4.88
6th Feature removed	0.30	3.64
7th Feature removed	0.34	3.68
8th Feature removed	0.68	3.31
9th Feature removed	0.62	3.74
10th Feature removed	0.59	3.35

Boosting SVM performed almost equally when one, two and three features were removed, and performed better when fourth features were removed but subsequently, removal of features reduced its accuracy (Fig. 3 and Table 2).

5 Conclusion

Classification of a disease like malaria fever is very crucial and thus, this study analyzed the performance of 250 patients' data collected from the University of Ilorin Teaching Hospital (UITH). The enhanced version of the algorithms in the determination of the level of disease was used. The result shows that the time taken by SVM is very fast in building its classification model, but not effective in classifying malaria fever as much as the boosted version of SVM. Because of the possible variance in the causes of malaria parasite to human body, getting a high accuracy is of crucial importance and from all the experiments removing four features (Vomiting,

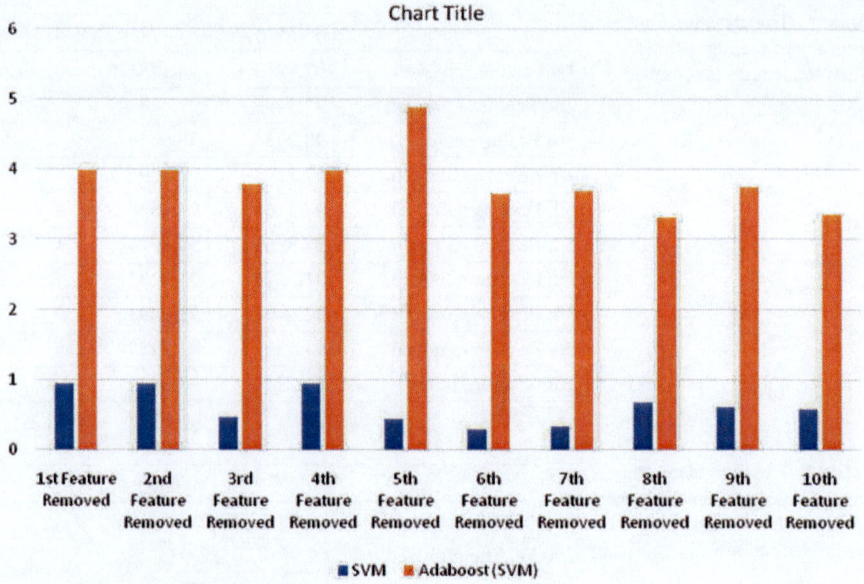

Fig. 3 Time taking for classification

Jaundice, enlarge liver, and loss of Appetite) as determined by the feature selector yields the highest classification accuracy overall from the boosted version of SVM, thus Boosting SVM with the four features removed is recommended for the classifications in this domain. In this study, the performance of the boosted version of SVM gave the highest accuracy, other methods that can be applied to improve the classification accuracy of SVM can be further investigated. Other classification algorithms such as Neural Network, KNN, and Naïve Bayes can also be considered for the purpose of comparison and generalization of our findings.

References

1. WHO (2013) World Malaria Report 2013. Geneva, World Health Organization
2. Awotunde JB, Jimoh RG, Oladipo ID, Abdulraheem M (2020) Prediction of malaria fever using long-short-term memory and big data. In: Communications in computer and information science, November, vol 1350. pp 41–53
3. Mutabingwa TK (2005) Artemisinin-based combination therapies (ACTs): best hope for malaria treatment but inaccessible to the needy! Acta Trop 95:305–315
4. Leslie T, Mikhail A, Mayan I, Anwar M, Bakhtash S, Nader M et al (2012) Over-diagnosis and mistreatment of malaria among febrile patients at primary healthcare level in Afghanistan: an observational study. BMJ 345:e4389
5. Ayo FE, Ogundokun RO, Awotunde JB, Adebiyi MO, Adeniyi AE (2020). Severe Acne Skin Disease: A Fuzzy-Based Method for Diagnosis. Lecture Notes in Computer Science (including

subseries Lecture Notes in Artificial Intelligence and Lecture Notes in Bioinformatics), July 2020, 12254 LNCS, pp. 320–334.

6. Awotunde JB, Matiluko OE, Fatai OW (2014) Medical diagnosis system using fuzzy logic. African J Comput ICT **7**(2):99–106. Published by IEEE Computer Society, Nigeria Section
7. Ayo FE, Awotunde JB, Ogundokun RO, Folorunso SO, Adekunle AO (2020) A decision support system for multi-target disease diagnosis: a bioinformatics approach. Heliyon 6(3):e03657
8. Awotunde JB, Folorunso SO, Bhoi AK, Adebayo PO, Ijaz MF (2021) Disease diagnosis system for IoT-based wearable body sensors with machine learning algorithm. Intell Syst Ref Libr 2021(209):201–222
9. Ameen AO, Olagunju M, Awotunde JB, Adebakin TO, Alabi IO (2017) Performance evaluation of breast cancer diagnosis using radial basis function. In: C4.5 and Adaboost, University of Pitesti scientific bulletin electronic and computer science series, 17(2):1–12. published by EdituraUniversitatii din Pitesti, Romania
10. Lebbe A, Saabith S, Sundararajan E, Bakar AA (2014) Comparative study on different classification techniques for breast cancer dataset. Int J Comput Sci Mob Comput 3(10):185–191
11. Johansson EW, Selling KE, Nsona H, Mappin B, Gething PW, Petzold M, Hildenwall H (2016) Integrated paediatric fever management and antibiotic over-treatment in Malawi health facilities: data mining a national facility census. Malar J 15(1):396
12. Bui QT, Nguyen QH, Pham VM, Pham MH, Tran AT (2019) Understanding spatial variations of malaria in Vietnam using remotely sensed data integrated into GIS and machine learning classifiers. Geocarto Int 34(12):1300–1314
13. Jain VK, Kumar S (2018) Effective surveillance and predictive mapping of mosquito-borne diseases using social media. J Comput Sci 25:406–415
14. Sow B, Mukhtar H, Ahmad HF, Suguri H (2019) Assessing the relative importance of social determinants of health in malaria and anemia classification based on machine learning techniques. Inform Health Soc Care 1–13
15. Sajana T, Narasingarao MR (2018) An ensemble framework for classification of malaria disease. ARPN J Eng Appl Sci Asian Res Publishing Net (ARPN) 13(9):3299—3307
16. Kouwaye B, Rossi F, Fonton N, Garcia A, Dossou-Gbété S, Hounkonnou MN, Cottrell G (2017) Predicting local malaria exposure using a Lasso-based two-level cross validation algorithm. PLoS ONE 12(10):e0187234
17. Taufik WM, Ghani NL, Drus SM (2019) Data mining techniques for disease risk prediction model: a systematic literature review. In: Proceedings of the 3rd international conference of reliable information and communication. pp 40–46. https://doi.org/10.1007/978-3-319-99007-1_4
18. Lashari SA, Ibrahim R, Senan N, Taujuddin NSAM (2018) Application of data mining techniques for medical data classification: a review. In: MATEC web of conferences, vol 150.https://doi.org/10.1051/matecconf/201815006003
19. Rabbi F, Uddin P, Ali A, Kibria F, Afjal I, Islam S, Nitu M (2018) Performance evaluation of data mining classification techniques for heart disease prediction. American J Eng Res 7(2):278–283
20. Ogundokun RO, Sadiku PO, Misra S, Ogundokun OE, Awotunde JB, Jaglan V (2021) Diagnosis of long sightedness using neural network and decision tree algorithms. J Phys: Conf Series **1767**(1):012021
21. Oladele TO, Ogundokun RO, Awotunde JB, Adebiyi MO, Adeniyi JK (2020) Diagmal: a malaria coactive neuro-fuzzy expert system. In: Lecture notes in computer science (including subseries Lecture Notes in Artificial Intelligence and Lecture Notes in Bioinformatics), July, vol 12254. LNCS, pp 428–441
22. Oladipo ID, Babatunde AO, Awotunde JB, Abdulraheem M (2020) An improved hybridization in the diagnosis of diabetes mellitus using selected computational intelligence. In: Communications in computer and information science, vol 1350. pp 272–285
23. Naraei P, Abhari A, Sadeghian A (2016). Application of multilayer perceptron neural networks and support vector machines in classification of healthcare data. In: 2016 Future technologies conference (FTC), December, IEEE, pp 848–852

24. Ren Y, Zhang L, Suganthan PN (2016) Ensemble classification and regression-recent developments, applications and future directions. IEEE Comput Intell Mag 11(1):41–53
25. Krawczyk B, Galar M, Jeleń Ł, Herrera F (2016) Evolutionary undersampling boosting for imbalanced classification of breast cancer malignancy. Appl Soft Comput 38:714–726
26. Galar M, Fernández A, Barrenechea E, Bustince H, Herrera F (2016) Ordering-based pruning for improving the performance of ensembles of classifiers in the framework of imbalanced datasets. Inf Sci 354:178–196
27. Salunkhe UR, Mali SN (2016) Classifier ensemble design for imbalanced data classification: a hybrid approach. Proc Comput Sci 85:725–732
28. Xia Y, Liu C, Li Y, Liu N (2017) A boosted decision tree approach using Bayesian hyper-parameter optimization for credit scoring. Expert Syst Appl 78:225–241
29. Hassan AR, Haque MA (2017) An expert system for automated identification of obstructive sleep apnea from single-lead ECG using random under sampling boosting. Neurocomputing 235:122–130
30. Zhou T, Han G, Xu X, Lin Z, Han C, Huang Y, Qin J (2017) δ-agree AdaBoost stacked autoencoder for short-term traffic flow forecasting. Neurocomputing 247:31–38
31. Wyner AJ, Olson M, Bleich J, Mease D (2017) Explaining the success of adaboost and random forests as interpolating classifiers. J Mach Learn Res 18(1):1558–1590
32. Baig MM, Awais MM, El-Alfy ESM (2017) AdaBoost-based artificial neural network learning. Neurocomputing 248:120–126
33. Lee W, Jun CH, Lee JS (2017) Instance categorization by support vector machines to adjust weights in AdaBoost for imbalanced data classification. Inf Sci 381:92–103

FNH—A Data Repository for Studying Fake News in Healthcare Domain

Isha Agarwal, Dipti Rana, Ch Surya Teja, and Nunna Naga Surya Sai Daivik

Abstract Although the Internet is a tremendous source of beneficial information, it has become tainted by the propagation of false information. Relying on such information can be disastrous. According to a study done by the World Health Organization (WHO), about 6000 people were hospitalized, and 800 people died as a result of fake news on COVID-19 in the first three months of 2020. As a result, recognizing fake news is critical in order to limit its harmful repercussions, particularly in the healthcare sector. This work presents an assembled dataset on fake news in the healthcare domain. Thus, an extensive dataset including labeled news material might aid in the diffusion, identification, and mitigation of fake news; so far, no datasets explicitly related to health care exist. As a result, in this study, a fake news data repository is presented: fake news on health care (FNH), which comprises labeled news items, the publishing date of news, source URL, and dynamic information to facilitate fake news-related research in the healthcare area. A detailed description of this dataset, an exploratory analysis of this data repository from several viewpoints, and the advantages of FNH for future applications in fake news research in the healthcare domain are presented in this work.

Keywords Fake news · Dataset · Health care · COVID-19 · Infodemic

1 Introduction

During the pandemic, WHO devised the term "Infodemic" to describe the spread of fake news, alleging that it was more dangerous than the virus itself [1]. Detecting and preventing the spread of fake news has become more important than ever as the world deals with the global epidemic COVID-19. Misinformation undermines people's faith in their leaders and destabilizes the economy of the country. The spread of incorrect

I. Agarwal (✉) · D. Rana · C. S. Teja · N. N. S. Sai Daivik
Sardar Vallabhbhai National Institute of Technology, Surat, Gujarat 395007, India
e-mail: isha.yash.agarwal@gmail.com

D. Rana
e-mail: dpr@coed.svnit.ac.in

© The Author(s), under exclusive license to Springer Nature Singapore Pte Ltd. 2023
J. K. Mandal and D. De (eds.), *Frontiers of ICT in Healthcare*, Lecture Notes in Networks and Systems 519, https://doi.org/10.1007/978-981-19-5191-6_4

information about lockdowns, vaccines, and death numbers heightened fear and anxiety. It has also had an effect on the supply chain for everyday items, resulting in a considerable rise in the purchase of foodstuffs, sanitizers, masks, and paper products. As a result, there was a shortage, supply chain imbalances exacerbated, and food insecurity intensified.
Furthermore, it has caused enormous losses in the price of oil and gasoline, as well as a dramatic decrease in the world economy [2]. The development of statistical methods for discriminating between fake and authentic news is a major task. These technologies might be used to assist organizations in fact-checking as well as categorizing and preventing the spread of fake news. As a result, they can assist people in avoiding potentially dangerous actions like self-medication with chloroquine phosphate, bleaching, or drinking too much alcohol [3]. As a result, in this work, we create and make available the FNH data repository, which presently comprises labeled news items, the date of publication, the source URL, and dynamic metadata. Various websites, such as Cable News Network (CNN), The Atlantic, and others, are scraped for this project, and a dataset dubbed "fake news in healthcare dataset" (FNH) is curated [4]. There are 7069 true news articles and 2424 fake news articles in this dataset. The newly built FNH repository has the potential to accelerate research into a variety of open research topics in health care, including fake news investigations.

2 Motivation and Contribution

Any fake news about health care that spreads across the Internet has the potential to harm people across the globe. There was an increase in fake news associated with COVID-19 and other health-related topics during the pandemic. Many individuals are still skeptical about COVID-19 guidelines and vaccine safety. Consuming incorrect healthcare information from online sources can have lethal consequences. At the global scale on which the Internet operates, it becomes critical to recognize any fake news regarding health care spreading on the Internet and to verify the credibility of sources.
The key contributions of this work include:

1. Fake news healthcare dataset (FNH) for the purpose of fake news detection in the healthcare domain.
2. Exploratory study on the FNH dataset from several perspectives to show the dataset's validity and identify their key features.

3 Background and Related Work

For the purpose of detection of fake news in health care, there is a significant need for a dataset. Many traditional fake news classification datasets primarily focus on general or political genres only. Several research studies used Twitter as a data source for

Table 1 Comparison of publicly available datasets

Dataset	Attributes	Limitations
Kaggle dataset [17]	Title, author, text	Consists of news articles relative to the politics subject only
FakeNewsNet [18]	Title, URLS, list of tweet ID	Specific to twitter social platform
LIAR [19]	Statement, speaker, speaker's job title, state	Consists of short articles only and non-relative to health care
HWB [20]	Content of articles	Consist of short text news article and no presence of headline or publishing date
ISOT [17]	Title, content, subject, date	Consists of news articles relative to the politics subject only

their work [5, 6]. Li et al. introduced MM-COVID, a news dataset containing around 11,000 instances [7]. This dataset consists of multi-dimensional and multilingual COVID-19 false news data. Ayoub et al. presented a dataset containing data obtained from various new sites (e.g., Aljazeera), fact-checking sites (e.g., Poynter), and other trustworthy sources such as CDC, WHO, and others [8]. Various datasets have been published by scraping fact-checked news articles from various authentic fact-checker websites and other resources including WHO [9].

A dataset constitutes either bi-class or multi-class targeted labels. Datasets included within the studies [10, 11] utilize the common classes for fake news detection—fake and real. Hossain et al. proposed COVID-19 lies which comprise stance-related labels and the fake news dataset is performed efficiently on it [12]. Multi-class targeted labels have been curate and covered in various studies [6, 9]. Each dataset provides an efficient performance score for fake news detection.

Various datasets are created by researchers with the objective of detecting fake news in different languages. Several studies focus on monolingual data [13, 14], while few others focus on multilingual data [7, 15, 16].

As observed, many datasets have been published in the field of fake news detection. Comparison of various datasets is presented in Table 1 relative to fake news is provided based on the features and their limitations within each dataset.

The objective of this report is to provide a dataset for fake news detection in the healthcare domain constituting all attributes across the globe.

4 Dataset Curation

In this section, the dataset integration process of the FNH Dataset is introduced. The block diagram showcases the flow from scraping data to removing redundant observations and creating the final FNH dataset (Fig. 1).

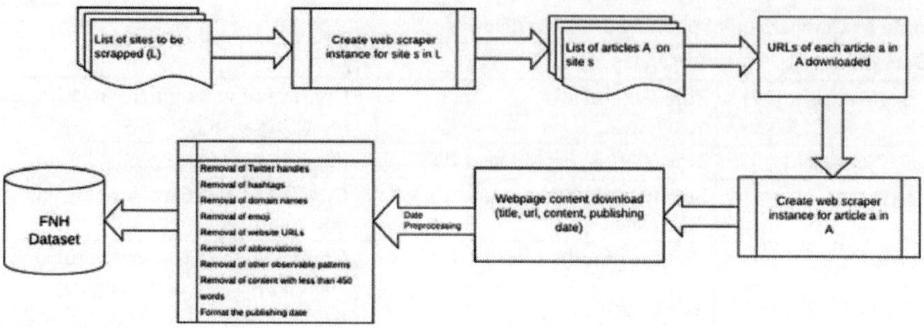

Fig. 1 Data scraping

The major problem associated with collecting the news content from the website is to find fake and truth-labeled websites. For this purpose, a document constituting the label associated with each website is used. The website with satire or fake labels within the document has been chosen for extracting the fake news. While for the truth news, websites such as CNN, BBC News, The Atlantic, and other well-known reliable websites have been used.

Each website has been filtered to provide news content relative to health care. Based on the filter, there are n pages with k articles on each page. The web scraper instance first extracts the title, publishing date, and the URL of the articles from each page. Once the URL of the k articles is extracted, the content of the article is extracted by initiating another web scraper instance for the specific URL. For each site, the implementation varies as the document object model (DOM) query is used for extracting instances that are different for each website.

Algorithm 1 Algorithm for data scraping

Require: List of news sites L
Ensure: Dataset with annotated news articles Ni {True, Fake}

```
Dataset D := {}
Create instance of WebScrapper(W)
for site s in L do
    n := number of pages in s
    for page p_i in s do, i ← 1 to N
        k := number of articles in p_i
        for article a_j in p_i do, j ← 1 to K
            Document d_ij := {}
            W.visit(a_j)
            d_ij.title := W.get(a_j.title)
            d_ij.content := W.get(a_j.content)
            d_ij.publishing_date := W.get(a_j.publishing_date)
            d_ij.url := W.get(a_j.url)
            d_ij.label := annotate(s, a_j)
            append(D, d_ij)
        end for
    end for
end for
return D
```

Table 2 FNH dataset distribution

	True	Fake
Count	2424	7069

After the data for individual websites is captured, the instances for the attributes are concatenated and formatted. Following this, data cleaning has been performed in the four steps. The first step is the removal of duplicate or irrelevant observations, then fixing structural errors and filtering unwanted outliers. Finally, missing data is handled using imputation methods and the final data is presented with the statistics given in Table 2.

5 Data Analysis

FNH has multi-dimensional information relative to the news content associated with the healthcare domain. In this section, we provide an in-depth quantitative analysis to illustrate the features of FNH and give an in-depth analysis relative to the context of news articles.

5.1 Assessing the Distribution of Classes

The FNH dataset has two classes associated with it, true and fake. For understanding the distribution of the classes, a bar chart and a donut chart have been analyzed. From the bar chart, a high imbalance is observed. True news encompasses 76.4% of the data, and fake news encompasses 23.6% of the data. The ratio of imbalance is given as the number of true news to fake news documents, and for FNH, the ratio of imbalance is 4:1. The dataset is extracted from the websites and is subjected to noisy and dirty data. Thus, preprocessing of the data to keep the data clean. For this purpose, each instance of the textual attribute in the dataset is subjected to lemmatization, normalization, removal of stop words, and redundant observations. Further analysis is performed on the clean data. The FNH dataset has two textual attributes, title and content (Fig. 2).

5.2 Character Count Distribution for the Textual Data

For each textual attribute, a character count has been performed for each document instance in the dataset.

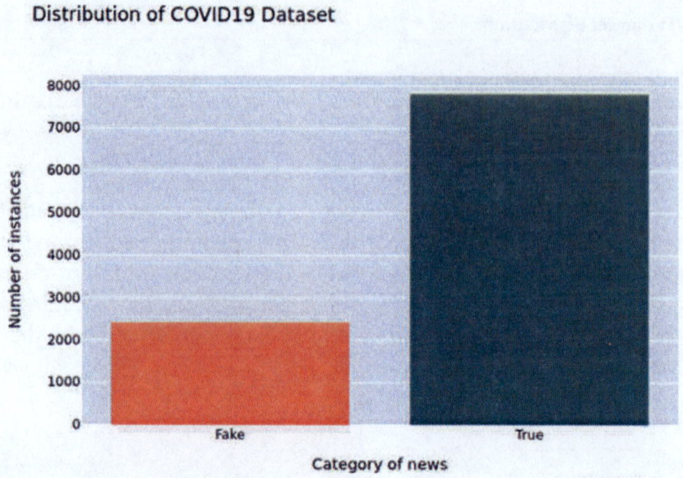

Fig. 2 Numerical distribution of dataset

Within Fig. 3, the analysis is performed for character count for content and title for each class. The character count is presented in two views—histogram and box plot view. Both plots provide visuals on the number of characters along with their frequency in the documents. For the character count for the content attribute, it is observed that the majority of the documents lie between 500 and 1000 characters. For the true class, the maximum observed is 10 thousand characters, and for the fake class, the maximum is 4000 characters. For the title attribute, the majority of documents lie between 40 and 60 characters. For the true class, the maximum observed is 111 characters and for the fake class, 100 characters. In conclusion, the character count of the true documents is higher than the fake documents.

5.3 Word Count Distribution for the Textual Data

For each textual attribute, a word count has been performed for each document instance in the dataset. Similar to character count, the analysis is performed for word count for content and title for each class. The word count is performed similarly to that of character count. For the word count for the content attribute of each document, it is observed that the majority of the documents lie between 50 and 100 words. For the true class, the maximum observed is 1500 words, while for the fake class, the maximum is 533 words. Similarly, for the title attribute, the majority of documents lie between 7 and 10 words, and for the true class, the maximum observed is 18 words and for the fake class, 13 words. Similar to character count, the word count of true news is greater than fake news.

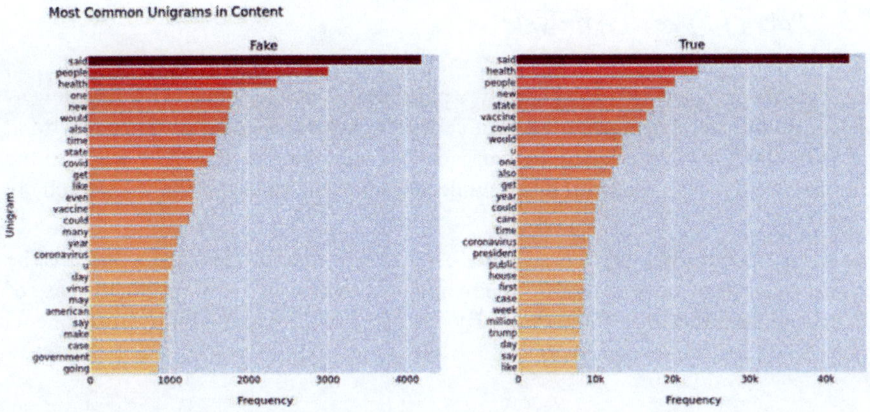

Fig. 3 Unigram distribution of content

5.4 N-gram Distribution for Content Attribute

N-grams have been utilized to understand the most common words or sequence of words utilized in the context of fake and true documents. For n-grams analysis, unigrams, bigrams, and trigrams are used.

Within the true documents, the unigrams majorly revolve around the words vaccine, people, and health, while in fake news, the unigrams majorly revolve around people and COVID. This signifies that during the COVID pandemic, the fake news revolved more around COVID, while the true documents covered in-depth documents around healthcare topics.

For the bigrams, the sequence of words revolves around the same words in both true and fake documents; however, the frequency of these bigrams differs. Within the fake documents, the words story, president trump, and public health are majorly used. For the true documents, the words fully vaccinated, health care are majorly used. This signifies that fake news revolves around telling a story related to health care in the USA.

For the trigrams, the sequence of words revolves around the same words in both true and fake documents; however, the frequency of these trigrams differs. Within the fake documents, the words story, New York Times, and center disease control are frequently used and in true documents, the words revolve around disease control and food drug administration. This signifies that fake news repeats the word story frequently in its context.

5.5 Part of Speech Analysis

The part of speech (POS) indicates how a particular word functions in the meaning as well as grammatical in a document. The spaCy library has been utilized to understand the POS and TAG variables of the words within a document. The POS provides the simple UPOS part of the speech tag, while TAG is the detailed part of the speech tag (Fig. 4).

In the fake documents, there is a higher use of verbs than proposition while it is the opposite case for true documents. The majority of the words are nouns, in the case of fake documents there are 150 thousand occurrences of nouns, and for true documents more than 1 million occurrences.

5.6 Topic Distribution for Context

Latent Dirichlet allocation (LDA) has been used to create a document-topic matrix and topic-word matrix from which the frequent nine topics are extracted. Representation has been done to see, which topic is majorly used within the fake and true documents (Figs. 5 and 6).
Within the fake documents, most topics are relative to people looking to make a new lifetime and vaccinations. This suggests that the majority of fake documents talk relative to individuals looking for a new perspective. Within the true documents, most topics are relative to new cases of COVID in hospitals and new healthcare programs (Fig. 7).

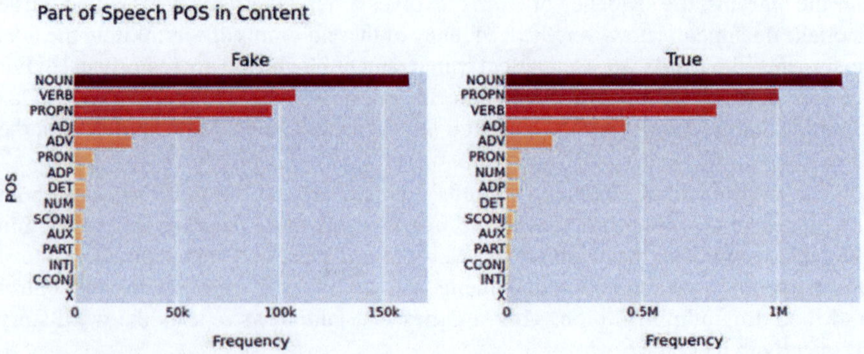

Fig. 4 Top 15 POS tags distribution

Topic Distribution for content (true)

Topic ID	Topic
0	Stop tobacco and vaping, excercise and be healthy
1	Voting campaign in US
2	Introducing new schools in city
3	People with new cases of covid in hospitals
4	LLC firm government business
5	People think time going in work
6	Chicago and china government economy
7	Covid vaccinates given by doctors
8	Risk of children studying at schools
9	Company came with new healthcare program

Fig. 5 Topics associated with true news

Topic Distribution for content (fake)

Topic ID	Topic
0	Coronovirus lockdown for people health
1	China cause outbreak, covid spread and virus causing death
2	President trump coming with healthcare solution for the democrat country
3	Research and study for treatment using drugs is on trial
4	Vaccinating the people to prevent covid
5	Police arrested woman for sexual abortion
6	People looking to make new life time
7	Mexican migrants cross border
8	Healthy food and water helps with the body health
9	Voting and election between biden and harris

Fig. 6 Topics associated with fake news

5.7 Word Cloud Distribution

Word clouds have been created for the content within fake and true documents. In the word cloud, the size of the word is proportional to the frequency of the word. For fake documents, the most frequent word is the vaccine, and for true documents, the most frequent word is health care (Fig. 8).

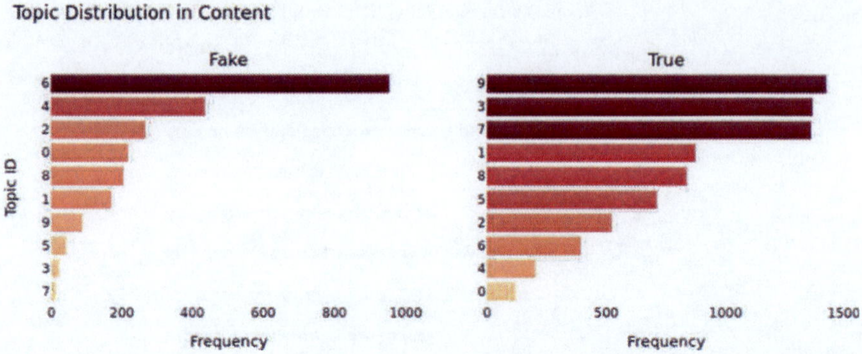

Fig. 7 Topics distribution for content

Fig. 8 Word cloud distribution

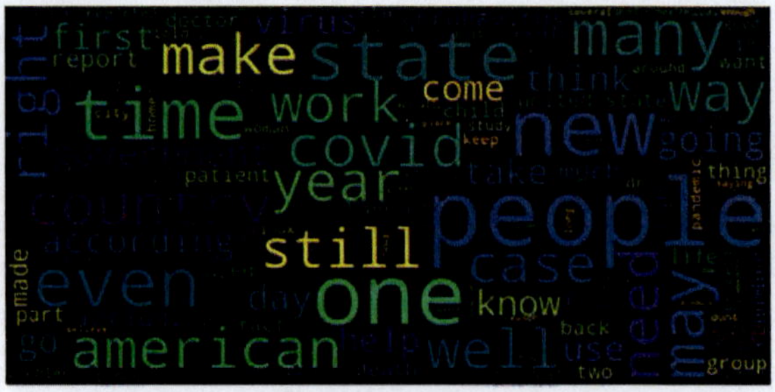

(a) Word cloud for fake news content

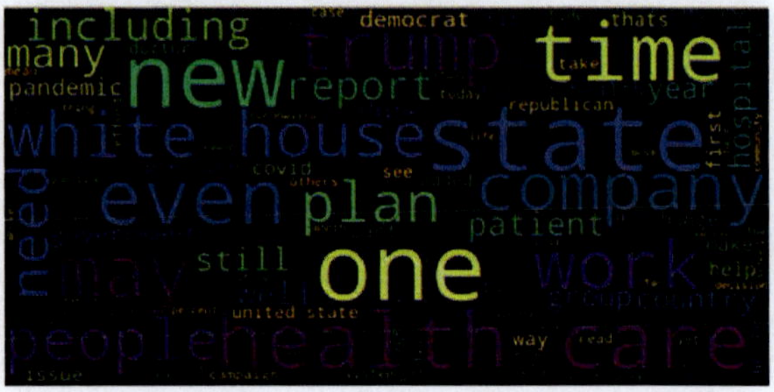

(b) Word cloud for true news content

5.8 Wildcard Distribution for Content

Wildcards are the repetitive redundant observations in the textual data. This includes Twitter handles, website URLs, hashtags, emoji, and other patterns. For both the classes, there is a significant number of wildcards.
Within the dirty FNH data, there is 2.33% of wildcards and on the removal of the wildcards, in the FNH cleaned dataset, there is 0% of the wildcards.

5.9 Publishing Date Analysis

A line chart has been plotted to observe the number of documents published in the years 2000–2099. It will showcase the rise and fall of the number of documents for both fake and true documents as the years pass.
For the fake news data, there has been an increase from the year 2014 and has been at the highest peak in the years 2020, 2021 during the COVID pandemic time. It has also been observed that there are few fake documents with the publishing year of 2097 and other future dates which is not the case for true documents.

5.10 Bivariate Analysis of Topic and Publishing Date

Using LDA, each document has been assigned the topic using the document-topic matrix. Based on that, the five most frequent topics have been analyzed for both fake and true documents. A line chart is plotted to understand the number of documents associated with a particular topic within the range of years 2000–2021. Within the fake documents, topic six has the majority of documents associated between the range 2014 and 2015 and it reduces in 2021 giving rise to topic four which is associated with vaccinating people to prevent COVID. Within the true documents, the topic three and seven have the majority of documents associated and both topics are highly associated with COVID and vaccination.

6 Potential Applications

FNH dataset can be used for multiple applications. It can be used for fake news detection and mitigation.

6.1 Fake News Detection

The FNH dataset provides various attributes such as title, length, content, source, and publishing date, which can help in the detection of fake news using various approaches.

6.2 Fake News Mitigation

FNH dataset provides rich information about various news related to health care that aids in the reduction of negative effects brought by the spread of fake news.

7 Conclusion and Future Work

In this paper, a data repository FNH is collected which consists of news content related to the healthcare domain. A principal strategy is proposed to collect relevant data from various sources. Moreover, a detailed analysis is done for the attributes of the dataset to understand the difference between fake and real news.
The current data repository includes the linguistic news content only, thus the future repository will include the extension to visual news content as well as news content from social media relative to health care.

References

1. Zarocostas J (2020) How to fight an infodemic. In: The lancet 395, no 10225, p 676
2. Albulescu C (2020) Coronavirus and oil price crash. In: Available at SSRN 3553452
3. Cinelli M et al (2020) The COVID-19 social media infodemic. Sci Rep 10(1):1–10
4. Agarwal I et al (2021) Fake news on COVID-19 healthcare. https://doi.org/10.21227/k0qs-bz38, https://dx.doi.org/10.21227/k0qs-bz38
5. D Kar (2021) No rumours please! a multi-indic-lingual approach for COVID fake-tweet detection. In: Grace Hopper Celebration India (GHCI), IEEE, pp 1–5
6. Dharawat A et al (2020) Drink bleach or do what now? Covid-HeRA: a dataset for risk-informed health decision making in the presence of COVID19 misinformation. In: arXiv preprint arXiv:2010.08743
7. Li Y et al (2020) Toward a multilingual and multimodal data repository for COVID-19 disinformation. In: 2020 IEEE international conference on big data (big data), IEEE, pp 4325–4330
8. Ayoub J, Yang XJ, Zhou F (2021) Combat COVID-19 infodemic using explainable natural language processing models. Inf Process Manage 58(4):102569
9. Ng LHX, Carley KM (2021) "The coronavirus is a bioweapon": classifying coronavirus stories on fact-checking sites. Comput Math Org Theor 27(2):179–194
10. Bandyopadhyay S, Dutta S (2020) Analysis of fake news in social medias for four months during lockdown in COVID-19

11. Kaliyar RK, Goswami A, Narang P (2021) MCNNet: generalizing fake news detection with a multichannel convolutional neural network using a novel COVID-19 dataset. In: 8th ACM IKDD CODS and 26th COMAD, pp 437–437
12. Hossain T (2021) COVIDLIES: detecting COVID-19 misinformation on social media. University of California, Irvine
13. WHO COVID19 Tweets (2021) https://www.kaggle.com/gpreda/covid19-tweets
14. Alqurashi S, Alhindi A, Alanazi E (2020) Large Arabic twitter dataset on covid-19. In: arXiv preprint arXiv:2004.04315
15. Qazi U, Imran M, Ofli F (2020) GeoCoV19: a dataset of hundreds of millions of multilingual COVID-19 tweets with location information. SIGSPATIAL Special 12(1):6–15
16. Chen E, Lerman K, Ferrara E et al (2020) Tracking social media discourse about the covid-19 pandemic: development of a public coronavirus twitter data set. JMIR Public Health Surveillance 6(2):e19273
17. Ahmad I et al (2020) Fake news detection using machine learning ensemble methods. In: Complexity 2020
18. Shu K et al (2018) Fakenewsnet: a data repository with news content, social context and spatialtemporal information for studying fake news on social media. In: arXiv preprint arXiv:1809.01286
19. Wang WY (2017) " liar, liar pants on fire": a new benchmark dataset for fake news detection. In: arXiv preprint arXiv:1705.00648
20. Anoop K, Deepak P, Lajish VL (2020) Emotion cognizance improves health fake news identification. In: IDEAS, vol 2020, 24th

Modeling and Simulation of Total Harmonic Distortion (THD) in Multilevel H Bridge Inverters for Healthcare

Akash Mourya and Mithlesh Gautam

Abstract Due to COVID-19 overhead on ICU, CCU is more demanding the high voltage backup solar PV inverters in healthcare. To fulfill high voltage requirement of the medical equipment in healthcare applications, many multilevel inverter designs have been proposed in recent times. Cascaded H Bridge (CHB) inverter is light weight and requires fewer components to design. The major concern in the inverter design is to compensate for the THD performance. It is obvious to have THD due to uses of large switches. Therefore, this paper has reviewed the FFT performance of various single and three phase inverting architectures using CHB. The paper first describes the basic single H bridge used for Solar PV inverter design. In this prime, focus is to design the GTO-based high voltage inverters. There are five level, seven level, nine level, and eleven level inverters considered for the evaluation of performance during the survey. The THD is considered for the evaluation parameter in the survey. The FFT analysis is considered for the performance comparison of the multilevels inverters. Various applications of the H bridge inverters are also considered for the paper to discuss. It is concluded that increasing the levels may reduce the harmonic distortions and may increase voltage performance of medical equipments.

Keywords Cascade H bridge · Multilevel inverter · FFT analysis · Total harmonic distortion (THD) · SPWM

1 Introduction

The H bridge inverters are frequently used in the solar panel to save voltage. Usually, the task of inverters is to used for the converting the DC energy to the AC lines directly operating the grid line. There are certain high voltages medical equipments required internal inverters, and every ICU needs power supply and inverters. With the invention

A. Mourya (✉) · M. Gautam
Truba College of Science and Technology, Bhopal, India
e-mail: akash2327@gmail.com

M. Gautam
e-mail: mithlesh.gautam@trubainstitute.ac.in

© The Author(s), under exclusive license to Springer Nature Singapore Pte Ltd. 2023
J. K. Mandal and D. De (eds.), *Frontiers of ICT in Healthcare*, Lecture Notes in Networks and Systems 519, https://doi.org/10.1007/978-981-19-5191-6_5

Fig. 1 Classification of multilevel inverters

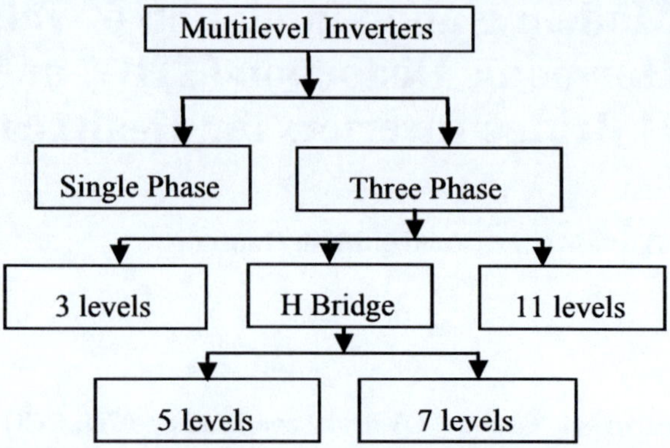

of the different electronic components, the quality and performances of the converters and inverters have been significantly improved in last two decades. Researchers have designed different inverter [1–3, 5] modules by modifying architectures. Therefore, it is required to analyze the performance of existing inverter architectures. The major role is to generate the AC voltage from the applied DC voltage source. If the input DC voltage varies, then AC output is also varying; therefore, the gain of the inverter remains constant. Due to availability of the various inverting architecture, it is difficult to get optimum results. It is required to evaluate performance for different inverting circuits. There are various types of the inverters available in the literature; thus in the beginning, the classification of the inverter design is presented in the Fig. 1.

The broadly inverting operation is classified as single phase and three phases. Then our main concern is to focus on cascaded H bridge (CHB) inverter. The inverters are classified base on the level of trace used in multilevel inverters. In this paper, our prime concern will be to compare the performance of each of these inverters based on the THD and FFT analysis. It is highly desired to minimize the THD in inverter designs.

These multilevel modes depend on the operating sequences and of the switches and the input of the switches. The three phase inverter is required to produce the three phase waveform as shown in the Fig. 2.

2 H Bridge Inverters

The single cell architecture of the cascade H bridge (CHB) inverter consists of the four switches. The main advantage is use of less capacitors and components for design. The single cell structure is used in the H bridge which is shown in the Fig. 3.

Usually, GTO has been opted for multilevel inverter design for the high voltage appliance. The basic construction of the GTO is shown in the Fig. 4.

The main advantage of using GTO for switching is high operating voltage and current ratings up to 1600 V and 250 A approx. The GTO basic construction or

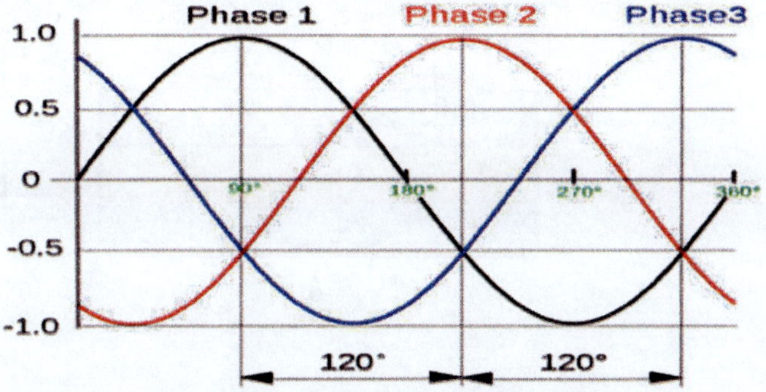

a) Normal three phase waveform of Voltages

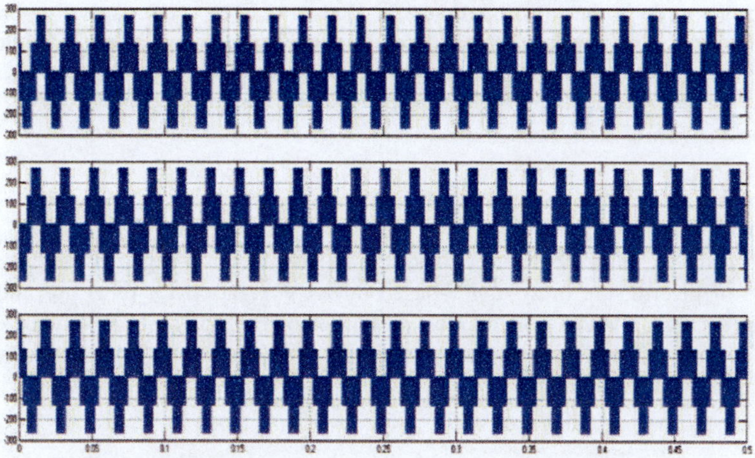

b) Simulation of Multilevel voltages of three phases inverters

Fig. 2 Wave form of three phases AC inverting output

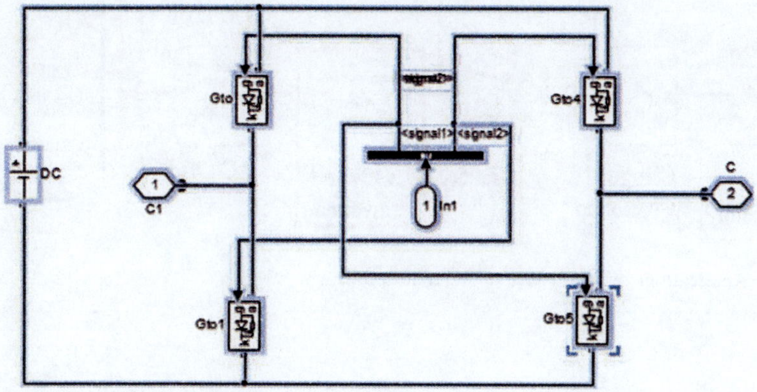

Fig. 3 Single cell H bridge model using switches

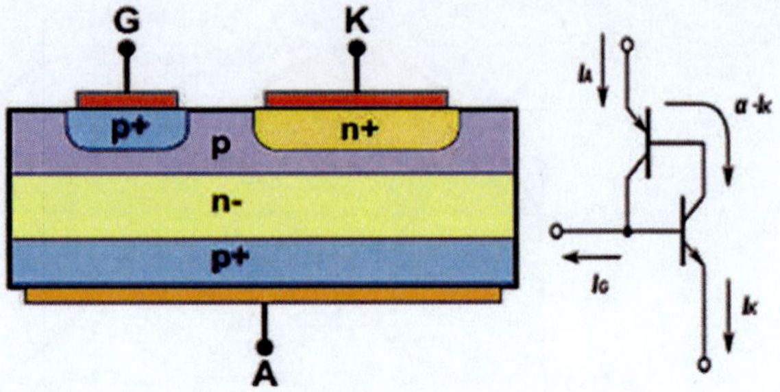

Fig. 4 GTO construction structure and circuit

structure and its equivalent circuit is shown in the Fig. 4. Using the high-power operating source in the most of industrial loads, it can be proven advantageous to high-power motors applications. But on the other side, it may damage additional loads in system. Using H bridge inverter, it may be suitable option in such cases.

2.1 Applications

Applications of solar PV inverters in hospitals are shown in Fig. 5. Usually, applications of inverter are in Solar PV-based power generation for rural hospitals for support during COVID-19 pandemic over burden on existing systems. The inverting AC mains may give support system during night to OT, ICU, CCU, and emergency of hospitals as mentioned.

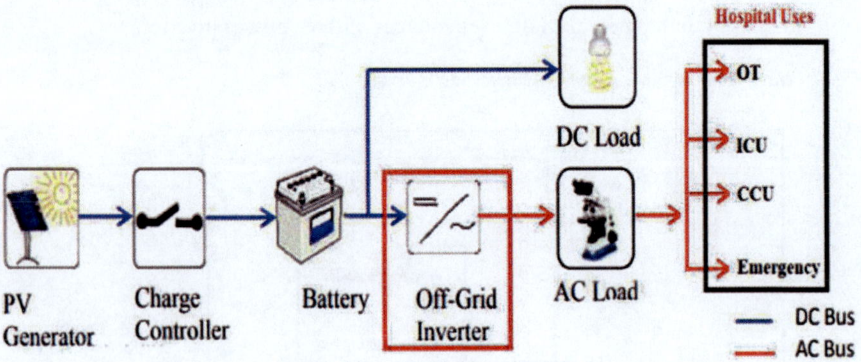

Fig. 5 Applications of solar PV inverters in hospitals

3 Reviews of Multilevel Inverters

The operation efficiency of the inverting operation depends on the performance of switches used for designing. Many architecture of cascaded H bridge (CHB) inverters was designed to improve the performance. Ali et al. [1] have used the pulse width modulation (PWM) for improving the performance of the multilevel CHB inverters.

Lee et al. [2] have opted the modified PWM8 approach with phase shifting to improve CHB inverting performance. The PWM is used for controlling performance of cascaded H bridge inverter. Rajesh et al. [3] have compared THD performances of 3 and 5 levels CHB inverters. They have reported THD of 26.3% for 3 level and THD of 15.04% for 5 level inverters at stator voltage. Singh et al. [4] have simulated 5 levels three phase CHB inverter using SPWM and reported 21.2% THD. Singh et al. [5] have presented good analysis of THD for various multilevel CHB inverters and concluded 23.54% for 9 level and 10.84% THD for 11 level CHB inverters. Gupta et al. [6] have presented the design of CHB inverter and presented minimum voltage THD of 28.9% for single phase 4 level inverter. Savanur [7] presented the state space model for CHB inverter of single phase. Shreya Bandil et al. [12] have designed the CHB-based 7 level inverter and also evaluated the THD performance for inverters. Chitha et al. [13] have proposed to evaluate the performance of the THD analysis of various 7 level inverters.

MLI with evolutionary algorithm-based switching, according to Menaka et al. [21], is a good alternative for medical electronic equipment used in hospitals to obtain quality power with low THD. Matías et al. [23] and George et al. [24] have designed the DC–DC converters for medical equipments. Table 1 keeps the summary of all reviewed papers.

4 Proposed Multilevel Inverting Models

In this paper, multilevel CHB inverter with 5 levels is designed and proposed to evaluate for 400 V high voltage uses. It is proposed to use GTO-based high switching high voltage inverter. It is proposed to increase inverting levels to produce the better approximate of the sine waves. The multilevel inverter may need filtering for harmonic distortion reduction. There are different types of multilevel inverters. The single phase five level multilevel inverter is shown in the Fig. 6.

Similarly, the three phase five level inverting cascaded architecture is represented in the Fig. 7 as designed by Singh et al. [4]. The five level three phase inverter proposed by Singh [4] offers the THD level of 21.2%.The THD performance is shown in the Fig. 7b). It can be observed that six H bridge blocks are used for the 3 phase inverter structure.

It is required to minimize the THD performance of CHB inverters. Therefore, this paper evaluates the performance of the multilevel cascaded H bridge inverters based on FFT analysis and comparing the THD performance.

Table 1 Summary of survey

S. no.	Authors	Type of inverter	Work
1	Ali et al. [1]	Multilevel CHB inverters	Used PWM for improving performance of the multilevel CHB inverters
2	Rajesh et al. [3]	3 and 5 levels CHB	Have compared THD performances of 3 and 5 levels CHB inverters
3	Singh et al. [4]	Three phase 5 level CHB inverter	Design using SPWM for five level CBH inverter
4	Singh et al. [5]	Single phase multilevel CHB inverters	Analyzed THD performance of various multilevel CHB inverters
5	Shreya Bandil et al. [12]	7 level inverter	7-level CHB inverter designed for PV cell applications using SPWM
6	Chitha et al. [13]	Multilevel inverters	Have evaluated performance of THD analysis of various 7 level inverters
7	Menaka et al. [21]	Multilevel Inverter	Inverter design of electronic medical equipments harmonic analysis
8	George et al. [24]	DC–DC converter	Have designed the DC–DC converters for medical equipments

5 Evaluations of Multilevel Inverter

This section presents performance evaluation of the various THD values achieved by the different CHB inverters. The waveform of the line voltage for the five level cascade inverters is shown in the Fig. 8.

The results of the proposed method are given sequentially below for line and phase voltages and shown in Fig. 9. The simulation of the MATLAB model is used for evaluating the harmonic performance of the CHB inverter for the healthcare applications. The simulated FFT analysis of five levels CHB inverter is shown in the Fig. 10.

5.1 Parametric Comparison

Total harmonic distortion (THD) as ref by Vadizadeh et al. [22] defines degree of closeness of the shape between output and its fundamental FFT component and is mathematically given as;

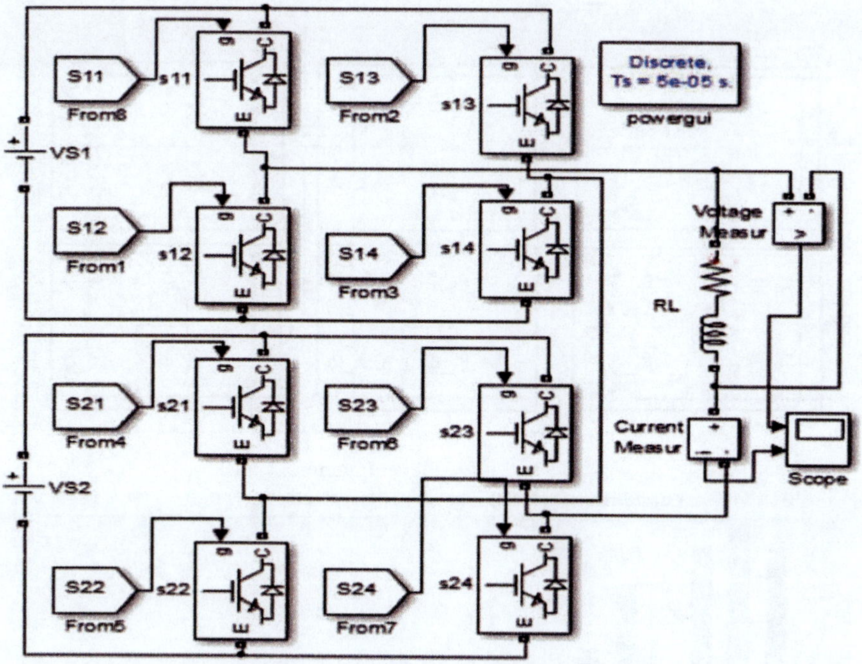

a) Single phase five level multilevel inverter

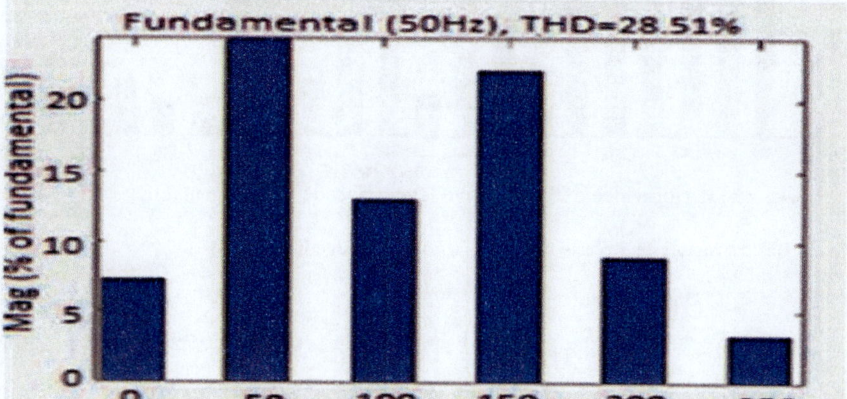

b) THD of the five level single phase Inverter [5]

Fig. 6 Single phase five level cascade H bridge inverter

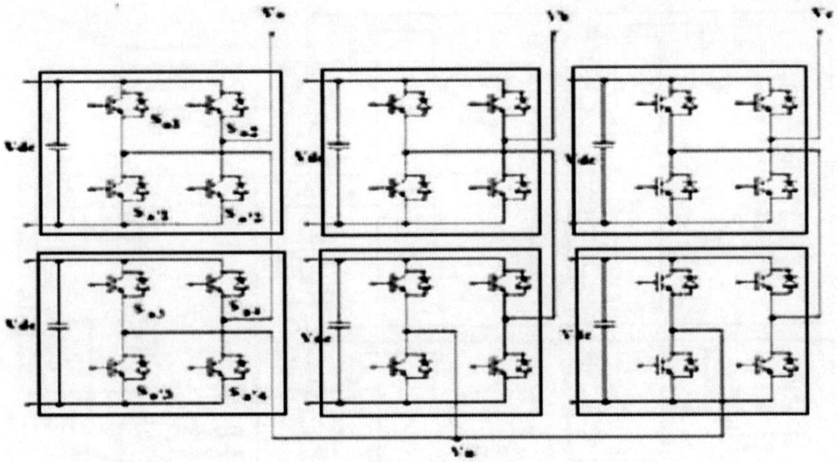

a) Five level Inverter.

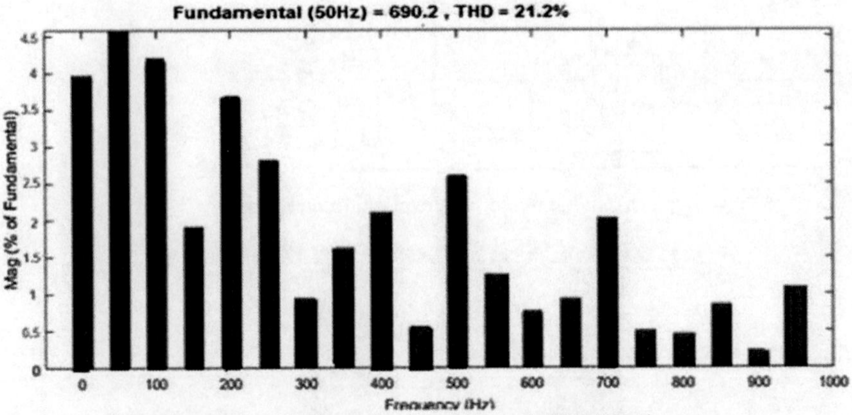

b) Performance of 3 phase five level Cascade H Bridge inverter

Fig. 7 Basic structure of 3 phase five level cascade H bridge inverter [4]

$$\mathrm{THD} = \frac{1}{V_{01}}\left(\sqrt{\sum_{n=2,3}^{\infty}(V_n)^2}\right) \quad (1)$$

where V_n is amplitude of harmonics, V_{ol} is line voltage

The tabular comparisons of the performance of the inverters have been given in the Table 2. It can be observed that 5 level three phase inverter performs better to minimize the THD performance.

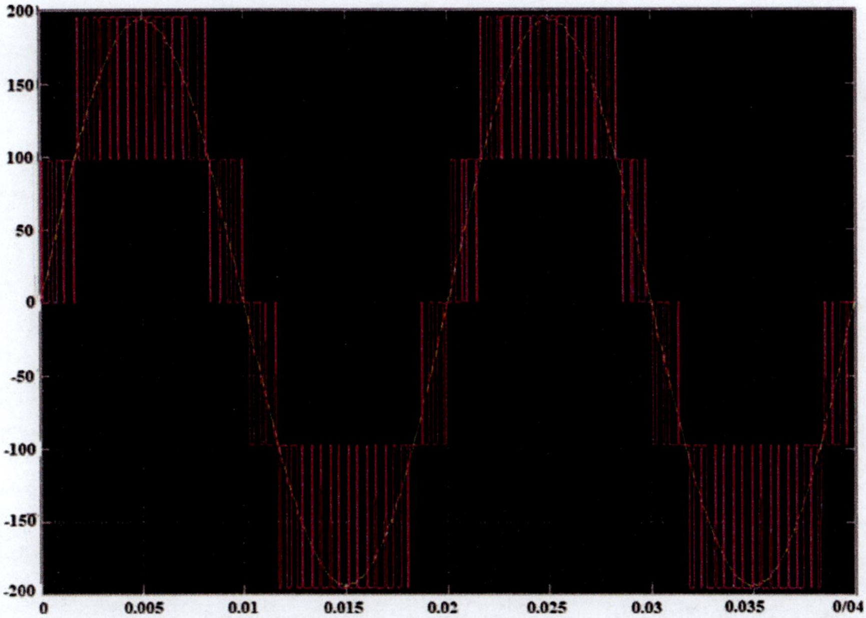

Fig. 8 Line voltage waveform for five level cascade inverters

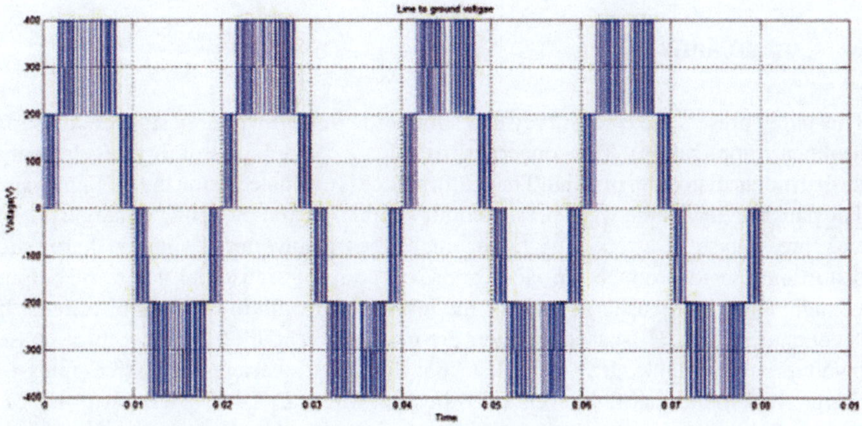

Fig. 9 Comparison of the validation of 5 level CHB inverter waveforms

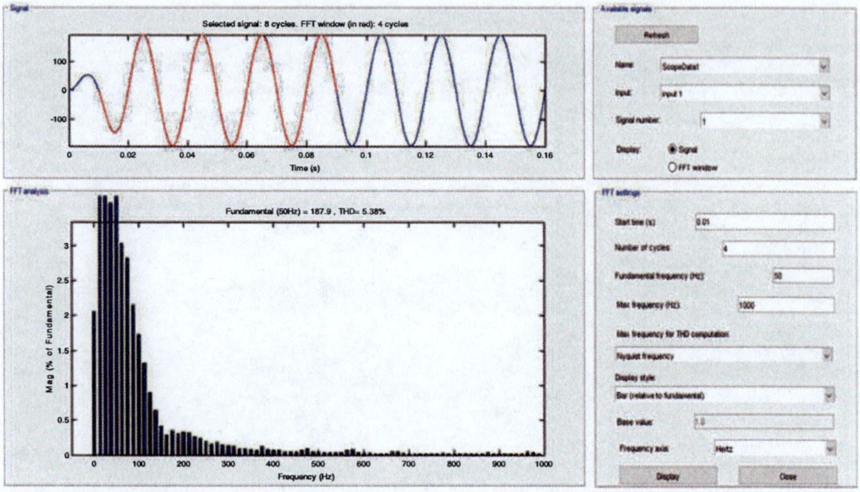

Fig. 10 FFT simulations for CHB inverter

Table 2 Comparison of THD with single phase performance of Rajesh et al. [3] with 5 levels

S. no	Single phase 5 level CHB inverter	Three phase 5 level CHB inverter
1	28.51 Rajesh et al. [3]	21.2

6 Conclusions

This paper presets the brief survey and simulation of the inverter designs models for healthcare applications. The concern is to evaluate performance of inverters keeping the harmonic distortion in mind. The performance is evaluated using the FFT analysis. The paper reviewed the work presented for simulation and modeling of single phase and three phase inverters. The major challenges in inverter design are harmonic distortion and to produce the close approximation of sinusoidal nature of output voltage. Paper is focused to reviews the inverters specific to CHB architectures. It is concluded that CHB-based inverters are more efficient, then the other three phase inverters are available. It is also clear that the CHB inverters are less complex in design. It is found that five levels CHB inverter offers 25% less THD performance. In future, the performance of the multilevel inverters will be evaluated and validated for minimizing the THD performances.

Acknowledgements Author here by acknowledges each and every individual who have supported directly or indirectly for the current research and helped the authors.

References

1. Ali A, Nakka J (2016) Improved performance of cascaded multilevel inverter. In: 2016 International conference on microelectronics, computing and communications (MicroCom), Durgapur, India, pp 1–5
2. Lee E, Kim S, Lee K (2020) Modified phase-shifted PWM scheme for reliability improvement in cascaded H-bridge multilevel inverters. IEEE Access 8:78130–78139
3. Rajesh B, Manjesh (2016) Comparison of harmonics and THD suppression with three and 5 level multilevel inverter-cascaded H-bridge. In: 2016 International conference on circuit, power and computing technologies (ICCPCT), Nagercoil, India, pp 1–6
4. Singh A, Mahanty RN (2017) Simulation of simplified SVM technique for three phase five-level cascaded H-bridge inverter. In: 2017 International conference on information, communication, instrumentation and control (ICICIC), Indore, India, pp 1–6
5. Singh G, Garg VK (2017) THD analysis of cascaded H-bridge multi-level inverter. In: 2017 4th international conference on signal processing, computing and control (ISPCC), Solan, India, pp 229–234
6. Gupta LK, Chaturvedi KT, Sharma ST, Srikakolapu J (2014) Simulation of a cascade connected H-bridge five level inverter. In: 2014 IEEE international conference on MOOC, innovation and technology in education (MITE), Patiala, India, pp 165–170
7. Savanur SR, Teli K (2018) Simulation and state space representation of single phase five level h-bridge inverter using MATLAB. In: 2018 International conference on recent innovations in electrical, electronics and communication engineering (ICRIEECE), Bhubaneswar, India, pp 1832–1837
8. Islam SM, Sharif GM (2009) Microcontroller based sinusoidal PWM inverter for photovoltaic application. In: First IEEE international conference development in renewable energy technology, December 2009, pp 1–4
9. Zope P, Bhangale P, Sonare P, Suralkar S (2012) design and implementation of carrier based sinusoidal PWM inverter. Int J Adv Res Electri Electron Instrum Eng 1:230–236
10. Senthilkumar R, Singaaravelu M (2012) design of single phase inverter using DSPIC30F4013. Int J Eng Res Technol (IJERT) 2:6500–6506
11. Chauhan D, Agarwal S, Suman MK (2013) Policies for development of photovoltaic technology:a review. Int J Softw Hardware Res Eng **1**:52–57
12. Qazalbash A, Amin A, Manan A, Khalid M (2009) Design and implementation of microcontroller based PWM technique for sine wave inverter. In: International conference on power engineering energy and electrical drives, March 2009, IEEE, pp 163–167
13. Chithaj M, Niteesh S, Sangeeta M (2019) Comparative analysis of conventional and modified H-bridge inverter configuration. research gate
14. Hassaine L, Olías E, Haddadi M, Malek A (2007) Asymmetric SPWM used in inverter grid connected. Revue des Energies Renouvelables 10:421–429
15. Isa MN, Ahmad MI, Murad AZ, Arshad MK (2007) FPGA based SPWM bridge inverter. Am J Appl Sci 4:584–586
16. Ahuja RK, Kumar A (2014) Analysis, design and control of sinusoidal PWM three phase voltage source inverter feeding balanced loads at different carrier frequencies using Matlab. Int J Adv Res in Electr Electron Instrum Eng 3(5)
17. Dutta A (2013) Some aspects on three phase bridge inverter. IJEI 3(4):18–21
18. Mathukiya MG (2017) three phase inverter with 180 and 120 conduction mode. IJMTER 4(3):113–118
19. Zope PH, Bhangale PG, PrashantSonare S, Suralkar R (2012) Design and Implementation of carrier based SPWM Inverter. IJAREEIE 1(4)
20. Ismail B, Taib S, Isa M, Daut I, Saad AM, Fauzy F (2013) Microcontroller Implementation of single phase inverter switching strategies. In: International conference on control, instrumentation and mechatronics engineering, May 2007, 2 May 2013 pp 104–107

21. Menaka S (2018) Application of evolutionary algorithms for harmonic profile optimization in symmetric multilevel inverter used in medical electronic equipments. Current Signal Transduction Therapy 13(1)
22. Vadizadeh H, Farokhniah N, Toodeji H, Kavousi A (2013) Formulation of line-to-line voltage total harmonic distortion of two-level inverter with low switching frequency. Power Electron IET 6:561–571. https://doi.org/10.1049/iet-pel.2012.0019
23. Miguez Matías R, Alfredo A, Alejandro Raúl O, Pedro J (2016). Step down DC/DC converter for micro-power medical applications. Analog Integr Circuits Signal Process 89(3):531–539
24. George L, Gargiulo GD, Lehmann T, Hamilton TJ (2016) A 0.04 mm buck-boost DC–DC converter for biomedical implants using adaptive gain and discrete frequency scaling control. IEEE Trans Biomed Circ Syst 10(3):668–678
25. Report IEA-PVPS T9-15: (2014) PV systems for rural health facilities in developing areas. International Energy Agency Photovoltaic Power Systems Programme

Classification of Melanoma Skin Cancer Using Inception-ResNet

Sumit Kumar Singh, Shubhendu Banerjee, Avishek Chakraborty, and Aritra Bandyopadhyay

Abstract Melanoma, often known as malignant melanoma, is the commonest yet deadliest kind of skin cancer. While melanoma can be prevented to some extent by educating, the public about safe sun activities like avoiding high radiation hours, wearing protective clothing, trying to apply sunscreen, and keeping a safe distance UV light sources that are generated artificially, early diagnosis and the exact treatment of illness can help to reduce the fatality rate. Efficient and early appropriate treatment of melanoma has been a priority for researchers and the doctors, numerous invasive and non-invasive approaches for melanoma diagnosis have come into focus from time to time. Easy access to skin exams increases the likelihood of accurate and timely identification of melanoma, according to an analysis of different approaches established over the years, and computer-assisted diagnosis (CAD) has played a vital part in achieving this goal. We have proposed a convolutional neural network with eight thick layers for the categorization of melanoma lesions in this research. Inception and Residual blocks are used to extraction of features at both local and global level. When tested on the International Skin Imaging Collaboration (ISIC) 2018, ISIC 2019, and ISIC 2020 datasets, the suggested classifier has a depth of 40 layers, allowing it to attain a high accuracy score.

Keywords Skin cancer · Melanoma · Skin lesion classification · Deep learning

S. K. Singh
Department of CSE, University of Essex, Colchester CO43SQ, UK

S. Banerjee
Department of CSE, Narula Institute of Technology, Kolkata 700109, India

A. Chakraborty (✉)
Department of Engineering Science, Academy of Technology, Adisaptagram, West Bengal 712502, India
e-mail: tirtha.avishek93@gmail.com

A. Bandyopadhyay
Department of CSE, Supreme Knowledge Foundation Group of Institutions, Mankundu 712139, India

© The Author(s), under exclusive license to Springer Nature Singapore Pte Ltd. 2023
J. K. Mandal and D. De (eds.), *Frontiers of ICT in Healthcare*, Lecture Notes in Networks and Systems 519, https://doi.org/10.1007/978-981-19-5191-6_6

1 Introduction

According to a World Health Organization (WHO) study, cancer is among the major causes of mortality worldwide [1]. It is predicted that the number of persons diagnosed with cancer would be double within next twenty years [2]. Cancer-related death rates may be lowered if the disease is discovered and treated early [3]. The major objective of researchers is to devote research resources to the development of cancer in its early detection technologies. Melanoma is still the most dangerous kind of skin cancer. It has been listed tenth on the list of the most frequent cancers. Every year, over 132,000 cases are diagnosed. According to a research issued in 2019 by The American Cancer Organization, 192,310 persons in the United States were identified with melanoma [4]. Melanoma occurrences, like all other cancer cases, have been steadily rising over the last 30 years. If melanoma is detected early enough, a small operation may improve the chances of recovery. Dermoscopy is among the most common imaging methods used by dermatologists. It amplifies the skin lesion's surface, making its structure more obvious to the dermatologist for assessment. However, since it is entirely dependent on the practitioner's visual acuity and expertise, this approach can only be performed efficiently by qualified doctors [5]. These difficulties encourage scientists to seek novel methods for seeing and diagnosing melanoma. Melanoma cancer is diagnosed using a computer-aided diagnostic (CAD) system. For inexperienced dermatologists, the CAD tool offers a user-friendly platform [6]. The evidence of a CAD diagnostic tool may be utilized as a second opinion in the diagnosis of melanoma cancer. With dermoscopy, a skilled dermatologist may obtain an accuracy rate of 65–75% [7]. Furthermore, for questionable situations, accuracy may be increased even further by utilizing a camera with a high-resolution lens and a magnifying lens for collecting dermoscopic images for visual inspection. During the picture capture process, the light is adjusted, which increases the transparency of deep layers of skin. With this technological assistance, the quality of a skin cancer diagnosis may be enhanced by up to 50% [8]. Using visual perception and dermoscopic pictures increased dermatologist accuracy [9]. Fully automated melanoma detection can help clinicians in their daily clinical practice by providing speedy and cost-effective access to life-saving diagnosis [10]. The above-mentioned concerns and obstacles highlight the need for the machine learning team to work on melanoma identification [11]. Machine learning is a set of statistical algorithms for understanding that first train and then test input by changing their parameters [12]. Before 2016, most of the research concentrated on the traditional machine learning process, which includes preprocessing, classification, segmentation, and feature extraction [13]. Furthermore, the feature extraction from malignant photos necessitates a reasonable amount of knowledge. Poor segmentation may result in poor feature extraction, lowering classification accuracy [9]. Melanoma and non-melanoma have a lot of visual similarities, which may lead to erroneous diagnosis of a lesion even by a qualified dermatologist.

In this paper, we have proposed a convolutional neural network which is equipped with eight dense layers for classification of melanoma lesion. It is inspired from the concept of Inception block [16] and Residual block, thereby making the layers more dense and deep. The proposed classifier has a depth of 40 layers, thereby enabling it to achieve high score of accuracy when evaluated on International Skin Imaging Collaboration (ISIC) 2018, ISIC 2019, and ISIC 2020 dataset. The above-mentioned publicly available datasets are used for training the proposed classifier with specific hyperparameters. The proposed method achieves higher value of sensitivity and specificity when compared with few well-established methods, because we have used a bottleneck softmax layer for classification along with Residual and Inception blocks which helps in training the parameters more effectively.

This article is encapsulated into three further subsection, Sect. 2 illustrates about the proposed methodology, whereas Sect. 3 deals with results analysis section where various classifiers are contrasted against our proposed classifier. This article is concluded in Sect. 4 where conclusion and future objectives are highlighted.

2 Proposed Method

The proposed architecture of the deep learning model for classification of malignant lesion is briefly explained in Sect. 2.1. Training the model under specific hyperparameter and input image is summarized in Sect. 2.2.

2.1 Network Architecture

We have investigated the use of Residual and Inception modules to address overfitting, vanishing gradient, and network saturation issues. The suggested network begins with a lightweight version from every module and progressively increases the proportion of convolutions and Residual-Inception blocks. The early layers create low-level abstraction, while the later layers give more high-level characteristics from the input. Rather than using highly deep stacks than each single module, the proposed scheme employs a small number of Residual-Inception stacks. It begins with the standard CNNs, as well as a lighter form of residual and an Inception module. Then, on top of the preceding layer, a Residual-Inception layer with a higher dimension is added. To obtain the final classification results, an average pooling, a dropout, a fully connected layer, and softmax are added at the end of the last Residual block. This block is also appended to the end of the previous set of Inception blocks. In this scenario, we can see which module produces the smallest losses throughout each training stage. A schematic perspective of the proposed design is shown in Fig. 3. The full architecture is also included in Table 1. All convolutions, including those within Residual and Inception modules, employ ReLU as an activation function. It is eliminated, however, after each element-by-element addition process [14]. To prevent overfitting, we utilize dropout [20] following average pooling. Three CNNs, 21 Residual layers, 8 Inception layers, and eight fully linked layers make up the

Table 1 Distribution of ISIC 2018, ISIC 2019, and ISIC 2020 dataset

Dataset	Training		Testing		Validation		Total		Total
	M	NM	M	NM	M	NM	M	NM	
ISIC18	779	7916	334	986	*	*	1113	8902	10,015
ISIC19	3603	10,239	450	1280	450	1280	4503	12,799	17,302
ISIC20	–	–	584	1996	*	*	584	1996	2580

total of 40 layers. The softmax layer consists of 8 fully connected dense layers with variable filter size; these layers are added after the dropout layer, and the model prevents overfitting. ReLU is employed as the activation function for each kernel, as it is fast, and backpropagation is much smoother than any other activation. Moreover, RMSProp is used as an optimizer which is used for calculation of weights and biases during back propagation. Variable kernel size is used to learn more features from the image and thereafter classify in the last output layer. Moreover, increase in kernel size from 128 to 256 (from 2nd to 3rd dense layer) allows the proposed model to learn minute details about large features. Pictorial representation of the proposed method is illustrated in Fig. 1. The proposed network shows that an architecture of 40 layers can achieve high accuracy for classification melanoma lesion without overfitting the model. Additionally, the training and inference time are also reduced, thereby allowing the model to be trained over higher epochs. Moreover, the model can also be deployed to edge device due to its small size.

2.2 *Training Proposed Model with ISIC 2018, ISIC 2019, and ISIC 2020 Dataset*

In the recent years, medical imaging has seen a significant advancement in the identification of melanoma lesions. Furthermore, it is a difficult effort to train the suggested algorithm using appropriate lesion pictures. Our suggested technique is being trained and tested on datasets that are freely available to the public, including ISIC 2018, 2019, and 2020. ISIC 2018 has 10,015 dermoscopic pictures, with 8695 and 1320 dermoscopic images assigned for training and testing, respectively, with grouped lesion images being 24-bit RGB images. The ISIC 2019 dataset contains a total of 17,302 lesion pictures, which are divided into 13,842 photos for training and 1730 images for testing and validating the algorithm. These are RGB photos with a 24-bit resolution ranging of 4499 × 6748 to 540 × 722 pixels. ISIC 2020 datasets are likewise 24-bit RGB pictures that serve as a holdout dataset in the proposed architecture and are therefore solely utilized to test the model. Table 1 represents division of numerous publicly available datasets into training, testing, and validation sets. The melanoma vs. non-melanoma training followed by testing between the two, and ultimately validation. Before making any further alterations, the resolutions were shrunk to 299 × 299px in order to make it suitable for training. Classifier was trained

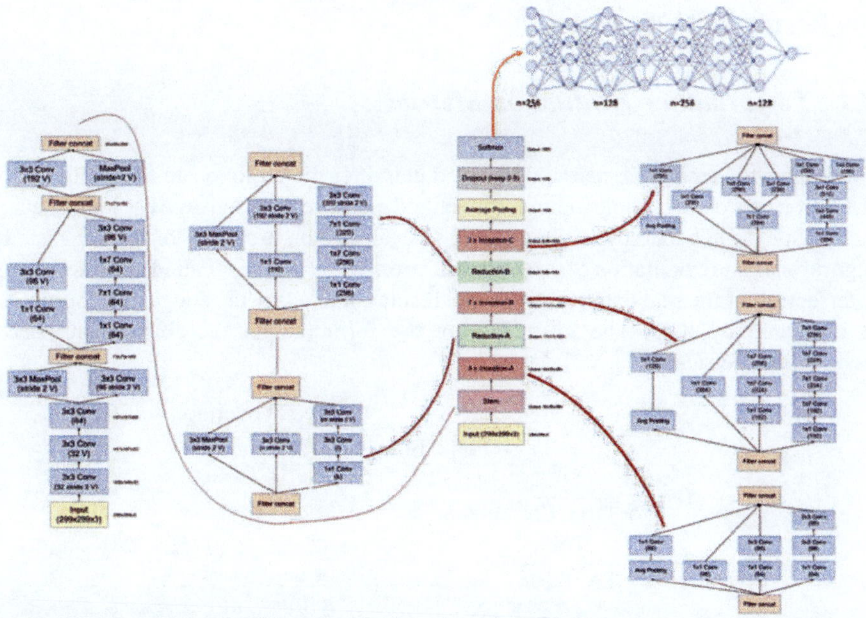

Fig. 1 Representation of proposed architecture for classification

with the following settings after suitable conversion to the necessary configurations: batch size = 32, momentum = 0.9, subdivisions = 16, a learning rate of 0.001, and decay = 0.05. Saving results of epoch after every 100 weights have indisputably demonstrated to effectively locate the position of the required lesion from dermoscopic pictures that were supplied and created, according to the findings obtained by training through 7000 epochs. Accuracy seems to be higher at 7000 epochs, and after this range, the models starts overfitting itself. Moreover, we have used higher number of epochs, as minute details like streak and other clinical features are also considered during training. We have noticed that the loss becomes minimum and fixed after 7000 epochs. RMSProp is used as optimizes as it updates the weight and biases most suitably for melanoma classification, moreover, binary cross entropy is used as loss function. ReLU activation is used throughout the layers except the output layer, where softmax is used for classification. ReLU is not only cost-efficient but also proves to be much more effective while back propagation.

3 Result and Discussion

3.1 Performance Evaluation Metrics

The suggested technique uses a developed classifier model to locate the location of the lesion on a dermoscopic picture. Predefined measures like sensitivity (Sen), specificity (Spe), and accuracy (AC) are used to evaluate the precision of the suggested algorithms. The calculation of total classification performance is called accuracy. The intersection of the real data result and the result obtained by the suggested approach is measured by IOU. The following are the formulae for the above-mentioned assessment metrics:

$$IoU = 2 * \frac{\mathrm{TP}}{\mathrm{TP} + \mathrm{FN} + \mathrm{FP}} = \frac{\text{Area of overlap}}{\text{Area of union}}$$

$$Sen = \frac{\mathrm{TP}}{\mathrm{TP} + \mathrm{FN}}$$

$$Spe = \frac{\mathrm{TN}}{\mathrm{TN} + \mathrm{FP}}$$

$$Ac = \frac{\mathrm{TP} + \mathrm{TN}}{\mathrm{TP} + \mathrm{FN} + \mathrm{TN} + \mathrm{FP}}$$

3.2 Result Analysis

The evaluation of the algorithms and techniques described in this work is the subject of this section. The outcome is evaluated based on the efficiency of site recognition and segmentation of dermoscopic pictures of the disease from publicly available datasets ISIC 2018, ISIC 2019, and ISIC 2020. The whole procedure was carried out using a personal computer with an i7 CPU, 16 GB of RAM, and a Windows 10 operating system. The suggested techniques were also developed using Python 3.5 and the OpenCV framework. The algorithm's and classifier's effectiveness was measured in terms of location detection with three key metrics: sensitivity, specificity, and IOU. The ISIC 2018 dataset has a sensitivity rate of 98.98%, a specificity rate of 99.83%, and an IOU metric of 99. On the ISIC 2019 dataset, the sensitivity, specificity, and IOU are 97.13%, 97.76%, and 97%, respectively. On the ISIC 2020 dataset, these measures show somewhat significantly higher rates, with sensitivity and specificity of 96.87% and 98.49%, respectively, and an IOU of 97. Table 2 summarizes the process of determining the position of dermoscopic pictures using the proposed classifier, and Fig. 2 depicts the whole process of the suggested model, where Fig. 2a shows the acquisition of image, and in Fig. 2b, the image is being preprocessed using histogram equalization, thereafter in Fig. 2c, the lesion is localized and a bounding box is formed across it.

Table 2 Analysis of skin lesion location detection

Datasets	Sen	Spe	IOU
ISIC 2018	98.98	99.83	99
ISIC 2019	97.13	97.76	97
ISIC 2020	96.87	98.49	97

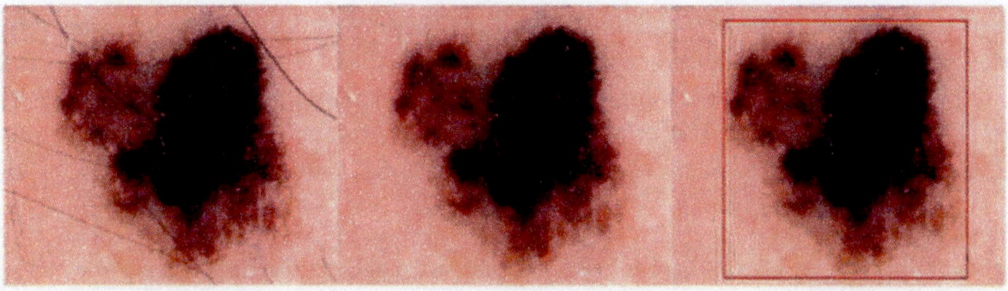

Fig. 2 **a** Input images **b** Preprocessed Image **c** location detection

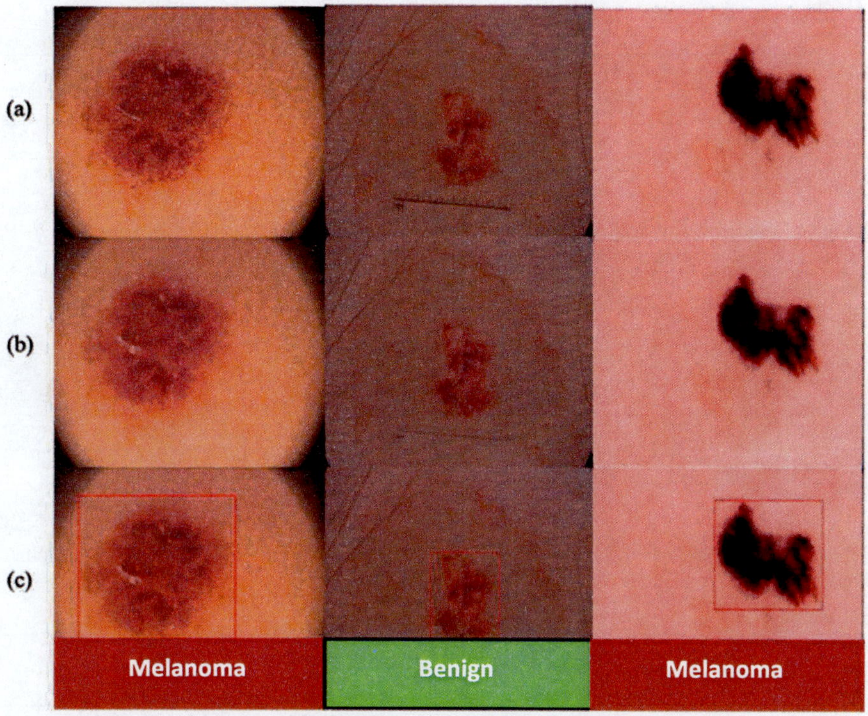

Fig. 3 **a** Input images **b** Preprocessed image **c** Classification of melanoma lesion

The proposed approach is compared to YOLO, SVM, KNN, and MLP, which are all well-known classifiers. On the basis of accuracy, specificity, sensitivity, and time, comparisons are made (in second). Tables 3, 4 and 5 demonstrate an analogical comparison of well-established classifiers for items from the ISIC 2020, ISIC 2019, and ISIC 2018 datasets. All of these classifiers are trained for 7000 epochs over same dataset and testing and validation conditions. The proposed method proves to perform better than the pre-existing classifiers, thereby indicating the supremacy of proposed classifier for diagnosis of melanoma lesion.

The use of proposed classification model for melanoma skin cancer categorization has improved diagnostic efficiency while also reducing detection time. The use of preprocessing methods for electronic hair removal, immediately followed by an

Table 3 Comparison of well-known classifiers and the suggested classifier for the ISIC 2018 dataset's skin lesion pictures classification

Classifier	Ac	Sen	Spe	Time(in sec)
YOLO	93.93	90.12	95.23	13.65
KNN	92.42	86.52	94.42	89.23
MLP	87.88	72.16	93.20	292.50
SVM	92.72	89.52	93.81	69.26
Proposed method	96.21	95.51	96.45	22.76

Table 4 Comparison of well-known classifiers and the suggested classifier for the ISIC 2019 dataset's skin lesion pictures classification

Classifier	Ac	Sen	Spe	Time(in sec)
YOLO	93.49	90.22	94.61	18.54
KNN	91.39	86.44	93.13	102.43
MLP	88.50	80.67	91.25	367.51
SVM	90.81	85.33	92.73	79.58
Proposed method	96.13	94.67	96.64	29.16

Table 5 Comparison of well-known classifiers and the suggested classifier for the ISIC 2020 dataset's skin lesion pictures classification

Classifier	Ac	Sen	Spe	Time(in sec)
YOLO	93.80	91.27	94.54	26.13
KNN	90.78	88.87	91.33	142.71
MLP	88.19	84.08	89.38	583.52
SVM	91.51	89.73	92.03	97.10
Proposed method	96.28	95.21	96.60	38.98

image refining procedure, helped to improve the method's overall accuracy. Classification results of the proposed method along with preprocessing stage are represented in Fig. 3.

4 Conclusion

Though the incidence of melanoma has increased in the previous decade, a new research from the American Cancer Society offers a ray of hope in the therapy of the condition, since the fatality rate seems to have reduced in recent years. According to reports, mortality among individuals under the age of 50 is declining at a rate of 7% each year, while deaths among adults above the age of 50 are declining at a rate of 5.7% per year. The progress in the area of melanoma detection and treatment has been aided by innovative concepts and cutting-edge approaches. By offering a self-designed method for classification, we hope to make a modest contribution to its prompt and accurate identification. The use of the concept of Inception block and Residual block, which is based on deep learning, speeds up the procedure without sacrificing the output's validity. Three distinct publicly accessible datasets—ISIC 2018, ISIC 2019, and ISIC 2020—were used for picture testing and training. We have employed Inception and Residual block with a bottleneck softmax layer which helps our classifier yield high score of accuracy. Moreover, the use to latest dataset pushes the bar of accuracy. The study is compared to other notable research efforts from today's period and performs somewhat better on most stated criteria than the rest. Though there has been a decrease in the death rate among melanoma patients, more sophisticated research is still needed to assist all patients, regardless of color, sex, ethnicity, or age.

References

1. Haenssle HA, Fink C, Schneiderbauer R, Toberer F, Buhl T, Blum A, Kalloo A et al. (2018) Man against machine: diagnostic performance of a deep learning convolutional neural network for dermoscopic melanoma recognition in comparison to 58 dermatologists. Annals of Oncology 29(8):1836–1842
2. Rathee G, Sharma A, Saini H, Kumar R, Iqbal R (2020) A hybrid framework for multimedia data processing in IoT-healthcare using blockchain technology. Multimedia Tools and Appl 79(15):9711–9733
3. Ashim LK, Suresh N, Prasannakumar CV (2021) A comparative analysis of various transfer learning approaches skin cancer detection. In: 2021 5th International conference on trends in electronics and informatics (ICOEI), IEEE, pp 1379–1385
4. Banerjee S, Singh SK, Chakraborty A, Das A, Bag R (2020) Melanoma diagnosis using deep learning and fuzzy logic. Diagnostics 10(8):577
5. Banerjee S, Singh SK, Chakraborty A, Basu S, Das A, Bag R (2021) Diagnosis of Melanoma lesion using neutrosophic and deep learning. Traitement du Signal 38(5)

6. Banerjee S, Singh SK, Das A, Bag R (2022) Diagnoses of Melanoma lesion using YOLOv3. In: Computational advancement in communication, circuits and systems, Springer, Singapore, pp 291–302
7. Nami N, Giannini E, Burroni M, Fimiani M, Rubegni P (2012) Teledermatology: state-of-the-art and future perspectives. Expert Rev Dermatol 7(1):1–3
8. Blum A, Giacomel J (2015) "Tape dermatoscopy": constructing a low-cost dermatoscope using a mobile phone, immersion fluid and transparent adhesive tape. Dermatol Pract Conceptual 5(2):87
9. Marchetti MA, Codella NCF, Dusza SW, Gutman DA, Helba B, Kalloo A, Mishra N et al. (2018) Results of the 2016 international skin imaging collaboration international symposium on biomedical imaging challenge: comparison of the accuracy of computer algorithms to dermatologists for the diagnosis of melanoma from dermoscopic images. J American Acad Dermatol 78(2):270–277
10. Esteva A, Kuprel B, Novoa RA, Ko J, Swetter SM, Blau HM, Thrun S (2017) Dermatologist-level classification of skin cancer with deep neural networks. Nature 542(7639):115–118
11. Oliveira RB, Papa JP, Pereira AS, Tavares JMRS (2018) Computational methods for pigmented skin lesion classification in images: review and future trends. Neural Comput Appl 29(3):613–636
12. Char DS, Shah NH, Magnus D (2018) Implementing machine learning in health care—addressing ethical challenges. N Engl J Med 378(11):981
13. David G, Codella NCF, Celebi E, Helba B, Marchetti M, Mishra N, Halpern A (2016) Skin lesion analysis toward melanoma detection: a challenge at the international symposium on biomedical imaging (ISBI) 2016, hosted by the international skin imaging collaboration (ISIC). arXiv preprint arXiv:1605.01397
14. Gross S, Wilber M (2016) Training and investigating residual nets. http://torch.ch/blog/2016/02/04/resnets.html, Retrieved at: 20 Nov 2016
15. Hinton GE, Srivastava N, Krizhevsky A, Sutskever I, Salakhutdinov RR (2012) Improving neural networks by preventing co-adaptation of feature detectors. arXiv preprint arXiv:1207.0580
16. Szegedy C, Liu W, Jia Y, Sermanet P, Reed S, Anguelov D, Erhan D, Vanhoucke V, Rabinovich A (2015) Going deeper with convolutions. In: Proceedings of CVPR, pp 1–9. arxiv.org/abs/1409.4842

Melanoma (Skin Cancer) Classifier Using RESNet

Naveen Kanuri, Bhaskar K. Uday, and Teegala Tejaswi

Abstract Skin cancer is a root for many problems in human beings. There is a need to identify the skin cancer in early stage so that skin cancer can be cured in better. Existing mathematical model in the image processing not reached this requirement; hence, there is a need to investigate and analyze the skin cancer in depth. Deep learning emerging field with possible solution to detect the cancer in early stage using advance methods. 0.976 is the ROC score achieved using ResNet 50 deep learning method.

Keywords Deep learning · Exploratory data analysis · One hot encoding · Image augmentation · ResNet

1 Introduction

Skin cancer can be classified in two types as malignant melanoma and non-melanoma. Malignant melanoma is found in people with blue eyes. Non-melanoma is detected mainly in face and neck and ears [1]. It is very important to identify and detect the problem as soon as possible. The benign tumor and malignant tumor can be observed as given in below figures with the help of cell representation. Benign swelling units are not cancerous and won't spread. Malignant swelling units are more danger because these cells affect the near cells badly with it internal structure. Machine learning methods adapted here to solve this problem [1–5]. The traditional image processing not achieved this process. So here, ResNet 50 is used to solve this problem. "Generally speaking, complete extraction (careful evacuation) prompts fitness. Going against the norm, a harmless growth has the ability to grow, however, it won't spread. With regards to harmless skin developments, knowing the normal signs and side effects of those that could be threatening is basic, as is looking for clinical consideration when skin developments show suspect. Harmless skin developments incorporate

N. Kanuri (✉) · B. K. Uday · T. Tejaswi
Department of Electronics and Communication, MLR Institute of Technology, Hyderabad, India
e-mail: naveenkanuri458@gmail.com

© The Author(s), under exclusive license to Springer Nature Singapore Pte Ltd. 2023

J. K. Mandal and D. De (eds.), *Frontiers of ICT in Healthcare*, Lecture Notes in Networks and Systems 519, https://doi.org/10.1007/978-981-19-5191-6_7

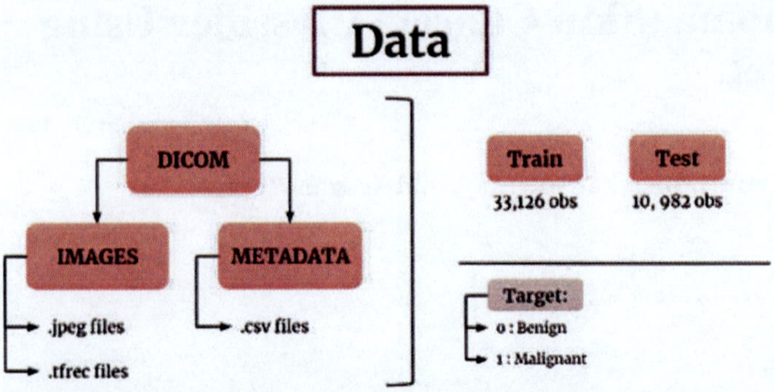

Fig. 1 DICOM portfolio break in educate (33,126) and check (10,982)

seborrhea keratoses, cherry angora's, dermat of fibromas, skin labels (Crichton), pathogenic granules, and pimples (epidermal considerations). Here, Fig. 1 describes disease types in people of various ages. Frequency rates growth consistently from around the age of 21–25 and all the more pointedly in males from around the age of 53–58. Females matured 90 and above had the best rates, while males matured 84–88 had the most minimal. Females have a lot more noteworthy paces of malignant growth than males in prior age gatherings, while females have fundamentally lower paces of disease in more seasoned age gatherings. The uniqueness is most prominent among males and females between the ages of 20 and 24, when young ladies have a 2.5-overlay more noteworthy age-explicit rate than males" [6].

1.1 Data Pre-processing

DICOM portfolio break in educate (33,126) and check (10,982) as Fig. 1 files present in the given dataset: (1) records (2) train.csv (3) train (4) test (5) test.csv (6) sample_submission.csv (7) jpeg 'train' and 'test' are folders containing images in form of dcm. Folder named 'jpeg' has the same images in jpeg format. 'train.csv' contains the csv data of the train dataset. This file contains result column which is not present in 'test.csv'. The results of test.csv are present in the file 'sample_submissions.csv' [3–5, 7–11].

Exploring CSV Files Train.csv has 33,126 rows and Test.csv has 10,982 rows. Head of Trans.csv: The given Table 1 describes head train data with age and sex and anatomy and diagnosis of skin cancer of different people. Table 3 gives a summary of all heading levels. Filling missing values visualize the missing values: Train Data: Sex: 65 missing values Age: 68 missing values Anatomy: 527 missing values Test Data: Anatomy: 351 missing values Train–Sex Variable: All missing values are benign, and the majority of the patients have the melanoma in the lower extremity, upper extremity, and torso. All values for diagnosis are unknown. Therefore, we

Table 1 Head test data

Dcmname	ID	Sex	Age	Anatomy
ISIC0052060	IP_{3}579734	Male	70	NAN
ISIC0052349	IP_{7}782715	Male	40	Lower extremity
ISIC0058510	IP_{7}960270	Female	55	Torso
ISIC0073313	IP_{6}375035	Female	50	Torso
ISIC0073502	IP_{0}589375	Female	45	Lower extremity

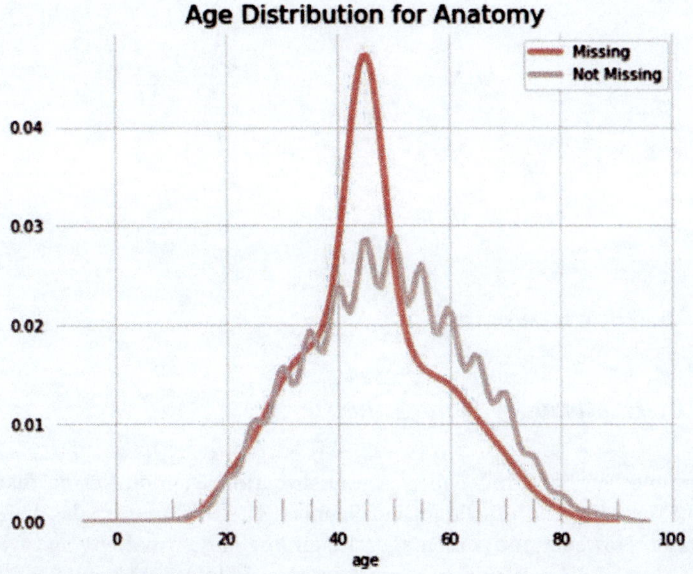

Fig. 2 Age distribution for anatomy

used the most predominant gender that appears in these values to impute the missing values. Train–Age Variable: The distributions and values are very similar with the missing pattern in sex variable. So, we imputed in the same manner. The mean and the median of the variable have the same value of 50, while the mode is 45. The distribution is normal, see we used median to impute. Train–Anatomy Variable: We need to keep in mind that in the missing data, there are 9 malignant cases, so we should treat the imputation separate for both benign and malignant. In terms of age and gender, both missing and not missing data seem to behave about the same. Test–Anatomy Variable: The majority of the people with missing anatomy have 70-year-old, so we used to anatomy with the biggest frequency for age 70 (Fig. 2).

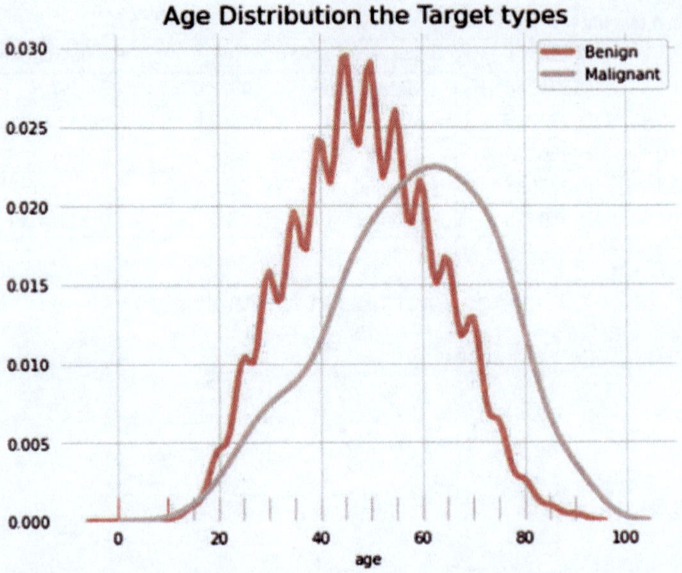

Fig. 3 Age distribution the target types

1.2 *EDA-Exploratory Data Analysis*

Target Variable: Very high imbalance. Age Distribution: Benign: Normal distribution Malignant: Skewed to the left. Target and Genders: There are more males than females in the dataset. However, the percentages are almost same. Anatomy and Diagnosis: Anatomy: Most of the melanomas are in the torso and lower extremities of the body. Diagnosis: For most patients, the diagnosis is unknown, but there are around 17 Anatomy and Target: Distributions are about the same for both benign and malignant cases (Fig. 3).

1.3 *Preprocess CSV Files*

One Hot Encoding: This is the process of converting all categorical values into numerical values so that the machine can take them as input. Sex, anatomy, and diagnosis need to be encoded benign_malignant column will be dropped.

```
Train .dcm number of images: 33126
Test .dcm number of images: 10982
Train .jpeg number of images: 33126
Test .jpeg number of images: 10982
----------------------
There is the same number of images as in train/ test .csv datasets
```

Fig. 4 Check the number of images in each format and compare them with the rows in csv files

1.4 Images

Sanity Check: Check the number of images in each format and compare them with the rows in csv files as given Fig. 4 describes that type of images and its count. "Profound brain networks assume a critical part in skin malignant growth discovery. They comprise a bunch of interconnected hubs. Their construction is like the human mind as far as neuronal interconnected. Their hubs work agreeably to take care of specific issues. Brain networks are prepared for specific assignments; in this way, the organizations fill in as specialists in the spaces in which they were prepared. In our review, brain networks were prepared to characterize pictures and to recognize different sorts of skin malignant growth. Various kinds of skin sore from international images dataset are introduced. We looked for changed strategies of learning, like KNN, and GAN for skin disease location frameworks. Research connected with every one of these profound brain networks is examined exhaustively in this segment" [12]. "The Kohonen self-arranging map is an exceptionally well known sort of profound brain organization. CNNs are prepared based on unaided realizing, and that implies that a KNN requires no engineer's mediation in educating system as well as need little data about the traits of the information. A KNN by and large comprises two layers. In the 2D plane, the principal layer is called an information sheet, while another is named a cutthroat sheet. Both of these layers are completely associated, and each association is from quick to second layer aspect. A KNN can be utilized for information grouping without knowing the connections between input information individuals. It is otherwise called a self-arranging map. KNNs don't contain a result layer; each hub in the serious layer likewise goes about as the result hub itself" [12].

1.5 Class Imbalance

This is a very important topic in image classification. Especially for this problem, as the 2 classes we are dealing with are highly imbalanced. 98 Solution: Oversampling Under sampling Data Augmentation: Data augmentation is a technique used to tackle oversampling. Different techniques are used on the available images to create new images and add them to the available data set [6, 12–16].

2 Method

2.1 Data Preparation

The data we worked on has a Train and Test folder with corresponding .jpg images. Number of data points also increased with external sources. Len Train: 37,648 Len Test: 10,982 A. PyTorch Dataset Setting up the dataset according to the input PyTorch models accept. When reading the images, custom augmentations that are shown in previous sections are applied. Train will have a complex transformation, while valid data will have no augmentations. Test data will have similar augmentations to Train data (Fig. 5 and 6).

2.2 Neural Networks

Table 3 gives a summary of all heading levels. ResNet 50 Fig. 8 shows the Result from pre-trained weights: EfficientNet. Figure 9 shows the Result from pre-trained weights Result from pre-trained weights (Table 2).

2.3 Proposed Training Loop

Figures 7 and 8 describe how training loop is functioning for the train and test data. This is the state-of-the-art, open-source training loop used for Image Classification

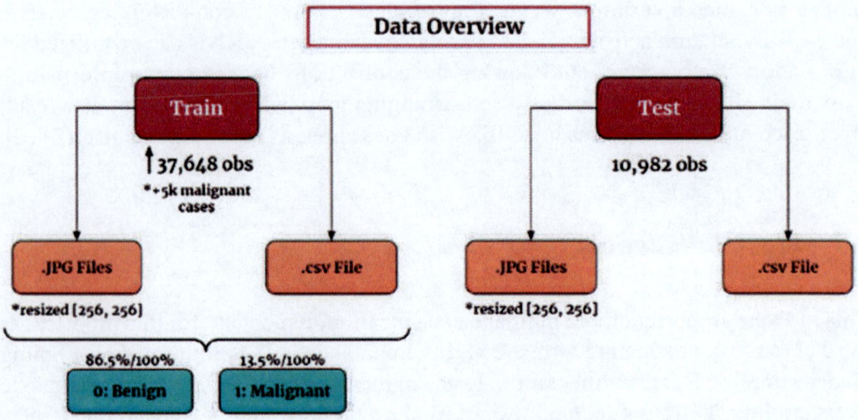

Fig. 5 Data preparation

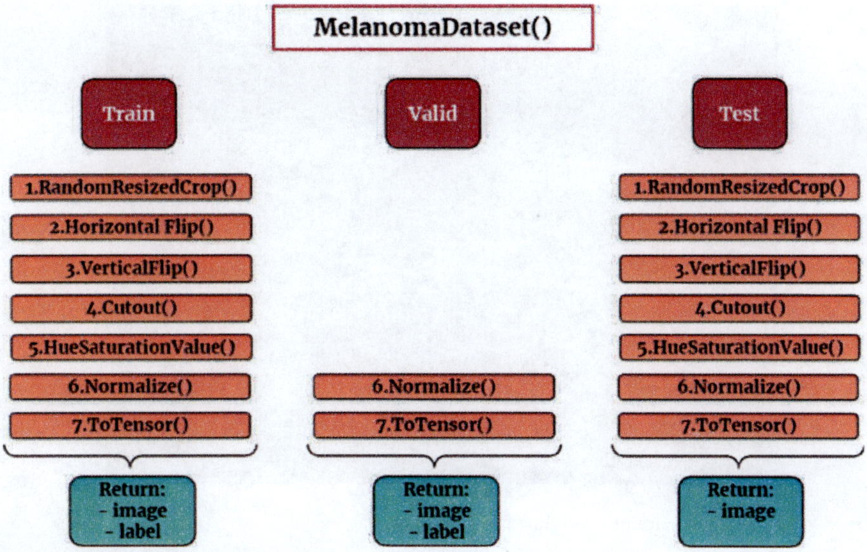

Fig. 6 PyTorch dataset

Table 2 Comparison between a few famous models

Model	Training accuracy	Validation accuracy
Resnet18	0.83	0.87
Resnet35	0.84	0.85
Proposed resnet	0.85	0.88

```
Data shape: torch.Size([3, 3, 224, 224]) |
 tensor([[0.0000, 0.9994, 0.0333],
        [0.0000, 0.9999, 0.0143],
        [0.0000, 0.9685, 0.2490]])
Label: tensor([0., 0., 1.])

Input Image shape: torch.Size([3, 3, 224, 224])
Input csv_data shape: torch.Size([3, 3])
Features Image shape: torch.Size([3, 1000])
CSV Data: torch.Size([3, 500])
Out shape: torch.Size([3, 1])
Loss: 1.1359907388687134
```

Fig. 7 Result from pre-trained weights

```
Data shape: torch.Size([3, 3, 224, 224]) |
 tensor([[0.0000, 0.9975, 0.0712],
        [0.0000, 0.9981, 0.0614],
        [0.0200, 0.9980, 0.0599]])
Label: tensor([0., 0., 1.])

Input Image shape: torch.Size([3, 3, 224, 224])
Input csv_data shape: torch.Size([3, 3])
Features Image shape: torch.Size([3, 1408, 7, 7])
Image Reshaped shape: torch.Size([3, 1408])
CSV Data: torch.Size([3, 250])
Out shape: torch.Size([3, 1])
Loss: 0.8280633091926575
```

Fig. 8 Result from pre-trained weights

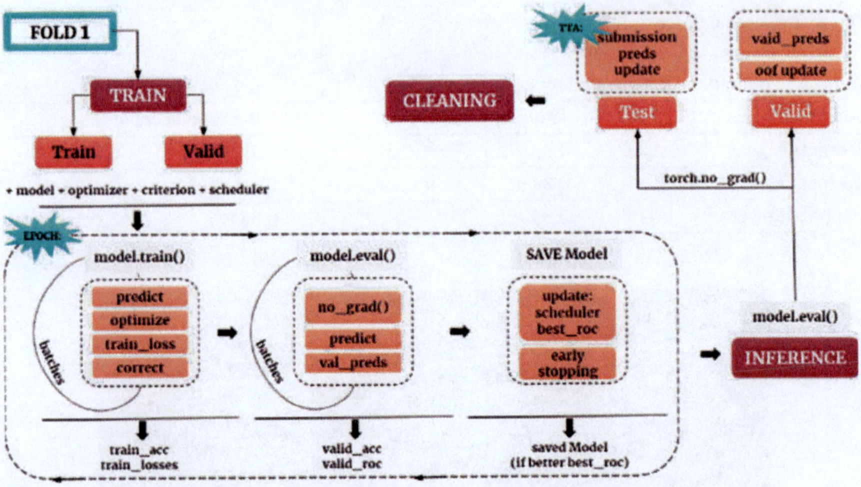

Fig. 9 Training loop

tasks of tasks with high Class Imbalance like the following.Different models can be applied using the same loop. We training a ResNet 50 model on the following dataset and commented the following models due to computational limitations.

3 Results and Discussions

Accuracy is a bad metric to measure the performance of these tasks. As the data is highly class imbalanced (98 ResNet 50), Figure 10 shows the result from each epoch of training data. "ResNet 50 is a leftover organization with 48 sheets and 25 million boundaries. In 2015, Microsoft presented the lingering organization, a profound complication brain mesh model. As opposed to learning highlights, the leftover organization gains from remaining, which are the deduction of elements learnt before the contributions of the layer. The skip association was utilized by ResNet to ship data across layers. The engineering of ResNet 50 is isolated into 4 phases, as found in the image given. A sense with a size that is products of 32 and a medium thickness of three can be acknowledged by the framework. For lucidity, we will guess the channel dimension is 224 by 224 with 3. For starter convolution and max-pooling" [6].

B. ROC Score This metric is derived from the area under the curve of graph drawn between True Positive, True Negative, False Positive, and False Negative. This is the official metric used in the following competition where the dataset was provided. ROC Score Achieved: 0.976 C. Confusion Matrix The below given table3 describes an important metric for the following task as the number of False Negatives need to be as minimum as possible. "A disarray lattice (otherwise called a blunder grid) is a quantitative way to deal with depicting picture arrangement precision, and a table sums up the consequences of an order model. The quantity of right and erroneous appraisals is counted and consumed with smoldering heat by class. The disarray network depends on evident negative (TN), misleading negative (FN), genuine positive (TP), and bogus positive (FP). The disarray framework (CM) assists with finding different outcomes all the more precisely" [6]. Table 3 gives a summary of all heading levels.

```
---------- Fold: 5 ----------
0:04:48 | Epoch: 1/15 | Loss: 206.1 | Train Acc: 0.925 | Valid Acc: 0.971 | ROC: 0.972
0:04:46 | Epoch: 2/15 | Loss: 206.7 | Train Acc: 0.925 | Valid Acc: 0.969 | ROC: 0.975
0:04:47 | Epoch: 3/15 | Loss: 198.9 | Train Acc: 0.929 | Valid Acc: 0.972 | ROC: 0.97
0:04:46 | Epoch: 4/15 | Loss: 202.3 | Train Acc: 0.927 | Valid Acc: 0.977 | ROC: 0.977
0:04:47 | Epoch: 5/15 | Loss: 201.2 | Train Acc: 0.927 | Valid Acc: 0.971 | ROC: 0.973
0:04:53 | Epoch: 6/15 | Loss: 197.1 | Train Acc: 0.93 | Valid Acc: 0.966 | ROC: 0.971
0:05:06 | Epoch: 7/15 | Loss: 191.2 | Train Acc: 0.93 | Valid Acc: 0.975 | ROC: 0.979
0:04:59 | Epoch: 8/15 | Loss: 191.2 | Train Acc: 0.931 | Valid Acc: 0.976 | ROC: 0.979
0:05:03 | Epoch: 9/15 | Loss: 191.3 | Train Acc: 0.932 | Valid Acc: 0.974 | ROC: 0.979
0:05:06 | Epoch: 10/15 | Loss: 188.6 | Train Acc: 0.932 | Valid Acc: 0.973 | ROC: 0.98
0:05:12 | Epoch: 11/15 | Loss: 186.3 | Train Acc: 0.933 | Valid Acc: 0.972 | ROC: 0.979
0:05:06 | Epoch: 12/15 | Loss: 187.8 | Train Acc: 0.932 | Valid Acc: 0.977 | ROC: 0.983
0:05:03 | Epoch: 13/15 | Loss: 183.6 | Train Acc: 0.934 | Valid Acc: 0.974 | ROC: 0.978
0:05:00 | Epoch: 14/15 | Loss: 186.1 | Train Acc: 0.932 | Valid Acc: 0.973 | ROC: 0.98
0:04:59 | Epoch: 15/15 | Loss: 183.3 | Train Acc: 0.933 | Valid Acc: 0.975 | ROC: 0.981
Early stopping (no improvement since 3 models) | Best ROC: 0.9830294890684985
---------- Fold: 6 ----------
0:05:00 | Epoch: 1/15 | Loss: 202.1 | Train Acc: 0.929 | Valid Acc: 0.974 | ROC: 0.983
0:05:00 | Epoch: 2/15 | Loss: 202.6 | Train Acc: 0.927 | Valid Acc: 0.981 | ROC: 0.986
0:04:59 | Epoch: 3/15 | Loss: 203.0 | Train Acc: 0.926 | Valid Acc: 0.977 | ROC: 0.984
0:04:59 | Epoch: 4/15 | Loss: 198.5 | Train Acc: 0.93 | Valid Acc: 0.982 | ROC: 0.987
0:05:00 | Epoch: 5/15 | Loss: 197.4 | Train Acc: 0.929 | Valid Acc: 0.981 | ROC: 0.986
0:05:00 | Epoch: 6/15 | Loss: 198.9 | Train Acc: 0.928 | Valid Acc: 0.972 | ROC: 0.983
0:05:00 | Epoch: 7/15 | Loss: 191.6 | Train Acc: 0.931 | Valid Acc: 0.979 | ROC: 0.984
Early stopping (no improvement since 3 models) | Best ROC: 0.9868998283213488
```

Fig. 10 Results from each epoch of training

Table 3 Confusion matrix

Benign	True Negative 32.344 85.9%	False Positive 198 0.5%
Malignant	False Negative 877 2.3%	True Positive 4229 11.2%
Type	Benign	Malignant

• True Negative: 32,334 (85.9 • False Positive: 198 (0.5 • False Negative: 887 (2.3 • True Positive: 4229 (11.2

4 Conclusion

As the doctors are always under numbered compared to the patients that need attention, doctors being able to examine each sample personally is an impossible task. While using this technique, the number of samples that needs to be examined decreases drastically. Following this, the doctors can examine the limited number of samples of take necessary following steps accordingly. Even one life saved due to early attention because of decreasing workload on doctors is a major victory.

Acknowledgements The authors are grateful to acknowledge the support from the MLR Institute of Technology. The authors would like to thank the anonymous reviewers for giving good insights for this article.

References

1. Deng J, Dong W, Socher R, Li L-J, Li K, Fei-Fei L (2009) ImageNet: a large-scale hierarchical image database. In: CVPR09 (2009)
2. Krizhevsky A (2010) Convolutional deep belief networks on cifar-10. Unpublished manuscript
3. Ara A (2012) Deserno TM (2012) A systematic review of automated melanoma detection in dermatoscopic images and its ground truth data. Proc SPIE Int Soc Opt Eng. 8318:1–6. https://doi.org/10.1117/12.912389. [CrossRef] [Google Scholar]
4. Gonzalez Diaz I (2018) Dermaknet: incorporating the knowledge of dermatologists to convolutional neural networks for skin lesion diagnosis. IEEE J Biomed Health Inf PP(99):1–1
5. Codella NCF, Cai J, Abedini M, Garnavi R, Halpern A, Smith JR (2015) Deep learning, sparse coding, and CNN for melanoma recognition in dermoscopy images. In: Machine learning in medical imaging, pp 118–126, MLMI 2015. 2
6. Sánchez J, Perronnin F (2011) High-dimensional signature compression for large-scale image classification. In: 2011 IEEE conference on computer vision and pattern recognition (CVPR). IEEE, pp 1665–1672
7. Breiman L (2001) Random forests. Mach Learn 45(1):5–32
8. Breiman L (2001) Random forests. Mach Learn 45(1):5–32
9. Fei-Fei L, Fergus R, Perona P (2007) Learning generative visual models from few training examples: an incremental bayesian approach tested on 101 object categories. Comput Vis Image Underst 106(1):59–70

10. Krizhevsky A (2009) Learning multiple layers of features from tiny images. Master's thesis, Department of Computer Science, University of Toronto
11. Jarrett K, Kavukcuoglu K, Ranzato MA, LeCun Y (2009) What is the best multi-stage architecture for object recognition? In: International conference on computer vision. IEEE, pp 2146–2153
12. LeCun Y, Huang FJ, Bottou L (2004) Learning methods for generic object recognition with invariance to pose and lighting. In: Computer vision and pattern recognition, 2004. CVPR 2004. In: Proceedings of the 2004 IEEE computer Society Conference on, vol 2, pp II-97. IEEE
13. Krizhevsky A (2010) Convolutional deep belief networks on cifar-10. Unpublished manuscript
14. Krizhevsky A, Hinton GE (2011) Using very deep autoencoders for content-based image retrieval. In: ESANN
15. https://www.hindawi.com/journals/jhe/2021/5895156/
16. https://www.ncbi.nlm.nih.gov/pmc/articles/PMC8160886/#:~:text=A%20deep%20CNN%2Dbased%20system,image%2C%20with%2086.67%25%20accuracy

Complementarity of Logistic Regression over the Nonparametric Classifications for Improved Decision-Making—A Case of Maternal Health Risk Data

Abhijit Roy

Abstract Nonparametric classification models are widely used in predictive analysis with multiple healthcare datasets. Even with high accuracy of different classifiers, we raise our concern that, in the field of health care, the cost of misclassification is supposed to be very high. Using maternal health risk data, the present paper proposes a complementary approach of combining parametric models along with sophisticated nonparametric classifiers to draw rich inferences about the causality of the associations between variables of importance. We present our case with the help of parametric model of binomial logistic regression. We clearly show how the inclusion of the parametric model improves the decision-making ability for better healthcare management.

Keywords Healthcare analytics · Random forest · Logistic regression · Maternal health risk

1 Introduction

Classification has been a major area in the filed of data science and advanced computational algorithms especially in the field of 'big-data'. There are several use cases where data classification algorithms have been successfully implemented. Health care is rapidly gaining momentum in this space. With the popularity of wearable biosensors, novel applications of individualized smart health technologies have emerged [1]. Different Internet of Health Things (IoHT)-based gadgets generate a lot of health data in real time to monitor and warn an individual's health risk. Fundamentally, this is a classification problem where the algorithms are trained with different parameters to classify the health risk of an individual in a particular category.

A. Roy (✉)
Dr. Bhupendra Nath Dutta Smriti Mahavidyalaya, Kalna Road, Purba Barddhaman, West Bengal 713407, India
e-mail: abhijitroy81@gmail.com

© The Author(s), under exclusive license to Springer Nature Singapore Pte Ltd. 2023
J. K. Mandal and D. De (eds.), *Frontiers of ICT in Healthcare*, Lecture Notes in Networks and Systems 519, https://doi.org/10.1007/978-981-19-5191-6_8

There is a major difference in the use of classification algorithms in healthcare applications vis-a-vis other areas of applications. This is because the cost of misclassifications in health care may be very high. Moreover, in a healthcare risk assessment problem, the users in many cases are medical practitioners and there is a subjective element in the decision-making which is based on experiential learning. In this scenario, the interdisciplinary interactions between smart technologies and medical expertise develop new avenues in healthcare risk monitoring [2]. Here, not only the classification of risk but the degree of association of different explanatory variables to cause a particular health risk is also important. Having said that we cannot ignore the strength of the nonparametric classification algorithms rather we propose to use the same as a strong filtering mechanism in stage one. In the stage two, we propose to implement parametric tests to further understand the degree of association between different healthcare variables. This will surely improve the decision-making process of healthcare professionals as well as individuals.

So, the objective of the paper is to show the complementarity of nonparametric classification algorithms and binomial logistic regression to improve the decision-making in healthcare risk management. Using maternal health risk data, we show the usefulness of different classification algorithms as robust filtering tools. Then, in next stage, we use the binomial logistic regression to understand the degree of association between different explanatory variables and maternal health risk.

2 Related Work

Classification of big-data in the area of health care has been steadily gaining prominence among researchers. Lakshmanaprabu et al. [3] use random forest (RF hereafter) classifier on IoT generated health data and report a 94.2% precision in classifications. Akbar et al. [4] apply predictive analytic model using RF algorithm to classify asthma severity of patients and report as high as 98.80% accuracy in the prediction of asthma disease. RF, logistic regression classifier and decision tree models are used to predict the re-admission rates of patients suffering from diabetes [5]. The study reports that the RF classifier has been most accurate to predict the re-admission rate of patients. In the similar area, Rallapalli and Suryakanthi [6] worked on the risk of diabetes studying the electronic health records. The authors report RF as the most accurate classifier among different alternatives. In another study, boosted RF algorithm is used on the Kaggle dataset of COVID-19 patients to predict their health risk [7]. The study reports the substantial accuracy of 94% in predicting COVID-19 related health risk. The efficacy of RF algorithm is further established by Fawagreh and Gaber [8] on three different medical dataset. On the other hand, Boukenze et al. [9] report the superiority of decision tree algorithm in predicting chronic kidney disease. Naive Bayes, decision tree and RF algorithms are used by Nagarajan and Kumar [10] for the prediction of risks from three different diseases, namely, heart disease, lung cancer and leukemia. The study reports substantial accuracy in classification. Support vector machine (SVM) has been another popular classifier that is also used in healthcare dataset.

Using electronic health records, Razzaghi [11] shows that multi-level SVM produces fast and accurate classification results. SVM along with other classifiers has been used in the prediction of lung cancer survivability [12], chronic kidney disease [13], diabetes disease [14], prevent and control of chronic diseases [15] among other areas.

As we have mentioned earlier, all these classification algorithms have been quite accurate on different healthcare datasets, but the problem we highlight in this paper is that, only classification brings limited information to the medical practitioners for management of healthcare risks. Along with classification, inferential statistics may be immensely helpful particularly in the healthcare sector. This has been further established in the unprecedented pandemic of COVID-19. In these kinds of unknown or less-known diseases, not only the classification but also drawing the inference about how different health conditions are impacting the risk of severity is highly important. So, in our paper, we propose the complementarity of inferential statistics in the form of binomial logistic regression along with nonparametric classification tools like RF, decision tree, SVM and Gaussian Naive Bayes algorithms. The rest of the paper is presented as follows: first, we present the materials and methods. Here, we describe the dataset, data preprocessing, descriptive statistics and model-based methodological aspects. Then, we describe the results of our study followed by discussions and conclusions.

3 Data and Methodology

3.1 Dataset

The dependencies of the study include several packages of 'R' and 'Python'. The major problem in the healthcare analytics is the privacy of the dataset. In most of the cases, health data are proprietory in nature. So a substantial number of studies are based on limited number of publicly available health datasets. In the present study, we use Kaggle dataset of maternal health risks collected from different hospitals, maternal healthcare centers, healthcare clinics through IoT-based systems. The dataset consists of 1014 observations of pregnant women with basic health parameters like age in number of years, systolic and diastolic blood pressure in 'mmHg', blood glucose level in molar concentration, heart rate in beats per minute and risk level. The labeling of risk level is done in three distinct categories, that is, low risk, moderate risk and high risk. There were no loss of data points due to missing values.

3.2 Data Preprocessing and Descriptive Analysis

As there were no loss of data points due to missing values, we could use the whole dataset for the purpose of classification and regression. Health risk is an ordinal data

Table 1 Correlation matrix

	Age	SystolicBP	DiastolicBP	BS	BodyTemp	HeartRate
Age	1.000	0.416	0.398	0.4732	−0.255	0.079
SystolicBP	0.416	1.000	0.787	0.425	−0.286	−0.023
DiastolicBP	0.398	0.787	1.000	0.423	−0.257	−0.046
BS	0.473	0.425	0.423	1.000	−0.103	0.142
BodyTemp	−0.255	−0.286	−0.257	−0.103	1.000	0.098
HeartRate	0.079	−0.023	−0.046	0.142	0.098	1.000

with labels of low, moderate and high risks. Other than health risk, all the variables carry discrete data points. For classification problems, we preprocess the health risk data as 1 for low risk, 2 for moderate risk and 3 for high risk. We use 75–25% split between training and testing datasets for training and backtesting of classification algorithms. For binomial logistic regression, we again preprocess the data in two categories. Here, we consider the value of high risk as 1 and club the cases of low and moderate risk and assign them the value of 0. For logistic regression analysis, we have used both original data as well as log-transformed data.

In Table 1, we show the correlation matrix. To better understand the intensity of association, we also present the correlation heat-map of all the variables in Fig. 1. The correlation heat-map includes the categorical variable also. We find that blood glucose level and systolic blood pressure show moderately high association with health risks.

Table 2 presents the descriptive statistics of the maternal health dataset used for the study. The average age of the subjects of the dataset is 29.87 years with a wide variations in age of the pregnant women with a high standard deviation of 13.47. The usefulness of the nonparametric models lies in the values of skewness and kurtosys. We know majority of the parametric models assume normal distribution that requires a skewness to be zero and kurtosys, three. None of the variables satisfies this requirements. Naturally, distribution-free nonparametric models are bound to be good-fit for the predictive analysis. Following the nature of the data and the problem in hand, we use binomial logistic regression as our parametric test that does not assume linear relationship between dependent and independent variables and the error terms are not required to be normally distributed. The scatteredness and the skewedness of the data are further evident in the histograms of individual variables shown in Fig. 2. Figure 3 shows the count of pregnant women according to the risk levels.

3.3 *Algorithms for Nonparametric Classifications*

In this subsection, we briefly mention different classification models that we use in the present study. We use SVM with polynomial kernel, decision tree, random forest

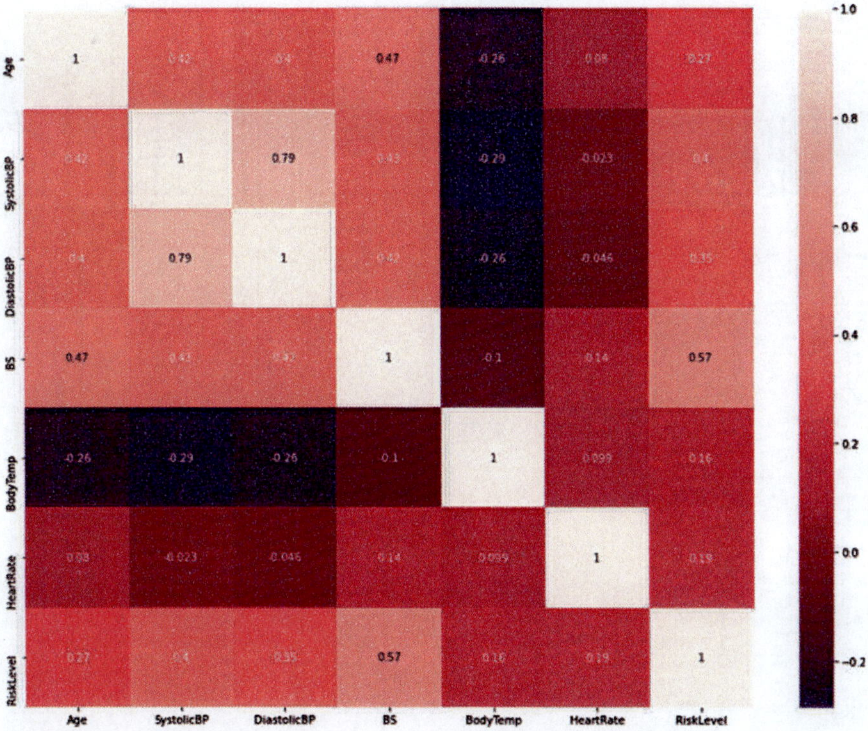

Fig. 1 Correlation heat-map

Table 2 Descriptive statistics

	Age	SystolicBP	DiastolicBP	BS	BodyTemp	HeartRate
Mean	29.871	113.198	76.460	8.725	98.665	74.301
Median	26.000	120.000	80.000	7.5000	98.000	76.000
Std. Dev.	13.474	18.403	13.885	3.293	1.371	8.088
Skewness	0.783	−0.251	−0.048	1.868	1.750	−1.043
Kurtosys	−0.391	−0.613	−0.948	2.303	1.451	8.398
25th Percentile	19.000	100.000	65.000	6.900	98.000	70.000
75th Percentile	39.000	120.000	90.000	8.000	98.000	80.000
Observations	1014	1014	1014	1014	1014	1014

and Gaussian Naive Bayes classifiers as nonparametric models and compared their results.

Support Vector Machine: This is a supervised machine learning model that is developed by Vladimir Vapnik with his colleagues in AT&T Bell Laboratories [16]. The model constructs hyperplanes in n-dimensional space that is used for the purpose

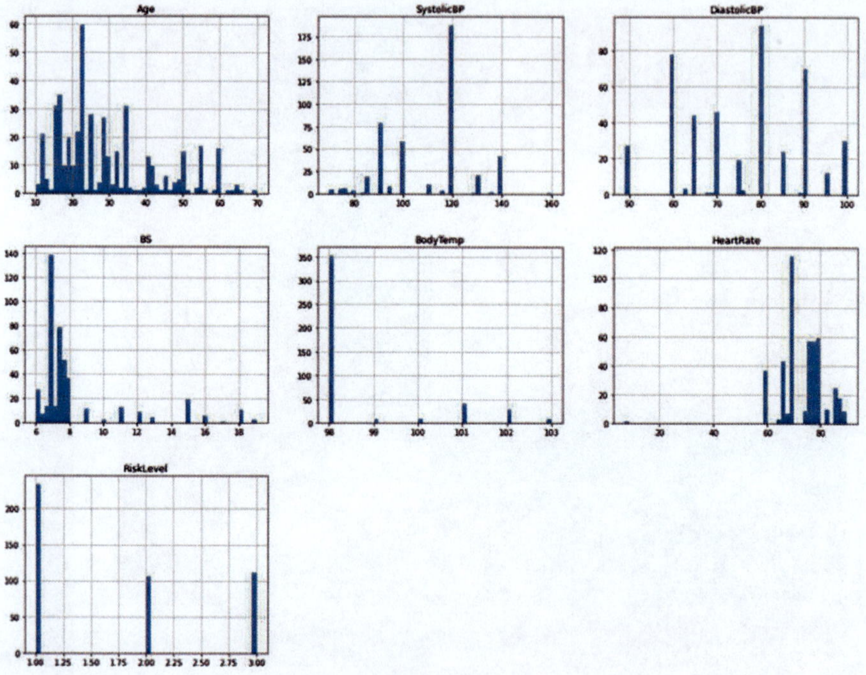

Fig. 2 Histogram of variables

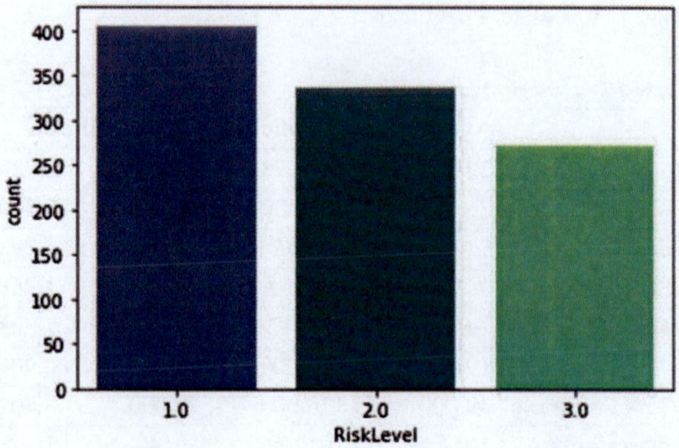

Fig. 3 Counts of pregnant women according to risk level. Label 1 = low risk, 2 = moderate risk and 3 = high risk

of classification. To reduce the computational load, the SVM model uses a Kernel function $K(x, y)$ according to the nature of the problem.

Decision Tree Algorithm: The objective of the algorithm is to predict the target variable based on the learning of the decision rules from the data features. That is, we present our dataset as (x, Y), where x is a vector of k features $(x_1, x_2, x_3, \ldots, x_k)$ and Y is the dependent variable or the target variable that we want to classify.

Random Forest Algorithm: Random forest (RF) is the collection of multiple decision trees that are associated with samples generated through bootstrapping from the original dataset. This model of random decision forest is first proposed by Ho [17]. The model is further developed by Amit and Geman [18] followed by Breiman [19]. The training of RF is based on bootstrap aggregating or bagging. In a training dataset of $X = x_1, x_2, x_3, \ldots, x_n$ with respective responses $Y = y_1, y_2, y_3, \ldots, y_n$, the bootstrap aggregation procedure selects random samples with replacement repetitively for b (where $b = 1\ to\ B$) times. After training, the prediction of random samples is aggregated. The bootstrapping procedure increases the accuracy of the classification as it reduces the variance of the model.

Gaussian Naive Bayes Classification: Naive Bayes classifier is a model of conditional probability where the independent variable X is a vector with n features as $X = (x_1, x_2, x_3, \ldots, x_n)$ and the probability of k possible outcomes of the class C_k is given as $p(C_k|x_1, x_2, x_3, \ldots x_n)$.

3.4 Evaluation Metrics

These metrics simply consider four data points after the classification is done, these are, true positive (TP), true negative (TN), false positive (FP) and false negative (FN). Using these four factors, we evaluate our classification models according to the following four parameters:

$$\text{Accuracy} = \frac{\text{TP} + \text{TN}}{\text{TP} + \text{TN} + \text{FP} + \text{FN}};\quad \text{where } 0.0 < \text{Accuracy} < 1.0$$

$$\text{Precision} = \frac{\text{TP}}{\text{TP} + \text{FP}}$$

$$\text{Recall} = \frac{\text{TP}}{\text{TP} + \text{FN}}$$

$$F_1\ \text{Score} = 2 \times \frac{\text{Ptrecision} \times \text{Recall}}{\text{Precision} + \text{Recall}}$$

3.5 Parametric Test

We use binomial logistic regression analysis as our parametric test procedure based on the problem and the nature of the data. Our dependent variable is categorical variable where logistic regression is an ideal choice for estimation. The dependent variable 'Risk Level' has three categories low risk, moderate risk and high risk. For simplicity and better accuracy, we have combined these three categories into two, that is, high risk and moderate/low risk. This allows us to apply binomial logistic regression model. The rationality behind applying binomial model is, in a health risk scenario drawing accurate inference on high-risk patients is much more important than multiple categorization of patients according to multiple risk factors. So, inference drawn from binomial logistic regression will be much more reliable for medical practitioners. Further, as our dataset does not follow normal distribution, logistic regression is an ideal choice where normality of residuals is not a prerequisite. To make the paper concise, we purposefully avoid the detail mathematical expressions of logistic regression.

4 Experimental Study and Results

In Table 3, we present the comparative analysis of different classification models. All the four classification models are supervised models and use train-test split of 75–25% of the total 1014 observations. Both Tables 3 and 4 report performance of the models using the parameters of evaluation metrics explained earlier. The results suggest that the overall accuracy of the RF model is better than other competing models

Table 3 Comparative study of classification models

Model	Type	Train-test split (%)	Test accuracy (%)
SVM-Polynomial kernel	Supervised	75–25	67.32
Decision tree	Supervised	75–25	79.13
Random forest	Supervised	75–25	81.49
Gaussian naive bayes	Supervised	75–25	61.02

Table 4 Model precision according to risk level

	Risk level	Precision	Recall	f1-score	Support
SVM-polynomial Kernel	Low	0.61	0.77	0.68	98
	Moderate	0.60	0.44	0.50	85
	High	0.86	0.83	0.84	71
Decision tree	Low	0.83	0.76	0.79	98
	Moderate	0.70	0.80	0.75	85
	High	0.87	0.83	0.85	71
Random forest	Low	0.85	0.80	0.82	98
	Moderate	0.75	0.79	0.77	85
	High	0.85	0.87	0.86	71
Gaussian naive bayes	Low	0.55	0.90	0.68	98
	Moderate	0.51	0.21	0.30	85
	High	0.83	0.69	0.75	71

closely followed by decision tree. This seems to be obvious as the RF algorithm is a modified and randomized version of the decision tree model. All the models, that is SVM, decision tree, RF and Gaussian NB in predicting high-risk patients which is desirable. The result is not satisfactory in the classification between low and moderate health risk categories. The evaluation metrics of 'Recall' are highly important in a health risk prediction scenario. 'Recall' measures the percentage of true positive (TP) over the total of TP and FN. That means, our best performing model RF is showing a recall value of 87% for high-risk patients which indicates that 13% of the patients are wrongly classified as moderate/low risk patients, which is dangerous. So it is always important in a health risk classification scenario to leave a space for subjective decision-making based on the causality of different explanatory and dependent variables. This will not only help medical practitioners to understand the causality of variables for health risk but also the intensity of the individual explanatory variables causing such risks. This motivates us to resort to parametric tests along with highly efficient classification models.

As we use binomial logistic regression, we re-classify our data into two categories, high risk and low or moderate risk. In the descriptive statistics in Table 2, the skewness and kurtosys data read with the histogram in Fig. 2, we find that the dataset does not follow any distribution pattern. This is further evident in the density function presented in Fig. 4. The density function below is broken according to the risk levels. The figure demonstrates high degree of differences between density function of high-risk patients and low/moderate risk patients.

The result of logistic regression models is reported in Table 5. We use both original dataset and log-transformed dataset for the logistic regression model. We find that apart from age, all other explanatory variables are showing highly significant

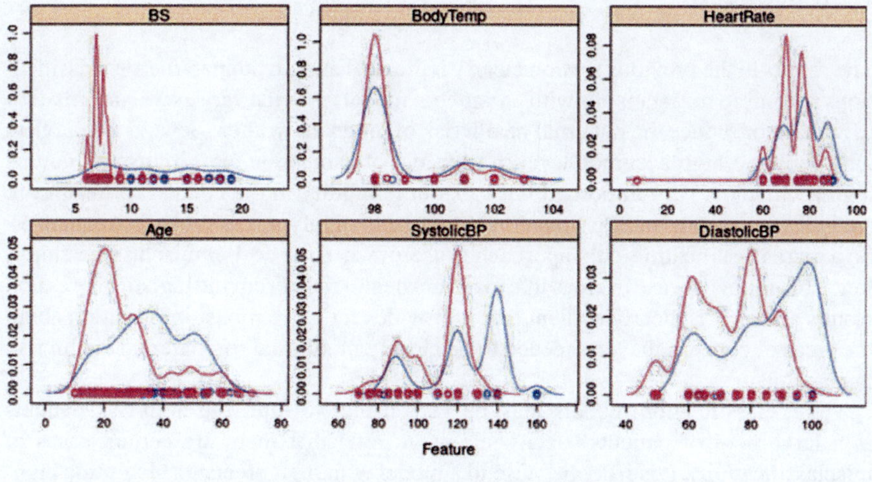

Fig. 4 Density distribution of explanatory variables broken-down by RiskLevel values ('High' for high risk and 'LowMod' for low to moderate risk)

Table 5 Results of logistic regression model

	Original dataset		Log-transformed	
	Estimates	Std. Error	Estimates	Std. Error
Age	0.016	0.009	0.401	0.306
SystolicBP	−0.028**	0.00 9	−2.634*	1.116
DiastolicBP	−0.046***	0.012	−3.515***	0.986
BS	−0.496***	0.045	−5.316***	0.439
BodyTemp	−0.561***	0.071	−55.094***	7.268
HeartRate	−0.051***	0.012	−3.272***	0.953
AIC	684.32		680.78	

Intercept terms are not reported. Significance Codes: ***0.001, **0.01, *0.05

association with health risk. We consider 0.1, 1 and 5% level of significance as the decision rule. As expected, the sign (+/−) of the associations is negative as the health parameters in the explanatory variables should remain within an acceptable range and the values above or below that range leads to higher health risk. As we see here for both the models, body temperature of the pregnant women is the most significant factor to be monitored to avoid the health risk. Next important factor to monitor is the glucose level in the blood (BS). In blood pressures, the variation in the diastolic blood pressure may cause more health risk than the variation of the systolic blood pressure. This result gives a clear insight that will improve the management of health risk.

5 Discussion

The results in the previous section clearly indicate that both nonparametric classifications and inferential statistics with parametric models provide very useful information to manage or reduce the maternal health risk of pregnant women. Several researchers have reported high accuracy level in different classification algorithms. While this high accuracy is very important but lacks in reliability in the context of healthcare analytics as a small misclassification may lead to highly undesirable consequences. So a mare classification-only approach is useful when the cost of misclassification is low. That is not the case in areas like maternal health risk. From the logistic regression results above, it is clearly evident that it provides far more robust information about the areas of concern that are needed to be closely monitored for maternal health risk management.

Here, classification models may be very useful to filter the high-risk patients in a large pool of patients' data keeping in mind that there are certain cases of misclassifications. It is risky because in a model with high precision also some high-risk patients will be classified as false negative (FN). So, while classification helps to easily filter high-risk patients for better monitoring, it leaves us with the job of finding out the false negatives. Here, the degree of causal association becomes very helpful as we can identify which health parameters are most important to observe closely. So, even if the false negatives happen, the patients with higher risks can be monitored from the second layer of observations of variables whose degree of association with the health risk is higher. Thus, in the present paper, we propose that in the field of healthcare analytics, parametric models should always be used to complement the nonparametric classification models for better healthcare management.

6 Conclusion and Scope for Future Research

Healthcare management is a critical factor as it requires awareness of the recipients of healthcare services as well as dissemination of accurate information and timely intervention of healthcare professionals. With the proliferation of health data through the systems like IoHT, it becomes imperative to utilize these data to get meaningful information and offer better healthcare services. Having said that, we must keep in mind that the machine learning-based algorithms on the healthcare data should be applied with care and responsibility. In a subject like health care, there will always be the space for subjective decision-making of healthcare professionals. So in one hand, when classification substantially reduces their workloads and helps them focus better on the management of health risk, the causality of health risk and other health parameters provide them with rich and meaningful insights for healthcare management. The findings of the present paper substantiate that the parametric causality test along with classification algorithm gives more reliable outcome. So, we conclude that specifically in the field of health care, inferential statistics with appropriate parametric tests should always complement each other.

The present paper is based on maternal health risk data. This complementary approach of combining parametric and nonparametric classification models may further be tested on other healthcare datasets.

References

1. Firouzi F, Rahmani AM, Mankodiya K, Badaroglu M, Merrett GV, Wong P, Farahani B (2018) Internet-of-things and big data for smarter healthcare: from device to architecture, applications and analytics (2018)
2. Eskofier BM, Lee SI, Baron M, Simon A, Martindale CF, Gaßner H, Klucken J (2017) Appl Sci 7(10):986
3. Lakshmanaprabu S, Shankar K, Ilayaraja M, Nasir AW, Vijayakumar V, Chilamkurti N (2019) Int J Mach Learn Cybernet 10(10):2609
4. Akbar W, Wu WP, Faheem M, Saleem S, Javed A, Saleem MA (2020) 2020 International conference on electrical, communication, and computer engineering (ICECCE), IEEE, pp 1–4
5. Bhatt V, Chakravorty T, Chakraborty S (2022) Proceedings of international conference on data science and applications. Springer, pp 743–754

6. Rallapalli S, Suryakanthi T (2016) 2016 international conference on advances in computing and communication engineering (ICACCE). IEEE, pp 281–284
7. Iwendi C, Bashir AK, Peshkar A, Sujatha R, Chatterjee JM, Pasupuleti S, Mishra R, Pillai S, Jo O (2020) Front Pub Health 8:357
8. Fawagreh K, Gaber MM (2020) Computing, 1–12
9. Boukenze B, Mousannif H, Haqiq A et al (2016) Comput Sci Inf Technol 1:1
10. Nagarajan V, Kumar V (2018) Int J Innov Res Sci Technol 4(10):79
11. Razzaghi T, Roderick O, Safro I, Marko N (2016) PloS one 11(5):e0155119
12. Pradeep K, Naveen N (2018) Proced Comput Sci 132:412
13. Charleonnan A, Fufaung T, Niyomwong T, Chokchueypattanakit W, Suwannawach S, Ninchawee N (2016) 2016 Management and innovation technology international conference (MITicon). IEEE, pp MIT–80
14. Mir A, Dhage SN (2018) 2018 fourth international conference on computing communication control and automation (ICCUBEA). IEEE, pp 1–6
15. Deepika K, Seema S (2016) 2016 2nd international conference on applied and theoretical computing and communication technology (iCATccT). IEEE, pp 381–386
16. Cortes C, Vapnik V (1995) Mach Learn 20(3):273
17. Ho TK (1995) Proceedings of 3rd international conference on document analysis and recognition, vol 1. IEEE, pp 278–282
18. Amit Y, Geman D (1997) Neural computation 9(7):1545
19. Breiman L (2001) Mach Learn 45(1):5

Towards Machine Learning-Based Emotion Recognition from Multimodal Data

Md. Faiyaz Shahriar, Md. Safkat Azad Arnab, Munia Sarwat Khan, Safwon Sadif Rahman, Mufti Mahmud, and M. Shamim Kaiser

Abstract Understanding human emotion is vital to communicate effectively with others, monitor patients, analyse behaviour, and keep an eye on those who are vulnerable. Emotion recognition is essential to achieve a complete human-machine interoperability experience. Artificial intelligence, mainly machine learning (ML), have been used in recent years to improve the model for recognising emotions from a single type of data. A multimodal system has been proposed that uses text, facial expressions, and speech signals to identify emotions in this work. The MobileNet architecture is used to predict emotion from facial expressions, and different ML classifiers are used to predict emotion from text and speech signals in the proposed model. The Facial Expression Recognition 2013 (FER2013) dataset has been used to recognise emotion from facial expressions, whilst the Interactive Emotional Dyadic Motion Capture (IEMOCAP) dataset was used for both text and speech emotion recognition. The proposed ensemble technique consisting of random forest, extreme gradient boosting, and multi-layer perceptron achieves an accuracy of 70.67%, which is better than the unimodal approaches used.

Keywords Emotion recognition · Machine learning · Multimodal · MobileNet · Prediction

---

Md. F. Shahriar · Md. S. A. Arnab · M. S. Khan · S. S. Rahman
Department of Information and Communication Technology, Bangladesh University of Professionals, Dhaka, Bangladesh, India

M. Mahmud (✉)
Department of Computer Science, Nottingham Trent University, Clifton, Nottingham NG11 8NS, UK
e-mail: muftimahmud@gmail.com

MTIF, Nottingham Trent University, Clifton, Nottingham NG11 8NS, UK

CIRC, Nottingham Trent University, Clifton, Nottingham NG11 8NS, UK

M. S. Kaiser
IIT, Jahangirnagar University, Savar 1342, Bangladesh, India

© The Author(s), under exclusive license to Springer Nature Singapore Pte Ltd. 2023

J. K. Mandal and D. De (eds.), *Frontiers of ICT in Healthcare*, Lecture Notes in Networks and Systems 519, https://doi.org/10.1007/978-981-19-5191-6_9

1 Introduction

Communication is essential to human survival, and we frequently encounter confusing circumstances,. For example, the remark "This is fantastic" may be used in both joyful and sad situations. In most cases, humans can resolve ambiguity because we can easily interpret information from many domains (referred to as modalities hereafter), notably speech, text, and visual. Multiple attempts to solve the problem have been made since the development of machine learning techniques.

Basically, in this research, emotion was recognised from the multimodal system. Three types of data were collected as input, i.e. Text, Speech Signal and Facial Expression and predicted emotion as output. Mobilenet architecture was used to predict emotion from facial expressions. Six different classifiers, i.e. Random Forest (RF), eXtreme Gradient Boosting (XGB), Multi-Layer Perceptron (MLP), Multinomial Naïve Bayes (MNB), Support Vector Machine (SVM) classifier and Logistic Regression (LR), were used to predict emotion from Text and Speech signal. The ensembled technique was used to improve the accuracy of combined classifiers. At last, the predicted results from text, speech signal and facial expression were concatenated together to introduce the multimodal emotion recognition system.

1. To propose a *multimodal*, system that can predict emotion.
2. To compare the *accuracy of each classifier*, used for predicting emotion.

The following section will discuss the methodology where MobileNet architecture and used classifiers are discussed, along with their respective block diagrams. In Sect. 4, the results of classifiers and architecture are to be discussed briefly. Several visual comparisons are shown with bar diagrams. At last, in Sect. 5, the conclusion is discussed.

2 Related Work

ML has been applied to different application domains, including anomaly detection [2, 3, 10–12, 21], disease detection [7, 9, 14, 20, 23–25, 28, 29] and smart data analytics [1, 6, 13, 15, 16, 26, 31, 32, 37]. Emotion recognition based on physiological signals has been a prominent issue in recent years, with applications in a variety of fields, including safe driving, health care, and social security [36]. In their research, we proposed a multimodal emotion recognition model with facial expression recognition, speech recognition, and text recognition. Firoz et al. [22] proposed a facial expression identification method using the k-Nearest Neighbours classification approach and used Cohn-Kanade (CK+), RaFD, and KDEFto assess the performance. Neha et al. [19] presented a Hybrid Convolution-Recurrent Neural Network approach for FER in images in this paper. The suggested network design consists of Convolution layers preceded by a Recurrent Neural Network (RNN). Two public datasets are used to verify the proposed hybrid model. Deepak et al. [18]

suggested a model where distinguish Deep Convolutional Neural Networks (DNNs) with convolution layers and deep residual blocks are used. The Extended CK+ and Japanese Female Facial Expression (JAFFE) Datasets were used to train this model. Daario et al. [5] proposed the growth of a real-time CNN model for detecting emotion in speech in his paper. On three key emotions, "Angry," "Happy," and "Sad," their CNN system achieved an overall accuracy of 66.1%. Saikat et al. [4] said in this paper, they employed a Convolution Neural Network (CNN) and Long Short-Term Memory (LSTM)-based strategy to classify 13 Mel Frequency Cepstral Coefficient (MFCC) features with 13 velocity and 13 acceleration components. For classification, they used the Berlin Emotional Speech dataset (EmoDB). On test data, they have an accuracy rate of around 80%. Aharon et al. [30] introduced a new method of emotion recognition based on para-lingual data in speech, which is applied directly to spectrograms and is built in a deep neural network. It was tested on IMOCAP, which obtains a prediction of 66%. Jonathan et al. [17] presented a paper where they suggested a new strategy that makes use of pre-trained, dense word embedding representations in this paper. Their studies used five different datasets for emotion recognition from various domains and found that the global average F1-score improved by 11.6% on average. Kush et al. [35] offered a sequence-based convolutional neural network (CNN) with word embedding in this paper. In the suggested model, an attention mechanism is used to allow CNN to concentrate on the texts that have the most impact on categorisation or the parts of the features that should be paid more attention to. Dibyendu et al. [33] detected emotions in the text using NLP by searching an emotion database for keywords. Chan et al. [8] used convolutional attention networks to propose a new way for learning about hidden representations in simply audio and text data in their research. The suggested attention model performs substantially better in the CMU-MOSEI dataset. Jilt et al. [34] focussed on cross-modal fusion strategies for emotion recognition from spoken audio and transcripts using deep learning models. For text-based emotion recognition, they evaluate the usage of a Recurrent neural network (RNN) with pre-trained word embedding and convolutional neural network (CNN) with utterance-level descriptors for long short-term memory (LSTM). The presented techniques are effective in speaker and session-independent testing on the IEMOCAP multimodal emotion identification dataset. Amol et al. [27] proposed a way for automatically detecting emotional duality and mixed emotional experience using multimodal audio-visual continuous data. The features were calculated using the OpenEar toolbox and the Face API. The overall accuracy was found to be 96.6% using multimodal mixed emotion recognition.

3 Methodology

The feature vectors from the three modalities are fused in the proposed technique (facial expression, speech signal, and text). Feature vectors were concatenated from facial expression, speech signal, and text to produce the fused feature vectors. We would be able to understand how much information is present in each of the modalities

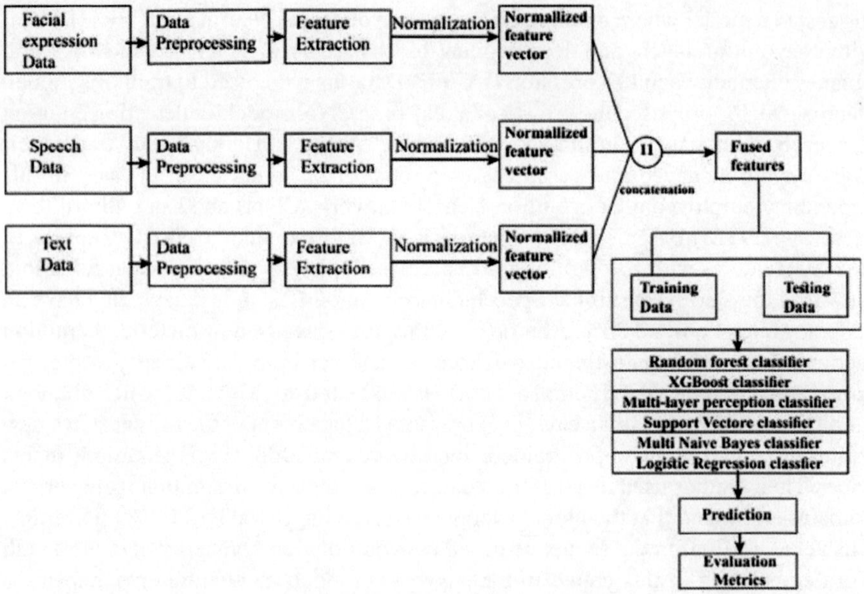

Fig. 1 Ensemble technique using average prediction for speech signal

and how fusion affects the model's performance using this strategy. Then after feature extraction, we need to normalise the feature vector to scale these vectors in the same size. After that, we concatenate these three-feature vectors by selecting axis=1, which means the concatenation will be done column-wise. Then finally, we get the fused feature vector. We split that into training and testing data, then train it on different classifiers and predict the emotion using testing data. We can evaluate the accuracy, precision, recall, and f score of the proposed technique. A simplified version of the multimodal system has been represented in Fig. 1. Here the basic steps of a multimodal system are shown in a sequential pattern.

3.1 Data Preprocessing

Before photos are utilised in model training, they go through a few preprocessing procedures to prepare them. The frequency analysis of the dataset shows that the emotion label "Disgust" has so few samples. So, we combined the instances from the "Angry" and "Disgust" classes. Then we utilised Keras ImageDataGenerator to augment the photos in real-time whilst the model was still training. This would not only make the model more robust but would also save space. For the augmentation $p[0, 1]$ using rescale. As a result, we may handle all photographs the same way: some have a large pixel range, whilst others have a low pixel range. The overall loss will be distributed more equally by scaling all photos to the same range [0, 1]. When we used rescaling with rotation, every pixel value is transformed from the range [0, 255].

According to preliminary frequency analysis, the dataset is not balanced. Up-sampling techniques were used to compensate for the under-representation of the emotions "fear" and "surprise." We then combined instances from the "happy" and "excited" classes since "happy" was underrepresented, and the two feelings were quite similar. Furthermore, we exclude cases labelled "others" since they match examples deemed unclear even for a human. The operations mentioned above yielded a total of 7837 samples.

At first, labels were extracted from the evaluation files, and all data were compiled in a single file. Then any special symbols were deleted once the transcriptions were adjusted to lowercase.

3.2 *Feature Extraction*

To extract relevant features, the face is first detected using Haar Cascade Classifier, and the image is outlined using NaN. Then the face is divided into several blocks, features are extracted from each block to create a feature vector.

As the waveforms generated by the voice chords alter based on emotions, the pitch is an important feature which can be calculated using several methods. The most widely used approach has been applied here, which relies on the autocorrelation of centre-clipped frames.

We can extract the feature from text data by measuring Term Frequency-Inverse Document Frequency (TFIDF) that indicates the relationship between a term and a document in a corpus.

3.3 *Ensemble Technique*

In the proposed ensemble technique, we take the prediction output from different classifiers, make the average prediction using that output, and select the highest measured value as the final prediction. Figure 2 shows the ensemble technique for speech signal. Classifiers with highest accuracy are the RF, XGB, and MLP. The predictions of six classes are taken individually for each classifier. Then the average is calculated from these three classifiers. From the average value of six classes, the highest value is picked as the final prediction. By following the same procedure, we ensemble the XGB, MLP, RF, MNB, and LR classifiers for only text data and the fused data.

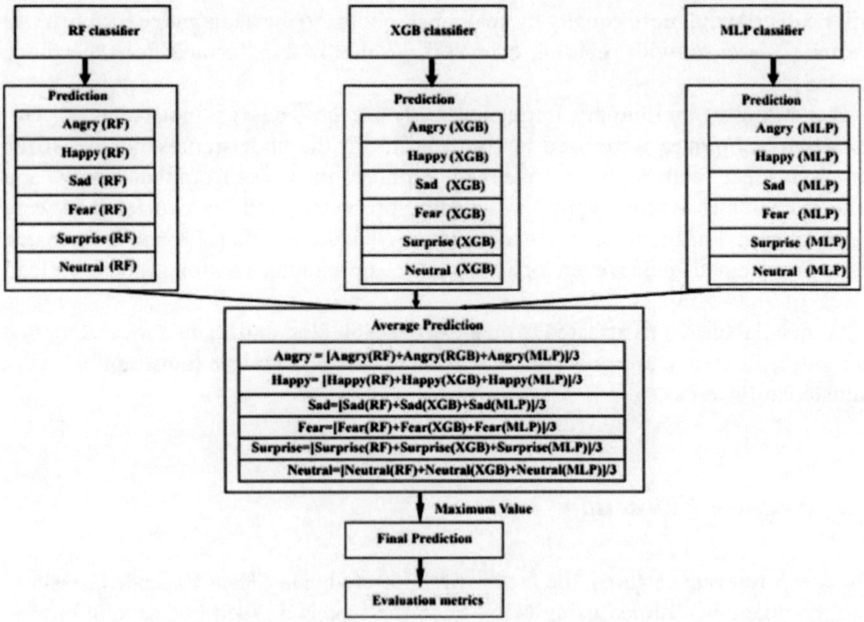

Fig. 2 Ensemble technique using average prediction for speech signal

4 Results and Discussion

In this section, Accuracy, Precision, Recall, and F-score are provided for individual CNN model and different classifiers, and, lastly, the result of ensemble models are also provided.

4.1 *Facial Expression Performance Analysis*

Table 1 shows the overall performance of the MobileNet model. The accuracy, precision, recall, and F-score is obtained from the confusion matrix shown in Fig. 3. Trained on 100 epochs, the model achieved an accuracy of 66%.

We received a good accuracy and a fair recall. But we got less precision compared to other performance parameters because we found high False Positives as shown in the confusion matrix in Fig. 3. The trained model can be improved by reducing the false positive and false negative classified data.

Table 1 The performance of mobileNet architecture

Factors	Performance (%)
Accuracy	66
Precision	58.48
Recall	82.35
F-score	68.39

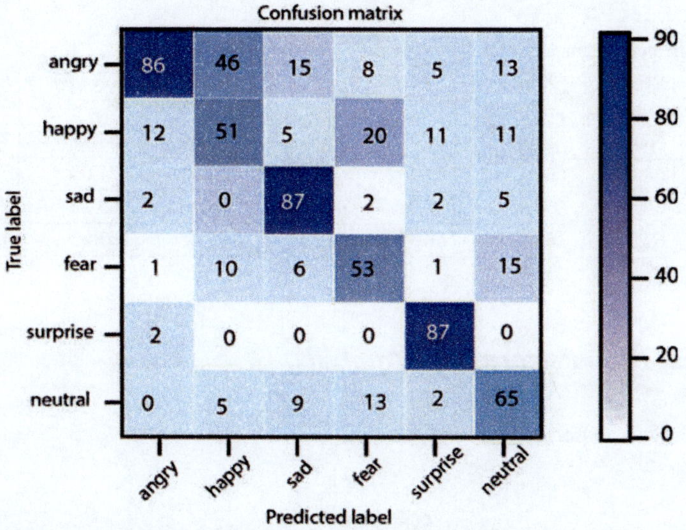

Fig. 3 Confusion matrix of trained model with MobileNet architecture

Table 2 The performance of classifiers for speech

	RF (%)	XGB (%)	SVC (%)	MNB (%)	MLP (%)	LR (%)	Ensemble (%)
Accuracy	57.54	55.79	42.12	30.05	42.2	32.08	64.17
Precision	55.22	52.7	53.87	54.25	54.3	40.92	70.04
Recall	61.72	66.14	50.57	40.24	48.03	42.47	66.48
F-score	58.29	58.66	52.16	46.2	50.97	41.94	68.21

4.2 Speech Signal Performance Analysis

Table 2 shows the accuracy, precision, recall, and F-score for individual classifiers for speech signal.

Table 3 The performance of classifiers with text data

	RF (%)	XGB (%)	SVC (%)	MNB (%)	MLP (%)	LR (%)	Ensemble (%)
Accuracy	60.08	53.91	63.23	59.83	64.83	63.54	66.13
Precision	68.33	58.73	73.23	66.81	63.14	67.27	68.27
Recall	67.49	58.93	61.35	62.16	69.55	67.94	70.47
F-score	67.91	58.82	66.89	64.4	66.19	67.6	68.29

Table 4 The performance of classifiers for multimodal data

	RF (%)	XGB (%)	SVC (%)	MNB (%)	MLP (%)	LR (%)	Ensemble (%)
Accuracy	66.4	64.07	64.32	60.28	68.69	64.77	70.67
Precision	68.65	69.1	69.7	71.39	68.91	71.09	72.04
Recall	66.19	64.97	67.99	61.05	68.13	65.13	72.25
F-score	67.39	66.91	68.83	65.81	68.5	67.98	72.14

4.3 *Text Data Performance Analysis*

Table 3 shows the performance of the text data.

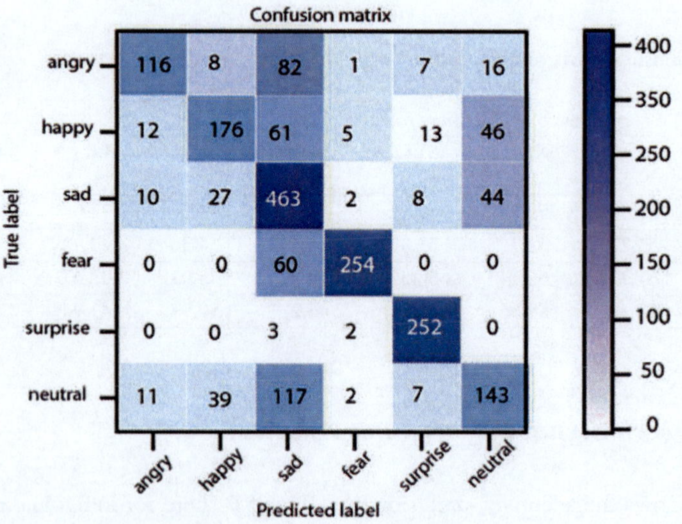

Fig. 4 Confusion matrix of multimodal data after ensembling

4.4 Performance Analysis of Multimodal System

The result of multimodal emotion recognition is shown in Table 4. If facial expression, speech signal, and text are merged, it can provide better accuracy in practical cases. After the fusion process, the same classifiers were used as previous. Figure 4 shows the confusion matrix after concatenating facial expression, speech signal, and text.

5 Conclusion

In the world of increasing digitalisation, we can find the dependency of AI-based systems as responsible for recognising emotion from different modes. Many of the systems reached a milestone of accuracy. Intelligent systems increasingly use emotion recognition models to better their interactions with people. This is significant because the systems may adjust their reactions and behavioural patterns in response to human emotions, making the encounter more genuine.

We mainly focussed on the prime modes of emotion recognition, and we found three modes, i.e. text, image, and speech. Individually from each mode, emotion can be detected, and we have tried to make our system predict from three of these modes to get the prediction as accurate as possible.

Acknowledgements MM and MSK are supported by the DIVERSASIA project (618615-EPP-1-2020-1-UKEPPKA2-CBHEJP) funded by the European Commission under the Erasmus+ programme.

References

1. Al Banna MH et al (2021) Attention-based bi-directional long-short term memory network for earthquake prediction. IEEE Access 9:56589–56603
2. Al Nahian MJ, Ghosh T et al (2020) Towards artificial intelligence driven emotion aware fall monitoring framework suitable for elderly people with neurological disorder. In: Proceeding of Brain Information, pp 275–286
3. Al Nahian MJ et al (2021) Towards an accelerometer-based elderly fall detection system using cross-disciplinary time series features. IEEE Access 9:39413–31
4. Basu S, Chakraborty J, Aftabuddin M (2017) Emotion recognition from speech using convolutional neural network with recurrent neural network architecture. In: Proceeding of ICCES, pp 333–336
5. Bertero D, Fung P (2017) A first look into a convolutional neural network for speech emotion detection. In: Proceeding of ICASSP, pp 5115–5119
6. Biswas M, Tania MH, Kaiser MS et al (2021) Accu3rate: a mobile health application rating scale based on user reviews. PloS one 16(12):e0258050
7. Biswas M et al (2021) An xai based autism detection: the context behind the detection. In: Proceeding of Brain Information, pp. 448–459
8. Choi WY, Song KY, Lee CW (2018) Convolutional attention networks for multimodal emotion recognition from speech and text data. In: Proceeding of challenge-HML, pp 28–34

9. Deepa B et al (2022) Pattern descriptors orientation and map firefly algorithm based brain pathology classification using hybridized machine learning algorithm. IEEE Access 10:3848–3863
10. Fabietti M, Mahmud M, Lotfi A (2021) Anomaly detection in invasively recorded neuronal signals using deep neural network: effect of sampling frequency. In: Proceeding of AII, pp 79–91 (2021)
11. Fabietti M, Mahmud M, Lotfi A (2022) Channel-independent recreation of artefactual signals in chronically recorded local field potentials using machine learning. Brain Inform 9(1):1–17
12. Fabietti M et al (2020) Artifact detection in chronically recorded local field potentials using long-short term memory neural network. Proceeding AICT 2020:1–6
13. Faria TH et al (2021) Smart city technologies for next generation healthcare. In: Data-driven mining, learning and analytics for secured smart cities, pp 253–274
14. Ghosh T et al (2021) Artificial intelligence and internet of things in screening and management of autism spectrum disorder. Sustain Cities Soc 74:103189
15. Ghosh T et al (2021) An attention-based mood controlling framework for social media users. In: Proceeding of brain information, pp 245–256
16. Ghosh T et al (2021) A hybrid deep learning model to predict the impact of covid-19 on mental health form social media big data. Preprints 2021(2021060654)
17. Herzig J et al (2017) Emotion detection from text via ensemble classification using word embeddings. In: Proceeding ICTIR, pp 269–272
18. Jain DK, Shamsolmoali P, Sehdev P (2019) Extended deep neural network for facial emotion recognition. Pattern Recognit Lett 120:69–74
19. Jain N et al (2018) Hybrid deep neural networks for face emotion recognition. Pattern Recognit. Lett. 115:101–106
20. Kumar I et al (2022) Dense tissue pattern characterization using deep neural network. Cogn Comput 1–24 (2022) [ePub ahead of print]
21. Lalotra GS, Kumar V, Bhatt A, Chen T, Mahmud M (2022) Iretads: an intelligent real-time anomaly detection system for cloud communications using temporal data summarization and neural network. Secur Commun Netw 2022:9149164
22. Mahmud F, Islam B, Hossain A, Goala PB (2018) Facial region segmentation based emotion recognition using k-nearest neighbors. In: Proceeding ICIET, pp 1–5 (2018)
23. Mahmud M, Kaiser MS, McGinnity TM, Hussain A (2021) Deep learning in mining biological data. Cognit Comput 13(1):1–33
24. Mahmud M et al (2018) Applications of deep learning and reinforcement learning to biological data. IEEE Trans Neural Netw Learn Syst 29(6):2063–2079
25. Mammoottil MJ, Kulangara LJ, Cherian AS, Mohandas P, Hasikin K, Mahmud M (2022) Detection of breast cancer from five-view thermal images using convolutional neural networks. J Healthc Eng 2022:4295221
26. Nawar A, Toma NT, Al Mamun S, et al (2021) Cross-content recommendation between movie and book using machine learning. In: Proceeding AICT, pp 1–6
27. Patwardhan AS (2017) Multimodal mixed emotion detection. In: Proceeding of ICCES, pp 139–143
28. Paul A et al (2022) Inverted bell-curve-based ensemble of deep learning models for detection of covid-19 from chest x-rays. Neural Comput Appl 1–15
29. Prakash N et al (2021) Deep transfer learning covid-19 detection and infection localization with superpixel based segmentation. Sustain Cities Soc 75:103252
30. Satt A, Rozenberg S, Hoory R (2017) Efficient emotion recognition from speech using deep learning on spectrograms. In: Interspeech, pp 1089–1093
31. Satu M et al (2020) Towards improved detection of cognitive performance using bidirectional multilayer long-short term memory neural network. In: Proceeding of Brain Information, pp 297–306
32. Satu MS et al (2021) Tclustvid: a novel machine learning classification model to investigate topics and sentiment in covid-19 tweets. Knowl-Based Syst 226:107126

33. Seal D, Roy UK, Basak R (2020) Sentence-level emotion detection from text based on semantic rules. In: Information and communication technology for sustainable development, pp 423–430
34. Sebastian J, Pierucci P et al (2019) Fusion techniques for utterance-level emotion recognition combining speech and transcripts. In: Interspeech, pp 51–55
35. Shrivastava K, Kumar S, Jain DK (2019) An effective approach for emotion detection in multimedia text data using sequence based convolutional neural network. Multimed Tools Appl 78(20):29607–29639
36. Shu L, Xie J, Yang M, Li Z, Li Z, Liao D, Xu X, Yang X (2018) A review of emotion recognition using physiological signals. Sensors 18(7):2074
37. Watkins J, Fabietti M, Mahmud M (2020) Sense: a student performance quantifier using sentiment analysis. In: Proceeding of IJCNN, pp 1–6

A Hybrid Approach for Stress Prediction from Heart Rate Variability

Md. Rahat Shahriar Zawad, Chowdhury Saleh Ahmed Rony, Md. Yeaminul Haque, Md. Hasan Al Banna, Mufti Mahmud, and M. Shamim Kaiser

Abstract Stress is a condition that causes a specific physiologicsal response. Heart rate variability (HRV) is a critical aspect in identifying stress. It is crucial for those who want to keep track of their wellness. Currently, numerous research is being conducted on stress prediction from HRV. The existing works in this field cover different data sets to identify stress, where significantly few models can predict stress with high accuracy. This work combines two well-known stress prediction data sets comprising HRV features named WESAD and SWELL-KW to compare twelve classical machine learning models and hybrid models. Finally, it proposes a hybrid stress prediction model that combines Artificial Neural Network (ANN) with Naive Bayes (NB). The proposed model performed auspiciously, having an accuracy of 95.75% within only 0.80 s. A stress prediction framework is also suggested based on the findings.

Keywords Stress · HRV · Machine learning · Hybrid method

Md. Rahat Shahriar Zawad, Chowdhury Saleh Ahmed Rony, Md. Yeaminul Haque : Equal Contributor.

Md. R. S. Zawad · C. S. A. Rony · Md. Y. Haque · Md. H. A. Banna
Bangladesh University of Professionals, Dhaka, Bangladesh

M. Mahmud (✉)
Department of Computer Science, Nottingham Trent University, Clifton, Nottingham NG11 8NS, UK
e-mail: muftimahmud@gmail.com

Medical Technologies Innovation Facility, Nottingham Trent University, Clifton, Nottingham NG11 8NS, UK

Computing and Informatics Research Centre, Nottingham Trent University, Clifton, Nottingham NG11 8NS, UK

M. S. Kaiser
IIT, Jahangirnagar University, Savar 1342, Dhaka, Bangladesh

© The Author(s), under exclusive license to Springer Nature Singapore Pte Ltd. 2023
J. K. Mandal and D. De (eds.), *Frontiers of ICT in Healthcare*, Lecture Notes in Networks and Systems 519, https://doi.org/10.1007/978-981-19-5191-6_10

1 Introduction

With the advancement of technology, our present way of life is growing more complex, which is of utmost concern for our everyday life. At the same time, mental health is one of the most overlooked and critical components of today's complex world [15, 16, 34]. A variety of physical and mental issues have resulted from uncontrolled human behaviour. Stress is a specific biological and psychological reaction that is an environmental stimulus generating stress in a body [8]. A moderate level of stress is beneficial and may encourage a person; however, excessive stress or a strong stress response can be harmful [14]. As a result, stress management has been a prevalent issue due to its enormous influence on our well-being. The increase of stress in our life leads to many problems such as heart disease, high blood pressure, depression, anxiety, and stroke [2, 30]. Presently, there is no globally accepted standard for stress assessment. Several research studies have examined biological markers (such as cortisol, amylase) and used established stress measuring methods. Heart rate variability (HRV) can be a reliable index to predict stress. HRV is defined as the variation in the duration of heartbeat intervals produced from an ECG measurement and assessed by measuring the time interval between two consecutive heartbeat peaks [8]. It rises during restful and recuperative activities and falls under stressful situations. Low HRV is linked to decreased autonomic nerve system (ANS) regulation and homeostatic functioning, lowering the body's capacity to cope with internal and external stimuli. In this way, for assessing the ANS in a clinical setting, HRV is a non-invasive electrocardiographic (ECG) approach. The contribution of this work is summarised as below:

- We combined two very well-known data sets (SWELL-KW and WESAD) to form a larger HRV data set for stress prediction.
- We used hybrid approaches, where ANN extracted features to speed up the prediction process.
- We used six different machine learning (ML) classifiers, namely Support Vector Machine (SVM), Logistic Regression (LR), Random Forest (RF), Naive Bayes (NB), XGBoost (XGB), and Decision Tree (DT) and made hybrid architectures with the same ML classifiers to figure out which model works best for the problem.
- We proposed a framework for stress prediction based on our work.

For the rest of the article, Sect. 2 surveys the literature and discusses the existing work. Section 3 describes the methodology, Sect. 4 lists the results and discusses them, and Sect. 5 concludes the article.

2 Literature Review

ML has been applied to different application domains, including anomaly detection [4, 5, 10–12, 20], disease detection [7, 9, 14, 19, 21–23, 27, 28] and smart data analytics [3, 6, 13, 15, 16, 25, 29, 30, 35]. For stress prediction, a variety of sensors have been utilised, including accelerometers (ACC), skin temperature (ST), electrodermal activity (EDA), blood volume pulse (BVP), galvanic skin response (GSR), heart rate (HR), and HRV. To predict stress, the majority of the studies used traditional ML techniques. Deep learning methodologies, on the other hand, have attracted the attention of this field's researchers [3, 21, 22]. Sriramprakash et al. [33] focused on a strategy for extracting the dominant and intersecting features from physiological sensors for stress and context identification in working people. They used the SWELL-KW data set where physiological features (like HR, HRV, and GSR) were extracted. SVM and KNN algorithms were used for classification where SVM with RBF kernel outperformed and got 72.83% accuracy. Koldijk et al. [17] concentrated on rating the modalities to find the ones that were most closely associated for predicting stress and mental effort. SWELL-KW was used as the data set, and the most useful data was gleaned from posture and facial expressions. SVM had the highest accuracy of 90.03% when inferring working conditions and mental states from a multimodal set of sensor data out of many ML approaches used. A study on stress level evaluation in virtual reality environments was published by Ahmad et al. [1]. They recorded a data set called Ryerson Multimedia Research Laboratory (RML) containing physiological signals and analysed ECG, GSR, and breathing signals of nine subjects. They translated the gathered data into 1D and 2D forms to generate a multimodal fusion of ECG data. They got 66.6% and 72.7 % in the RML and WESAD data sets, respectively, using this multimodal deep fusion model with RF, K-Nearest Neighbours (KNN), SVM, and XGB classifier algorithms. McDonald et al. [24] employed real-time heart rate data to detect the development of post-traumatic stress disorder (PTSD) triggers. For the missing heart rate data, the authors utilised the Kalman filter imputation technique and to assess the performance, the Receiver Operating Characteristic (ROC) curve (AUC) was utilised. They utilised five ML algorithms, with CNN, SVM, and RF being the most effective. The AUC of the SVM using the radial basis kernel was the highest at 0.67. Neurological techniques were proposed by Stewart et al. as a strategy for creating tailored models and addressing individual interactions with physiological stress. They used leave-one-participant cross-validation to construct stress classifiers that were compared on two public data sets, DRIVEDB and WESAD. Multiple sensor recordings, including ECG and GSR, were obtained using the DRIVEDB and WESAD databases. They used ML models that were only a few layers deep (like KNN, SVM, and LR). Also, when stress and baseline circumstances were provided as background, neural processing models outperformed them, with the precision of 0.957 (average precision) for WESAD and 0.804 (average precision) for DRIVEDB. Siirtola et al. [32] investigated alternative user-independent sensor combinations for accurately detecting stress. They used commercial smartwatches with various sensors to detect stress in different window sizes. The scientists employed linear discriminant analysis (LDA), quadratic discriminant analysis (QDA), and RF classifiers with various sensors, including ACC, ST, EDA, BVP, HR, and HRV. With the LDA classifier, the combination of skin temperature, BVP, and heart rate had the best accuracy (87.4%). Using physiological samples obtained from a broad population, Nkurikiyeyezu et al. [26] suggested a cost-effective approach for individualised stress prediction models. They built a generic model containing HRV and EDA features from the WESAD and SWELL-KW data sets, then an RF hybrid model with 10-fold cross-validation. The generic model's accuracy was just 42.5%. The accuracy level was enhanced to roughly 95.2 ± 0.5% with only 100 calibration samples.

3 Methodology

3.1 Proposed Framework

This paper proposes a stress prediction architecture that includes a wristband and a mobile application server. The wristband was connected to the mobile application server for continuous monitoring and data storage. Sensor data from the wristband was sent to the server, which will store it in the cloud server as well as do processing of the data [13]. The wristband is the output device in our framework. After the stress detection, it will present the user with an alarm to rest or take preventive measures in the event of stress. Figure 1 shows the proposed framework for stress prediction.

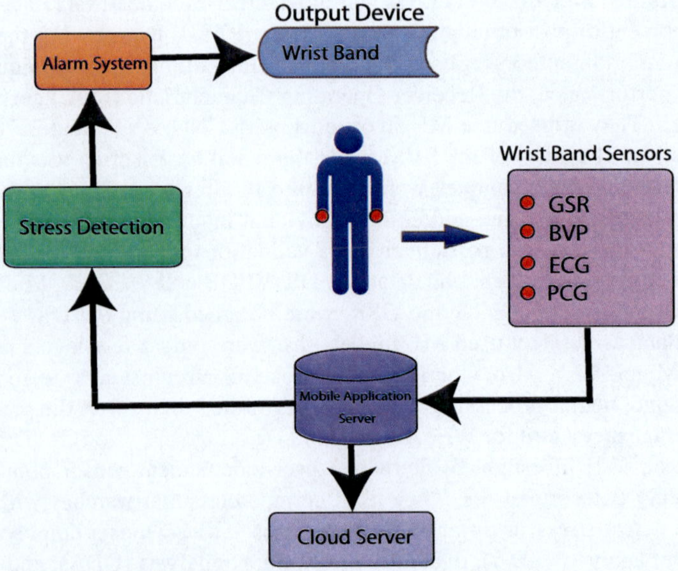

Fig. 1 Proposed stress prediction framework

Table 1 Description of the data sets

Data set name	Participants	No. of samples	Features
WESAD	15	3,91,638	67
SWELL-KW	25	1,35,650	69
Combined	40	5,27,288	64

3.2 Data Set Description

For model building and training, two multimodal data sets named WESAD [31] and SWELL-KW [18] have been used. The processed HRV was collected from Kaggle on which the HRV features were calculated by Nkurikiyeyezu et al. [26]. In the SWELL-KW data set, the conditions are marked as 'no stress', 'time pressure', and 'interruption'. On the other hand, in WESAD, the conditions are 'baseline', 'amusement', and 'stress'. Combining the two data sets derived common HRV features, we treated the 'no stress', 'baseline', and 'amusement' conditions as 'no stress' in the combined data set. 'Stress', 'time pressure', and 'interruption' are considered as 'stress' situations. The table contains information on the data sets. Table 1 shows the description of the data sets.

3.3 Feature Selection

The combined data set had 64 HRV features and 527288 samples in it. We used correlation-based feature selection methods to select the best and more suitable features for stress prediction out of them. For this, we used the Pearson correlation. We compare the correlation between features and remove highly correlated features higher than 0.9.

3.4 Classical ML Models

We used six classical ML models for our first part of the model building and training process. LR, NB, SVM, and DT were used to predict trees from the data set. Two ensemble methods, RF and XGB, were also built in this level. In all the cases, 70% of the data set was used for training and 30% was used for testing the model.

3.5 ANN Model Building

An optimised ANN was built using test and trial methods to construct the hybrid architectures. The ANN had 11 layers in total, including two dropout layers. All the

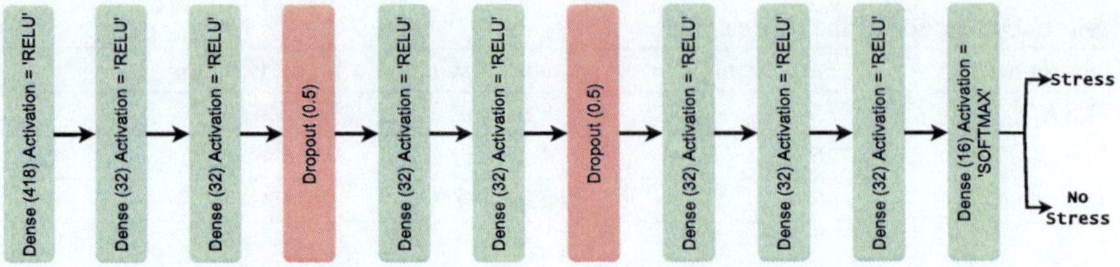

Fig. 2 Optimised ANN for the data set

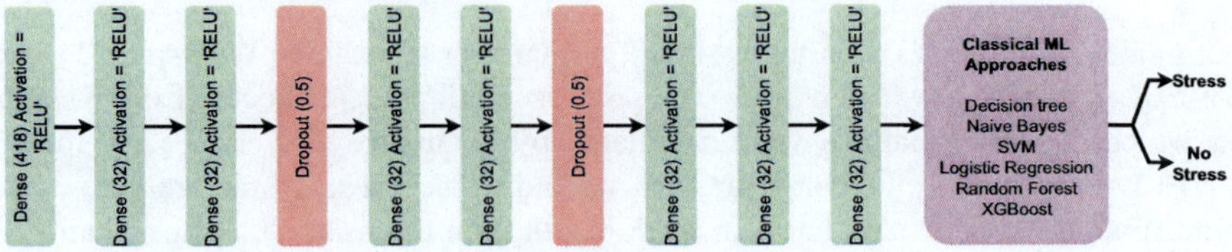

Fig. 3 Hybrid models that uses the optimised ANN

layers of the ANN were dense layers and used the RELU activation function except the last one, which used the softmax activation function. The structure of optimised ANN is shown in Fig. 2.

3.6 Hybrid Model Building

The hybrid architectures were a combination of ANN and classical ML models. ANNs use their last layer for the classification of the data sets provided. The ANN we built used the softmax activation function to classify the results as stress or no stress. We removed the last layer of the ANN and used the remaining layers as the feature extractor for the classical ML models using the pre-trained weights we had while building the ANN. After the last dense layer was removed from the network, the output from the last layer was unclassified high-level features for classical ML models. So, after the features extraction, the extracted features were used in the classical ML models to predict stress. Figure 3 shows the structure of proposed hybrid models.

4 Results and Discussion

The classical ML models we used worked on different levels of accuracy on our data set. The performance of the classical ML, such as DT, NB, SVM, RF, XGB and LR, is given in Table 2. NB achieved the lowest accuracy of 50.99% but within 0.76 s. On the other hand, DT and XGB achieved high accuracies of 88.40 and 89.62%. Though

Table 2 Performance of the classical ML models

Metrices	DT	NB	SVM	RF	XGB	LR
Accuracy (%)	88.40	50.99	77.84	80.91	89.62	63.72
Precision (%)	88.76	64.73	85.32	84.21	89.86	63.15
Recall (%)	88.40	50.99	77.84	80.91	89.62	63.72
F-measure (%)	88.76	45.38	75.23	79.70	89.50	61.29
Time (s)	15.228	0.76	165.52	148.08	96.09	84.94

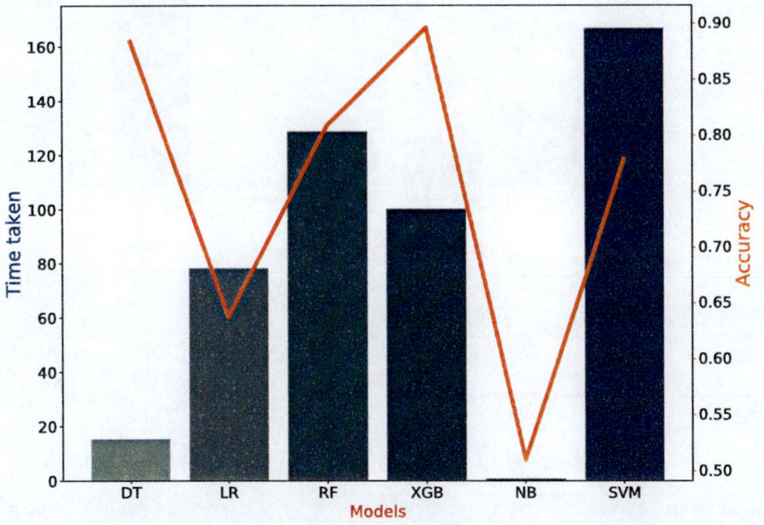

Fig. 4 Performance comparison of the classical ML models

these two algorithms achieved high accuracy, they didn't cross the 90% accuracy level and took a considerable amount of time to provide the results. Performance comparison of ML approaches is shown in Fig. 4.

When we went on to work with the hybrid architectures comprising our optimised ANN model and classical ML approaches, the findings were significantly better, which is shown in Fig. 5. In the case of hybrid models, all the classifiers achieved an accuracy of more than 95%. ANN and DT combination achieved the lowest accuracy, which is also 95.18% within 12.10 s. ANN, XGB and ANN, NB combination were the cases with two of the best accuracy with 95.72 and 95.75%. But ANN and NB combination achieved this accuracy within only 0.80 s, which is less than a second and can be considered real time. The performances of hybrid models are given in Table 3.

If we compare the performances of classical ML models and hybrid architectures, we can easily observe the increase in accuracy in the case of hybrid architectures. The consumption of time increased slightly in the case of hybrid structures, but that was

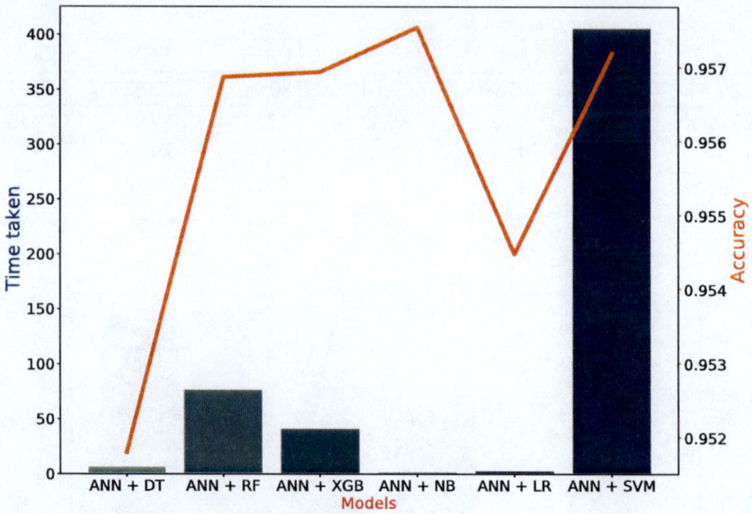

Fig. 5 Performance comparison of the hybrid models

Table 3 Performance of the hybrid models

Metrices	ANN+ DT	ANN+ NB	ANN+ SVM	ANN+ RF	ANN+ XGB	ANN+ LR
Accuracy (%)	95.18	95.75	95.72	95.69	95.69	95.52
Precision (%)	95.18	95.75	95.72	95.69	95.69	95.45
Recall (%)	95.18	95.75	95.72	95.69	95.70	95.46
F-measure (%)	95.17	95.75	95.72	95.69	95.69	95.46
Time (s)	12.10	0.80	403.08	97.74	37.06	1.97

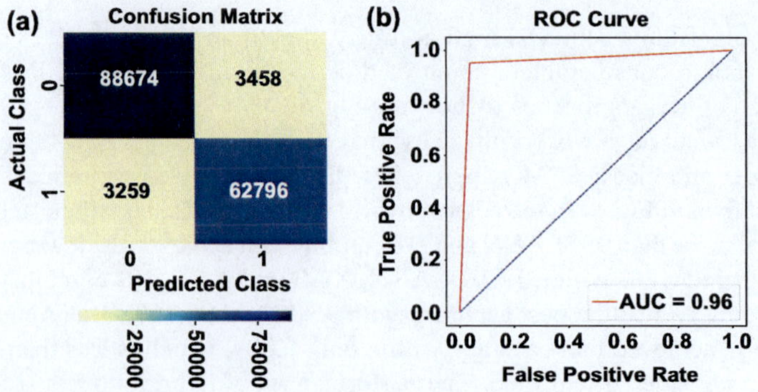

Fig. 6 **a** ROC curve and **b** Confusion matrix for ANN and NB model

acceptable as the best performing models achieved a staggering 95.75% accuracy within only 0.80 s, all other performance metrics like precision, recall, etc. F-measure also supports this statement. The confusion matrix and ROC curve in Fig. 6 show the performance characteristics of ANN and NB combination models.

5 Conclusion

In recent years, technological innovation has aided us in every aspect of our lives. Machines now can assist humans in real-life situations thanks to AI-based technologies. On the other hand, workplace pressure and stress have become inevitable for people from all walks of life. AI-assisted stress prediction can help in this area by offering advanced warning and accelerating preventative steps. In this paper, we proposed a hybrid deep learning approach with a combination of ML classifiers. The models we proposed could work in real time with excellent performance. Our best model, a combination of ANN and NB, predicts stress with 95.75% accuracy within only 0.80 s. We finally proposed a framework based on our findings to help people in real-life stress situations. In future, we hope to extend our approach for stress level prediction in individuals.

Acknowledgements MM and MSK are supported by the DIVERSASIA project (618615-EPP-1-2020-1-UKEPPKA2-CBHEJP) funded by the European Commission under the Erasmus+ programme.

References

1. Ahmad Z et al (2021) Multi-level stress assessment from ECG in a virtual reality environment using multimodal fusion. arXiv 2107.04566
2. Ahuja R, Banga A (2019) Mental stress detection in university students using machine learning algorithms. Procedia Comput Sci 152:349–353
3. Al Banna MH et al (2021) Attention-based bi-directional long-short term memory network for earthquake prediction. IEEE Access 9:56589–56603
4. Al Nahian MJ, Ghosh T et al (2020) Towards artificial intelligence driven emotion aware fall monitoring framework suitable for elderly people with neurological disorder. In: Proceedings of Brain Informatics, pp 275–286
5. Al Nahian MJ et al (2021) Towards an accelerometer-based elderly fall detection system using cross-disciplinary time series features. IEEE Access 9:39413–31
6. Biswas M, Tania MH, Kaiser MS et al (2021) Accu3rate: a mobile health application rating scale based on user reviews. PloS One 16(12):e0258050
7. Biswas M et al (2021) An xai based autism detection: the context behind the detection. In: Proceedings of Brain Informatics, pp 448–459
8. Dalmeida KM, Masala GL (2021) HRV features as viable physiological markers for stress detection using wearable devices. Sensors 21(8):2873
9. Deepa B et al (2022) Pattern descriptors orientation and map firefly algorithm based brain pathology classification using hybridized machine learning algorithm. IEEE Access 10:3848–3863

10. Fabietti M, Mahmud M, Lotfi A (2021) Anomaly detection in invasively recorded neuronal signals using deep neural network: effect of sampling frequency. In: Proceedings of AII, pp 79–91
11. Fabietti M, Mahmud M, Lotfi A (2022) Channel-independent recreation of artefactual signals in chronically recorded local field potentials using machine learning. Brain Inform 9(1):1–17
12. Fabietti M et al (2020) Artifact detection in chronically recorded local field potentials using long-short term memory neural network. In: Proceedings of AICT 2020, pp 1–6
13. Faria TH et al (2021) Smart city technologies for next generation healthcare. In: Data-driven mining, learning & analytics for secured smart cities, pp 253–274
14. Ghosh T et al (2021) Artificial intelligence and internet of things in screening and management of autism spectrum disorder. Sustain Cities Soc 74:103189
15. Ghosh T et al (2021) An attention-based mood controlling framework for social media users. In: Proceedings of Brain Informatics, pp 245–256
16. Ghosh T et al (2021) A hybrid deep learning model to predict the impact of Covid-19 on mental health form social media big data. Preprints 2021 (2021060654)
17. Koldijk S, Neerincx MA, Kraaij W (2016) Detecting work stress in offices by combining unobtrusive sensors. IEEE Trans Affect Comput 9(2):227–239
18. Koldijk S, Sappelli M et al (2014) The swell knowledge work dataset for stress and user modeling research. In: Proceedings of ICMI, pp 291–298
19. Kumar I et al (2022) Dense tissue pattern characterization using deep neural network. Cogn Comput, pp 1–24 (ePub ahead of print)
20. Lalotra GS, Kumar V, Bhatt A, Chen T, Mahmud M (2022) iReTADS: an intelligent real-time anomaly detection system for cloud communications using temporal data summarization and neural network. Secur Commun Netw 2022:9149164
21. Mahmud M, Kaiser MS, McGinnity TM, Hussain A (2021) Deep learning in mining biological data. Cogn Comput 13(1):1–33
22. Mahmud M et al (2018) Applications of deep learning and reinforcement learning to biological data. IEEE Trans Neural Netw Learn Syst 29(6):2063–2079
23. Mammoottil MJ, Kulangara LJ, Cherian AS, Mohandas P, Hasikin K, Mahmud M (2022) Detection of breast cancer from five-view thermal images using convolutional neural networks. J Healthc Eng 2022:4295221
24. McDonald AD, Sasangohar F, Jatav A, Rao AH (2019) Continuous monitoring and detection of post-traumatic stress disorder triggers among veterans: a supervised machine learning approach. IISE Trans Healthc Syst Eng 9(3):201–211
25. Nawar A, Toma NT, Al Mamun S et al (2021) Cross-content recommendation between movie and book using machine learning. In: Proceedings of AICT, pp 1–6
26. Nkurikiyeyezu K, Yokokubo A, Lopez G (2019) The effect of person-specific biometrics in improving generic stress predictive models. arXiv 1910.01770
27. Paul A et al (2022) Inverted bell-curve-based ensemble of deep learning models for detection of Covid-19 from chest x-rays. Neural Compu Appl, pp 1–15
28. Prakash N et al (2021) Deep transfer learning Covid-19 detection and infection localization with superpixel based segmentation. Sustain Cities Soc 75:103252
29. Satu M et al (2020) Towards improved detection of cognitive performance using bidirectional multilayer long-short term memory neural network. In: Proceedings of brain informatics, pp 297–306
30. Satu MS et al (2021) TClustVID: a novel machine learning classification model to investigate topics and sentiment in Covid-19 tweets. Knowl-Based Syst 226:107126
31. Schmidt P, Reiss A, Duerichen R, Marberger C, Van Laerhoven K (2018) Introducing wesad, a multimodal dataset for wearable stress and affect detection. In: Proceedings of ICMI, pp 400–408
32. Siirtola P (2019) Continuous stress detection using the sensors of commercial smartwatch. In: Proceedings of ubiquitous computing, pp 1198–1201
33. Sriramprakash S, Prasanna VD, Murthy OR (2017) Stress detection in working people. Procedia Comput Sci 115:359–366

34. Walambe R, Nayak P, Bhardwaj A, Kotecha K (2021) Employing multimodal machine learning for stress detection. J Healthc Eng 2021
35. Watkins J, Fabietti M, Mahmud M (2020) Sense: a student performance quantifier using sentiment analysis. In: Proceedings of IJCNN, pp 1–6

Machine Learning in Healthcare

A Method of Genome Sequence Comparison Based on a New Form of Fuzzy Polynucleotide Space

Soumen Ghosh, Jayanta Pal, Bansibadan Maji, and Dilip Kumar Bhattacharya

Abstract Genome sequence similarity targeted to actual biological taxa is one of the foremost challenging tasks. Several attempts are taken to represent whole-genome sequences using standard fuzzy polynucleotide metric spaces. Nevertheless, in this space, intuitively similar sequences are found to be dissimilar under the NTV metric and all the metrics do not behave similarly in all genome sequences. In this paper, a new form of sixteen-dimensional fuzzy polynucleotide space is proposed over a unit hypercube. Furthermore, to measure similarity/dissimilarity between these fuzzy polynucleotides a modified form of the standard NTV metric is introduced. The method is verified on whole-genome sequences of Corynebacterium diphtheriae, Haemophilus influenza, Halobacterium sp. and Xylella fastidiosa. The proposed technique produces consistent and satisfactory results in all such cases. The results indicate that this new form of fuzzy polynucleotide space with the modified form of NTV metric is satisfactory for genome sequence comparison.

Keywords Genome sequence comparison · NTV metric · Fuzzy polynucleotide space

1 Introduction

Two types of methods, alignment-based and alignment-free are used in sequence comparison, in general, and genome sequence comparison, in particular. There is no doubt that alignment-based methods are more accurate than alignment-free methods. But the former type of methods has limitations. So the latter type is of current choice. The basic thing of alignment-free methods is to first represent the sequence

S. Ghosh (✉) · J. Pal
Narula Institute of Technology, Kolkata, India
e-mail: soumenghosh.kolkata@gmail.com

S. Ghosh · J. Pal · B. Maji
National Institute of Technology, Durgapur, India

D. K. Bhattacharya
University of Calcutta, Kolkata, India

© The Author(s), under exclusive license to Springer Nature Singapore Pte Ltd. 2023
J. K. Mandal and D. De (eds.), *Frontiers of ICT in Healthcare*, Lecture Notes in Networks and Systems 519, https://doi.org/10.1007/978-981-19-5191-6_11

of nucleotides numerically. The numerical representation may be one-dimensional [1–3], two-dimensional [4, 5], three-dimensional [6–11], more-dimensional [12–14], complex-valued [15] or quaternion-valued [16]. For visualization purposes, the representations which are one, two, or three-dimensional and even which are complex-valued are all right. The rest is not so. Sometimes the representation is not 1–1. This is called a degenerate form of geometrical representation and it is not helpful for sequence comparison [17–19]. A non-degenerate geometrical descriptor [20] and a matrix form of descriptor [6, 21–25] are well-known. A descriptor based on graph theory is given in [26]. There is a 4-dimensional binary representation where the nucleotides T, C, A, G are represented by (1,0,0,0), (0,1,0,0), (0,0,1,) and (0,0,0,1) four-component vectors for each base [13]. On the represented series FFT is performed. Finally in the frequency domain, the comparison is made by two types of descriptors (1) descriptors based on the Inter Coefficient distance (ICD) method [27] and (2) descriptors based on the moment vector method [28]. The above type of 4D binary representation is important for its contribution to the introduction of the very concept of fuzzy polynucleotide. The fuzzy set theory is directly accessible to the sequence analysis and their comparison in the year 1990 [29–31]. Several papers since 2003 [32–35] have obtained similar 12-dimensional unit hypercube for the representation of genome sequences. They have used similar notions of distance function and also have given the same name fuzzy polynucleotide space for this 12-dimensional unit hypercube I12. It may be observed that although a codon is represented only at the 12 corners of a 12-dimensional unit hypercube, a multi-codon is always represented as a fuzzy vector on a 12-dimensional unit hypercube.

Example: UACUGU (tyrosine/cysteine).

Representation of di-codon UACUGU is (1, 0, 0, 0, 0, 0, 0.5, 0.5, 0.5, 0.5, 0, 0)$\in$ I^{16} as shown in Table 1.

It is a fuzzy representation. The method may be extended for the representation of any multi-codon and even for whole-genome sequences. Naturally, under such a representation, the descriptor for every genome sequence is a 12-component fuzzy vector only. As a result, under this representation, the comparison may be made easily between genome sequences of equal and unequal lengths, however large the lengths may be, provided the metric applied on the descriptors is fuzzy NTV metric given by

Table 1 Representation of UACUGU when $N = 3n$, $n = 2$

	Number of nucleotides				Total	Fraction of nucleotides			
	U	C	A	G		U	C	A	G
1st Bases	2	0	0	0	2	1	0	0	0
2nd Bases	0	0	1	1	2	0	0	0.5	0.5
3rd Bases	1	1	0	0	2	0.5	0.5	0	0

$$d_{NTV}(P, Q) = \frac{\sum_{i=1}^{12} |p_i - q_i|}{\sum_{i=1}^{12} \max(p_i, q_i)} \tag{1}$$

This is why this method of representation is so much popular.

In this space, metrics other than the NTV metric are also introduced [32]. All of these formulae can be justified from a mathematical point of view. These are given by

$$d_1(p, q) = \frac{d(p, q)}{1 + d(p, q)} \tag{2}$$

$$d_2(p, q) = \frac{\sqrt{\sum_{i=1}^{12} (p_i - q_i)^2}}{\sqrt{12}} \tag{3}$$

$$d_3(p, q) = \frac{d_2(p, q)}{1 + d_2(p, q)} \tag{4}$$

$$d_4(p, q) = \frac{\sum_{i=1}^{12} |p_i - q_i|}{12} \tag{5}$$

$p = (p_1, p_2, p_3, \ldots, p_{12}), q = (q_1, q_2, q_3, \ldots, q_{12}) \in I^{12}$ are two different points.

Naturally, it is expected that genome sequences may be compared conveniently on this 12-dimensional fuzzy unit hypercube under the use of any one of the above metrics. But the following drawbacks of this space are pointed out.

The first limitation is pointed out in [29]. It says that in this space intuitively similar DNA sequences are found to be dissimilar and conversely under the use of the NTV metric. The authors consider two RNA sequences UACAGU and UGUUAC and by using the NTV metric they calculate the similarity to the extent of 0.833 and dissimilarity to the extent of 0.167. Thus the sequences are found to have more similarity and less dissimilarity. But intuition gives the opposite result, as the sequences have only one element common in the first place, the rest are all different. So the very concept of the above fuzzy polynucleotide space is at stake. The authors [29] remark that "FPNS Nieto—Torres is irremediably faulty".

They also suggest the alternative as the 4n-dimensional (n being the length of the sequence) representation based on the aforesaid 4D Binary representation of the nucleotides. They show that this representation is free from the above limitations. But this representation misses the very essence of 12-dimensional fuzzy representation, which reduces the comparison of genome sequences of any length (equal or unequal) to that of 12 component fuzzy vectors only. Instead of reducing the length, it increases it to 4 times its original length. Moreover, it is no longer a fuzzy representation. It is again a crisp representation. So this space is not a proper alternative to the 12-dimensional polynucleotide space of Torres and Nieto.

The second limitation is pointed out in [36]. It is found in Nieto et al. [33] that the pair of whole-genome sequences of *M. tuberculosis* and *A. Aeolicus, M. tuberculosis* and *E. coli*, *E.coli* and *A. Aerolicus* do behave similarly. But as the sequences under comparison are only three, so a question is raised in [36], whether the result is general or not! The authors could cite counterexamples of other genome sequences to show that the assertion is not true in general. As the NTV metric is a standard metric on fuzzy unit hypercube and as all other metrics are derivable mathematically from the NTV metric, so the very formation of 12-dimensional fuzzy nucleotide space is again at stake. The authors settles the problem by introducing the notion of polynucleotide space of Intuitionistic fuzzy logic based on the Intuitionistic fuzzy set theory. Thus Intuitionistic fuzzy polynucleotide space may be a better alternative to the fuzzy polynucleotide space of Torres and Nieto. But this space is much more complicated than the fuzzy polynucleotide space of Torres and Nieto. Naturally, the real challenge is to develop such a fuzzy polynucleotide space, which is as simple as the 12-dimensional fuzzy polynucleotide space of Torres and Nieto but at the same time is free from all the limitations as mentioned above. The present paper is mainly motivated to develop such a fuzzy polynucleotide space for genome sequence comparison.

2 Methodology

The proposed methodology is divided into two parts. First of all, the genome sequence is represented by a new form of base-4 nucleotide representation. After representation, sequences are compared using a modified form of NTV metrics.

2.1 *Representation of Genome Sequences*

The genome sequence is represented using their four different bases. It may be noted that under this representation scheme any genome sequence of length N is expressed as $N = 4n$, $4n + 1$, $4n + 2$, $4n + 3$, $n > 1$ being a positive integer. This is illustrated by considering a sample of nucleotide sequences for $n = 2$. The representation may be obtained similarly for any $n > 1$. For our experiment, a sample sequence UACUGUAG is considered, where $n = 2$ and the length of the sequence $(N) = 8$.

Based on our proposed representation technique the 16-component vectors of UACUGUAG is $(0.5, 0, 0, 0.5, 0.5, 0, 0.5, 0, 0, 0.5, 0.5, 0, 0.5, 0, 0, 0.5) \in I^{16}$ as shown in Table 2.

Next one more nucleotide is increased in the previous sequence. The sequence becomes UACUGUAGC, where $N = 4n + 1$. Representation of the polynucleotide is $(0.33, 0.33, 0, 0.33, 0.5, 0, 0.5, 0, 0, 0.5, 0.5, 0, 0.5, 0, 0, 0.5) \in I^{16}$ as shown in Table 3.

Now one more nucleotide is added to the previous sample. The sequence becomes UACUGUAGCA, where $N = 4n + 2$. Representation of polynucleotide

Table 2 Representation of UACUGUAG when $N = 4n, n = 2$

	Number of nucleotides				Total	Fractions of nucleotides			
	U	C	A	G		U	C	A	G
1st Bases	1	0	0	1	2	0.5	0	0	0.5
2nd Bases	1	0	1	0	2	0.5	0	0.5	0
3rd Bases	0	1	1	0	2	0	0.5	0.5	0
4th Bases	1	0	0	1	2	0.5	0	0	0.5

Table 3 Representation of UACUGUAGC when $N = 4n + 1, n = 2$

	Number of nucleotides				Total	Fractions of nucleotides			
	U	C	A	G		U	C	A	G
1st Bases	1	1	0	1	3	0.33	0.33	0	0.33
2nd Bases	1	0	1	0	2	0.5	0	0.5	0
3rd Bases	0	1	1	0	2	0	0.5	0.5	0
4th Bases	1	0	0	1	2	0.5	0	0	0.5

UACUGUAGCA is (0.33, 0.33, 0, 0..33, 0.33, 0, 0.67, 0, 0, 0.5, 0.5, 0, 0.5, 0, 0, 0.5) $\in I^{16}$ as shown in Table 4.

Next, the sequence "UACUGUAGCAC" is considered, where $N = 4n + 3$.

Representation of polynucleotide UACUGUAGCAC is (0.33, 0.33, 0, 0.33, 0.33, 0, 0.67, 0, 0, 0.67, 0.33, 0, 0.5, 0, 0, 0.5)$\in I^{16}$ shown in Table 5.

Table 4 Representation of UACUGUAGCA when $N = 4n + 2, n = 2$

	Number of nucleotides				Total	Fractions of nucleotides			
	U	C	A	G		U	C	A	G
1st Bases	1	1	0	1	3	0.33	0.33	0	0.0.33
2nd Bases	1	0	2	0	3	0.33	0	0.67	0
3rd Bases	0	1	1	0	2	0	0.5	0.5	0
4th Bases	1	0	0	1	2	0.5	0	0	0.5

Table 5 Representation of UACUGUAGCAC when $N = 4n + 3, n = 2$

	Number of nucleotides				Total	Fractions of nucleotides			
	U	C	A	G		U	C	A	G
1st Bases	1	1	0	1	3	0.33	0.33	0	0.0.33
2nd Bases	1	0	2	0	3	0.33	0	0.67	0
3rd Bases	0	2	1	0	3	0	0.67	0.33	0
4th Bases	1	0	0	1	2	0.5	0	0	0.5

From the above experiment, 16-dimension fuzzy representation is obtained on a sequence of length $N = 4n$. This representation may be extended to length $N = 4n + 1, 4n + 2, 4n + 3$.

2.2 *Modified Form of NTV Metric*

The Modified NTV metric on this space is defined as

$$d_{NTV}(P, Q) = \frac{\sum_{i=1}^{16}|p_i - q_i|}{\sum_{i=1}^{16} \max(p_i, q_i)} \tag{6}$$

Modified forms of other Metrics

$$d_1(p, q) = \sum_{i=1}^{16} \frac{d(p, q)}{1 + d(p, q)} \tag{7}$$

$$d_2(p, q) = \frac{\sqrt{\sum_{i=1}^{16}(p_i - q_i)^2}}{\sqrt{16}} \tag{8}$$

$$d_3(p, q) = \frac{d_2(p, q)}{1 + d_2(p, q)} \tag{9}$$

$$d_4(p, q) = \frac{\sum_{i=1}^{16}|p_i - q_i|}{16} \tag{10}$$

3 Results

To meet the queries in [29] on 12-dimensional fuzzy polynucleotide spaces, three sequences are considered. Each sequence consists of 12 nucleotides shown in Table 6. 12-dimensional representation of these three sequences are shown in Table 7.

Representation of seq. 1 is (0.5, 0, 0.5, 0, 0, 0.5, 0.25, 0.25, 0.25, 0, 0.25, 0.5) $\in I^{12}$.

Table 6 Three sample sequences

	1	2	3	4	5	6	7	8	9	10	11	12
Sequence 1	U	A	G	A	C	U	A	G	G	U	C	A
Sequence 2	U	C	G	A	C	G	A	G	G	U	C	A
Sequence 3	U	C	G	U	C	G	A	G	C	U	G	A

Table 7 Representation based on I^{12} on sample sequences

		No. of nucleotides				Total	Fraction of nucleotides			
		U	C	A	G		U	C	A	G
Sequence 1	1st Base	2	0	2	0	4	0.50	0.00	0.50	0.00
	2nd Base	0	2	1	1	4	0.00	0.50	0.25	0.25
	3rd Base	1	0	1	2	4	0.25	0.00	0.25	0.50
Sequence 2	1st Base	2	0	2	0	4	0.50	0.00	0.50	0.00
	2nd Base	0	3	0	1	4	0.00	0.75	0.00	0 .25
	3rd Base	0	0	1	3	4	0.00	0.00	0.25	0.75
Sequence 3	1st Base	3	0	1	0	4	0.75	0.00	0.25	0.00
	2nd Base	0	2	0	2	4	0.00	0.50	0.00	0.50
	3rd Base	0	1	1	2	4	0.00	0.25	0.25	0.50

Table 8 Representation based on I^{16} on sample sequences

		No. of nucleotides				Total	Fractions of nucleotides			
		U	C	A	G		U	C	A	G
Sequence 1	1st Base	1	1	0	1	3	0.33	0.33	0.00	0.33
	2nd Base	2	0	1	0	3	0.67	0.00	0.33	0.00
	3rd Base	0	1	1	1	3	0.00	0.33	0.33	0.33
Sequence 2	1st Base	0	0	2	1	3	0.00	0.00	0.67	0.33
	2nd Base	1	1	0	1	3	0.33	0.33	0.00	0.33
	3rd Base	1	1	0	1	3	0.33	0.33	0.00	0.33
Sequence 3	1st Base	0	1	1	1	3	0.00	0.33	0.33	0.33
	2nd Base	0	0	2	1	3	0.00	0.00	0.67	0.33
	3rd Base	1	2	0	0	3	0.33	0.67	0.00	0.00

Representation of seq. 2 is $(0.5, 0, 0.5, 0, 0, 0.75, 0, 0.25, 0, 0, 0.25, 0.75)\in I^{12}$.
Representation of seq. 3 is $(0.75, 0, 0.25, 0, 0, 0.5, 0, 0.5, 0, 0.25, 0.25, 0.5)\in I^{12}$.
Representation of sequence 1 is

$$(0.33, 0.33, 0, 0.33, 0.67, 0, 0.33, 0, 0, 0.33, 0.33, 0.33, 0, 0, 0.67, 0.33) \in I^{16}$$

Representation of sequence 2 is

$$(0.33, 0.33, 0, 0.33, 0.33, 0.33, 0, 0.33, 0, 0.33, 0.33, 0.33, 0, 0, 0.67, 0.33) \in I^{16}$$

Representation of sequence 3 is

$$(0.33, 0.67, 0, 0, 0.33, 0.33, 0, 0.33, 0, 0, 0.33, 0.67, 0.33, 0, 0.33, 0.33) \in I^{16}$$

Table 9 Comparison using NTV metric on sample data

	Comparison	Mismatch
Apparent View	Sequence 1 versus Sequence 2	2
	Sequence 2 versus Sequence 3	3
	Sequence 1 versus Sequence 3	5
	Comparison	Dissimilarity
Comparison of I^{12}	Sequence 1 versus Sequence 2	0.285714
	Sequence 2 versus Sequence 3	0.400000
	Sequence 1 versus Sequence 3	0.400000
Comparison of I^{16}	Sequence 1 versus Sequence 2	0.286638
	Sequence 2 versus Sequence 3	0.403614
	Sequence 1 versus Sequence 3	0.591150

It is seen in Table 9 that results on similarity/dissimilarity on I^{12} do not always agree with the intuitive results. This challenges the very construction of 12-dimensional fuzzy polynucleotide space. But results in I^{16} shows that no such counter-intuitive results occur at all. Hence the above example shows that the 16-dimensional fuzzy polynucleotide space constructed in this paper is free from the limitations as pointed out in [20].

To meet the queries in [36] on 12-dimensional fuzzy polynucleotide spaces, four different species are considered. Details of the species are given in Table 10. Sequences are collected from www.ncbi.nlm.nih.gov.

At first, all four sequences are represented on the 12-dimensional unit hypercube.
(i) $d_{NTV}(1, 2) = d_{NTV}(3, 4)$ (ii) $d_1(1, 2) > d_1(3, 4)$
(iii) $d_3(1, 2) < d_3(3, 4)$ (iv) $d_4(1, 2) = d_4(3, 4)$

It is seen in the above example (Table 11) that the dissimilarity between (a) Corynebacterium diphtheria and (b) Haemophilus influenza and the dissimilarity between (c) Halobacterium sp. and (d) Xylella fastidiosa are the same for metrics

Table 10 Description of the species

Sequence no	Species name	Accession no
a	*Corynebacterium diphtheriae*	BX248353.1
b	*Haemophilus influenza*	CP000057.2
c	*Halobacterium salinarum*	AE004437.1
d	*Xylella fastidiosa*	AE003849.1

Table 11 Results of comparison in [36] based on the use of different metrics

Genome	d_{NTV}	d_1	d_2	d_3	d_4
(a) versus (b)	0.265	0.210	0.077	0.071	0.076
(c) versus (d)	0.265	0.209	0.077	0.072	0.076

Table 12 Results on 16-dimensional new fuzzy polynucleotide space under different metrics

Genome	d_{NTV}	d_1	d_2	d_3	d_4
Genome (a) versus Genome (b)	0.266506	0.210426	0.076878	0.071390	0.076870
Genome (a) versus Genome (c)	0.220789	0.180858	0.062057	0.058431	0.062047
Genome (a) versus Genome (d)	0.048530	0.046284	0.013397	0.013220	0.012434
Genome (b) versus Genome (c)	0.434851	0.303063	0.138924	0.121978	0.138917
Genome (b) versus Genome (d)	0.252773	0.201771	0.073540	0.068502	0.072335
Genome (c) versus Genome (d)	0.235028	0.190302	0.067681	0.063390	0.066581

d_{NTV}, d_2 and d_4, while the dissimilarity between (a) and (b) is more than the dissimilarity between (c) and (d) for metric d_1 and the dissimilarity between (a) and (b) is less than the dissimilarity between (c) and (d) for the metric d_3.The dissimilarity cannot be judged under metrics d_2 and d_4. Results of comparison show that all the metrics do not behave similarly on a 12-dimensional unit hypercube.

Representations of the same sequences on 16-dimensional unit hypercube.

For genome (a) the fuzzy set of frequencies is (0.232, 0.233, 0.266, 0.269, 0.231, 0.233, 0.267, 0.269, 0.232, 0.233, 0.267, 0.268, 0.232, 0.233, 0.267, 0.268) $\in I^{16}$

For genome (b) the fuzzy set of frequencies is (0.310, 0.307, 0.191, 0.192, 0.310, 0.309, 0.189, 0.192, 0.310, 0.309, 0.190, 0.191, 0.310, 0.308, 0.190, 0.192) $\in I^{16}$

For genome (c) the fuzzy set of frequencies is (0.170, 0.170, 0.331, 0.329, 0.171, 0.171, 0.330, 0.329, 0.170, 0.171, 0.329, 0.330, 0.169, 0.171, 0.329, 0.331) $\in I^{16}$

For genome (d) the fuzzy set of frequencies is (0.226, 0.248, 0.277, 0.250, 0.226, 0.248, 0.277, 0.249, 0.226, 0.248, 0.277, 0.249, 0.226, 0.248, 0.276, 0.250) $\in I^{16}$

i. $d_{NTV}(1,2) > d_{NTV}(3,4)$ ii. $d_1(1,2) > d_1(3,4)$ iii. $d_2(1,2) > d_2(3,4)$.
iv. $d_3(1,2) > d_3(3,4)$, v. $d_4(1,2) > d_4(3,4)$.

It is seen in the above example (Table 12) that the dissimilarity between (a) and (b) is more than the dissimilarity between (c) and (d) under comparison of sequences based on all the metrics d_{NTV}, d_1, d_2, d_3 and d_4.

4 Discussion

(a) On 16-dimensional new fuzzy polynucleotide space, intuitively similar sequences are also similar under the modified NTV metric but this is not true on 12-dimensional fuzzy polynucleotide space.

(b) On 16-dimensional new fuzzy polynucleotide space, all the modified forms of NTV metric behave similarly for genome sequence comparison. But the similar behavior of the metrics fails in 12-dimensional fuzzy polynucleotide space.

5 Conclusion

Fuzzy representation of 12-dimensional fuzzy polynucleotide space is a good tool to compare two genomes of any length. But there are some limitations. In this space, intuitively similar sequences, are found to be dissimilar for some cases. This means the method is not relevant in general. Even all the metrics do not behave similarly for all genome sequences in this space. The present paper establishes that the 16-dimensional new fuzzy polynucleotide space is a good replacement for the 12-dimensional fuzzy polynucleotide space. The proposed method is verified on three sample sequences and sequences of four different species. It is found that the 16-dimensional new fuzzy polynucleotide spaces always produce satisfactory results. Further, it is free from all challenges made against the 12-dimensional fuzzy polynucleotide space, as mentioned above. Therefore, 16-dimensional new fuzzy polynucleotide space with the revised form of NTV metric is a well-organized technique for genome sequence comparison.

References

1. Akhtar M, Epps J, Ambikairajah E (2008) Signal processing in sequence analysis: advances in eukaryotic gene prediction. IEEE J Selected Topics in Signal Process 2(3):310–321
2. Chakravarthy N, Spanias A, Iasemidis LD, Tsakalis K (2004) Autoregressive modeling and feature analysis of DNA sequences. EURASIP J Adv Signal Process 2004(1):952689
3. Zhou H, Yan H (2006) Autoregressive models for spectral analysis of short tandem repeats in DNA sequences. In: 2006 IEEE international conference on systems, man and cybernetics, October, vol 2. IEEE, pp 1286–1290
4. Wu Y, Liew AWC, Yan H, Yang M (2003) DB-Curve: a novel 2D method of DNA sequence visualization and representation. Chem Phys Lett 367(1–2):170–176
5. Liao B, Xiang X, Zhu W (2006) Coronavirus phylogeny based on 2D graphical representation of DNA sequence. J Comput Chem 27(11):1196–1202
6. Randić M, Vracko M, Nandy A, Basak SC (2000) On 3-D graphical representation of DNA primary sequences and their numerical characterization. J Chem Inf Comput Sci 40(5):1235–1244
7. Liao B, Wang TM (2004) 3-D graphical representation of DNA sequences and their numerical characterization. J Mol Struct (Thoechem) 681(1–3):209–212
8. Das S, Choudhury NR, Tibarewala DN, Bhattacharya DK (2018) Application of Chaos game in tri-nucleotide representation for the comparison of coding sequences of β-globin gene. In: Industry interactive innovations in science, engineering and technology,). Springer, Singapore, pp 561–567
9. Zhang X, Luo J, Yang L (2007) New invariant of DNA sequence based on 3DD-curves and its application on phylogeny. J Comput Chem 28(14):2342–2346
10. Qi XQ, Wen J, Qi ZH (2007) New 3D graphical representation of DNA sequence based on dual nucleotides. J Theor Biol 249(4):681–690

11. Wąż P, Bielińska-Wąż D (2014) 3D-dynamic representation of DNA sequences. J Mol Model 20(3):2141
12. Randić M, Balaban AT (2003) On a four-dimensional representation of DNA primary sequences. J Chem Inf Comput Sci 43(2):532–539
13. Chi R, Ding K (2005) Novel 4D numerical representation of DNA sequences. Chem Phys Lett 407(1–3):63–67
14. Tan C, Li S, Zhu P (2015) 4D Graphical representation research of DNA sequences. Int J Biomath 8(01):1550004
15. Anastassiou D (2001) Genomic signal processing. IEEE Signal Process Mag 18(4):8–20
16. Brodzik AK, Peters O (2005) Symbol-balanced quaternionic periodicity transform for latent pattern detection in DNA sequences. In: Proceedings.(ICASSP'05). IEEE international conference on acoustics, speech, and signal processing, March vol 5. IEEE, pp v-373
17. Gates MA (1986) A simple way to look at DNA. J Theor Biol 119(3):319–328
18. Nandy A (1996) Graphical analysis of DNA sequence structure: III. Indications of evolutionary distinctions and characteristics of introns and exons. Current Sci 661–668
19. Leong PM, Morgenthaler S (1995) Random walk and gap plots of DNA sequences. Bioinformatics 11(5):503–507
20. Yao YH, Nan XY, Wang TM (2006) A new 2D graphical representation—Classification curve and the analysis of similarity/dissimilarity of DNA sequences. J Mol Struct (Thoechem) 764(1–3):101–108
21. Randić M, Vračko M, Lerš N, Plavšić D (2003) Novel 2-D graphical representation of DNA sequences and their numerical characterization. Chem Phys Lett 368(1–2):1–6
22. Randić M, Vračko M, Lerš N, Plavšić D (2003) Analysis of similarity/dissimilarity of DNA sequences based on novel 2-D graphical representation. Chem Phys Lett 371(1–2):202–207
23. Das S, Das A, Mondal B, Dey N, Bhattacharya DK, Tibarewala DN (2020) Genome sequence comparison under a new form of tri-nucleotide representation based on bio-chemical properties of nucleotides. Gene 730:144257
24. Randić M, Witzmann F, Vračko M, Basak SC (2001) On characterization of proteomics maps and chemically induced changes in proteomes using matrix invariants: application to peroxisome proliferators. Med Chem Res 10(7–8):456–479
25. Luo J, Guo J, Li Y (2010) A new graphical representation and its application in similarity/dissimilarity analysis of DNA sequences. In: 2010 4th international conference on bioinformatics and biomedical engineering, June, IEEE, pp 1–5
26. Qi X, Wu Q, Zhang Y, Fuller E, Zhang CQ (2011) A novel model for DNA sequence similarity analysis based on graph theory. Evolutionary Bioinform 7:EBO-S7364
27. King BR, Aburdene M, Thompson A, Warres Z (2014) Application of discrete Fourier intercoefficient difference for assessing genetic sequence similarity. EURASIP J Bioinf Syst Biol 2014(1):8
28. Hoang T, Yin C, Zheng H, Yu C, He RL, Yau SST (2015) A new method to cluster DNA sequences using Fourier power spectrum. J Theor Biol 372:135–145
29. Sadegh-Zadeh K (2000) Fuzzy genomes. Artif Intell Med 18(1):1–28
30. Sadegh-Zadeh K (2007) The fuzzy polynucleotide space revisited. Artif Intell Med 41(1):69–80
31. Kosko B (1992). Neural networks and fuzzy systems: a dynamical systems approach to machine intelligence (No. QA76. 76. E95 K86)
32. Nieto JJ, Torres A, Vázquez-Trasande MM (2003) A metric space to study differences between polynucleotides. Appl Math Lett 16(8):1289–1294
33. Nieto JJ, Torres A, Georgiou DN, Karakasidis TE (2006) Fuzzy polynucleotide spaces and metrics. Bull Math Biol 68(3):703–725
34. Torres A, Nieto JJ (2003) The fuzzy polynucleotide space: basic properties. Bioinformatics 19(5):587–592
35. Torres A, Nieto JJ (2006) Fuzzy logic in medicine and bioinformatics. J Biomed Biotechnol
36. Das S, De D, Dey A, Bhattacharya D (2013) Some anomalies in the analysis of whole genome sequence on the basis of Fuzzy set theory. Int J Artif Intell Neural Netw 3(2):38–41

Identification of Humans by Using Machine Learning Models on Gait Features

Jayati Ghosh Dastidar, Souvik Samanta, Arghya Basu, and Santanu Purkait

Abstract In this paper, an attempt has been made to make a low-cost, marker-less, distance independent biometric identification system that will be able to analyze gait parameters from the walking video sequence of a person at a variable distance from the camera, train itself and later will be able to identify the same person by observing his/her gait pattern with the knowledge it has been trained with. Gait parameters analyzed in this system are heel strike angle, toe-off angle and stride angle. The system is based on three models: support vector machine (SVM), K-nearest neighbors (KNN) and random forest. A comparison of the result of these three classification models has also been made. Also, the effect of individual parameters upon the classification has been shown.

Keywords Gait · Heel strike · Toe-off · Silhouette · Biometric · Identification · Classification · SVM · KNN · Random forest · Machine learning

1 Introduction

In the last few years, artificial intelligence (AI) and machine learning (ML) have been an important topic of interest for researchers. With petabytes of data that are being generated in different sectors, the application of ML in various fields has been skyrocketing. Researchers are constantly working on ML models to improve their reliability in areas like the stock market, weather forecasting, health care, sentiment analysis and recognition systems. Coming to the healthcare sector, the assistance of ML in diagnosing diseases and recommending treatment can be path breaking. Since ML can process genetic data, it can also be used for diagnosis and prediction

J. Ghosh Dastidar (✉) · A. Basu
St. Xavier's College (Autonomous), Kolkata, India
e-mail: j.ghoshdastidar@sxccal.edu

S. Samanta
Deloitte US-India, Kolkata, India

S. Purkait
National Institute of Technology, Raipur, India

© The Author(s), under exclusive license to Springer Nature Singapore Pte Ltd. 2023
J. K. Mandal and D. De (eds.), *Frontiers of ICT in Healthcare*, Lecture Notes in Networks and Systems 519, https://doi.org/10.1007/978-981-19-5191-6_12

of various diseases that are carried through genes. Biometric identification has been one of the biggest security goals. Some of the major biometric identification mechanisms nowadays are fingerprint, iris, retina, voice and face identification. Fingerprint sensors, cameras and microphones are now common in almost every mobile device because of the reliability shown by their implementations. Iris and retina scanners have been put to use in many high-security areas. Other parameters are also quite good and even better in some situations, but the absence of a reliable implementation is holding them back from being used commercially. Gait cycle analysis has been in the field study for many years since the advancement of technologies. Human identification using gait analysis is suitable in places where a strong security measurement is required. For example, in banks, military bases, airports, ATM counters or secured areas when a person walks toward the target place, his/her gait sequence is used to identify him/her, and authorization can be given to grant the access. One can analyze the gait cycle in various methodologies like kinematics analysis, temporal and spatial analysis, marker-less gait capture, dynamic electromyography, etc. This paper presents a marker-less gait-based identification system designed using the concepts of computer vision, image processing and machine learning. There are many parameters using which a person's gait can be defined. Some of them are step length, stride length, cadence, velocity, dynamic base, progression line, foot angle and hip angle. A combination of two or more of these features may be used to uniquely identify a person. The identification scheme presented in this paper uses heel strike angle, stride angle and toe-off angle as parameters. Heel strike angle is the foot's angle with the heel while walking when the heel strikes the ground. Stride angle is the angle between 2 legs in the heel strike stage. Toe-off angle is the foot's angle with the toe while walking when the toe goes off the ground. The gait cycle can be divided into six stages [1] (see Fig. 1), which are heel strike (HS), foot flat (FF), mid-stance (MS), heel off (HO), toe-off (TO) and mid-swing (MSW). The afore-mentioned parameters can be measured in one of these cycles.

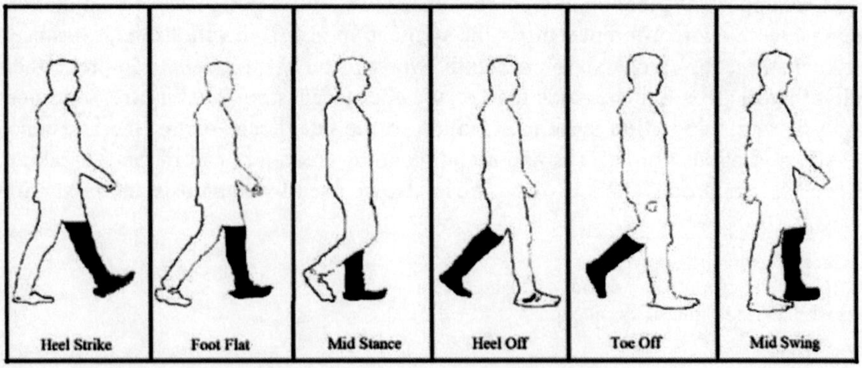

Fig. 1 Six stages of the human gait cycle

2 Literature Survey

Durward et al., in their paper [1], elucidated the steps in a person's gait as well as the kinematics related with each of the steps. Wang et al., in their paper [2], for the first time presented an approach of gait recognition task by deriving the binary silhouette of a walking person. Yam et al., in their paper [3], performed the analysis of the bottom-up model-based methodology for extricating the most relevant dynamic gait features for recognizing individuals. Wang et al., in their paper [4], extended the work of Yam by adding extraction of the static features of the gait motion by using a model-based approach. Tafazzoli et al., in their paper [5], put forth a model-based approach for human gait recognition, which is built on scrutinizing the leg and arm actions. In that paper, they showed an anthropometric model in which the whole body is fragmented into four sections, viz., head (13% of bounding box height), torso (34%), upper legs (24%) and lower legs (29%). Tao et al., in their paper [6], argued and showed that wearable systems are suitable and exact schemes for gait exploration. In this method, wearable sensors are brought in contact to body parts to gather gait-related data and then study them. These sensors can quantify different gait characteristics as signals, which can be analyzed. Murray, et. al. in their paper [7] observed that the step lengths, stride times, velocity, etc., varies for every individual. Kundu et al., in their paper [8], argue why occasionally an unassuming and speedy algorithm is essential to detect someone's presence and motion with a low inaccuracy in a controlled setting for safety causes. They proposed a lightweight algorithm that sounds a warning on detecting a person's presence and his/her motion in a certain direction. The algorithm used fixed angle CCTV camera images shot progressively and relied upon skeleton transformation of continual images and calculated the difference in their coordinates. Nieto-Hidalgo et al., in their paper [9], made efforts to identify frailty and senility syndromes using gait analysis. They have proposed a vision-based gait approach that uses a smartphone camera to record gait sequences extracted by the smartphone to acquire spatiotemporal attributes that are then stored in the cloud to analyze and liken them to a pre-stored database to generate diagnostic. Ghosh Dastidar et al., in their paper [10], attempt to identify an individual distinctively by observing their gait without the use of wearable sensors. The extracted silhouette is used to form a proper skeleton to extract gait attributes. The features are represented using pattern vectors, and similarity indices are computed using cosine distance with attributes pre-stored in the database causing identification/rejection. Davenport et al. in their paper [11] have explained how multiple types of AI techniques (e.g., NLP, RPA, image processing, neural networks and deep learning) have been in use in different sectors of health care (e.g., diagnosis, treatment, patient engagement and administration). Singh et al. in their paper [12] presented a survey of the current progress made in vision-based recognition of human using gait parameters. Chen et al. in their paper [13] presented a method to identify a person while walking with multiple people using gait attributes. Takemura et al. in their paper [14] presented a large gait database with a wide variation to be applied in a reliable performance evaluation of vision-based gait recognition. Bari et al. in their paper [15] have introduced two new geometric features (joint relative triangle area and joint relative cosine dissimilarity) with a new architecture designed using deep learning neural network (DLNN), which has improved the recognition performance.

3 Methodology

3.1 Overview

In this paper, a low-cost, marker-less, camera to subject distance independent identification system has been proposed that will be able to identify a person by observing his/her gait cycle. Three angular values have been used as identification features. Since it is difficult to measure angles directly from an image, the lengths of several subject body parts have been calculated, and the angles are determined using trigonometry and geometry. By using principal component analysis (PCA), one can show that the angles, thus computed are dependent variables, i.e., dependent upon length variables. Also, the value of the angle will lose some of its precision during its determination. It is undesirable to use the angle instead of two length variables that are directly coming from the data, but the measurement of lengths of several parts of a subject in an image depends on the average distance between the camera and the subject. An attempt has been made to keep the system independent of the distance between the subject and camera; angles have been taken as classification attribute instead of lengths. Also, three different classification models have been used: K-nearest neighbors (KNN), random forest and support vector machine (SVM). A comparison of the performance of these three models has also been performed. Lastly, the effects of individual attributes upon the classification of the subjects have been shown.

3.2 Extraction Process of Gait Parameters

To extract the gait parameters, first, a silhouette of the subject in the video is created with the help of background subtraction, binary thresholding, opening morphological operation, Gaussian blurring and optional flipping and cropping to remove extra space in the video where the subject never reaches. Figure 2 shows the process of silhouette generation.

Once the silhouette of the subject has been created, in order to extract the necessary parameters, it is first necessary to identify the frames of the video which contain the event of heel strike and toe-off. The heel strike and stride angles are calculated in each heel strike frame; and the toe-off angles are calculated in each toe-off frame. To identify these frames of the video, it has to be ensured that the subject is inside the frame by keeping a check on a threshold of the number of white pixels in the frame.

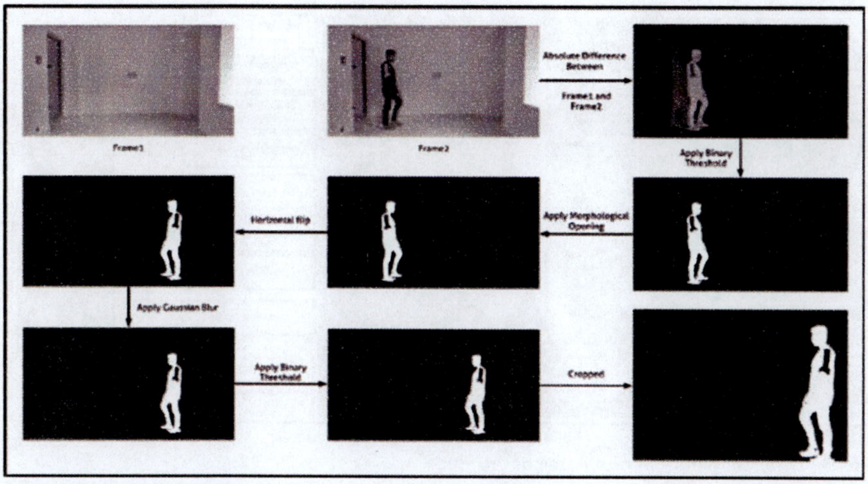

Fig. 2 Silhouette generation process

After that, a bounding box [9] is drawn around the silhouette in such a way that the following conditions are fulfilled:

a. Y-coordinate of the top bounding line = topmost point of the silhouette
b. Y-coordinate of the bottom bounding line = bottommost point of the silhouette
c. X-coordinate of the left bounding line = leftmost point of the silhouette
d. X-coordinate of the right bounding line = rightmost point of the silhouette

Noise avoiding algorithms have been used at appropriate places to avoid any noise while creating the bounding box. After the bounding box is created, the lower-leg part is extracted by taking the 29% height of the subject [5]. Next, the whole silhouette is divided horizontally into two halves. The bottom left subsection is identified as the front_leg_frame, as the front leg of the walking subject will always be in this subsection; and the bottom right subsection is identified as back_leg_frame, as the back leg of the walking subject will always be in this subsection (see Fig. 3).

The heel strike or toe-off happens only when the legs are spread, not when they are closed to each other (in mid-stance or mid-swing). In other words, when the difference between the leftmost point and the rightmost point is greater than a threshold, only then the heel strike or toe-off can occur. This is done to reduce the number of frames to be searched for the heel strike and toe-off frames. It has been observed that heel strike always occurs on the subject's front foot, and toe-off occurs on the subject's back foot. This way, both, heel strike and toe-off can be kept track of, across frames. It can be seen that the distance between front foot heel and toe, along Y-axis, is maximum during heel strike. Also, during toe-off, the distance between back foot heel and toe, along Y-axis is maximum. The diagrams in Figs. 4 and 5 show the graph of the frame number in the video versus the Y-axis difference between heel and toe of the corresponding video in the front_leg_frame and back_leg_frame, respectively.

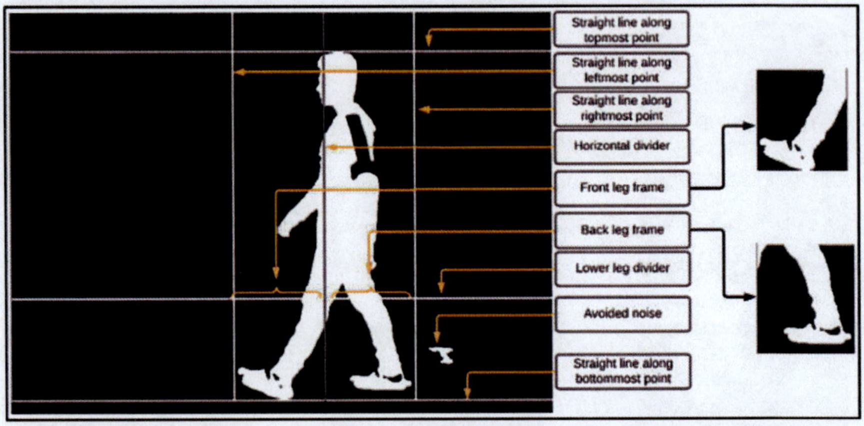

Fig. 3 Different partitions of a frame of the video

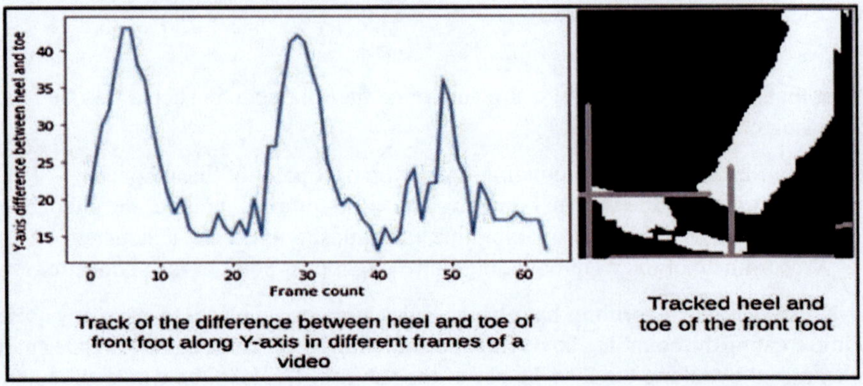

Fig. 4 Graph of the *Y*-axis difference between heel and toe of the front foot in various frames

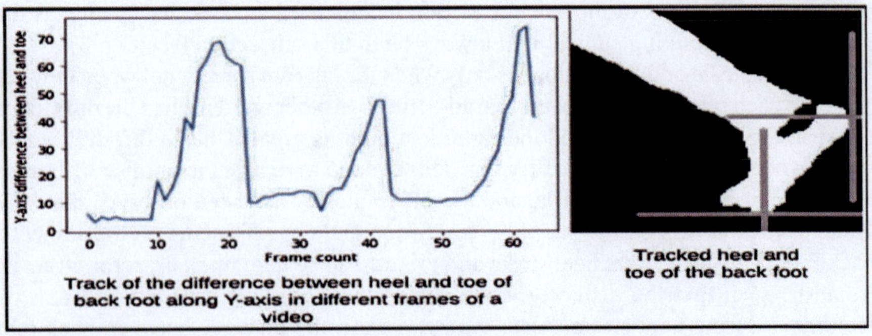

Fig. 5 Graph of the *Y*-axis difference between heel and toe of the back foot in various frames

So, if those frames can be taken in which the Y-axis difference has the local maximum values in the graph, it can be surely said that those frames are the heel strike and toe-off frames of that video. Now, as the search domain and the number of frames to be searched have been reduced; each frame's front_leg_frame and back_leg_frame subsection is taken and stored in two different arrays. To identify the heel and toe of the feet for each frame, skeletonization has been applied to the foot and the coordinates of the heels and toes have been determined. The array, array_of_Front_leg_coordinates [] stores the coordinates of each of the skeletonized front leg's toe (X_1, Y_1) and heel (X_2, Y_2). The array, array_of_Back_leg_coordinates [] stores the coordinates of each of the skeletonized back leg's heel (X_3, Y_3) and toe (X_4, Y_4). Now, the calculation of the difference between heel and toe along the Y-axis is done, against each frame of the video from these two arrays. In Figs. 3 and 4, we have already shown the graph of the Y-axis differences along with all the frames. From the graphs, the X-coordinates of those local maximum Y values are taken out. The X-axis of those graphs signifies the frame count. So, in other words, the index of the arrays where heel strike and toe-off take place has been extracted. There are two coordinates in the heel strike frame: (X_1, Y_1) and (X_2, Y_2). For calculating the heel strike angle, the following calculations are performed:

$$y\_\text{diff} = (Y_2 - Y_1) \tag{1}$$

$$x\_\text{diff} = (X_2 - X_1) \tag{2}$$

$$\text{heel\_strike\_angle} = \tan^{-1}(y\_\text{diff}/x\_\text{diff}) \tag{3}$$

For calculating the stride angle, first the stride length which is the expanse between the front foot heel and the back foot heel is calculated in the heel strike frame. The index of the heel strike frame (say, it is the ith index of array_of_Front_leg_coordinates []) is taken and the back leg heel coordinate from the same index (i) of array_of_Back_leg_coordinates [] array which is (X_3, Y_3), is considered. Now, the following calculations are performed to obtain the stride length:

$$\begin{aligned}&\text{front\_leg\_frame\_heel\_difference}\\&\quad = (\text{width of the front\_leg\_frame}) - X_2\end{aligned} \tag{4}$$

$$\text{back\_leg\_frame\_heel\_position} = X_3 \tag{5}$$

$$\begin{aligned}\text{stride\_length} &= \text{front\_leg\_frame\_heel\_difference}\\&+ \text{back\_leg\_frame\_heel\_position}\end{aligned} \tag{6}$$

Next, to calculate the length of the back leg, two imaginary lines are drawn: a horizontal line is drawn along the back foot heel (keeping Y_3 fixed), and an imaginary vertical line is drawn that goes through the intersection of the two legs. Here, the rear leg is a hypotenuse of a right-angled triangle. To draw the vertical line passing through the intersection, the point where the two legs meet in the silhouette needs to be identified. To determine that point, the height of continuous black pixels is checked starting from X_2 (front foot heel) till X_4 (back foot toe) along the last pixel row of the frame. The X-coordinate with the maximum height of black pixel is the X-coordinate of the point where the two legs cross each other (say X_5). By calculating the height of the consecutive black pixels, the Y-coordinate of the point (say Y_5) can also be determined. The height and the base of the right-angled triangle are thus obtained. By applying the Pythagorean theorem, the length of the leg (hypotenuse) can be obtained. Once the length of the leg (r) and the stride_length (s) has been calculated, an approximate value for the stride angle (ɵ) can be obtained by applying the formula $s = r \times ɵ$, considering the stride length as an approximated arc of length, s of a circle that has a radius, r; creating an angle of ɵ at the center (see Fig. 6). The calculations performed are as follows:

$$\text{Coordinate of the point where the 2 legs meet} = (X_5, Y_5) \tag{7}$$

$$\text{Coordinate of the back foot heel} = (X_3,\ Y_3) \tag{8}$$

$$\text{Height of the triangle} = (Y_5 - Y_3) \tag{9}$$

$$\text{Base of the triangle} = (X_3 - X_5) \tag{10}$$

$$\text{Hypotenuse of the triangle} = \text{Length of Leg } (r)$$
$$= \sqrt{}\left((Y_5 - Y_3)^2 + (X_3 - X_5)^2\right) \tag{11}$$

$$\text{Determined Stride Length (s)} = \text{stride\_length} \tag{12}$$

$$\text{stride\_angle } (\Theta) = s/r \tag{13}$$

Since the stride length (s) has been approximated as an arc, it may result in some negative errors in measurement of the stride angle (ɵ) initially. But this negative error will occur for every stride angle calculation of each of the videos (as the same method for calculating the stride angle is followed) and the classification result will not be affected by that.

In the toe-off frame, there are two pairs of coordinates: (X_3, Y_3), (X_4, Y_4). For calculating the toe-off angle (see Fig. 7), the following calculations are performed:

$$\text{y\_diff } = (Y_4 - Y_3) \tag{14}$$

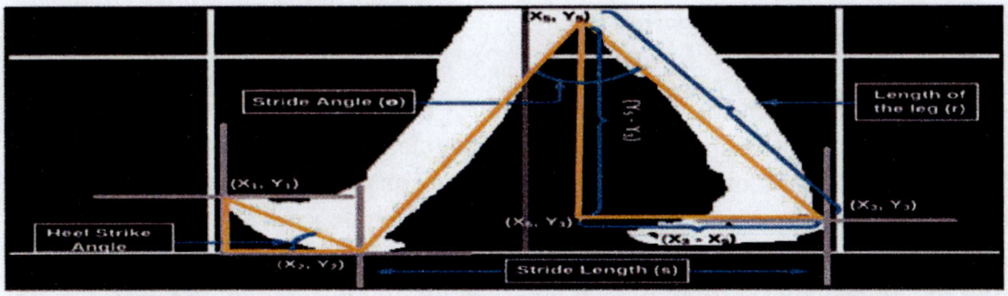

Fig. 6 Measurements of the heel strike angle and stride angle in the heel strike frame

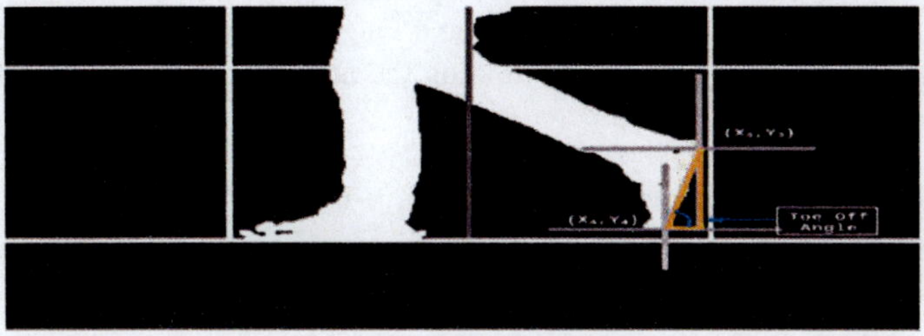

Fig. 7 Measurements of the toe-off angle in the toe-off frame

$$x\_\mathrm{diff} = (-1) \times (X_4 - X_3) \tag{15}$$

$$\mathrm{toe\_off\_angle} = \tan^{-1}(y\_\mathrm{diff}/x\_\mathrm{diff}) \tag{16}$$

3.3 *Classification of the Subjects*

Once the three attributes have been obtained, the datasets are created. These datasets are used to train the classification models. A linear kernel for support vector machine (SVM) has been assumed for two subjects. The K value for K-nearest neighbor (KNN) has been taken to be five. Since there is no pre-defined statistical method to determine a favorable value of K, trials were performed different values of K. With a value of $K = 3$, led to unstable decision boundaries. Therefore, the value of K was increased gradually. At $K = 5$, the classification showed smooth decision boundaries with a minimum error rate. For this reason, $K = 5$ is the optimal chosen value in this model. The number of decision trees in the random forest has been fixed at 20. A total of 12 tests have been conducted, i.e., three individual model tests for the merged attributes and three individual model tests for three individual attributes.

4 Results and Discussion

In some designs where the count of attributes is relatively big, it is beneficial to diminish the attribute dimension to escalate the classification precision. This paper considers a maximum of three features have been considered, so reduction of feature dimension is unnecessary. The features are extracted independently from the videos, and for this reason, the total number of heel strike angles and toe-off angles obtained from the videos are not the same. While creating the merged dataset, some of the values are discarded to create a dataset with no null values. Each of the attributes has been tested separately to utilize all the data gathered from the videos.

The performance has been quantified by computing the total number of True Positives, False Positives, True Negatives and False Negatives. The behavior of the different models was then judged by finding the accuracy, precision, recall and F-score for each model as follows:

$$\text{Accuracy} = (\text{TP} + \text{TN})/(\text{TP} + \text{TN} + \text{FP} + \text{FN}) \tag{17}$$

$$\text{Precision} = \text{TP}/(\text{TP} + \text{FP}) \tag{18}$$

$$\text{Recall} = \text{TP}/(\text{TP} + \text{FN}) \tag{19}$$

$$\text{F-Score} = \text{TP}/[\text{TP} + 0.5(\text{FP} + \text{FN})] \tag{20}$$

TP is the total number of True Positives, FP, the total number of False Positives, TN, the total number of True Negatives and FN, the total number of False Negatives.

Table 1 shows the accuracy of the three chosen models for different datasets, and Table 2 shows the detailed insight into the performance of the models for different datasets.

A null-hypothesis testing with a 95% confidence interval (using normal distribution) done on the precision obtained on a sample size of 40 for the three different classification techniques, gave a result of 0.1026 for SVM with a standard deviation of 0.18. The same test gave a 95% confidence interval result of 0.05 with a standard deviation of 0.095 for KNN. Finally, the random forest gave a result of 0.090 with a standard deviation of 0.1599. It can be easily concluded that KNN performs the

Table 1 Accuracy of the models for different datasets

	SVM	KNN	Random forest
Merged dataset	0.5	1.0	1.0
Heel strike angle	0.583334	0.833334	0.416667
Stride angle	0.583334	0.916666	0.583334
Toe-off angle	0.625	1.0	1.0

Table 2 Detailed insight into the performance of the models for different datasets

		SVM			KNN			Random forest		
		Precision	Recall	F-score	Precision	Recall	F-score	Precision	Recall	F-score
Merged dataset	Sub1	0.50	1.00	0.67	1.00	1.00	1.00	1.00	1.00	1.00
	Sub2	0.00	0.00	0.00	1.00	1.00	1.00	1.00	1.00	1.00
Heel strike angle	Sub1	0.00	0.00	0.00	0.80	0.80	0.80	0.33	0.40	0.36
	Sub2	0.58	1.00	0.74	0.86	0.86	0.86	0.50	0.43	0.46
Stride angle	Sub1	0.00	0.00	0.00	1.00	0.80	0.89	0.00	0.00	0.00
	Sub2	0.58	1.00	0.74	0.88	1.00	0.93	0.58	1.00	0.74
Toe-off angle	Sub1	0.62	1.00	0.77	1.00	1.00	1.00	1.00	1.00	1.00
	Sub2	0.00	0.00	0.00	1.00	1.00	1.00	1.00	1.00	1.00

best with a p-value of 0.05. It implies that the probability of occurrence of random results is as low as 0.05.

5 Conclusion

KNN has been proven the best classifier among the three classifying models. For individual features, toe-off angle has been established as the best identification attribute among the three. The SVM has a consistently poor accuracy throughout all the datasets. The random forest shows both high and low accuracy. The limitation of this system is that the generated silhouette always may not be accurate. Due to harsh lighting conditions, hard shadows may stay in the silhouette and result in a huge error. One can upgrade this system by integrating with other identification systems, using other advanced classification schemes and making the process less time-consuming by implementing multi-threading with GPU support. The system clubbed with other identification scheme(s) may prove to be fail-safe.

References

1. Durward BR, Baer GD, Rowe PJ (1999) Functional human movement: measurement and analysis. Boston, Mass, Butterworth-Heinemann, Oxford
2. Wang L, Tan T, Ning H, Hu W (2003) Silhouette analysis-based gait recognition for human identification. IEEE Trans Pattern Anal Mach Intell 25(12):1505–1518
3. Yam CY, Nixon MS, Carter JN (2004) Automated person recognition by walking and running via model-based approaches. Pattern Recogn Soc Elsevier 37.5:1057–1072
4. Wang L, Tan T, Ning H, Hu W (2004) Fusion of static and dynamic body biometrics for gait recognition. IEEE Trans Circuits Syst for Video Technol 14(2):149—158
5. Tafazzoli F, Safabakhsh R (2010) Model-based human gait recognition using leg and arm movements. Eng Appl Artif Intell 23(8):1237–1246
6. Tao W, Liu T, Zheng R, Feng H (2012) Gait analysis using wearable sensors. Sensors (Basel) 12(2):2255–2283. https://doi.org/10.3390120202255 PMID:22438763
7. Murray MP, Drought AB, Kory RC (1964) Walking patterns of normal men. J Bone Joint Surgery 46(2):335–360
8. Kundu M, Sengupta D, Ghosh Dastidar J (2014) Tracking direction of human movement—an efficient implementation using Skeleton. J Ref: Int J Comput Appl 96(13):27—33. https://doi.org/10.5120/16855-6722
9. Nieto-Hidalgo M, Ferrández-Pastor FJ, Valdivieso-Sarabia RJ, Mora-Pascual J, García-Chamizo JM (2018) Gait analysis using computer vision based on cloud platform and mobile device. Mobile Inform Syst 7381264
10. Ghosh Dastidar J, Chakraborty D, Mukherjee S, Bhattacharjee AK (2019) Analysis of human gait for designing a recognition and classification system. In: A book chapter in intelligent innovations in multimedia data engineering and management, Hershey, PA, IGI Global, pp 186–200. Copyright year (2019). ISBN13:9781522571070, ISBN10:1522571078, EISBN13:9781522571087
11. Davenport T, Kalakota R (2019) The potential for artificial intelligence in healthcare. Future Healthcare J 6(2):94–98. https://doi.org/10.7861/futurehosp.6-2-94

12. Singh JP, Jain S, Arora S, Singh UP (2018) Vision-based gait recognition: a survey. IEEE Access 6:70497–70527. https://doi.org/10.1109/ACCESS.2018.2879896
13. Chen X, Weng J, Lu W, Xu J (2018) Multi-gait recognition based on attribute discovery. IEEE Trans Pattern Anal Mach Intell 40(7):1697–1710. https://doi.org/10.1109/TPAMI.2017.2726061
14. Takemura N, Makihara Y, Muramatsu D (2018) Multi-view large population gait dataset and its performance evaluation for cross-view gait recognition. IPSJ Trans Comput Vision Appl 10:4. https://doi.org/10.1186/s41074-018-0039-6
15. Bari ASMH, Gavrilova ML (2019) Artificial neural network based gait recognition using kinect sensor. IEEE Access 7:162708–162722. https://doi.org/10.1109/ACCESS.2019.2952065

Efficient Heart Disease Prediction Using Modified Hybrid Classifier

Rishabh Pipalwa, Abhijit Paul, Tamoghna Mukherjee, and Ashika Jain

Abstract Cardiovascular diseases, popularly known as heart disease leading to heart attack, kill nearly 17.9 million humans. Heart disease is found in three out of five patients in critical care unit. The complexity of this disease lies in the fact that it suddenly fails the functioning of human and then Standard Operating Plan (SOP) is required; if not provided on time, patients' life is in danger. Proper healthcare system takes time to detect the cause and effectively start the diagnosis, whereas our proposed system efficiently and accurately tells the client weather a patient has a heart disease or not. It also tells whether the patient will face such kind of disease in near future or not. The system is developed based on machine learning techniques such as Naive Bayes, XGBoost gradient classifier, support vector machine (SVM), and decision tree. Some external factors were also considered which may lead to heart disease in the future. Furthermore, integrated web application has been developed which alert and gives a user-friendly interface for the recognition and prediction. Thirteen diagnostic factors and five environmental factors are analyzed. The proposed diagnosis system attained a good precision as compared to previous methods recommended earlier. In addition, system can easily be implemented in public domain to spread awareness regarding heart disease, and it also talks about the possibility of the heart disease in near future.

Keywords Heart disease · Cardiovascular disease · Clinical diagnostic system · Hybrid classifier

All the authors have contributed equally to this paper.

R. Pipalwa (✉) · A. Paul · A. Jain
Department of Information Technology, Amity University, Kolkata, India
e-mail: rishabhpipalwa@gmail.com

T. Mukherjee
Department of CSE, Amity University, Kolkata, India

© The Author(s), under exclusive license to Springer Nature Singapore Pte Ltd. 2023

J. K. Mandal and D. De (eds.), *Frontiers of ICT in Healthcare*, Lecture Notes in Networks and Systems 519, https://doi.org/10.1007/978-981-19-5191-6_13

1 Introduction

The heart being the essential and critical role of the physical body as it is in control for the flow of blood in different parts of the body which helps in adequate oxygen supply and nutritious elements to be supplied to the required part. Any life is dependent totally on a proper flow of blood, in human life hurt is the pumping room of blood. Any disturbance in the flow or the function of hurt may lead to death within seconds [1]. According to the World Health Organization, 17,000,000 people die every year; among those 3,000,000 are dying before the age of 60 from heart diseases. In the year 2008, percentage of untimely deaths from heart diseases ranges from 4% in high-income countries to 42% in low-income countries [2].

When heart receives a limited blood for a longer period of time, it is called ischemic heart disease. Search conditions develop through a course of time which can be periodically monitored and cured with the help of expert supervision. There is the time when an ischemic heart patients have an heart attack, and after that the chances of survival also reduces, as the disease has been developing across a longer period of time, and the heart is habituated or accustomed with limited blood flow. For such things, early predictions or alertness helps in the long run.

Identification of heart disease is conventionally done by reading the medical history of the patient, medical examination report, and assessment of concerned symptoms by a doctor of medicine. Though the study obtained from this diagnostic method is not so much accurate in identifying the patient of heart disease. Additionally, it is high priced and computationally challenging to analyze [3]. We have proposed a machine learning-based diagnosis approach for identification of the disease. In this research, machine learning prediction model includes four classifiers namely Naive Bayes, SVM, decision tree, and eXtreme gradient boosting algorithm. The standard state of these models has been maintained for analysis purposes. Stalog, Hungarian, Switzerland, Long Beach VA, and Cleveland dataset combinedly used in this article. We have designed a web-based application what is access to the model for general public use.

Firstly, the authors have tried to address the problem of predicting the possibility of a heart disease. Here, standard feature extraction and profound algorithm classifiers appropriate features were extracted and analyzed with expert guidance from medical's experts which game a good result in analysis and accuracy of the algorithm proposed. Secondly, the author tries to predict the future possibility of the heart disease by understanding the environmental factors and common habits which may lead to heart disease. Finally, the authors combined all this into a single Python-based framework known as flask for giving the model a front-end part. Therefore, any non-technical or layman can easily detect the heart disease.

2 Literature Survey

Here, various automatic learning algorithm-based diagnosis techniques are analyzed by the scholars to detect heart disease. Analysis presents some machine learning-based algorithms which help understand the proposed method efficiently. Detrano et al. [4] develop heart disease classification system algorithm using machine learning techniques showed the exactitude of 77.00% in terms of precision end result. The dataset that was used with the system with multi-layer kit architecture to extract the features. Another researcher Gudadhe et al. [5] formed a diagnosis technique using multi-layer operational design and SVM classifier for heart disease labeling and attained precision of 80.411%. Humar et al. [6] devised heart disease classification system by developing a neural network along with Fuzzy logic. The classification system attained precision of 87.40%. Li et al. [7] created an ANN troupe-based identification technique for heart disease. In addition to numerical measuring system, it attained precision of 89.01%. Akil et al. [8] devised a machine learning centered heart disease identification system. ANN-DBP system along with FS algorithm and execution was worthy. Palaniappan et al. [9] recommended a professional health diagnosis system for heart disease recognition. In enhancement of the system, the prognostic model of ML such as decision tree (DT), Navies Bayes (NB), and Neural Networks was used. The attained precision of 86.12% precision was achieved by Navies Bayes, ANN accurateness 88.12%, and decision tree Algorithms attained precision of 80.40%. Olaniyi et al. [10] built a three-layer method using on the neural network technique for prediction of heart disease and attended 88.89% accuracy. Liu et al. [11] recommended a heart disease categorization system using respite and tough set procedures. The method attained precision of 92%. Samuel et al. [12] established an amalgamated a medical assistance system based on Fuzzy AHP and artificial neural network for identification of heart disease. The performance of the recommended method in terms attained precision is 91%. In one of the research papers of Mohan et al., [13] intended a heart disease forecast method which was used by cross machine learning techniques. They also recommended a new method for extensive characteristic assortment from the data for efficient training and testing of ML classifier. They have been recorded attained precision of 88.07%. In [14], selection and classification of algorithm have been proposed: Sequential Backward Selection Algorithm for Features Selection. The proposed method got high-level accuracy. Geweid et al. [15] considered heart disease detection methods by using advanced support vector machine-based dichotomy optimization system. Previous experiment of heart disease diagnosis method's had some restraint, and recompenses have been summarized for better understanding of the importance of our proposed approach. Among all the to be had strategies used by numerous methods to identify the coronary heart disorder at early stage. The important issues in those previous strategies are decrease precision and high computation time, and these might be due using inappropriate functions in dataset. The prediction desires to be improved for extra accuracy of detection and wishes similarly development for efficient and correct detection at early stages for better treatment and healing.

In an effort to tackle these issues, new approaches are had to locate coronary heart disease accurately. The improvement in prediction accuracy is a large assignment and research gap.

3 Proposed Method

Hybrid classifier refers to the system being a composite mapping of four algorithms (Naive Bayes, decision tree, support vector machine, and XGBoost gradient classifiers). The mapping referred to design of system in an additive form such that accuracy of system gets increased and the error rate reduces because too many systems to run against.

3.1 Dataset

Stalog, Hungarian, Switzerland, Long Beach VA, and Cleveland dataset combinedly used in this article, featuring the following variables with its description. For training purpose, 648 data are used, and for testing purposes, 412 data have been used. In all the classifiers, same testing and training ratio has been maintained to get optimal result. Dataset consists of 13 features dataset where one is the output label output level has 2 possibilities one being presence of heart disease second been the absence of her disease. Table 1 gives the description of 13 features of the dataset with the feature code (Tables 2, 3 and 4).

Heatmap shown in Fig. 1 clearly reflects about the variable weightage which helps in understanding the relevance of each

4 Proposed Algorithm

Step 1: It starts with training of dataset, in which 624 data are trained to each algorithm classifiers.

a. There are four algorithm classifiers in the model namely decision tree, Navies Bayes, support vector machine, and XGBoost.
b. Decision tree is a graphical representation for getting all possible solutions to a decision making situation on a given condition. It follows supervised learning technique, where internal nodes represent the feature of a dataset, and branches represent the decision rules, and each leaf node represents the possible outcome.

Table 1 Features of dataset with their description

Sl. no	Feature name	Feature code	Description
1	Age	AGE	Age in years
2	Gender	SEX	Female = 0, Male = 1
3	Chest pain	CPT	Atypical angina = 1 Typical angina = 2 Asymptomatic = 3 Non-anginal pain = 4
4	Resting blood pressure	RBP	In Mm hg
5	Serum cholesterol	SCH	In Mg/dl
6	Fasting blood sugar > 120 mg/dl	FBS	True = 1 False = 0
7	Resting electrocardiogram	RES	Normal = 0 ST T = 1 Hypertrophy = 2
8	Maximum heart rate	MHR	Numeric
9	Exercise induced angina	EIA	Yes = 1 No = 0
10	Old peak = ST depression induced by exercise relative to rest	OPK	In Numeric
11	The slope of peak exercise ST segment	PES	Up sloping = 1 Flat = 2 Down sloping = 3
12	No. of major vessels colored by fluoroscopy	VCA	(0–3)
13	Thallium scan	THA	Normal = 3 Fixed defect = 6 Reversible defect = 7
14	Label	LB	Patient has heart diseases = 1 Healthy person = 0

Table 2 External factors with their description

Factors	Feature code	Description
Body mass index	BMI	True = has higher BMI False = BMI normal
History of diseases	Phist	Yes = factor present No = Factor not present
Family history of diseases	Fhist	Yes = factor present No = Factor not present
Alcohol	Alchol	Yes = factor present No = Factor not present

Table 3 Classifier algorithms with their description

Classifiers	Description
Navies Bayes algorithm	This is used for classifying problems related to anxiety disorders. There is a training dataset present which is used by the algorithm to compute the value of the conditional probability of vector for a given class. The conditional probability value is evaluated for each vector following which the new vector class is evaluated based on the same
Support vector machine algorithm	This is a supervised learning model with associated learning algorithms that analyze data for classification and regression analysis. This algorithm is mostly used for classification problems because of its exceptional performance
Decision tree algorithm	A decision tree consists of leaf node or addition node. In decision tress there are internal and external nodes linked to each other. The decision−making part of internal node takes the decisions and informs the child node to visit the next node
eXtreme gradient boosting algorithm	XGBClassifier of gradient boosting algorithm provides a wrapper class to allow models to be treated like classifier or regressor

Table 4 Classifier algorithms with their limitation, advantage, and accuracy

Classifiers	Limitation	Advantage	Accuracy in percentage (%)
Heart disease diagnosis using a single machine learning classifier	Accuracies are very low and system errors can occur very easily	Computation is less complex	70–80
kNN + decision tree	Accuracies are low Comparatively	Computation is less complex	74
Decision tree + SVM	More exaggeration time required to generate the result	Accuracy is comparatively high	82.01
SVM + kNN + k-Means	Computationally complex and performance time is very High	accuracy is high	87.4
System based on Navies Bayes + decision tree + ANN	Computationally complex and ANN performance is low	Navies Bayes and decision tree achieved a high performance in terms of accuracy	84.33
Random forest + XGBoost + decision tree	Random forest showed less accuracy in comparison to other classifier	XGBoost showed high accuracy	88.21
Navies Bayes + decision tree + Support vector machine	High execution time is required to generate results	All the classifiers showed high individual results	92.25
Navies Bayes + decision tree + Support vector machine + XGBoost	More execution time is required to generate results	Performance is high and accurate. It suggests that high performance in extreme situations	98.73

c. Navies Bayes is a probabilistic classifier that predicts the possibilities given by a probability of an object. It applies Bayes law which is based on probability of a hypothesis with prior knowledge.

d. In support vector machine, we plot each data item into a point in 'n' dimension space where 'n' represents number of features available in the dataset. Then, classification is performed on the hyperplane that differentiates two classes properly.

e. XGBoost or eXtreme gradient boost is an advanced version of gradient boosting classifiers. Major difference lies in the fact XGBoost is a regularized model formalized to control overfitting which gives a better performance.

Step-2: Extracted feature is computed after training of dataset for every algorithm classifier upon which each variable can be used for the model.

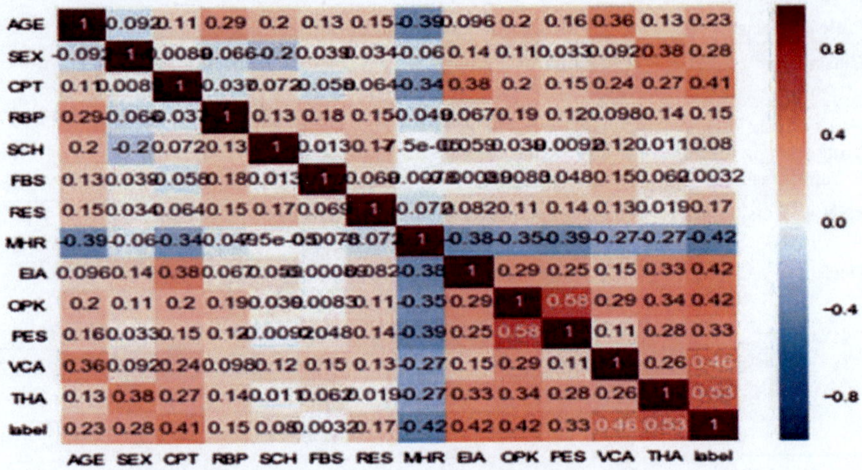

Fig. 1 Heatmap of dataset reflecting weightage of each variable

Step-3: All the extracted features are sent to four different ML algorithms, and a resultant output is obtained without any ambiguity.

Step-4: If there is any ambiguity between the four different algorithms, the system alerts its reserved feature of taking the most accurate method among the all.

Step-5: The resulted output shall we checked with 420 data for testing purposes and reliability of the model proposed.

Step-6: The resulting output is converted into a model which segregates prediction of heart disease and future possibilities of a heart disease.

Step-7: When a user enters a new data, it follows a certain pattern to label it into categories.

Step-8: Features are extracted from the new data. Then, it is passed to the proposed model.

Step-9: Then, a prediction is made about the possibility of having heart disease or not. If a person does not have a heart disease at present, then future possibilities are also looked upon.

Step-10: User gets a message about the present condition and consultations for future

Figure 2b explains the manner of prediction done on each new input arrival. Each new input is taken to individual classifiers namely Naive Bayes, decision tree, SVM, and XGBoost. Then, each of the classifier's results, with individual output are predicted which are verified for any ambiguous data or any system error, then it is converted into a model.

In the model verification and validation, results are calculated, and then, the results are categorized into positive and negative. If a patient has a negative result, it redirects

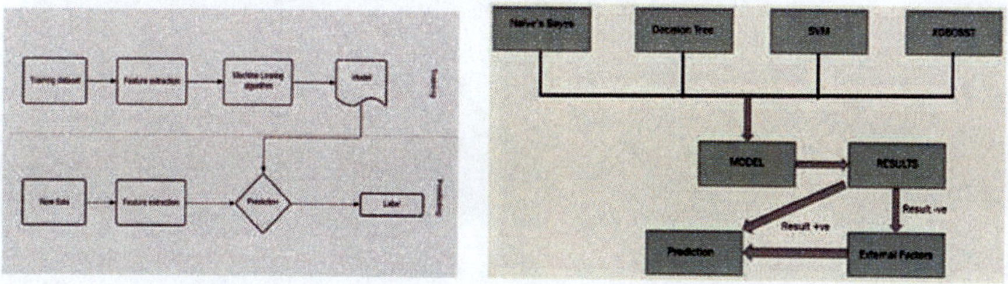

(a) (b)

Fig. 2 **a** Flow diagram of proposed algorithm. **b** Flow diagram of the proposed algorithm

to take external factors and then make a prediction according to it, whereas in positive results, a warning message is shown and consultation with a specialist is advised.

5 System U/I Design

See Fig. 3.

6 Result and Discussion

Table 5 clearly shows that all the four methods used have resulted very accurately in training and testing areas. The training and testing are done on the ratio of 60 and 40. Some data are kept reserved for model evaluation and application testing at the later stage to evaluate a proper idea of the system errors. While testing at the latest stage, no error was found neither at system end nor at web end. The resultant accuracy with the proposed algorithm (modified hybrid classifier) of the system proposed is 98.73% which is comparatively far better in the context of previous research (Fig. 4).

This graph (Fig. 5) tells about the various features entered in the line graph form, and the blue dot represent patients results; blue dot at 0 means heart diseases not found and blue dot at 1 means heart diseases detected. (Note that this is the sample testing done on 216 data for better understanding of system results and get overall view.)

The graph (Fig. 6) shows us about various algorithms which are present in the industry and their accuracy against the proposed method. The blue dotted lines suggest the industry standards line of accuracy.

The purpose of this experiment was to analyze and predict a possibility of heart disease with high precision which benefits directly to the human society. Result shown in the process of prediction suggest about the high accuracy and less system failures. The on-ground implementation of the project has been successfully deployed with

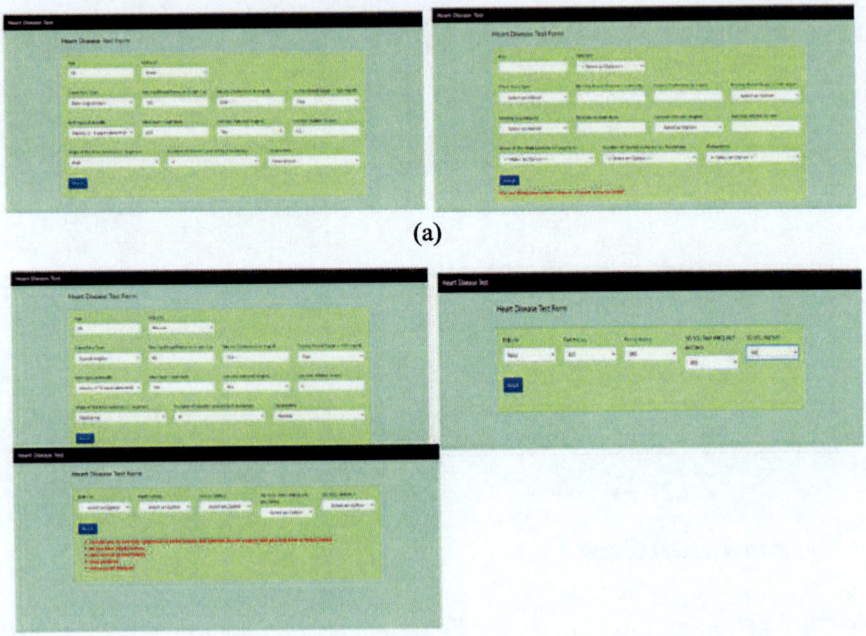

(a)

(b)

Fig. 3 **a** Positive result of heart disease symptoms **b** Result of a negative heart disease but having external factors positive

Table 5 Training and testing results

Classifiers	Training accuracy (%)	Testing accuracy (%)
Naive Bayes	85	78
Decision tree	100	96
Support vector machine	100	84
eXtreme gradient boosting	100	97
Modified hybrid classifier	100	98.73

accurate precision. At no point of time, no conclusive system error has occurred neither at system end nor at web application end.

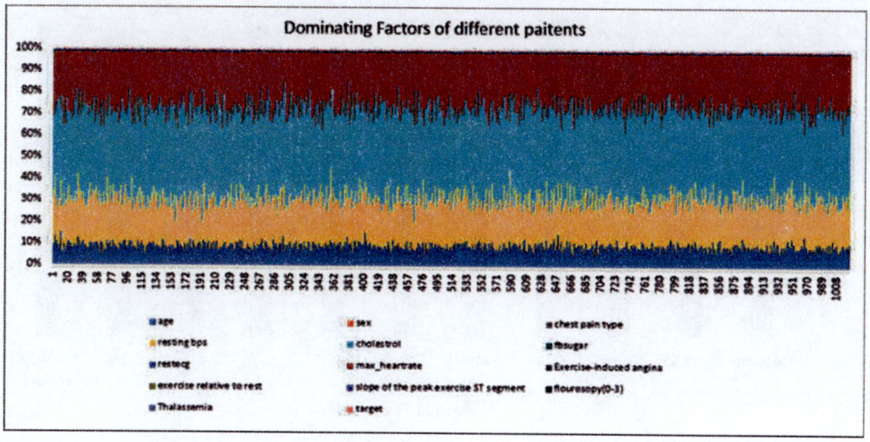

Fig. 4 Representation of performance parameter

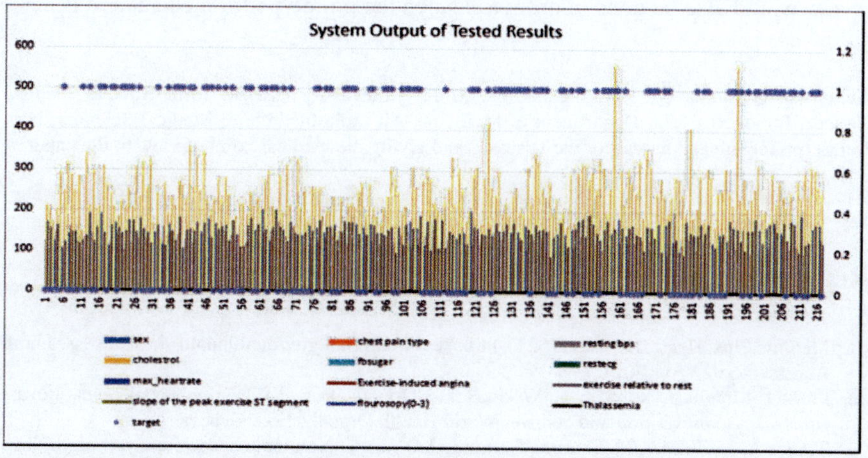

Fig. 5 Output of tested results for various parameters

7 Conclusion and Future Scope

The neural network system accepts 13 clinical data and 5 environmental data, and it is trained using back propagation algorithms. Proposed model can find out presence or absence of a heart disease in a patient and the accuracy achieved is 98.73% which is comparatively exceedingly high to the existing systems present in the market. We presented user-friendly application which helps a patient to easily access their present condition and act accordingly.

Integrated multiple disease prediction-based models would be designed in the future so that a user can analyze any condition according to their choice. A market

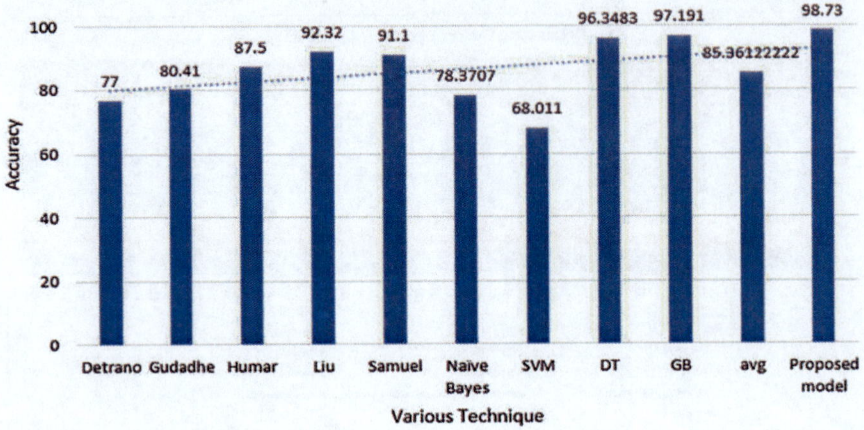

Fig. 6 Comparative analysis of algorithms

review would also be done in order to launch the prototype for medical and general public use.

Acknowledgements We would thank Dr. Mohit Chowdhary (MBBS form Kolkata Medical College, Junior Resident, Department of Medicine, All India Institute of Medical Sciences, New Delhi) for Technical Analysis of the Diseases and giving the medical point of view to the paper.

References

1. Medline Plus: Heart Diseases (2021). http://www.nlm.nih.gov/medlineplus/heartdiseases.html Accessed on 22 Apr 2021
2. Puska P, Mendis S, Norrving B, World Health Organization (2011) Global atlas on cardiovascular disease prevention and control. World Health Organization, Geneva
3. Tsanas A, Little MA, McSharry PE, Ramig LO (2011) Nonlinear speech analysis algorithms mapped to a standard metric achieve clinically useful quatacaine of average Parkinson's disease symptom severity. J Roy Soc Interface 8(59):842–855
4. Detrano R, Janosi A, Steinbrunn W, Pfisterer M, Schmid J-J, Sandhu S, Guppy KH, Lee S, Froelicher V (1989) International application of a new probability algorithm for the diagnosis of coronary artery disease. Amer J Cardiol 64(5):304–310
5. Gennari JH, Langley P, Fisher D (1989) Models of incremental concept formation. Artif Intell 40(1–3):11–61
6. Li Y, Li T, Liu H (2017) Recent advances in feature selection and its applications. Knowl Inf Syst 53(3):551–577
7. Li J, Liu H (2017) Challenges of feature selection for big data analytics 32(2):9–15
8. Xu Z, Hu H (2010) Projection models for intuitionistic fuzzy multiple attribute decision making. IEEE Intell Syst 32(2):9–15
9. Zhu L, Shen J, Xie L, Cheng Z (2017) Unsupervised topic hyper graph hashing for efficient mobile image retrieval. IEEE Trans Cybern 47(11):3941–3954
10. Raschka S (2018) Model evaluation, model selection, and algorithm selection in machine learning. arXiv:1811.12808 [Online]. Available http://arxiv.org/abs/1811.12808

11. Olaniyi EO, Oyedotun OK, Adnan K (2015) Heart diseases diagnosis using neural networks arbitration. Int J Intell Syst Appl 7(12):72
12. Palaniappan S, Awang R (2008) Intelligent heart disease prediction system using data mining techniques. In: Proceedings IEEE/ACS international conference computing systems, pp 108–115
13. Samuel OW, Asogbon GM, Sangaiah AK, Fang P, Li G (2017) An integrated decision support system based on ANN and Fuzzy_AHP for heart failure risk prediction. AExp Syst Appl 68:163–172
14. Das R, Turkoglu I, Sengur A (2009) Effective diagnosis of heart disease through neural networks ensembles. Expert Syst Appl 36(4):7675–7680
15. Kumar AVS (2012) Diagnosis of heart disease using fuzzy resolution mechanism. J Artif Intell 5(1):47–55

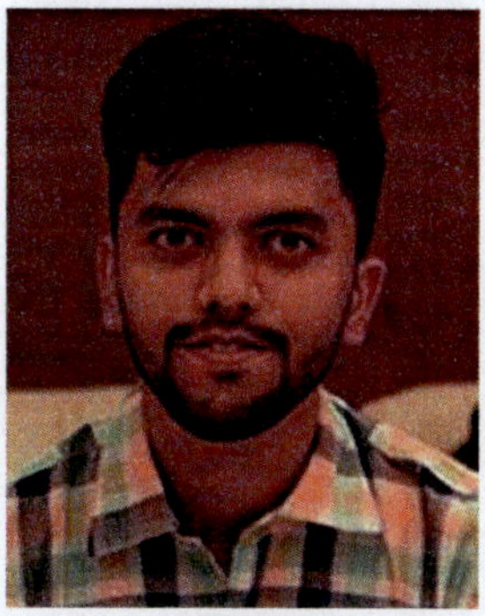

Rishabh Pipalwa is a student, pursuing Bachelor's and Master's in Computer Application in an integrated dual course from Amity University Kolkata. He has a keen interest in the research areas. His research area is Sensor network, Internet of things, Machine Learning in the field of Health Informatics. He has publications in many Journals and Conference proceedings. He is working on many research areas with the various professor at Amity University Kolkata and IIT Kharagpur on various topics.

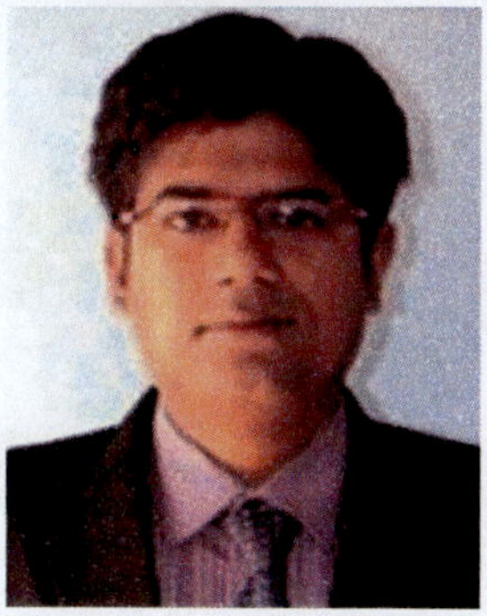

Abhijit Paul did his Ph.D. in Computer Science from Assam University, Silchar, India. He is currently associated with Department of Information Technology in Amity University Kolkata. His research area is Sensor network, Ad hoc network, Internet of things etc. He has publication in many Journals and Conference proceedings. He is also a member of Reviewer committee of IEEE Internet of Things journal. He teaches all Data communication and Computer networks related papers. UG and PG students are pursuing their research under his guidance.

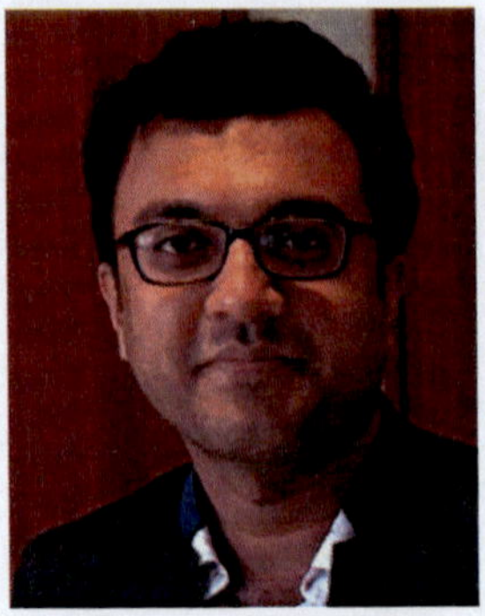

Tamoghna Mukherjee did his MTech in Computer Science and Engineering from West Bengal University of Technology, Kolkata, West Bengal, India. He is currently associated as Assistant Professor, Department of Computer Science and Engineering, Amity School of Engineering and Technology, Amity University Kolkata. His research area is Machine Learning in the field of Health Informatics. He has publications in different Journals and Conference proceedings. He is also a member of Reviewer committee of IEEE Internet of Things journal. The courses taught by him includes Data Structure, Artificial Intelligence, Soft Computing, Statistics etc. UG and PG students of Amity University Kolkata are pursuing their research under his guidance.

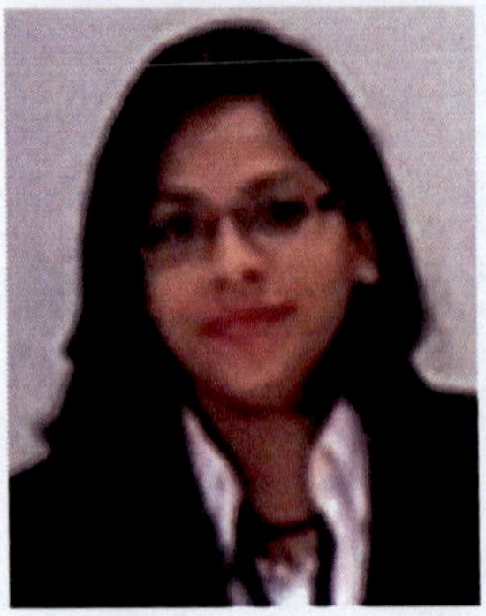

Ashika Jain is a student, pursuing Master's in Computer Application from Amity University Kolkata. She has a keen interest in software development and research areas.Her research area is Artificial Intelligence, Machine Learning, Data Mining and Internet of Things. She is having a good knowledge in application development.

An Unstructured Mammogram Analysis for Feasible Classification and Detection of Breast Cancer Using a Convolutional Approach

Debkumar Chowdhury, Tirtharaj Sinha, Arnobrata Ghosh, Anurag Unnikannan, Susmit De, Kartik Sau, and Sanjukta Mishra

Abstract Currently, different methods are available for the purpose of breast cancer classification and detection. Most of these techniques are well appreciated by society and in response to the demand of society, almost every year the different techniques are introduced by different researchers, but it does not satisfy the demand of current requirements. Under such a situation, we are going to propose a new breast cancer classification and detection algorithm using a convolutional approach. This technique starts with the mammogram preprocessing step. It is followed by the convolutional model architecture design step. In the next step, the segregation of the dataset into the training and testing phase is performed. Then, the convolutional model architecture is trained using the training dataset and pre-masked images. After that our proposed algorithm predicts, the breast cancer detection and classification result. We have found that our proposed algorithm can be used for breast tumor detection and classification from mammogram images with the average approximate accuracy of 98.5% and the average approximate F1 score of 0.98. Novel preprocessing steps and modifications in the convolutional architecture make the proposed methodology unique. Due to high performance, novelty, ease of use, our proposed method is useful to develop any mobile or web application in the future.

Keywords Breast cancer · Mammogram · Pre-masked image · Convolutional · Accuracy score · F1 score

1 Introduction

Breast cancer is considered to be most common nowadays. According to the December 2020 statistics of the World Health Organization (WHO), among 24.5% of world's female cancer population is affected by this disease. It starts spreading

D. Chowdhury (✉) · T. Sinha · A. Ghosh · A. Unnikannan · S. De · K. Sau · S. Mishra
University of Engineering and Management, Kolkata, India
e-mail: debkumar.cse@gmail.com

K. Sau
e-mail: kartik.sau@uem.edu.in

© The Author(s), under exclusive license to Springer Nature Singapore Pte Ltd. 2023
J. K. Mandal and D. De (eds.), *Frontiers of ICT in Healthcare*, Lecture Notes in Networks and Systems 519, https://doi.org/10.1007/978-981-19-5191-6_14

from breast. At the early stage of this disease, the cancerous cells we may be found as a tumor or lump, which is clearly visible from the X-ray images. Most of the breast tumors are found as non-cancerous in nature and often observed that they do not spread outside the breast, whereas malignant breast tumors are cancerous in nature and may spread outside the breast. Patients of this disease are often suffered from symptoms like breast or nipple pain, swelling of all or part of a breast, skin dimpling, nipple retraction, reddish nipple or breast skin, nipple discharge, swollen lymph nodes, etc. Among many types of this disease ductal carcinoma in situ (DCIS) and invasive carcinoma are considered to be the most common and phyllodes tumors and angiosarcoma are considered as rare.

Hence, it is considered as a serious issue of society and an automated computer-based method is required to detect and classify breast cancer with precision from mammogram images. This method helps the medical practitioner to start early treatment and also helps to reduce the fatality rate. The inconclusive, incomplete and dissatisfactory results of the previously proposed techniques encourage us to develop a novel breast cancer classification and detection algorithm using a convolutional approach that works on unstructured data such as mammogram images. It displays the classified output using convolutional model architecture along with the satisfactory accuracy rate and F1 score.

Our paper is divided into various sections. In Sect. 2, we explain the advantages and disadvantages of some pre-existing techniques; in Sect. 3, we explain our proposed methodology, which consists of the main architecture of the method and the algorithm, whereas the experiment result and analysis are explained in Sect. 4.

2 Literature Survey

This section represents various pre-existing methods [7–9], along with their advantages and disadvantages as shown in the survey table (Table 1). All these methods are well appreciated, but in context with our problem they are producing inclusive, incomplete and dissatisfactory results. In-depth analysis of these methodologies has proven to be very competent to identify the downsides. Identification of these drawbacks helps us to update and modify our algorithm and code and to calculate the accuracy rate. The survey table is given below:

3 Proposed Methodology

Our proposed methodology is focused on breast cancer classification and detection from an unstructured dataset (BUSI) [10] using breast mammogram classification and detection algorithm using a convolutional approach. We have proposed a block diagram to show the main concept of the methodology at a glance as shown in Fig. 1.

Table 1 Existing methodology analysis table

Methodology	Advantages	Disadvantages
Decision tree [1]	Decision trees require less effort for data preparation during preprocessing	A small change in the data can cause a large change in the structure. According to our problem, it causes instability
K-nearest neighbor [2]	No assumption about data	KNN needs a huge amount of memory
Random forest classifier [3]	Random forest minimizes the overfitting issue and tries to increase the accuracy score	This method needs high computational power and resources
Support vector machine [4]	It is effective in high-dimensional spaces	Due to a huge time consumption issue, the performance of this method is not satisfactory when we apply this strategy in a large dataset
Gaussian Naïve Bayes [5]	Naive Bayes is more appropriate for categorical input variables than numerical variables. In the context of our problem, this property is suitable	It presumes that every feature of the dataset is independent. This property limits the application of this technique in real-world cases
Multi-scale fusion U-Net [6]	It solves the problem of multi-scale variation in breast lesions and boundary pixel blurring	For the different modes of images, segmentation effects will be reduced

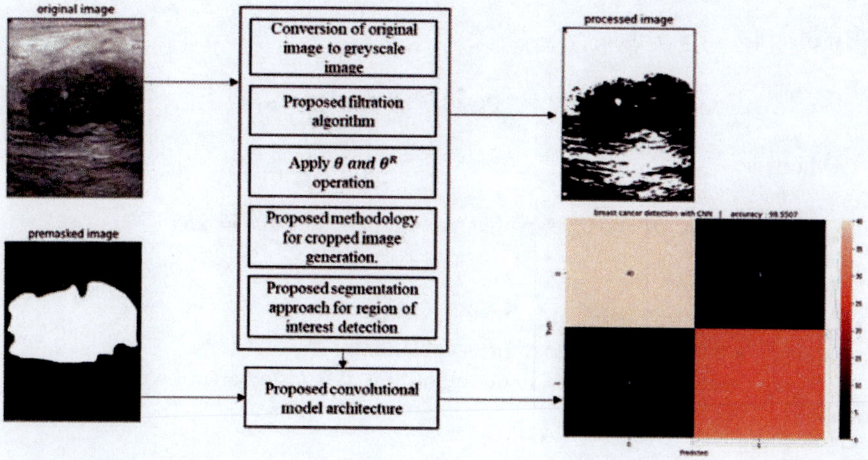

Fig. 1 Built-in architecture of mammogram classification and detection algorithm using a convolutional approach

3.1 Algorithm

Our algorithm is divided into 16 steps. The algorithm takes a mammogram image, $I(u, v)$ as an input from the dataset [10] and produces a binary output (Yes/No) and the accuracy rate. The algorithm is as follows:

Algorithm: mammogram classification and detection algorithm using a convolutional approach.

Input: $I(u, v)$

Output: Yes/No and the accuracy rate

1. Read an image $I(u, v)$ from the dataset.
2. Convert the image to a grayscale image, $G(u, v)$.
3. Preprocessed $G(u, v)$ using the following formula and 5×5 kernel:

$$G_1(u, v) = \frac{1}{2\pi d^2} e^{\frac{-u^2 + v^2}{2d^2}} \tag{1}$$

where,
$G_1(u, v) =$ Processed Image.
$d =$ Standard Deviation.
$u = u$ th row in the grayscale image.
$v = v$ th column in the grayscale image.

4. Perform segmentation on $G_1(u, v)$ using the following equation:

If pixel $(u, v) \geq \tau$ then,

$$(u, v) \leftarrow 1,$$

Otherwise,

$$(u, v) \leftarrow 0, \text{ provided maximum pixel value} = 255$$

Where,
$G_1(u, v) =$ grayscale image.
$(u, v) =$ a pixel of an image in (u, v) position.
$\tau =$ selected threshold value in our algorithm. It is tested after the trial-and-error method.
$1 =$ Light.
$0 =$ Dark.

5. Apply θ operation on each pixel (u, v) of $G(u, v)$ using a 3×3 kernel window, to probe and reduce the shape stored in $G(u, v)$.

$$G_2(u, v) \leftarrow G_1(u, v)\ \theta\ \Delta(u, v) \leftarrow \{\Phi \in \varepsilon \mid \Delta\ (u, v)\varphi\ subset\ of\ G_1(u, v)\} \quad (2)$$

where,

$\varepsilon \leftarrow$ A Euclidean space.

$G_1(u, v) \leftarrow$ a binary image in ε.

$\Delta(u, v)_\varphi \leftarrow \Phi$ is the translation of Δ by the vector Φ.

6. Apply θ^R operation on each pixel (u, v) of $G_2(u, v)$ as follows:

$$G_3(u, v) \leftarrow G_2(u, v)\theta^R\Delta(u, v) \bigcup_{\gamma\varepsilon G_1(u,v)} \Delta(u, v)_\gamma \quad (3)$$

where,

$\varepsilon \leftarrow$ A Euclidean space and $G_2(u, v)$ a binary image after θ operation in ε.

$\Delta(u, v) \leftarrow$ The structuring element.

$\Delta(u, v)_\gamma \leftarrow$ The Translation of $\Delta(u, v)$ by γ.

7. Find the best-bounded box of image $G3(u, v)$ using the following function.

7.1.

$$C_{u,v} \rightarrow \rho(G_3(u, v), \alpha(u, v), \beta(u, v) \quad (4)$$

where,

$C_{(u,v)} \rightarrow$ collection of boundary points.

$\rho() \rightarrow$ a method used for boundary points generation.

$G_3(u, v) \rightarrow$ processed image after step 6.

$\alpha(u, v) \rightarrow$ a method to retrieve outer boundary.

$\beta(u, v) \rightarrow$ a method to store the endpoints of the horizontal, vertical and diagonal boundary.

7.2 Merge all the boundary points together & produce the final boundary box.

8. Calculate the extreme left, right, top, and bottom-most corner points.
9. Create a cropped image $G_5(u, v)$ by segregating the blank area from the image $G_4(u, v)$ using the following equation.

$$G_5 \leftarrow C(t(u, v), b(u, v), l(a, v), r(u, v)) \quad (5)$$

where,

$C() \rightarrow$ a method to convert cropped images.

$t(u, v) \rightarrow$ a method to extract the extreme topmost corner point.

$b(u, v) \rightarrow$ a method to extract the extreme bottommost corner point.

$l(u, v) \rightarrow$ a method to extract the leftmost corner point.

$r(u, v) \rightarrow$ a method to extract the rightmost corner point.

$(u, v) \rightarrow$ the u th row and v^{th} column.

10. Apply τ operation on $G_5(u, v)$ using the following equation:

$$G_5(u, v) \leftarrow \tau(G_5(u, v), \text{selected } \tau \text{ value, maximum } \tau \text{value}, \tau_1\beta(u, v)) \quad (6)$$

where,

$G_5(u, v) \rightarrow$ a processed image.
$\tau() \rightarrow$ a thresholding method.
$G_5(u, v) \rightarrow$ a cropped image.
selected τ value $\leftarrow$ 100 in our algorithm.
maximum τ value $\leftarrow$ 255 in our algorithm.
$\tau_1 \leftarrow$ if a pixel $(u, v) \geq$ Selected τ value then $(u, v) \leftarrow 1$, otherwise $(u, v) \leftarrow 0$.
$\beta(u, v) \leftarrow$ a method to store the endpoints of horizontal, vertical, and diagonal boundary points.

11. Read the pre-masked image $\rho(u, v)$ from the dataset (D).
12. Resize $G_4(u, v)$ into a 128 X 128 image.
13. Declaring $A[n][2]$ list for each image for storing true and false sample values.

$n \leftarrow$ total number of images
$end\_of\_iterations \leftarrow n - 1$
$i \leftarrow no\_of\_iterations \leftarrow 0$
While ($i \leq end\_of\_iterations$) then,

If $G_6(u, v)$ is a tumourous image then

$G_6(u, v) \leftarrow$ True.
$A[i][0] \leftarrow 1$ and $A[i][1] \leftarrow 0$.
Go to Otherwise

If $G_6(u, v)$ is a non-tumorous image then,

$G_6(u, v) \leftarrow$ False.
$A[i][0] \leftarrow 0$ and $A[i][1] \leftarrow 1$.
Go to Otherwise

Otherwise
$i \leftarrow i + 1 + 1$.
Go to While.
End If

,
End While

14. The proposed convolutional architecture each has an input x of size 128 × 128 × 3 which is used to feed into it. In the convolutional architecture, following layers are observed:

    a. One two-dimensional convolution layer with kernel size 2 × 2
    b. One two-dimensional convolution layer with kernel size 2 × 2 and a rectified linear activation function
    c. One batch normalization layer
    d. One two-dimensional max pooling layer with pool size 2 × 2
    e. One dropout layer
    f. One two-dimensional convolution layer of 64-bit input and a rectified linear activation function
    g. One two-dimensional convolution layer of 64-bit input and a rectified linear activation function
    h. One batch normalization layer to calculate the mean output (close to 0) and the standard deviation output (close to 1)
    i. One two-dimensional max pooling layer with pool size 2 × 2
    j. One dropout layer
    k. One flatten layer
    l. One dense layer and activation layer
    m. One dropout layer
    n. One dense layer with an activation softmax function

15. Segregate the whole dataset [10] into two sections. We select 80% mammogram images from the dataset (BUSI) [10] for training purposes and 20% mammogram images from the dataset (BUSI) [10] for testing purposes.
16. We feed the training and testing data into the designed convolutional model architecture to generate result.

3.2 Model Architecture

Mammogram training and testing phase can be explained with the help of a model architecture as shown in Fig. 2. The architecture accepts preprocessed mammogram image and pre-masked image as output and displays predicted sample results and accuracy for the same.

4 Experimental Results

We consider the mammogram image dataset (BUSI) [10], which consists of 410 malignant and 130 non-malignant images collected from the dataset [10] and 209 malignant and 133 non-malignant pre-masked images to calculate the performance of mammogram classification and detection algorithm using a convolutional approach.

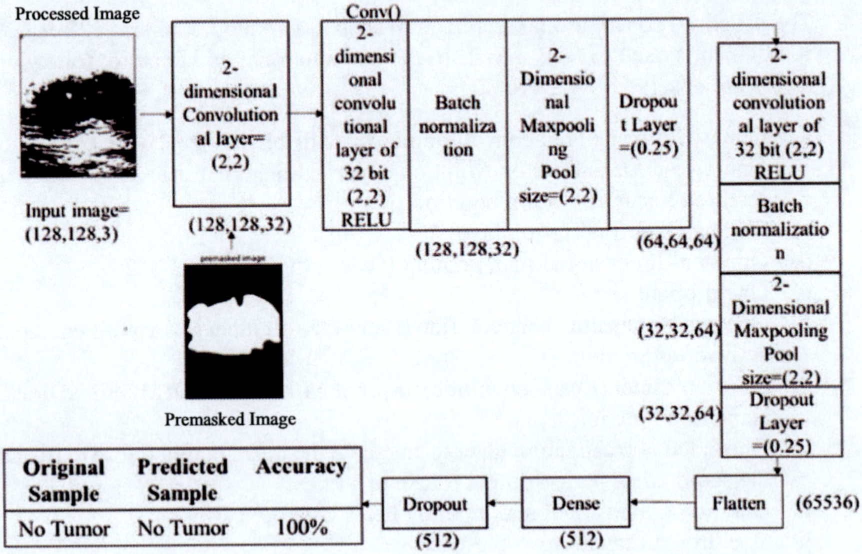

Fig. 2 Mammogram training and testing phase using proposed model architecture

The size, color and format of breast tumor images in the dataset [10] are similar in nature, whereas the resolutions of the images are different. The format of the mammogram images are ".png" by nature.

We have applied our algorithm in the Python environment, version 3.8, with the hardware configuration of the Intel Core i3 fifth generation processor, 4 GB DDR3 primary memory (RAM) and an integrated graphics card. Anaconda as a distributor of Python version 3.8 is used. Jupyter Notebook version 6.3.0 as an open web interface is used as a programming platform for the implementation of our algorithm.

After reading the images from the local machine, we partitioned them into two categories, i.e., "yes" (malignant) and "no" (normal) and we have achieved the following results as shown in Figs. 3. and 4.

After reading all the images from the dataset, each image will pass through the various steps of the algorithm as shown in Fig. 5.

We are splitting our dataset (BUSI) [10] into training and testing sets. 80% of the mammogram images are used for training, and the rest is used for testing. After the execution of our proposed algorithm, we observed that the number of training samples are 344, number of testing samples are 69, whereas training shape values are (344, 128, 128, 3) and (344, 1). Our proposed convolutional layered architecture is trained. It is used to train on n number of samples (344 in our case). With the changes of several iterations or epochs, the total time consumed by the algorithm is calculated (Table 2).

After calculation of accuracy and loss during the testing and validation phase, we have discovered two graphs, as shown in Figs. 6 and 7, respectively.

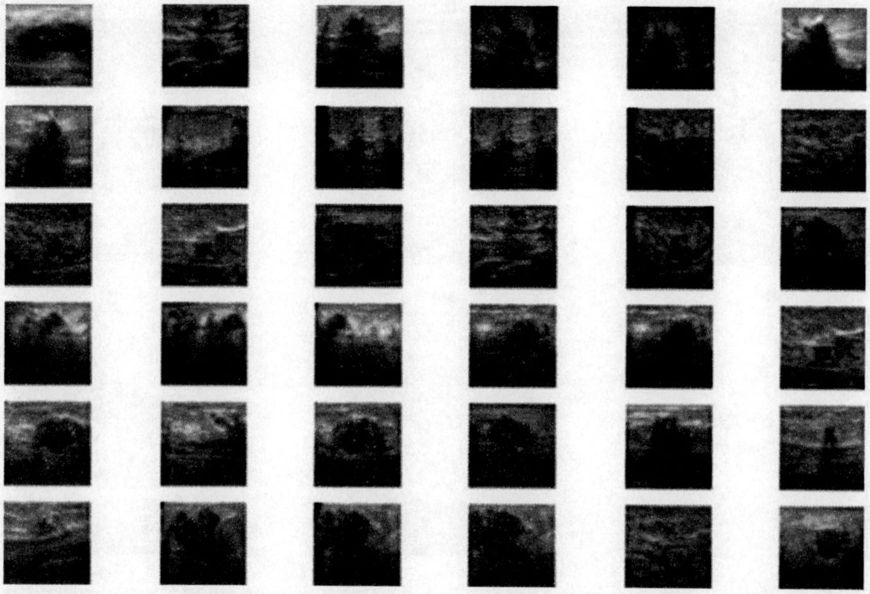

Fig. 3 Malignant images

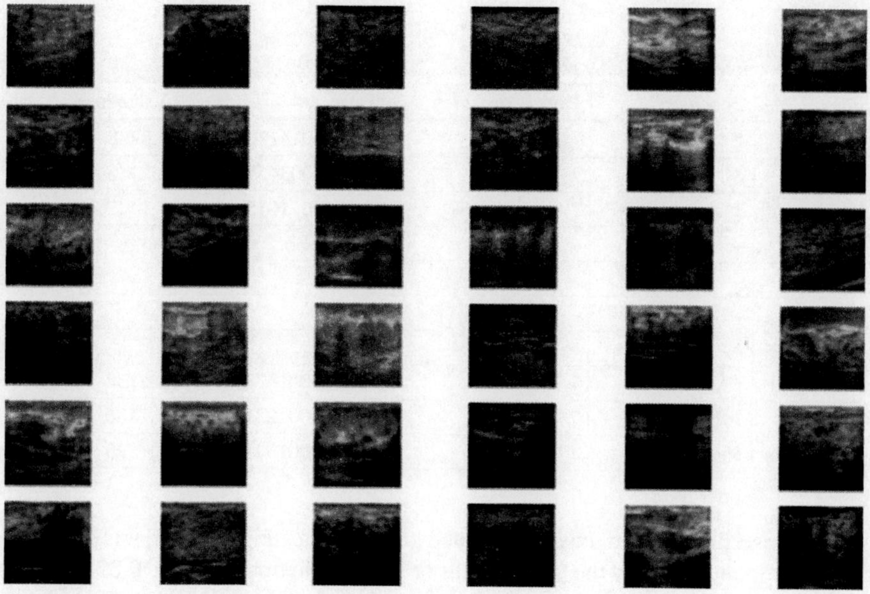

Fig. 4 Non-malignant images

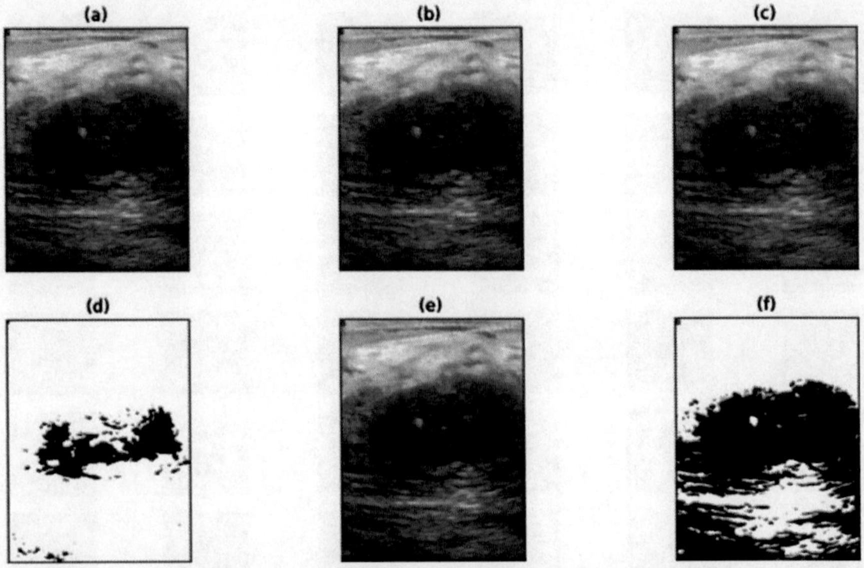

Fig. 5 **a** Original image, **b** grayscale image, **c** image after applying proposed filtration method, **d** image after applying θ and θ^R operation, **e** cropped image after applying proposed image cropping methodology and **f** proposed segmentation approach for the region of interest detection

Table 2 Example of the training phase

S. no	Epoch no	Time taken (s)	Loss	Value loss
1	1	7.989	0.0000014170	1.0888
2	2	7	0.0000003455	1.1316
3	3	7	0.0000011035	1.1742
–	–	–	–	–
–	–	–	–	–
–	–	–	–	–
–	–	–	–	–
13	13	7	0.0000001478	1.2158
14	14	7	0.0000001231	1.2586
15	15	7	0.0000001321	1.2025

After inserting the previously calculated amount of testing samples, it is observed that the amount of loss in the test samples or false prediction cases are 0.02 whereas 0.98 or 98% accuracy or right prediction is received from our algorithm. It has been observed that the average F1 score is 0.98.

Table 3 displays 69 randomly selected original samples from the dataset, corresponding predicted sample results and the accuracy score. In the end, we have found

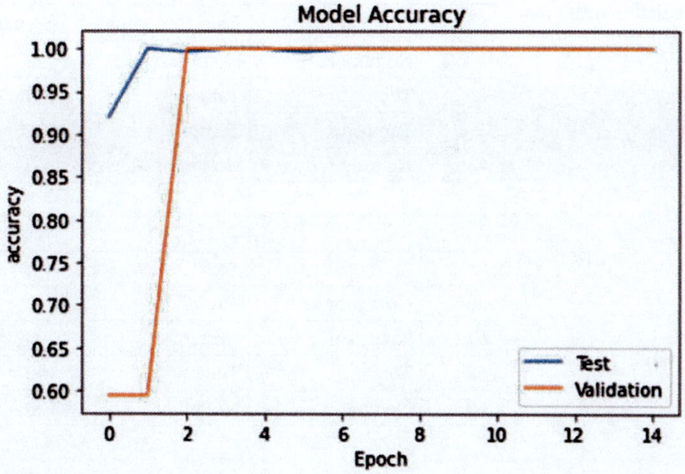

Fig. 6 Accuracy graph

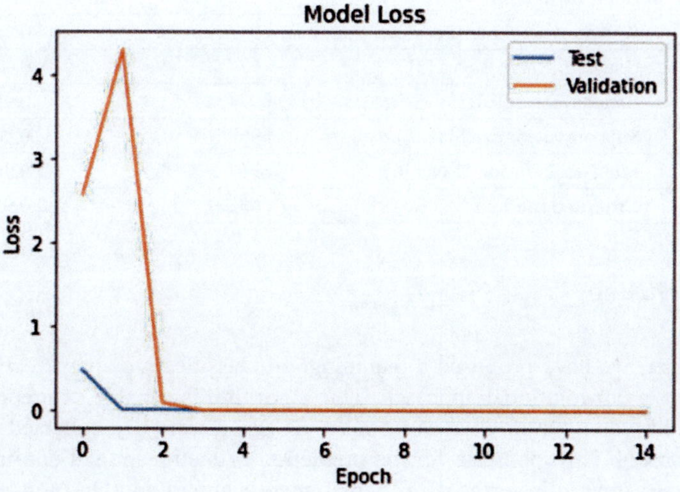

Fig. 7 Loss graph

that our proposed algorithm can be used for breast tumor detection and classification from mammogram images with an average approximate accuracy of 98.5%. As the data is balanced, we are considering the results to be satisfied. Comparing it with other existing methodologies, a satisfactory result is observed as shown in Table 4. We can conclude that our proposed methodology overpowers the existing classification algorithms [7–9] in terms of F1 and accuracy score.

Table 3 Prediction result and accuracy calculation

S. no	Original sample	Predicted sample	Accuracy (%)
1	No tumor	No tumor	100
2	Tumor	Tumor	100
3	Tumor	Tumor	100
4	No tumor	No tumor	100
–	–	–	–
–	–	–	–
–	–	–	–
66	No tumor	Tumor	0
67	No tumor	No tumor	100
68	Tumor	Tumor	100
69	No tumor	No tumor	100

Table 4 Comparison chart

Serial no	Name of the classification algorithm	Accuracy score (%)	F1 score
1	Decision tree [1]	97	0.97
2	K-nearest neighbor [2]	94.2	0.94
3	Gaussian Naïve Bayes [3]	97	0.97
4	Random forest [4]	97	0.95
5	Support vector machine [5]	96	0.96
6	Multi-scale fusion U-Net [6]	96	0.96
7	**Proposed method**	**98.5**	**0.98**

5 Conclusion

In this paper, we have proposed a mammogram classification and detection algorithm using a convolutional approach. This algorithm is capable of preprocessing unstructured mammogram images from the BUSI dataset [10], collected from the web resource. It is responsible for the prediction of malignant and non-malignant mammogram images in terms of Yes (malignant sample) and No (non-malignant sample) values. It also generates an accuracy and F1 score through, which we can compare our proposed method with existing methods [7–9]. The experimental result shows that after applying the proposed and existing methods [7–9] on the BUSI dataset [10], and our technique is producing approximately 98.5% accuracy and 0.98 F1 scores on average. This result is considered to be satisfactory and based on this result, we can say that the proposed algorithm overpowers the efficiency of the existing method as described in Table 4. Novel preprocessing steps and modifications in the convolutional architecture using multiple layers make the proposed methodology unique. Due to high performance, novelty, ease of use, our proposed method is useful to develop any mobile or web applications in the future. Our method can be tested on various mammogram datasets to identify the generic performance of the proposed method in the future. The performance of our method may be increased by making necessary modifications in algorithm and code.

References

1. Yi L, Yi W (2017) Decision tree model in the diagnosis of breast cancer. In: 2017 International conference on computer technology, electronics and communication (ICCTEC), 2017, pp 176–179. https://doi.org/10.1109/ICCTEC.2017.00046
2. Moh'd H, Abdulsalam A, Mohannad A (2016) Breast cancer detection using K-nearest neighbor machine learning algorithm. pp 35–39. https://doi.org/10.1109/DeSE.2016.8
3. Dai B, Chen R-C, Zhu S-Z, Zhang W-W (2018) Using random forest algorithm for breast cancer diagnosis. In: 2018 International symposium on computer, consumer and control (IS3C), 2018, pp. 449–452. https://doi.org/10.1109/IS3C.2018.00119
4. Gao S, Li H (2012) Breast cancer diagnosis based on support vector machine. In: 2012 2nd International conference on uncertainty reasoning and knowledge engineering, 2012, pp 240–243. https://doi.org/10.1109/URKE.2012.6319555
5. Kamel H, Abdulah D, Al-Tuwaijari JM (2019) Cancer classification using gaussian naive bayes algorithm. In: 2019 international engineering conference (IEC), 2019, pp 165–170. https://doi.org/10.1109/IEC47844.2019.8950650
6. Li J, Cheng L, Xia T, Ni H, Li J (2021) Multi-scale fusion U-net for the segmentation of breast lesions. IEEE Access 9:137125–137139. https://doi.org/10.1109/ACCESS.2021.3117578
7. Ara S, Das A, Dey A (2021) Malignant and Benign breast cancer classification using machine learning algorithms. In: 2021 international conference on artificial intelligence (ICAI), 2021, pp 97–101. https://doi.org/10.1109/ICAI52203.2021.9445249
8. Amrane M, Oukid S, Gagaoua I, Ensarİ T (2018) Breast cancer classification using machine learning. In: 2018 Electric electronics, computer science, biomedical engineering's meeting (EBBT), 2018, pp 1–4. https://doi.org/10.1109/EBBT.2018.8391453
9. Bılgıç B (2021) Comparison of breast cancer and skin cancer diagnoses using deep learning method. In: 2021 29th signal processing and communications applications conference (SIU), pp 1–4. https://doi.org/10.1109/SIU53274.2021.9477992
10. Al-Dhabyani W, Gomaa M, Khaled H, Fahmy A (2020) Dataset of breast ultrasound images. Data in Brief. https://doi.org/10.1016/j.dib.2019.104863

Emotion Recognition from EEG Data Using Hybrid Deep Learning Approach

Trishita Dhara and Pawan Kumar Singh

Abstract Emotion recognition from EEG signals is a challenging task. Researchers over the past few years have been working extensively to achieve high accuracy in emotion recognition from physiological signals. Several feature extraction methods, as well as machine learning models, have been proposed by earlier studies. In this paper, we propose a hybrid CNN-LSTM model for multi-class emotion recognition from EEG signals. The experiment is conducted on the standard benchmark DEAP dataset. The proposed model gives test accuracies of 96.87% and 97.31% on valence and arousal dimensions, respectively. Furthermore, the proposed model also succeeds in achieving state-of-the-art accuracy in both valence and arousal dimensions.

Keywords Emotion recognition · Electroencephalogram (EEG) signals · DEAP dataset · Deep learning

1 Introduction

Emotions are an important factor in our life. It controls our physical and psychological changes. Emotions can be positive or negative. Some positive emotions include happiness, hope, pride, etc., while some examples of negative emotions are regret, sadness, hatred, and guilt. Emotion models can be of two types, discrete models, and dimensional models. The former categorize emotions into discrete entities like sadness, frustration, happiness, anger, fear, etc. According to the dimension model, there are three dimensions of emotion, namely, valence, arousal, and dominance. High valence indicates positive emotion, and low valence indicates negative emotion. Arousal indicates the level of enthusiasm developed in the person. Excited, happy, and tensed are some examples of high arousal, and depressed, calm, and tired are some examples of low arousal. Dominance is the level of control associated with an emotion. A pictorial representation of valence-arousal space is depicted in Fig. 1.

T. Dhara · P. K. Singh (✉)
Department of Information Technology, Jadavpur University, Kolkata-700106, West Bengal, India
e-mail: pawansingh.ju@gmail.com

© The Author(s), under exclusive license to Springer Nature Singapore Pte Ltd. 2023

J. K. Mandal and D. De (eds.), *Frontiers of ICT in Healthcare*, Lecture Notes in Networks and Systems 519, https://doi.org/10.1007/978-981-19-5191-6_15

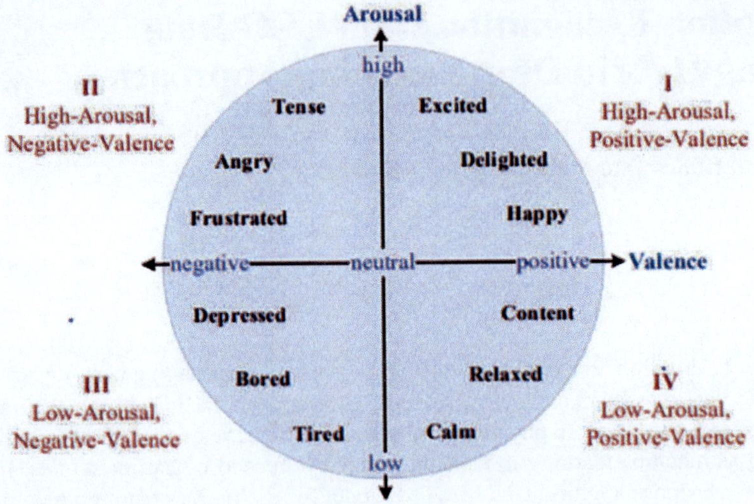

Fig. 1 Diagrammatic representation of a two-dimensional valence-arousal space [2]

Electroencephalogram (EEG) captures the electrical activity of the brain [1]. During the procedure, electrodes with thin wires are pasted on our scalp, which detects voltage fluctuations in brain neurons. These physiological signals are used for the recognition of emotion. The steps involved in the process are data preprocessing, feature extraction, classification, and evaluation. In this paper, we performed emotion recognition from EEG signals using a hybrid combination of convolution neural network (CNN) and long short-term memory (LSTM) models. The testing is done on the benchmark DEAP dataset. The flowchart of the proposed work is depicted in Fig. 2.

The paper is organized in the following manner. The literature survey is described in Sect. 2, whereas the dataset description is presented in Sect. 3. Experimental setup for recognition of emotions from EEG signals is presented in Sect. 4, and the detailed results are shown in Sect. 5, followed by conclusion and the scope for future work in Sect. 6.

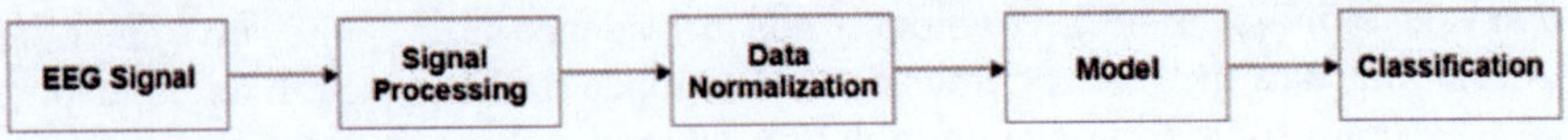

Fig. 2 Flowchart of our proposed work

2 Related Work

A number of researches have been conducted in the field of EEG-based emotion recognition. The most common approach is the extraction of features from preprocessed EEG data over a specific time window, followed by classification using supervised machine learning models. Wang et al. [3] compared wavelet features, power spectral density (PSD), and nonlinear dynamic features using support vector machine (SVM). You and Liu [4] used the DEAP dataset. The data was sliced into 5 s segments. For each piece of data, some time-domain features such as mean value, variance, and a second-order differential mean value were extracted. They reached the highest classification accuracy greater than 80% using an autoencoder neural network. Zhan et al. [5] extracted PSD of four frequency bands from EEG. It achieved an accuracy of 84.07 and 82.95% on arousal and valence, respectively, in the DEAP dataset, using a shallow depth-wise parallel CNN. Parui et al. [6] extracted several features from EEG signals and optimized them using correlation matrix, information gain calculation, and recursive feature elimination method. An XGBoost classifier was used for classification. The model achieved an accuracy of 75.97%, 74.206%, 75.234%, and 76.424% for valence, arousal, liking, and dominance, respectively. Aggarwal et al. [7] combined two gradient boosting machines (GBMs) based on supervised learning, XGBoost, and light GBM, for emotion classification on the DEAP dataset and obtained an accuracy of 77.11% for valence. Bagzir et al. [8] used discrete wavelet transform to change the EEG signals, which were decomposed into gamma, beta, alpha, and theta bands, to extract the frequency spectrum characteristics of each frequency band. Then, an SVM, k-nearest-neighbor (KNN), and an artificial neural network (ANN) were used for classification. The best accuracy rates on valence and arousal were 91.1% and 91.3%, respectively.

In recent years, deep learning has drawn the attention of many researchers besides traditional machine learning approaches to obtain a state-of-the-art accuracy in the realm of EEG-based emotion recognition.

3 DEAP Dataset

In this paper, the DEAP dataset [9] is used for emotion recognition. The dataset consists of EEG signals of 32 subjects. Each subject watched 40 music videos of one-minute duration containing different emotions, while their EEG was recorded. Each subject also rated the level of valence, arousal, liking, and dominance for each video. The data is stored in 32 files, one file for each participant. Each file consists of a total of 40 channels out of which 32 channels contain EEG data. The data is preprocessed and available in both Python (.dat) and MATLAB (.mat) format. Our experiment is conducted using the.dat files. The dataset also contains frontal face video recordings for 22 subjects which can be used for the multi-modal emotion

Table 1 Categorization of valence and arousal ratings

Valence rating	Valence label	Arousal rating	Arousal label
1–2	0	1–2	0
2–3	1	2–3	1
3–4	2	3–4	2
4–5	3	4–5	3
5–6	4	5–6	4
6–7	5	6–7	5
7–8	6	7–8	6
8–9	7	8–9	7

recognition task. The DEAP dataset is used as a standard benchmark dataset for emotion recognition by researchers across the world.

4 Proposed Methodology

4.1 Data Preparation

The time waves of EEG data were carefully observed and analyzed. Out of 32 channels containing EEG data 14 channels were selected for the emotion recognition task. The 14 channels are Fp1, AF3, F3, F7, T7, P7, Pz, O2, P4, P8, CP6, FC6, AF4, and Fz [9]. The EEG data is windowed as there is a possibility of quick detection of emotional states. Therefore, raw EEG data is sliced to 2 seconds temporal windows with 1 second overlap. Out of the four labels, the valence and arousal labels were considered for our study. The rating of each label had a value between 1 and 9. We developed a multi-class classification model, and the labels were categorized into eight classes each for valence and arousal. The categorization of labels is presented in Table 1. Finally, all data is normalized and the data is split into three sets train set, test set, and validation set. The train set consists of 60% data, whereas the validation and test set each consist of 20% data.

4.2 Convolutional Neural Network (CNN)

CNN is one of the most widely implemented deep learning models. It is a type of feed-forward artificial neural network. A CNN layer consists of a convolution layer, followed by a nonlinearity operation (commonly ReLU) which is generally followed by a pooling layer. The general architecture of CNN is demonstrated in Fig. 3. 2D CNN is commonly used in computer vision applications as it has the ability to learn complex spatial patterns from images. However, 2D CNN cannot be applied

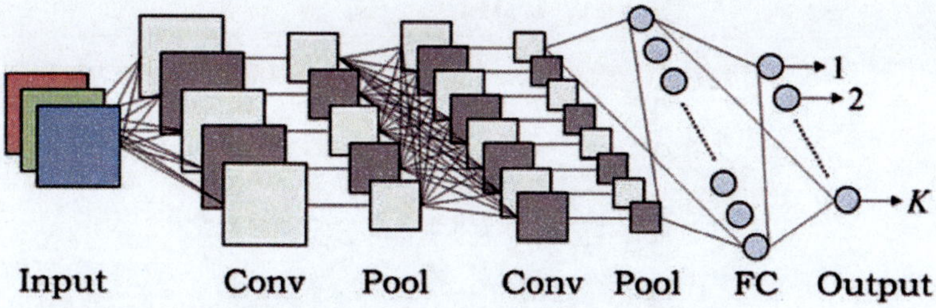

Fig. 3 General CNN architecture [11]

in all fields of application. For analysis of 1D signals, 1D CNN is very efficient and it has been successfully applied in biomedical data classification, structural health monitoring, etc. [10]. In our study, we have used 1D CNN to extract meaningful features from the EEG data.

4.3 Long Short-Term Memory (LSTM)

LSTM is a special type of recurrent neural network (RNN) [12]. The major disadvantage of RNN is short-term memory. To overcome this difficulty, LSTM is implemented which has various gates to regulate the flow of data and it is very efficient in learning long sequences of data and making predictions. The various gates are input gate, output gate, and forget gate. The input and output gates regulate the flow of data, and the forget gate determines if the data is to be kept or discarded. Finally, the output from the different gates is used to calculate the cell state. The architecture of LSTM with its different gates is represented in Fig. 4. The LSTM is widely used for speech recognition, text classification, sentiment analysis, and so on. While CNN is efficient in extracting spatial features, LSTM is good at analyzing temporal signals.

4.4 Proposed Hybrid CNN-LSTM Model

In our study, we used a hybrid model combining 1D-CNN and LSTM, followed by fully connected layers. The input is passed to the model in batches of size 256. The first layer is a 1D-CNN layer with 128 filters having kernel size 3. The CNN is followed by a max-pooling layer and dropout. The next layer is LSTM having 64 units followed by dropout. The output from the LSTM layer is flattened and passed to a fully connected layer having 32 units which are also followed by dropout. Finally, the output from the first fully connected layer is passed to another fully connected layer with 8 units, and softmax is applied to obtain the final output. All dropouts were implemented with a probability of 0.2 as it helped us to achieve optimal results. The

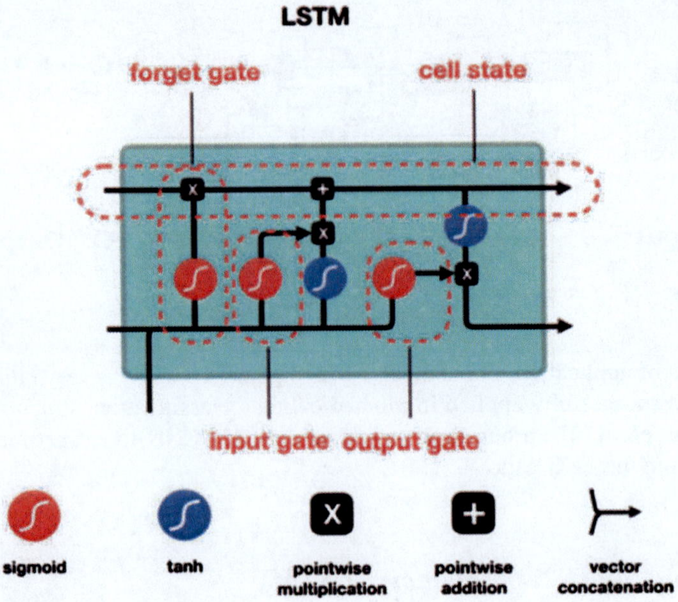

Fig. 4 Schematic diagram of the LSTM architecture [12]

activation function used in the convolution layer, and the first fully connected layer is ReLU. The ReLU adds sparsity and reduces the chances of vanishing gradient problems. The following is the expression for ReLU:

$$F(x) = \max(0, x) \tag{1}$$

The proposed hybrid CNN-LSTM model is presented in Fig. 5. The model is trained for 50 epochs.

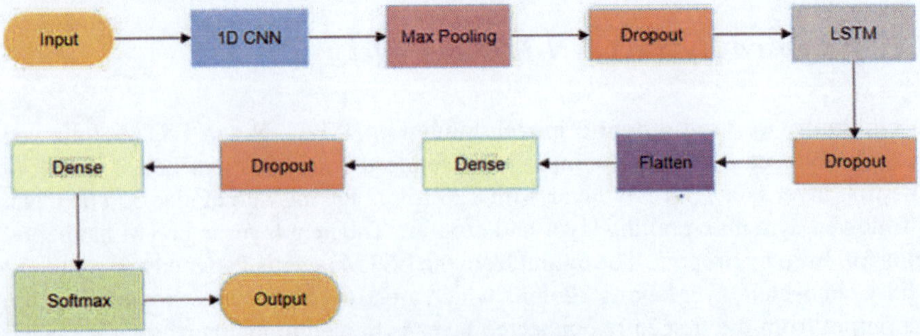

Fig. 5 Workflow of our proposed hybrid CNN-LSTM model

5 Results

In the proposed work, the EEG data for emotion recognition is collected from the benchmark DEAP dataset and a hybrid deep learning model is used to get better results as compared to existing works. As mentioned earlier in Sect. 4.1, we performed a multi-class classification on the arousal and valence dimensions. We tested our model on 20% of the entire data. In the study, we have obtained an accuracy of 97.32% and 96.89% on arousal and valence dimensions, respectively. We have also tried with different train, test, and validation ratios such as 50:25:25 and 50:20:30; however, best results were obtained for the 60:20:20 ratio and those results are presented in Table 2.

The results obtained from our study have been compared with results obtained by some of the existing models on the DEAP dataset. Performance comparison of the proposed model with some recent state-of-the-art models is presented in Table 3, and it indicates that our model has outperformed the existing models.

The graphs showing the variations of validation accuracy versus validation loss with respect to epoch on the arousal and valence dimensions are presented in Figs. 6. and 7, respectively. It can be seen from Figs. 6 and 7 that the loss initially decreases steeply and ultimately gets flattened near 50 epochs which indicates that the model has been completely trained at 50 epochs.

Table 2 Results were obtained by using our proposed work on the DEAP dataset

Parameter	Valence	Arousal
Test loss	0.2187	0.2094
Test accuracy	96.87%	97.31%
Train loss	0.1799	0.1770
Train accuracy	97.85%	98.25%
Validation loss	0.2185	0.2091
Validation accuracy	96.83%	97.25%

Table 3 Comparison of existing models with the proposed model

Reference	Model	Valence accuracy (%)	Arousal accuracy (%)
Zhan et al. [5]	CNN	82.95	84.07
Parui et al. [6]	XGBoost	75.97	74.206
Bazgir et al. [8]	SVM	91.1	91.3
Garg et al. [13]	GoogleNet	92.19	61.23
Alhagry et al. [14]	LSTM	85.45	85.65
Proposed work	CNN + LSTM	96.87	97.31

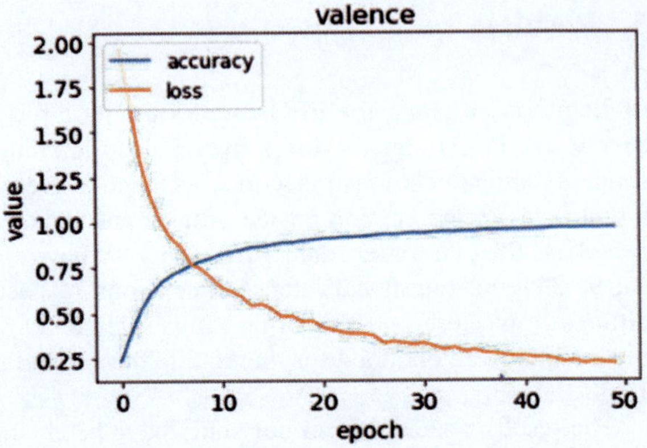

Fig. 6 Variation of validation loss versus validation accuracy with epoch for valence dimension

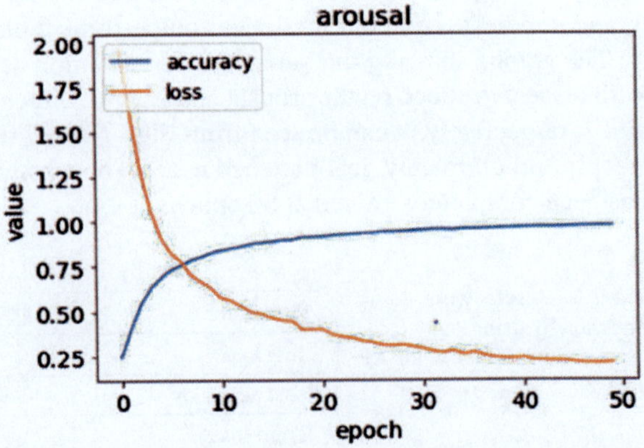

Fig. 7 Variation of validation loss versus validation accuracy with epoch for arousal dimension

The confusion matrices for valence and arousal dimensions are presented in Figs. 8 and 9, respectively. It can be observed that label 2 in valence has the lowest number of mismatches, whereas label 3 in arousal has low mismatches. Hence, from Table 1, an emotional state having a valence level between 3 and 4, and an arousal level between 4 and 5 can be most accurately predicted by the proposed model.

6 Conclusion and Scope for Future Work

Recognition of emotion from EEG signals is a challenging task as accurate prediction is necessary. Emotion recognition is applied for patient monitoring and medical diagnosis, therefore, inaccurate prediction can lead to the wrong diagnosis, which may lead to wrong treatment. The proposed model gives impressive recognition accuracies of 96.87% and 97.31% on the test set for both valence and arousal dimensions, respectively, on the DEAP dataset. The performance of the proposed model

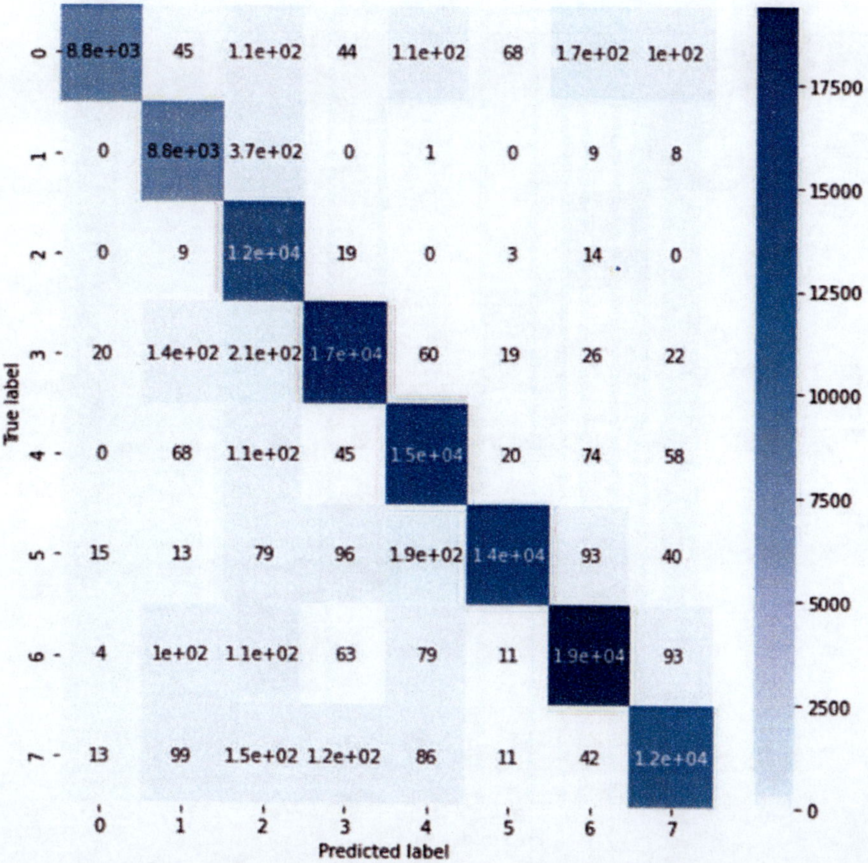

Fig. 8 Confusion matrix generated by the proposed model for valence dimension

has surpassed most of the previous works in the field of EEG-based emotion recognition. We have proposed a multi-class emotion classification model so that both the valence and arousal levels can be predicted more precisely than traditional binary classification.

Researchers have already applied ensemble learning by combining supervised machine learning models. In the future, ensemble deep learning models can be developed to achieve state-of-the-art accuracy in emotion recognition from EEG signals. Also, the models should be tested on different datasets to ensure the model is robust and not sensitive to any particular dataset.

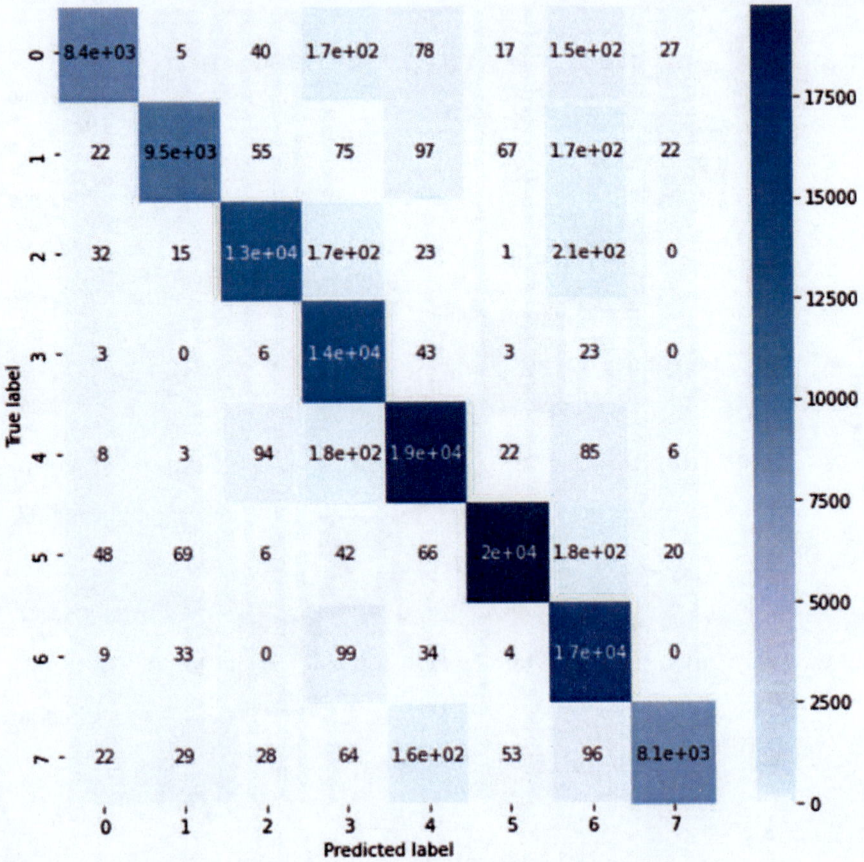

Fig. 9 Confusion matrix generated by the proposed model for arousal dimension

References

1. Electroencephalogram (EEG) (2021). https://www.hopkinsmedicine.org/health/treatment-tests-and-therapies/electroencephalogram-eeg. Accessed on 12 Oct 2021
2. Yu L-C, Lee L-H, Hao S, Wang J, He Y, Hu J, Lai KR, Zhang X (2016) Building chinese affective resources in valence-arousal dimensions. https://www.researchgate.net/publication/304124018
3. Wang X-W, Nie D, Lu B-L (2014) Emotional state classification from EEG data using machine learning approach. Neurocomputing 129. https://doi.org/10.1016/j.neucom.2013.06.046
4. You SD, Liu C (2020) Classification of user preference for music videos based on EEG recordings. In: Proceedings of the IEEE 2nd global conference on life sciences and technologies (LifeTech), Kyoto, Japan, Mar 2020
5. Zhan Y, Vai MI, Barma S, Pun SH, Li JW, Mak PU (2019) A computation resource friendly convolutional neural network engine for EEG-based emotion recognition. In: 2019 IEEE international conference on computational intelligence and virtual environments for measurement systems and applications (CIVEMSA). IEEE, pp 1–6, June 2019

6. Parui S, Bajiya AKR, Samanta D, Chakravorty N (2019) Emotion recognition from EEG signal using XGBoost algorithm. In: 2019 IEEE 16th India council international conference (INDICON). IEEE, pp 1–4, Dec 2019
7. Aggarwal S, Aggarwal L, Rihal MS, Aggarwal S (2018) EEG based participant independent emotion classification using gradient boosting machines. In: Proceedings of the IEEE 8th international advance computing conference (IACC), pp 266–271, Greater Noida, India, Dec 2018
8. Bazgir O, Mohammadi Z, Habibi SAH (2018) Emotion recognition with machine learning using EEG signals. In: Proceedings of the 25th national and 3rd international iranian conference on biomedical engineering (ICBME), 5p, Qom, Iran, June 2018
9. Koelstra S, Muhl C, Soleymani M, Lee JS, Yazdani A, Ebrahimi T, Pun T, Nijholt A, Patras I (2012) DEAP: a database for emotion analysis using physiological signals. IEEE Trans Affect Comput 3:18–31
10. Kiranyaz S, Avci O, Abdeljaber O, Ince T, Gabbouj M, Inman DJ (2021) 1D convolutional neural networks and applications: a survey. Mech Syst Sign Process. https://doi.org/10.1016/j.ymssp.2020.107398
11. Hidaka A, Kurita T (2017) Consecutive dimensionality reduction by canonical correlation analysis for visualization of convolutional neural networks. In: Proceedings of the ISCIE international symposium on stochastic systems theory and its applications, vol 2017, pp 160–167. https://doi.org/10.5687/sss.2017.160
12. Illustrated guide to LSTM's and GRU's: a step by step explanation. https://towardsdatascience.com/illustrated-guide-to-lstms-and-gru-s-a-step-by-step-explanation-44e9eb85bf21. Accessed on 21 Oct 2021
13. Garg D, Verma GK (2020) Emotion recognition in valence-arousal space from multi-channel EEG data and wavelet based deep learning framework. Procedia Comput Sci. https://doi.org/10.1016/j.procs.2020.04.093
14. Alhagry S, Aly A, El-Khoribi R (2017) Emotion recognition based on EEG using LSTM recurrent neural network. Int J Adv Comput Sci Appl 8(10)

Colon Cancer Prediction with Transfer Learning and K-Means Clustering

Tina Babu and Rekha R. Nair

Abstract The automatic diagnosis of colon cancer is important for patients and their prognosis through the analysis of histopathological images. Traditional feature extraction methods extract low-level image features, and prior knowledge is required to choose meaningful features, which may be modified significantly by humans. Hence, unsupervised and supervised deep convolutions neural networks were utilized to analyze histopathological images of colon cancer. To overcome the impact of the unbalanced histopathology images in sub-classes, the balanced sub-classes are turned right and left, up and down, and rotated counter clockwise by 90° and 180°. The proposed experimental findings for supervised histopathological image classification of colon cancer demonstrate that $Inception\_V3$ and $Inception\ ResNet\_V2$ outperform current algorithms. These findings suggest that the $Inception\_ResNet\_V2$ network is superior deep learning architecture for analyzing histopathological images for diagnosis colon cancers. As a result, in order to perform unsupervised image analysis, $Inception\_ResNet\_V2$ is utilized to extract features from colon cancer histopathology images. In addition, a new autoencoder network was created to convert the features collected by $Inception\_ResNet\_V2$ to a low-dimensional space for image clustering analysis. The test results demonstrate that the proposed autoencoder network outperforms the $Inception\_ResNet\_V2$ network in terms of clustering.

Keywords Autoencoder · Colon cancer · Clustering · Histopathological images · Transfer learning · Classification

T. Babu (✉)
Department of Computer Science and Engineering, School of Engineering,
Dayananda Sagar University, Bengaluru, Karnataka, India
e-mail: tinababup@gmail.com

R. R. Nair
Department of Computer Applications, School of Engineering, Dayananda Sagar University,
Bengaluru, Karnataka, India
e-mail: rekhasanju.sanju@gmail.com

© The Author(s), under exclusive license to Springer Nature Singapore Pte Ltd. 2023
J. K. Mandal and D. De (eds.), *Frontiers of ICT in Healthcare*, Lecture Notes in Networks and Systems 519, https://doi.org/10.1007/978-981-19-5191-6_16

1 Introduction

Colon cancer is among the most prevalent and lethal cancers in women (170,000 incident cases, 14.9 million disability-adjusted life years and 535,000 deaths) [1]. As a result, early detection of colon cancer has become critical. Biopsy techniques are still the most commonly used methods for correctly diagnosing colon cancer. The analysis of histopathological images, on the other hand, is a time-consuming and difficult task that necessitates the expertise of professionals. Furthermore, the level of experience of the pathologists involved may have an impact on the research outcome. As a result, computer-aided examination of histopathological images is becoming increasingly crucial in the diagnosis and prognosis of colon cancer [2].

Traditional feature extraction methods rely on supervised information, like local binary pattern (LBP), gray-level co-occurrence matrix (GLCM), and histogram [3, 4]. Apart from that, in order to identify relevant features, prior knowledge of the data is essential, which decreases feature extraction efficiency and increases computational cost. Only a few low-level and unrepresentative histopathological image features were retrieved in the end of the process. As a result, the final model may produce poor classification results.

Image analysis has been used to identify colon cancer for more than 40 years, and there have been numerous major scientific successes in the field. Based on their techniques, these studies may be divided into two types: those that use traditional machine learning methods and those that use deep learning methods. A multistep segmentation based on cytological images was proposed as a colon cancer diagnosis system [5]. There were four categorization models used:: multilayer perceptron(MLP) with backpropagation algorithm, learning vector quantization (LVQ), support vector machines (SVM), and probabilistic neural network (PNN).

Deep learning algorithms can retrieve information from data, extract features, and develop advanced abstract data representations automatically [6]. Deep learning algorithms can solve traditional feature extraction challenges and have been used successfully in computer vision, biomedical science, and a variety of other fields [7, 8]. Deep learning (DL) and other cutting-edge artificial intelligence (AI) approaches excel at classification and prediction. Multiple major applications of DL, mainly convolutional neural network (CNN), analysis of WSI for breast [9], lung cancer [10], skin [11], and prostate [12] tumors, have been reported. The majority of recent CNN for CRC WSI analysis focused on pathology work after cancer identification, like grade classification, tumor cell classification [13], and detection and survival prediction [14]. Despite their high degree of accuracy, their research sample sizes were limited and did not properly represent the various histologic types of CRC described. Tubular, mucinous, and signet ring cells are among the variants. When applied to different independent samples, these limitations increase prediction error. Meanwhile, the majority of DL models were constructed using a single data source without significant validation using independent data [15]. They estimated patch accuracy without assessing WSIs or patients.

This research utilizes deep learning approaches to analyze histological images of colon cancer, based on the significant feature extraction benefits of deep learning and the limitations in histopathology image analysis of colon cancer. To begin, advanced deep convolutional neural networks, such as $Inception\_ResNet\_V2$ [16], $Inception\_V3$ [17], were used, combined with techniques in transfer learning to classify the histopathological images of colon cancer [18]. Later, deep learning was combined with clustering, and the autoencoder network's dimension-reduction functionality was used. Thus, using the $Inception\_ResNet\_V2$ network, proposed a new autoencoder network structure in which nonlinear transformations are used to extract features from histopathological images of colon cancer. The extracted features are effectively mapped to a lower-dimensional space as a result of this. The newly created features are then used as input for the traditional clustering approach known as K-means, which is used to perform clustering analysis on colon cancer histology images.

2 Methodology

The $Inception\_ResNet\_V2$ network is used to extract features for clustering analysis of histopathological images of colon cancer because of its excellent performance in classifying these images and the benefit of automatically eliminating features. Each histopathological image of colon cancer can be well represented by the extracted features of the 1536-dimension vector formed by the $Inception\_ResNet\_V2$ network before its final classification layer. The collected feature vectors are fed into a clustering algorithm, which performs clustering analysis on colon cancer histopathology pictures, as illustrated in Fig. 1.

The $Inception\_ResNet\_V2$ network is used to extract features for clustering analysis of histopathological images of colon cancer and performance well when classifying these images. It also automatically removes the features from the images. Each extracted features of colon cancer histopathological image with 1536-dimension vector formed by the $Inception\_ResNet\_V2$ network before its final classification layer. The collected feature vectors are fed into a clustering algorithm, which performs clustering analysis on histological images of colon cancer, as illustrated in Fig. 1.

In this research, the simple and quick clustering technique K-means is used to perform the clustering analysis. Silhouette Score (SSE) is used to find the best K. The retrieved features by the Inception $ResNet\_V2$ network for each colon cancer histological images are considered a description images, and the K-means clustering method utilized to cluster colon cancer histopathological images. In addition, to improve clustering outcomes and clustering findings, a novel autoencoder network was created to convert the 1536-dimension vector to a two-dimensional vector via a nonlinear transformation. The proposed technique displays colon cancer histopathological images in a deep-dimensional space. There are two encode layers with neuron sizes of 500 and 2 and two matching decode layers to recreate the original input. The

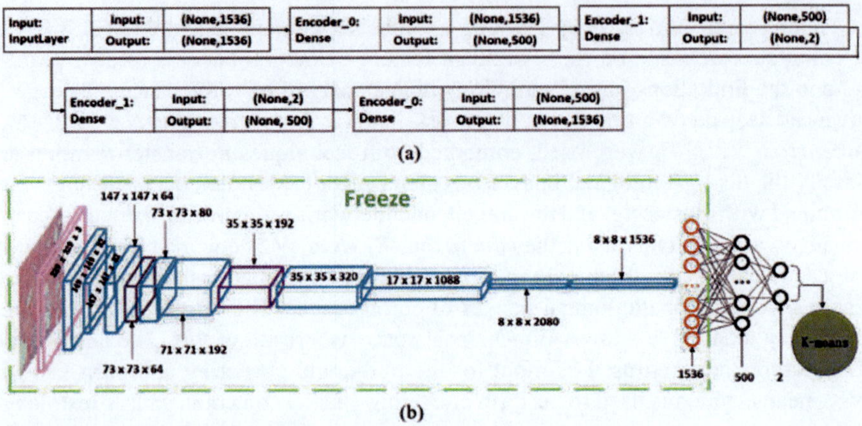

Fig. 1 Proposed framework with autoencoder with $Inception\_ResNet\_V2$, **a** Autoencoder network, **b** $Inception\_ResNet\_V2$ with autoencoder network

1536-dimension feature vector generated from a colon cancer histopathology image by the $InceptionResNetV2$ network will be transformed to a two-dimensional feature vector by training the layers indicated in Fig. 1a. The two-dimensional feature vector is then fed into K-means, which performs grouping analysis on colon cancer histopathology images. The whole network is seen in Fig. 1b.

3 Dataset Experimented

The framework is evaluated utilizing colon-pathological imaging data from Ishita Pathology Center (IPC), Allahabad (India), on different magnifications of the tissue sample. The H&E stained-colon biopsy slide was observed at 4×, 10×, and 40× magnifications, and obtained images with 640 × 480 resolution. There are many 100 and 150 images for normal and malignant under a specific magnification. The images were taken with a Magcam CD5 with Olympus CX33. Dr. Ranjana Srivastava evaluated the H&E slides, IPC Senior Consultant, prepared the ground truth labels and data set.

4 Performance Measures

Specificity, sensitivity, kappa, diagnostic odds ratio (DOR), positive predictive value (PPV), area under the receiver operating characteristic curve (AUC), F1 score, and accuracy are used to evaluate the classification findings. Equations 1–8 show the descriptions of the assessments.

$$\text{Accuracy} = \frac{\text{TP} + \text{TN}}{\text{TP} + \text{TN} + \text{FP} + \text{FN}} \quad (1)$$

$$\text{Sensitivity} = \frac{\text{TP}}{\text{TP} + \text{FN}} \quad (2)$$

$$\text{Specificity} = \frac{\text{TN}}{\text{TN} + \text{FP}} \quad (3)$$

$$\text{PPV} = \frac{\text{TP}}{\text{TP} + \text{FP}} \quad (4)$$

$$\text{DOR} = \frac{\text{TP} * \text{TN}}{\text{FP} + \text{FN}} \quad (5)$$

$$\text{F1}_{\text{Score}} = \frac{2 * \text{precision} * \text{recall}}{\text{precision} + \text{recall}} \quad (6)$$

$$\text{recall} = \frac{\text{TP}}{\text{TP} + \text{FN}} \quad (7)$$

$$\text{Kappa} = \frac{p_0 - p_e}{1 - p_e} \quad (8)$$

$$p_0 = \frac{N_{\text{rec}}}{N_{\text{all}}} \quad (9)$$

$$p_e = \frac{\Sigma N_{\text{true}_i} * N_{\text{pre}_i}}{N_{\text{all}} * N_{\text{all}}} \quad (10)$$

When the linked classifier is optimal, DOR will reach infinity. According to reports, a diagnosis system is efficient if the Specificity $\geq$ 95%, Sensitivity $\geq$ 80%, DOR$\geq$ 100, and PPV$\geq$ 95%. AUC values vary from 0 to 1, with higher scores indicating greater model performance. The picture level test accuracy is determined by P_0, and P_e is the proportion of the aggregate of the combination of the quantity of the actual scans within every group as well as the expected quantity of scans within this group to the square of the aggregate cases reported. This determines Kappa value.

The variables used in the adjusted random index (ARI) are p (prior to and following clustering, the quantity of sets containing specimens in the similar group), q (groups of specimens in a similar cluster that have been segmented into different sets using the technique of clustering), r (samples across different clusters that were incorrectly grouped into a similar set by that of the approach of clustering), and s (the clustering algorithm incorrectly clustered samples from different clusters into the same cluster). Adjusted mutual information (AMI) is based on R, the initial partition, and T, which is clustering method. E MI (R, T) indicates the anticipated MI across the original partition R and the clustering T, and MI(R, T) denotes the mutual information between two divisions R and T. $H(R)$, $H(T)$ are the entropies of the actual source partition R with the approach of T, individually. AMI is indeed a type of similarity measure that would be used to compare a clustering method's clustering T with the sample's actual structure R. This eliminates any consensus impact caused by the difference in clustering and the initial structure. This is analogous to what the Rand index is updated by the adjusted Rand index. The studies used functions from the skilearn library (a Python package), such like ARI, silhouette_score (SSE), AMI, and linear_assignment (ACC).

$$\text{ARI} = \frac{2 * (\text{ps}) - (\text{qr})}{(p+q)(q+s) + (p+r)(r+s)} \tag{11}$$

$$\text{AMI}(R, T) = \frac{\text{MI}(R, T) - \text{EMI}(R, T)}{\max H(R), H(T) - \text{EMI}(R, T)} \tag{12}$$

5 Experiment Result and Analysis

The work has been tested on Windows 10 using MATrix LABoratory (MATLAB) R2019a and the Intel(R) Core(TM)i5-6200U processor @ 2.30 GHz 2.40 GHz with 8 GigaByte (GB) Random Access Memory (RAM). Irrespective of how the attributes were collected, the optimum SSE value was calculated when the number of clusters was two. This shows that colon cancer pathological images must be divided into two categories: benign and malignant tumors, which corresponds to the real-life situation. The proposed framework with autoencoders and K-means clustering was experimented with Inception V3 and Inception Resenet V2 and is illustrated in Table 1. The Inception Resenet V2 was shown to outperform when compared to Inception V2. 4× magnification has given the highest performance in terms of accuracy, specificity, and sensitivity of 98.89, 97.01, and 97.89.

Figure 2 depicts the Inception_ResNet_V2s' loss function for such two-class classification of pathological images of colon cancer on the original and augmented data, accordingly. Table 2 shows that the results achieved from of the Inception_ResNet_V2 model do have a favorable ranking of most of the research identified previously regarding the categorization of pathological scans of colon cancer on extended datasets for the classification concerning two classes. The Inception ResNet V2 network's performance on raw datasets is superior to that of other models. As a result, the Inception_ResNet_V2 deep learning network with residual blocks is ideal for categorizing histopathology images of colon cancer. Additionally, more augmented histopathology imaging databases for colon cancer can help with categorization and diagnosis better (Fig. 3).

The following findings can be drawn from the proposed research: (1) Regarding ARI, SSE, AMI, and ACC for every dataset with varied magnification factors, the clustering performance of IRV2, AE, and K-means is superior to that of IRV2 K-means. This suggests that by capturing the features retrieved by the Inception_ResNet_V2 network, our suggested AE network may provide significantly more

Table 1 Performance of the proposed framework on various magnifications

Network	Measures	Magnification factors		
		4×	10×	40×
Inception V3	Accuracy	96.80	96.77	96.61
	Specificity	94.43	93.53	91.52
	Sensitivity	98.11	98.39	99.10
	F1 score	97.68	97.60	97.34
	PPV	97.50	96.51	95.79
	DOR	80,342	97,297	105,678
	Kappa	92.70	92.71	91.89
	AUC	99.51	99.10	99.30
Inception Resnet V2	Accuracy	98.89	97.01	97.99
	Specificity	97.01	93.02	93.79
	Sensitivity	97.89	97.89	98.98
	F1 score	97.85	96.77	98.01
	PPV	97.02	97.04	95.98
	DOR	186,885	117,883	146,673
	Kappa	94.74	91.99	94.01
	AUC	98.66	97.79	98.87

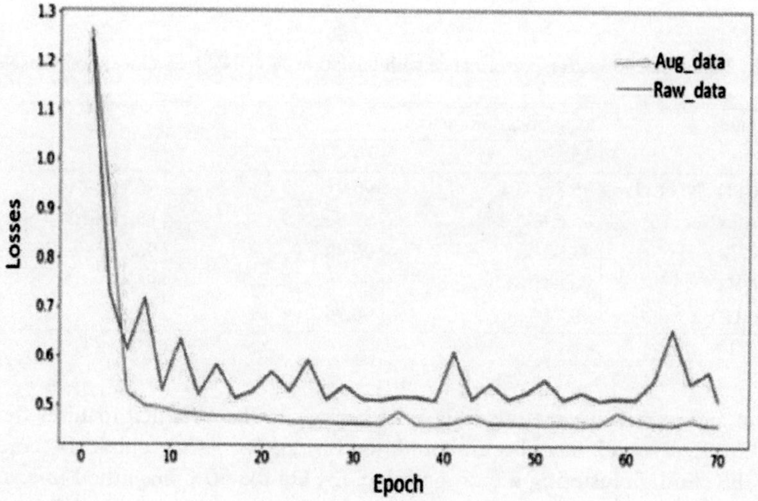

Fig. 2 Loss function change when trained with raw and augmented data on Inception_ResNet_V2 4× magnification for 2-class classification

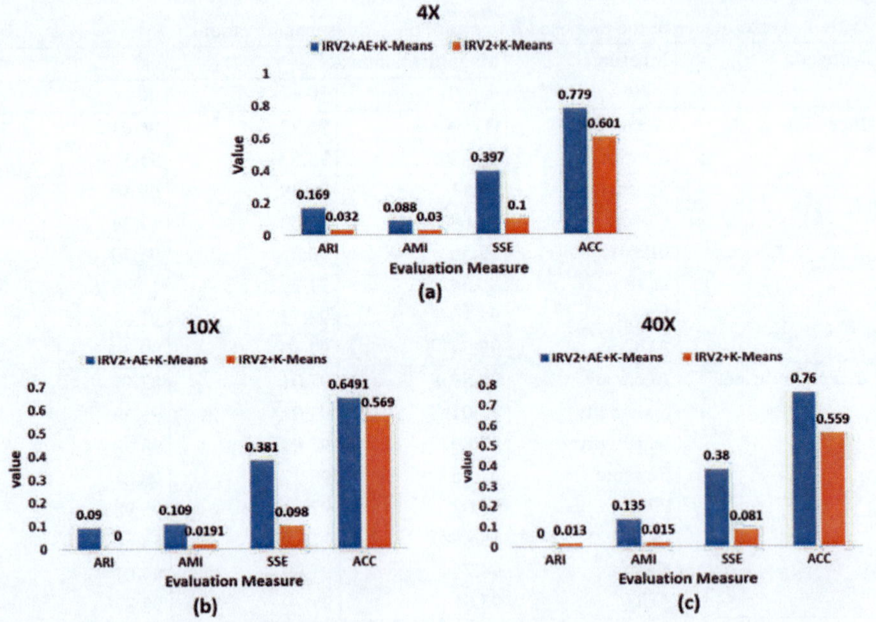

Fig. 3 Clustering results based on ARI, AMI, SSE, and ACC with **a** 4×, **b** 10×, **c** 40× magnification factors

Table 2 2-class categorization performance with Inception_V3 (INV3) and Inception_ResNet_V2 (IRV2)

Techniques	Magnification factors		
	4×	10×	40×
Raw_CSDCNN (29)	95.8 ± 3.1	96.9 ± 1.9	96.7 ± 2.0
Raw_AlexNet (25)	85.6 ± 4.8	83.5 ± 3.9	83.1 ± 1.9
Raw_RV2	97.90	96.88	96.98
Raw_NV3	96.84	96.76	96.49
Augm_IRV2	**98.74**	**98.76**	**98.60**

abstract and expressive features. (2) Whether or not the obtained features through Inception ResNet V2 have been altered, the SSE, ARI, ACC, and AMI scores for much the similar clustering are progressive. (3) On the 40× magnified images, the best clustering efficiency (ACC) is 59.3% with features produced by the Inception ResNet V2 network, and 76.4 percent with features generated by the proposed AE network utilizing extracted features as from Inception ResNet V2 network. In conclusion, features combining IRV2, AE, K-means, and IRV2, K-means have the superior ACC results of 76.4 and 59.3%, correspondingly.

The suggested framework is compared with the previous techniques on the dataset in Table 3. It is shown the proposed overcomes the current with 98.89% accuracy. The

Table 3 Proposed methods' comparison with the existing approaches

Dataset	Techniques used	Accuracy (%)
Babu et al. [19]	Inception V3/Bayesian optimized SVM	98.33
Babu et al. [4]	2DReCA Segmentation/Features/Random Forest	98.52
Babu et al. [20]	Wavelet features, salp swarm optimized neural network	98.50
Proposed	Inception ResNet V2, autoencoders, K-means clustering	98.89

existing methods were more into the segmentation and classification with optimized classifiers. Also, tuned segmentation techniques were also utilized to find the region of interest. Thus, the proposed method with transfer learning and autoencoders gives better performance.

6 Conclusion

Using the deep CNN-based Inception_ResNet_V2 built with transfer learning methods, this research offered methods for assessing pathological scans of colon cancer. The clustering conclusions drawn by that of the K-means employing characteristics derived from Inception_ResNet_V2 and adjusted using the presented AE seem to be significantly superior in AMI, ACC, ARI, and SSE than those obtained simply from Inception_ResNet_V2 features. The research also indicated that the findings of our experiments are superior to those discovered in other investigations. The Inception_ResNet_V2 network is better suited for analyzing colon cancer pathological images than the Inception_V3 network. As a future aspect, grading the cancerous colon tissues can be tried with transfer learning. A further generalized framework for various histopathological images classification can be developed.

References

1. Sung H, Ferlay J, Siegel R, Laversanne M, Soerjomataram I, Jemal A, Bray F (2021) Global cancer statistics 2020: Globocan estimates of incidence and mortality worldwide for 36 cancers in 185 countries. CA: Cancer J Clinicians 71(3):209–249
2. Babu T, Gupta D, Singh T, Hameed S, Zakariah M, Alotaibi YA (2021) Robust magnification independent colon biopsy grading system over multiple data sources. Comput Mater Continua 69(1):99–128
3. Babu T, Gupta D, Singh T, Hameed S, Nayar R, Veena R (2018) Cancer screening on Indian colon biopsy images using texture and morphological features. In: 2018 International Conference on Communication and Signal Processing (ICCSP), pp 0175–0181
4. Babu T, Singh T, Gupta D (2020) Colon cancer prediction using 2DReCA segmentation and hybrid features on histopathology images. IET Image Process 14:4144–4157(13)

5. Rathore S, Iftikhar MA, Chaddad A, Niazi T, Karasic T, Bilello M (2019) Segmentation and grade prediction of colon cancer digital pathology images across multiple institutions. Cancers 11(11)
6. Nair RR, Singh T, Sankar R, Gunndu K (2021) Multi-modal medical image fusion using lmf-gan-a maximum parameter infusion technique. J Intell Fuzzy Syst (Preprint):1–12
7. Nair RR, Singh T (2021) Mamif: multimodal adaptive medical image fusion based on B-spline registration and non-subsampled shearlet transform. Multimedia Tools Appl 80(12):19079–19105
8. Nair RR, Singh T (2021) An optimal registration on shearlet domain with novel weighted energy fusion for multi-modal medical images. Optik 225:165742
9. Bejnordi BE, Veta M, Va Diest JP, Beca F, Albarqouni S, Cetin-Atalay R, Qaiser T, Gracia IS, Shaban M, Kalinovsky A, Matsuda H, Seno S, Kartasalo K, Racoceanu D (2017) Diagnostic assessment of deep learning algorithms for detection of lymph node metastases in women with breast cancer. JAMA 318:2199–2210
10. Coudray N, Ocampo P, Sakellaropoulos T, Narula N, Snuderl M, Fenyö D, Moreira A, Razavian N, Tsirigos A (2018) Classification and mutation prediction from non-small cell lung cancer histopathology images using deep learning. Nat Med 24:10
11. Yu L, Chen H, Dou Q, Qin J, Heng P-A (2017) Automated melanoma recognition in dermoscopy images via very deep residual networks. IEEE Trans Med Imaging 36(4):994–1004
12. Bulten W, Pinckaers H, Boven H, Vink R, Bel T, Ginneken B, Laak J, van de Kaa CH, Litjens G (2020) Automated deep-learning system for gleason grading of prostate cancer using biopsies: a diagnostic study. Lancet Oncol 21
13. Ahmad C, Camel T (2017) Texture analysis of abnormal cell images for predicting the continuum of colorectal cancer. Anal Cell Pathol (Amst) 8428102
14. Skrede O-J, De Raedt S, Kleppe A, Hveem T, Liestøl K, Maddison J, Askautrud H, Pradhan M, Nesheim J, Albregtsen F, Farstad I, Domingo E, Church D, Nesbakken A, Shepherd N, Tomlinson I, Kerr R, Novelli M, Kerr D, Danielsen H (2020) Deep learning for prediction of colorectal cancer outcome: a discovery and validation study. The Lancet 395:350–360
15. Xie J, Liu R, Luttrell J, Zhang C (2019) Deep learning based analysis of histopathological images of breast cancer. Front Genetics 10
16. Szegedy C, Vanhoucke V, Ioffe S, Shlens J, Wojna Z (2015) Rethinking the inception architecture for computer vision
17. Szegedy C, Ioffe S, Vanhoucke V, Alemi AA (2017) Inception-v4, inception-resnet and the impact of residual connections on learning. In: Proceedings of the thirty-first AAAI conference on Artificial Intelligence, AAAI'17. AAAI Press, pp 4278–4284
18. Spanhol FA, Oliveira LS, Petitjean C, Heutte L (2016) A dataset for breast cancer histopathological image classification. IEEE Trans Biomed Eng 63(7):1455–1462
19. Babu T, Singh T, Gupta D, Hameed S (2021) Colon cancer prediction on histological images using deep learning features and Bayesian optimized SVM. J Intell Fuzzy Syst 41:5275–5286
20. Babu T, Singh T, Gupta D, Hameed S (2022) Optimized cancer detection on various magnified histopathological colon images based on dwt features and FCM clustering. Turkish J Electrical Eng Comput Sci 30:1–17

Lightweight Authentication Protocol for E-Healthcare Systems Using Fuzzy Commitment Scheme

Jhuma Dutta, Subhas Barman, Rathit Bandyopadhyay, and Moumita Ghosh

Abstract Authentication schemes are now getting importance in the field of the medical system. Medical data are private and sensitive to a patient, therefore, during sharing of data, privacy preservation is very crucial issues in electronic healthcare systems. An authentication protocol is required to ensure mutual authentication between a patient and a medical server before data communication. Single server-based authentication schemes require a separate registration of patients for every medical server. Moreover, most of the existing schemes do not consider error correction mechanism for disorderly biometrics. Further, the schemes have limitations like lack of user anonymity, non-diversification of biometric data, and being vulnerable to attacks if the smart card is stolen and also susceptible to user impersonation attacks. To overcome these shortcomings, we have proposed an authentication protocol for multi-server-based medical systems considering multi-factors to generate the key. In the proposed scheme, patient name is integrated with a cancelable biometric template and a randomly generated key to generate the patient ID. Then, that integrated ID is combined with an application-specific server ID and is used for authentication. The well-known security analysis tool, AVISPA tool has been used for formal security verification. The informal security has been analyzed and shows that the proposed scheme resists other familiar attacks.

Keywords Authentication · Electronic healthcare systems · Biometric · Multi-server environment · Formal security · Informal security · AVISPA tool

---

J. Dutta · S. Barman (✉)
Jalpaiguri Government Engineering College, Jalpaiguri, India
e-mail: subhas.barman@gmail.com

R. Bandyopadhyay
Siliguri Government Polytechnic, Siliguri, India

M. Ghosh
Siliguri Institute of Technology, Siliguri, India

© The Author(s), under exclusive license to Springer Nature Singapore Pte Ltd. 2023

J. K. Mandal and D. De (eds.), *Frontiers of ICT in Healthcare*, Lecture Notes in Networks and Systems 519, https://doi.org/10.1007/978-981-19-5191-6_17

1 Introduction

Recently, Information and Communication Tools are widely used in various online services of our day to day life, like teaching, health care, banking, tourism, shopping, etc. Several countries already started to use E-Healthcare and telemedicine services. Nowadays, due to easy access of web directory and IoT devices, E-Healthcare and telemedicine system becomes more friendly to use for a patient from any remote location. Patients send request to medical servers according to their requirements and the medical servers provide the services to the patients. Therefore, a secured session of communication should be established between the patient and the server through authentication protocols [9]. Li et al. [18] designed and implemented a telecare information platform so that patients get healthcare services through Internet. Chen et al. [10] considered dynamic ID for authentication protocol in telecare medical information system. Password-based authentication scheme is the oldest and widely used authentication system.

Lamport [16] in 1981 proposed password-based authentication scheme maintaining a password table, and the scheme is susceptible to stolen-verifier attack. Now, password-based authentication scheme has been improved by addressing the mentioned problems [15, 23] considering two factors, smart card and password for authentication. Token and knowledge are combined to yield a two factor-based authentication scheme for better security. In the literature, [13, 30] are two factor-based authentication schemes for telecare medicine information systems. Unfortunately, token (i.e., smart card) may be either changed or stolen out by the attacker. So, stored information may be revealed with side channel attacks or power analysis attacks. Moreover, different types of known attacks are found in the existing authentication protocols. Smart card-based remote authentication scheme [28] is sensitive to impersonation attacks and insider attacks with the compromised smart card. Subsequently, in 2012, He et al. proposed an authentication scheme [13] and state that their scheme is more secured, but it is vulnerable to the off-line password guessing attack. Zhu et al. [30] proposed a new authentication protocol based on RSA-cryptosystem.

Later on, three-factor-based authentication schemes [17, 21] have been introduced where user's biometric (e.g., finger print, iris, face, voice, etc.) is incorporated to an authentication system along with the smart card and the password to increase the security level. Three-factor-based authentication scheme proposed by Lee et al. [17] considered smart card, password, and fingerprint minutiae to enhance the level of security in authentication, but this scheme is vulnerable to masquerade attacks, server spoofing attacks [21]. Many researchers worked on three-factor-based authentication scheme [3] for telecare medicine information systems where level of communication security has been improved. In any remote user authentication scheme, user anonymity is highly expected to preserve the privacy of user's identity. But, many telecare medicine information schemes [13, 26, 30] overlooked the patient's privacy as patient's identity is transmitted openly to the server. In [10], Chen et al. addressed these problems. In 2015 [14], Giri et al.in 2015 proposed an efficient authentication protocol for telecare medical information systems for remote user based on RSA algorithm. There are several three-factors-based authentication schemes [11, 22, 25, 29] based on multi-server environment. However, [22] has limitation that the smart card may be robbed of, so suffered from attacks. In 2018, Barman et al. [5] proposed a multi-factor-based authentication scheme for multi-server environment. Recently, fuzzy commitment scheme is used to design a multi-server authentication systems using cancelable biometric data [4, 6]. Barman et al. [7] proposed an authentication scheme for e-healthcare system using fuzzy commitment for multi-server-based environment.

Here, we have proposed a multi-factor-based authentication scheme for medical system using fuzzy commitment for multi-server environment. In the proposed scheme, patient's biometric data in the form of cancelable biometric template [27] are combined with an encoded random number generated in each session. Therefore, it is quite difficult to reveal patient's credentials. We have also considered our scheme for multi-server environment. In this approach, all the medical servers are registered to be an authenticated server through a registration center. Patients are also registered. Only the registered patients and registered servers may establish a secured session for communication between them.

The work has been represented as follows. We have explained the proposed methodology in Sect. 2. In Sect. 3, the security of the proposed scheme has been analyzed and the performance of our scheme is compared with the existing schemes. Finally, we have drawn the conclusions in Sect. 4.

2 Proposed Scheme

The different steps of registration, login, authentication, and key agreement phases have been discussed in this section. The updating of the biometric data and password is also discussed here. Different notations along with their specification, we have used through the paper are listed in Table 1.

2.1 Registration Procedure

Before any communication between a patient and a medical server for any service, both the patient and the server have to be registered first so that a secured way of communication can be established between them. In this section, the detailed steps of registration procedure are discussed.

2.1.1 Medical Server Registration

Every server, available in the network should be registered first so that registered patients can communicate to an authenticated server. For each of the registered server,

Table 1 Notations and their specification

Notation	Specifications
$PNAME_{reg}$	Patient name during registration
PWD_{reg}	Password during registration
$PBIO_{reg}$	Patient's biometric information during registration
$PNAME_{log}$	Patient same during login
PWD_{log}	Password during login
$PBIO_{log}$	Patient's biometric information during login
MS_j	Medical server j
$MSID_j$	Identification of jth medical server
MSK_j	Key generated for j^{th} registered medical server
$E_{en}(), E_{dec}()$	Encoding and decoding functions for error correction
HD_p	Patient's helper data
X,R_n,N,n	Random numbers
$h(.)$	Hash function
RC	Registration center
SD	Smart device
$\oplus$, $\|\|$	Bitwise XOR and string concatenation operator

unique server ID ($MSID_j$) is generated. Now, an unique key MSK_j is computed for each registered medical server using a random number (X) chosen for each server. Registration center (RC) computes the following:

1. $MSK_j = h(MSID_j||X)$, for $1 \leq j \leq m$ where m is the number of available medical servers in the system.

2.1.2 Patient Registration

Patients provide their credentials, like patient name($PNAME_{reg}$), password (PWD_{reg}), and biometrics ($PBIO_{reg}$). A cancelable template (PCT_{reg}) is generated by using a one-way transformation function with the help of a transformation parameter(TP_i). Patient's registration procedure is illustrated as follows:

1. Patient (P_i) inputs $PNAME_{reg}$, PWD_{reg}, and $PBIO_{reg}$
2. Registration center (RC) computes a cancelable biometric template $PCT_{reg} = f(PBIO_{reg}, TP_i)$
3. Registration center selects a random number(R_n) as key and do the following steps:
   (a) Encodes the key with a error correction code as, $R_{ne} = E_{en}(R_n)$
   (b) Generates patient's helper data in the fuzzy commitment scheme as, $HD_p = PCT_{reg} \oplus R_{ne}$
   (c) Computes the following parameters:

i. $pid = h(R_n||PNAME_{reg}||PCT_{reg})$
ii. $M_1{}^j = pid \oplus h(MSK_j)$
iii. $SV_j = h(MSID_j||MSK_j)$
iv. $pwd = h(PWD_{reg}||R_{ne})$

HD_p, $h(R_{ne})$,$h(pid)$, $M_1{}^j$, SV^j, $h(pwd)$, $h(.)$, $E_{en}()$, and $E_{de}()$ are stored in a smart device (SD) and shared to patient through a secured channel.

2.2 Login Procedure

In this section, we have discussed about the login procedure. For any service from a medical server, the patient has to login first using patient name, password, and the biometric. The medical server then checks whether the patient is an enrolled patient or not. The detailed steps are given below:

1. Patient enters name $(PNAME_{log})$ and password (PWD_{log})
2. Patient scans his/her biometric $(PBIO_{log})$
3. Cancelable template PCT_{log} is generated, that is, $PCT_{log} = f(PBIO_{log}, TP_i)$
4. SD extracts $R_{log} = HD_p \oplus PCT_{log}$ and decodes R_{log} as $R_{log\,dec} = E_{dec}(R_{log})$
5. Now compares $h(R_{log_{dec}})$ with $h(R_n)$, i.e., check whether hash value of the randomly selected key is revealed correctly by using helper data and biometric. If it is not matched, then the session is terminated. Else, follow the steps:
6. Medical server computes, patient ID as pid_{log},
   where $pid_{log} = h(R_{log\,dec}||PCT_{log}||PNAME_{log})$
   if pid_{log} does not match with pid, then the session terminates. Otherwise,
7. Server computes pwd_{log}, where $pwd_{log} = h(PWD_{log}||R_{log})$, now compares pwd_{log} with pwd. If matches, then login is successful, otherwise, terminates the session. When login is successful, then the medical server computes the authentication and key agreement parameters using the following steps:
   (a) Server selects two random numbers N_1 and n
   (b) Computes the following parameters:
   $PID = h(pid_{log}||n)$
   $h(MSK_j) = M_1{}^j \oplus pid_{log}$
   $PID_i = h(PID \oplus h(MSK_j))$
   $M_2 = pid_{log} \oplus h(MSK_j)$
   $M_3 = h(SV_j||pid_{log}) \oplus N_1$

Smart device saves the parameters: PID, M_2, M_3, PID_i.

2.3 Mutual Authentication and Key Agreement Procedure

Here, we have discussed about the mutual authentication between patient and the specific medical server. After successful login of a patient, the authenticity of medical server is verified. If the server is being successfully authenticated, then a key is established for the session between the patient and the specific medical server. The authentication and key agreement protocol is discussed below:

1. The medical server MS_j receives (PID, M_2, M_3, PID_i) and computes $PID_i' = h(PID \oplus h(MSK_j))$. If $PID_i \neq PID_i'$, then the server terminates the session, otherwise, it follows the steps:
   1. Medical Server computes the following parameters:
      (a) $pid' = M_2 \oplus h(MSK_j)$
      (b) $N_1' = M_3 \oplus h(SV_j||pid')$
      (c) Server choose a random number, N_2 and generates the following:
      (d) $M_4 = h(SV_j||PID||N_1') \oplus N_2$
      (e) $n_0 = h(N_2 \oplus pid')$ and computes a key, $k = h(pid_{log}'||N_1'||N_2)$ for the session established between patient and the medical server.
   2. Server sends (n_0, M_4) to patient
2. The patient computes, $N_2' = M_4 \oplus h(SV_j||pid_{log}||N_1)$ and checks whether, $n_0 = h(N_2' \oplus pid_{log})$, if not, then the medical server is failed to proof its authenticity and the patient terminates the session, otherwise, the patient generates the key, $k = h(pid_{log}||N_1||N_2')$.

2.4 Biometric Update Procedure

Biometric update is required periodically in any biomeric-based system for better security. In our scheme, we have used cancelable biometric. For this purpose, a revocable transformation function is used to generate cancelable biometric. The function generates new template by changing the transformation parameter. The biometric update procedure is illustrated below:

1. Patient enters a new instance of biometric data, $PBIO_{new}$
2. Patient enters $PNAME_{log}, PWD_{log}, TP_i$
3. SD computes $PCT_{upd} = f(PBIO_{new}, Tp_i)$
4. SD extracts the key as, $R_{log}' = E_{dec}(HD_p \oplus PCT_{upd})$
5. If $h(R_{log}') = h(R_{log})$, then computes $pid_{log}' = h(R_{log}'||PNAME_{log}||PCT_{upd})$
6. If $h(PID_{log}') = h(PID_{log})$, then computes $pwd' = h(PWD_{log}||R_{log}')$
7. If $h(pwd') = h(pwd_{log})$, then continue, otherwise, terminates the session
8. If login is successful, the patient P_i selects a new parameter $TP_{i_{new}}$ randomly

9. SD computes $PCT_{upd} = f(PBIO_{new}, TP_{inew})$, $HD_p{}^{new} = PCT_{upd} \oplus R_{log}{}'$, $pid_{new} = h(R_{log}{}' || PNAME_{log} || PCT_{upd})$, $h(MSK_j) = M_1{}^j \oplus R_{log}{}'$ and $M_1{}^j(new) = pid_{new} \oplus h(MSK_j)$
10. The HD_p, $h(pid)$, $M_1{}^j$, TP_i are updated as $HD_p = HD_p{}^{new}$, $h(pid) = h(pid_{new})$ and $M_1{}^j = M_1{}^j(new)$, $TP_i = TP_{inew}$.

2.5 *Password Update Procedure*

In this section, we have discussed about the password update procedure by a patient. To update password, patient has to login first. The detailed steps are given below:

1. Patient inputs $PNAME_{log}$, PWD_{log}, $PBIO_{log}$ and use smart device for login
2. Computes $PCT_i = f(PBIO_{log}, TP_i)$, $R_{new} = E_{dec}(HD_p \oplus PCT_i)$
3. If $h(R_{new}) = h(R_{log})$, then reveals login ID as $pid' = h(R_{new} || PNAME_{log} || PCT_i)$
4. If $pid' = pid_{log}$, then reveals password as $pwd' = h(PWD_{log} || R_{new})$
5. If $h(PWD_{log}) = h(pwd')$, then login successful, otherwise, SD terminates the password changing phase
6. Patient selects a new password PWD_{new}, and it is integrated with the encoded random number, that is, $PWD_{upd} = h(PWD_{new} || R_{new})$ and PWD_{upd} is now becomes the updated password.

3 Security Analysis

To analyze the security, we have considered both the methods (i) informal security analysis (ii) formal security analysis as discussed below:

3.1 *Informal Security Analysis*

The informal security of our scheme has been analyzed by considering the same informal security analysis as Lin and Lai [21], Chang [8], Juang [15], Liao and Wang [20], and Yang and Yang [29].

3.1.1 Anonymity

In our scheme, actual patient ID is not stored in registration center and also is not shared with server. Patient ID is generated from patient's name and biometric integrated with a randomly generated key, i.e., $pid = h(R_n || PNAME_{reg} || PCT_{reg})$ and is stored as token in a smart device(SD). SD transmits $PID (PID = h(pid||n))$ and PID_i where $PID_i = h(PID \oplus h(MSK_j))$ through insecure channel. The values of PID and PID_i changed in each session depending on the random number, n. However, user identity may be disclosed to the attacker from either intercepted message or stolen smart card for the scheme in [8, 11, 15, 29].

3.1.2 Biometric Protection

Here, first, a cancelable template is generated for patient's biometric using a transformation function $PCT_{reg} = f(PBIO_{reg}, TP_i)$. Then, the transformed biometric data is concealed with an encoded randomly generated number using fuzzy commitment scheme, $HD_p = PCT_{reg} \oplus R_{ne}$. Therefore, it is quite difficult to extract the cancelable template PCT_{reg} from HD_p without the complete knowledge of R_n or R_{ne}. Even, due to the one-way transformation of the biometric data, the original biometric information of the patient can not be revealed from the cancelable template PCT_{reg}.

3.1.3 Password Protection

In the proposed scheme, the server does not store the password itself. The patient's password is integrated with an encoded randomly generated number using fuzzy commitment scheme $pwd = h(PWD_{reg}||R_{ne})$. Therefore, an encoded password is generated for each session and is not derivable from any old password.

3.1.4 Mutual Authentication

In our scheme, patient and the medical server mutually authenticate each other. The medical server authenticates the patient and the patient checks the authenticity of the server before establishing a secure communication.

3.1.5 Resistance to Replay Attacks:

We have used some random nonce to protect our scheme from replay attack. But, some existing multi-server-based authentication schemes [19, 22, 25] are not able to defeat replay attack.

3.1.6 Session Key Agreement

A session key is generated before setting up a session between patient and application server after successful mutual authentication on every session. In our proposed scheme, the session key k is generated using two random numbers and patient's ID where $k = h(N_1||N_2||pid)$). Hence, the session key is different for each session and the adversary is unable to derive the key from the generated messages. The schemes [22, 25, 29] do not achieve this security requirement to establish a secure session between user and the server for communication.

3.1.7 Resistance to Modification Attacks:

The authentication messages may be intercepted and modified by an adversary but in the proposed scheme, it is difficult to alter the messages without knowing the registered medical server identity and patient's identity as $M_2 = pid_{log} \oplus h(MSK_j)$, $M_3 = h(h(MSID_J||MSK_J)||pid_{log}) \oplus N_1$. If any credentials are changed, then the medical server can detect it easily.

3.1.8 Ephemeral Secret Leakage(ESL) Attack

The patient generates M_3 with random number N_1, $M_3 = h(SV_j||pid_{log}) \oplus N_1$. The patient shared M_3 to the medical server. Now, the server takes another random number N_2 and encodes it into M_4 then computes the session key, that is, $k = h(pid_{log}||N_1||N_2)$. Now, we have two cases:

1. Case 1: Attacker knows N_1 and N_2, but it is quite difficult to compute the key without knowing the pid_{log}.
2. Case 2: Attacker knows patient ID and the specific medical server ID, then also it is quite impossible to generate the key without the random numbers N_1 and N_2.

3.2 *Formal Security Analysis*

We have used the most widely-accepted tool, Automated Validation of Internet Security Protocols and Applications (AVISPA) to analyze formal security of our proposed authentication protocol [2]. AVISPA tool provides the following back ends that implements various automatic analysis techniques with most recent ideas. These are

1. On-the-fly model-checker (OFMC)
2. Constraint-logic-based attack searcher (CL-AtSe)
3. SAT-based model-checker (SATMC) and
4. Tree automata based on automatic approximations for the analysis of security protocols (TA4SP)

In AVISPA, a target protocol is specified using HLPSL [24]. HLPSL is built on the basis of two different roles firstly, basic role represents the role of each participant, secondly, composition role represents the cases of basic roles. Any protocol designed with HLPSL is compiled into an intermediate format(IF) and after execution of the IF file, one of the back end produces the output format (OF). Once a protocol is successfully executed it gives an output with attack or safe.

3.2.1 HLPSL Implementation in Proposed Protocol

HLPSL implemented using three basic roles:

1. patient P_i role
2. medical service registration center RC role
3. medical server MS_j role

In this application, three secrecy goals and two authentication properties used as below:

1. secrecy-of sub1: patient name $(PNAME)$, password (PWD), cancelable template (PCT), and random number(R_n) are kept secret between patient P_i and medical server MS_j
2. secrecy-of sub2: registered medical server key (MSK_j) is kept secret between medical service registration center and medical server
3. secrecy-of sub3: randomly generated key(R_n) is kept secret in registration center
4. authentication_on patient_medical server_N1: The medical server receives N_1 from patient and authenticates patient based on N_1.
5. authentication_on medical server_patient_N2: The patient receives N_2 from medical server and authenticates the medical server based on N_2.

The results of simulation using AVISPA on the proposed scheme for back ends OFMC and CL-AtSe confirm the safety of the proposed scheme.

3.3 Performance Comparison with Existing Schemes

We have compared the performance of our proposed scheme with some multi-server-based telemedicine systems such as Amin et al. [1], Das et al. [12], Chaudhry et al. [9], and Barman et al. [7] with respect to computational cost. The comparison is shown in Table 2. We see that our scheme has lower communication cost compared to other schemes. The corresponding graph in Fig. 1 shows that our scheme is efficient due to light weight computational cost with respect to other schemes. Following notations we have used to represent the cost of executing a particular operation such as

1. C_h : execution cost of an one-way hash function
2. C_{fe} : execution cost of a fuzzy extractor function
3. C_{fcs} : execution cost of fuzzy commitment scheme
4. c_{spm} : execution cost of symmetric/asymmetric encryption/decryption

In this cost computation, we assume that $C_{spm} \approx C_{fe} \approx C_{fcs}$ and $C_h \approx 0.0023$ms, $C_{spm} \approx 2.226$ ms as reported in [6].

Table 2 Performance comparison with existing multi-server-based telemedicine schemes

Schemes	Login phase	Authentication phase	Total
Amin et al. [1]	$C_{spm}+5C_h$	$14C_h$	$19C_h$
Das et al. [12]	$C_{fe}+4c_h$	$14c_h$	$C_{fe}+18c_h$
Chaudhry et al. [9]	$5c_h$	$7c_h+2c_{spm}$	$12c_h+2c_{spm}$
Barman et al. [7]	$C_{fcs}+3c_h$	$11c_h$	$C_{fcs}+14c_h$
Proposed scheme	$C_{fcs}+3C_h$	$10C_h$	$C_{fcs}+13C_h$

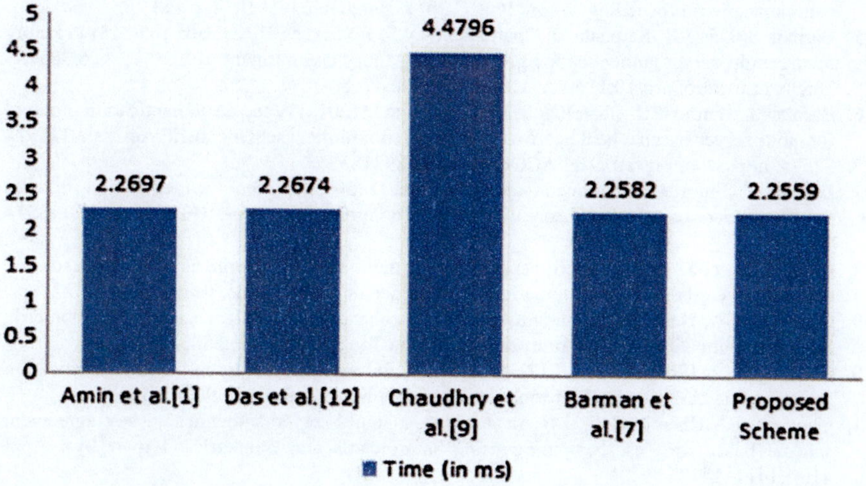

Fig. 1 Computational cost

4 Conclusions

We have proposed an improved authentication protocol for E-healthcare system in multi-server-based environment. In this authentication protocol, the mutual authentication between patient and medical server is established before initiation of data communication for different types of services. The security of the proposed authentication protocol is ensured with three factors like knowledge, token, and biometric. This protocol can detect error in any factor immediately with early error detection features. The security of our scheme is proved in terms of formal and informal security analysis. The performance comparison of the proposed scheme with existing authentication protocol in telemedicine systems shows that our multi-factor-based authentication scheme for E-healthcare system is more efficient.

References

1. Amin R, Biswas G (2015) A novel user authentication and key agreement protocol for accessing multi-medical server usable in tmis. J Med Syst 39(3):1–17
2. Armando A, Basin D, Cuellar J, Rusinowitch M, Viganò L (2006) Avispa: automated validation of internet security protocols and applications. ERCIM News 64(January)
3. Arshad H, Nikooghadam M (2014) Three-factor anonymous authentication and key agreement scheme for telecare medicine information systems. J Med Syst 38(12):1–12
4. Barman S, Chaudhuri A, Chatterjee A, Raza MR (2020) An elliptic curve cryptography-based multi-server authentication scheme using cancelable biometrics. In: Intelligent computing and communication: proceedings of 3rd ICICC 2019, Bangalore, vol 1034, p 153
5. Barman S, Das AK, Samanta D, Chattopadhyay S, Rodrigues JJPC, Park Y (2018) Provably secure multi-server authentication protocol using fuzzy commitment. IEEE Access 6:38578–38594. https://doi.org/10.1109/ACCESS.2018.2854798
6. Barman S, Shum HPH, Chattopadhyay S, Samanta D (2019) A secure authentication protocol for multi-server-based e-healthcare using a fuzzy commitment scheme. IEEE Access 7:12557–12574. https://doi.org/10.1109/ACCESS.2019.2893185
7. Barman S, Shum HP, Chattopadhyay S, Samanta D (2019) A secure authentication protocol for multi-server-based e-healthcare using a fuzzy commitment scheme. IEEE Access 7:12557–12574
8. Chang CC, Lee JS (2004) An efficient and secure multi-server password authentication scheme using smart cards. In: 2004 International conference on cyberworlds. IEEE, pp 417–422
9. Chaudhry SA, Naqvi H, Khan MK (2018) An enhanced lightweight anonymous biometric based authentication scheme for tmis. Multimedia Tools Appl 77(5):5503–5524
10. Chen HM, Lo JW, Yeh CK (2012) An efficient and secure dynamic id-based authentication scheme for telecare medical information systems. J Med Syst 36(6):3907–3915
11. Chuang MC, Chen MC (2014) An anonymous multi-server authenticated key agreement scheme based on trust computing using smart cards and biometrics. Expert Syst Appl 41(4):1411–1418
12. Das AK, Odelu V, Goswami A (2015) A secure and robust user authenticated key agreement scheme for hierarchical multi-medical server environment in tmis. J Med Syst 39(9):1–24
13. Debiao H, Jianhua C, Rui Z (2012) A more secure authentication scheme for telecare medicine information systems. J Med Syst 36(3):1989–1995
14. Giri D, Maitra T, Amin R, Srivastava P (2015) An efficient and robust rsa-based remote user authentication for telecare medical information systems. J Med Syst 39(1):1–9
15. Juang WS, Chen ST, Liaw HT (2008) Robust and efficient password-authenticated key agreement using smart cards. IEEE Trans Ind Electron 55(6):2551–2556
16. Lamport L (1981) Password authentication with insecure communication. Commun ACM 24(11):770–772
17. Lee J, Ryu S, Yoo K (2002) Fingerprint-based remote user authentication scheme using smart cards. Electron Lett 38(12):554–555
18. Li SH, Wang CY, Lu WH, Lin YY, Yen DC (2012) Design and implementation of a telecare information platform. J Med Syst 36(3):1629–1650
19. Li X, Xiong Y, Ma J, Wang W (2012) An efficient and security dynamic identity based authentication protocol for multi-server architecture using smart cards. J Netw Comput Appl 35(2):763–769
20. Liao YP, Wang SS (2009) A secure dynamic id based remote user authentication scheme for multi-server environment. Comput Stand Interfaces 31(1):24–29
21. Lin CH, Lai YY (2004) A flexible biometrics remote user authentication scheme. Comput Stand Interfaces 27(1):19–23
22. Sood SK, Sarje AK, Singh K (2011) A secure dynamic identity based authentication protocol for multi-server architecture. J Netw Comput Appl 34(2):609–618

23. Sun DZ, Huai JP, Sun JZ, Li JX, Zhang JW, Feng ZY (2009) Improvements of Juang's password-authenticated key agreement scheme using smart cards. IEEE Trans Ind Electron 56(6):2284–2291
24. Von Oheimb D (2005) The high-level protocol specification language HLPSL developed in the EU project AVISPA. In: Proceedings of the APPSEM 2005 workshop. Tallinn, Finland, pp 13–15
25. Wang B, Ma M (2013) A smart card based efficient and secured multi-server authentication scheme. Wirel Pers Commun 68(2):361–378
26. Wei J, Hu X, Liu W (2012) An improved authentication scheme for telecare medicine information systems. J Med Syst 36(6):3597–3604
27. Wu L, Meng L, Zhao S, Wei X, Wang H (2021) Privacy-preserving cancelable biometric authentication based on RDM and ECC. IEEE Access 9:90989–91000
28. Wu ZY, Lee YC, Lai F, Lee HC, Chung Y (2012) A secure authentication scheme for telecare medicine information systems. J Med Syst 36(3):1529–1535
29. Yang D, Yang B (2010) A biometric password-based multi-server authentication scheme with smart card. In: 2010 International conference on computer design and applications, vol 5, pp V5–554. IEEE
30. Zhu Z (2012) An efficient authentication scheme for telecare medicine information systems. J Med Syst 36(6):3833–3838

Performance Analysis of Machine Learning Algorithms for Prediction of Cerebral Attack (Stroke)

Diganta Sengupta, Subhash Mondal, Yash Raj Singh, and Amartya Pandey

Abstract In this study, we have analysed the behaviour and performance of twelve machine learning (ML) algorithms in prediction of cerebral attack (stroke). The ML algorithms used were light gradient boosting machine (LGBM), histogram-based gradient boost (HGB), random forest (RF), gradient boost classifier (GBC), XGBoost (XGB), AdaBoost (AB), decision tree (DT), support vector machine (SVM), K-nearest neighbours (KNN), logistic regression (LR), Bernoulli Naïve Bayes and Gaussian Naïve Bayes. The dataset comprised of 5110 entries, which were subjected to pre-processing prior to deployment in the ML algorithms. We observed an accuracy of 97.36% for RF classifier which was the highest among the twelve algorithms under consideration. Post hyper-parameter tuning, GBC reflected an accuracy of 97.73%. Stacking resulted in an accuracy of 98.85% having GBC as the meta model and XGB, RF, SVM, KNN, DT, AB and LR as the base models. Hence, form our observation, we conclude that GBC performs best in predicting stroke among all the ML algorithms.

Keywords Stroke prediction · Machine learning · Hyper-parameter tuning · Cerebral attack

D. Sengupta (✉) · S. Mondal · Y. R. Singh · A. Pandey
Department of Computer Science and Engineering, Meghnad Saha Institute of Technology, Kolkata 700150, India
e-mail: sg.diganta@ieee.org

S. Mondal
e-mail: subhash@msit.edu.in

Y. R. Singh
e-mail: yash_s.cse2019@msit.edu.in

A. Pandey
e-mail: amartya_p.cse2019@msit.edu.in

D. Sengupta
Department of Computer Science and Business Systems, Meghnad Saha Institute of Technology, Kolkata 700150, India

© The Author(s), under exclusive license to Springer Nature Singapore Pte Ltd. 2023

J. K. Mandal and D. De (eds.), *Frontiers of ICT in Healthcare*, Lecture Notes in Networks and Systems 519, https://doi.org/10.1007/978-981-19-5191-6_18

1 Introduction

A stroke results when our brain cannot get abundant oxygen and required supplements, commonly most strokes (87%) are ischaemic strokes. An ischaemic stroke takes place when blood flow by the artery that supplies oxygen-rich blood cells to the brain emerge as blocked. Each year, approximately 795,000 people in the USA have suffer a stroke, around 610,000 of these are first or new strokes. The after effects of stroke might involve failure of muscular coordination, transient or lasting paralysis, vision problem in one or both eyes and desperate straits in eating or speaking [1].

We can minimize the chance of having a stroke by keeping a check on our blood pressure, blood glucose, and cholesterol levels. Stroke can further be checked through food having high nutrient values, physical activity and, medicines in cases of severity. Chances of stroke in patients addicted to smoking can be further reduced if they quit smoking [2].

Machine learning via pattern perceiving at present is the most trusted way to cure and predict the oncoming disease. Cost of curing strokes in USA could soar to $180B annually by 2030 [3]. We can try to reduce 14–18% of this cost by building a well-trained machine learning model which can predict precisely whether a particular patient will suffer a stoke or not. In this research, we have analysed different machine learning models such as KNN, SVM, random forest, LGBM classifier and many more, out of these, we selected some models for stacking which will gives us the final result. The detailed work of this research has been mentioned in "workflow" section and subsection. The twelve machine learning algorithms used are provided in Table 1 along with the acronyms.

The paper is organized by having Related Work section after the Introduction followed by our proposal in Sect. 3. Section 4 provides the result and comparative analysis with Sect. 5 concluding the study.

Table 1 Machine learning algorithms used and their acronyms

Machine learning algorithms	Acronym
Random forest	RF
Histogram gradient boosting classifier	HGBC
LGBM classifier	LGBM
XGB classifier	XBG
Gradient boosting classifier	GBC
AdaBoost classifier	AB
Decision tree	DT
SVM	SVM
KNN	KNN
Logistic regression	LR
Bernoulli NB	BNB
Gaussian NB	GNB

2 Related Work

We present an exhaustive literature survey in this section. In [4], the authors proposed initially important features ranked by Shapiro-Wilk algorithm where recursive feature elimination was extensively used. Missing data and outliners were removed to test efficiency of RFEC method as aforesaid. The RFECV algorithmic approach was deviated with highest accuracy of 0.69 due to immature data and lack of other essential features.

Kashi et al. [5] proposed a ML-based automatic model which is used to gather precise info on the compensatory movements that a person makes. A total of 18 movements were considered for this and used RF algorithm. Various human movement data were collected that were considered for locomotion activities. In [6], the authors proposed SMOTE termed oversampling method with LR, RF and XGBoost which is applied to the prescribed dataset. The outlier data present in the dataset which is an imbalanced data is handled using SMOTE. Due to the presence of various missing values in the prescribed dataset, one of the important handling techniques called "mean value imputation" is applied and from the *Scikit-learn* library [7] a module named simple imputer is accompanied along. Further, grid search CV algorithm is applied for finest parameters. Thus, the overall accuracy of 99.07% is achieved with the RF and 99% precision.

In [8], the authors laid emphasis over the cardiovascular health study where there is through study of Cox proportional hazards model. The model comprises of one of the automatic feature selector algorithms in order to select the best feature. Missing entries are calculated with the imputation through linear regression and regularized expectation maximization. The major ML algorithms used are support vector machines and the margin-based censored regression. Sailasya et al. [9] proposed an approach that takes various physiological factors in its prescribed dataset to detect stroke in the brain. Several ML algorithms are used. Further, label encoding followed by handling various imbalanced data to get the best result ware achieved. The Naïve Bayes algorithms performed the best with overall accuracy of 82%.

In [10], the authors proposed a model consisting of ML algorithms like SVM, RF, AB and the multinomial Naïve Bayes to detect subtype ischaemic stroke. Further, some important features were taken in accounts which were further indexed using the Shapiro-Wilk algorithm. Recursive feature elimination with cross-validation (RFECV) was used that consisted of all the aforementioned algorithms. Further, data pre-processing with label encoding was performed. The performance of RFECV with selected feature with each of the mentioned algorithm was plotted based on the features that were indexed by Shapiro ranking. It was concluded that the RFECV method was better in accuracy score of 81.5%. The authors in [11] presented a prototype model for stroke classification to combine the extensive use of data mining techniques in order to precisely track information's along with ML algorithms like artificial neural networks, SVM, boosting and bagging and RF were applied. More emphasis on ANN was given which is constructed with around 22 inputs with one hidden layer. AdaBoost and RF gave accuracy of 90.9%, while the best performance was given by ANN algorithm with accuracy score of almost 95%.

In [12], the authors proposed an approach based on server-side resource utilization where the analysis and prediction is done using the Microsoft Azure ML, a cloud-based platform. Authors used two-class decision jungle. Further, confusion matrix and ROC graph are drawn for all the features. F1-score, precision and accuracy are calculated. They concluded results with accuracy 96.8%. In [13], the authors classify different type of stroke using different machine learning algorithms. The algorithms used are Naive Bayes, J48, kNN and RF. Dataset was cleaned using WEKA. Further, all the prediction parameters like accuracy, recall, F1-score and precision are calculated, for each of the above-mentioned algorithms a respective confusion matrix also calculated. In the given dataset, the Naïve Bayer could not performed well as expected. RF was the only algorithm with constant score across all accuracy parameters.

Krishna et al. [14] presented a detailed comparative analysis of ML algorithms consisting of K-nearest neighbour, LR, RF classifier and SVC. Using these algorithms, a model is built which is further built a GUI using FLASK framework, which becomes useful for any people (end user) to check prediction of brain stroke using the details of their health in the website. K-nearest neighbour has highest accuracy of 99.35% followed by DT, RF and SVM, then the least accurate being LR and a bar diagram is plotted of all the aforesaid algorithms with respect to accuracy. In [15], the authors presented a survey by considering 39 articles related to ML algorithms for brain stroke. The most widely used models were SVM, deep learning (DL), k-nearest neighbours, ANN, LR and the RF. The authors in [16] considered some certain importance arena of machine learning in neuroimaging especially for the region of acute ischaemic in stroke. The authors have expressed current as well as future challenges in machine learning for the treatment of acute ischaemic stroke. In [17], the authors proposed a model comprising of three hidden layers along with the fifteen ANN units for the DT algorithm approximately three hundred DTs were used. Further, ASTRAL score was taken into account to evaluate the accuracy of the model.

The authors in [18] trained the different classifiers by selecting best feature classification algorithms. Further, a heat-map was plotted for target variable against features present in the dataset. Among all the weighted voting classifier performed the best with measured an accuracy score of 97%. The XGBoost classifier and the Gradient Boosting classifier resulted in an accuracy of 96% each, with the least accuracy being observed via Gaussian Processes Classifier. In [19], the authors proposed the use of ML Algorithms. Dempster-Shafer method is used with gradient descent classifier. Abedi et al. in [20] proposed a model for prediction of recurrence long term stroke by using six ML algorithms. SMOTE was used for up-sampling of the data. In [21], the authors proposed model comprising of ML algorithms used support vector machine, LR, Gaussian NB, K-nearest neighbours, Bernoulli and linear regression. Pre-processing the data was achieved, and further, label encoding was performed. The DT classifier was best achieved accuracy score of 93%, and the linear regression performed worst with accuracy of just 0.095%.

Zhang et al. in [22] proposed the use of support vector machine which is further added with the glow-worm swarm optimization algorithm on the selected features of last five years. The combinational of algorithms fetched an accuracy of around 82.58% from 18 of the selected features form the given dataset. In [23], the authors proposed a unique singleton ML algorithm support vector machine where SVM is implemented with various Kernel mathematical functions. Here, the dataset was collected directly from international database of stroke diseases. The Kernel functions of SVM used are linear quadratic RBF and polynomial. Among the Kernel used linear Kernel gave best performance of 91% along with all other performance parameters much higher than rest whereas the RBF accountant to least accuracy of just close to 59%. In [24], the authors proposed model for predicting ischaemic stroke functional outcomes. Model training was done using LR, DT, SVM, RF and XGBoost.

3 Proposed Work

In this section, we discuss about the dataset acquisition which is being considered, the feature engineering that is applied on the dataset, model training and propose ensemble or stacking of the classifiers which are used for the classification of stroke prediction. The proposed workflow model is provided in Fig. 1.

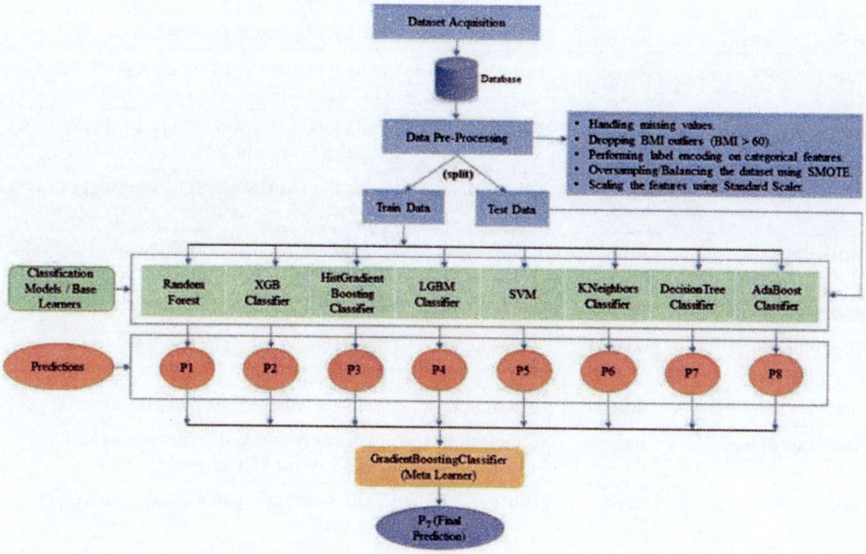

Fig. 1 Workflow model for proposed work

3.1 *Dataset Acquisition*

The dataset in this research work is taken from an open-source stroke prediction dataset downloaded from Kaggle [25]. This dataset is formed by conducting the study on 5110 patients and judged them on 11 features. Table 1 presents the features/attributes on which patients were judged.

3.2 *Feature Engineering*

Generally, input data consists of features which are usually represented by structured columns. Many times, it has been observed that in order to achieve excellent accuracy without getting any failure such as low accuracy or overfitting, we pre-processed the data by removing unwanted noise, outliers and handling missing values from the dataset. After analysing the entire dataset, we concluded that this dataset contains some issues that were resolved using techniques mentioned in Table 2.

Table 2 Feature details of the dataset and patient judgement

Feature/column name	Data type	Column nature	Feature/column description
gender	string	Categorical	Tells gender of patient "Male", "Female" and "Other"
age	float64	Continuous	Tells the age of the patient
hypertension	int64	Binary	Tells whether the patient is hypertensive (1) or not (0)
heart_disease	int64	Binary	Tells whether a patient has any heart disease (1) or not (0)
ever_married	string	Categorical	Tells the martial status of a patient ("Yes") or ("No")
work_type	string	Categorical	"children", "Govt_job", "Never_worked", "Private" or "Self-employed"
residence_type	string	Categorical	"Urban" or "Rural"
avg_glucose_level	float64	Continuous	Tells the average glucose level of the patient
bmi	float64	Continuous	Tells the BMI of the patient
smoking_status	string	Categorical	"Formerly smoked", "never smoked", "smokes" or "Unknown"
stoke	int64	Binary	Tells whether a patient had a stroke (1) or not (0)
Gender	string	Categorical	Tells gender of patient "Male", "Female" and "Other"

Handle Missing Values

We observed 201 missing values in bmi column which was handled by using gender specific median.

Outlier Detection

In bmi and gender column, we noticed some outliers. We dropped those instances related to bmi and gender column. The final instance count was 5096 after application of outlier detection technique.

Encoding Technique

To manage the string type categorical features, we have applied one hot encoding technique to convert the categorical data into integer without considering the dummy variable trap.

Balancing Imbalanced Data

We have used the famous technique SMOTE to handle the imbalance of the target class. After oversampling, our dataset contains total 9694 instances. The values pre- and post-balancing are presented in Table 3.

Scaling Features to Common Range

After applying the above discussed data pre-processing techniques, we have split the both old (before SMOTE) and new (after SMOTE) dataset into train and test separately with ratio of 0.80:0.20, respectively. The values are presented in Table 4.

Table 3 Imbalance data balancing

	Before SMOTE	After SMOTE
Label 0 count from stroke column	4847	4847
Label 1 count from stroke column	249	4847

Table 4 Dataset splitting in training and testing set pre and post SMOTE balancing

	Dataset split before SMOTE	Dataset split after SMOTE
Count of training instances	4076	7755
Count of test instances	1020	1939

Table 5 Test accuracy comparisons between balanced and imbalanced datasets

	Best accuracy (%)	Algorithm name
Test accuracy from imbalanced dataset	95.29	K-nearest neighbours
Test accuracy from balanced dataset	97.31	RF

3.3 Model Training

In initial phase of our study, we tested our both balanced and imbalanced processed test data on LR, SVM, K-nearest neighbours classifier, Gaussian NB, Bernoulli NB, DT classifier, RF classifier, XGBoost classifier, AB, GBC, histogram GBC and LGBM classifier, respectively. After analysing the above trained ML models result, we concluded that KNN classifier gives the best result for imbalanced test data with an accuracy of 95.29% and RF classifier gives the best result for balanced test data with an accuracy of 97.31 as shown in Table 5. Hence, it is proved that balancing the dataset is a very important step in pre-processing.

3.4 Ensemble/Stacking Algorithm

Ensemble learning is a machine learning paradigm where multiple models (often called "weak learners") are trained to solve the same problem and combined to get better results. In stacking, an algorithm takes the outputs of sub-models as input and attempts to learn how to best combine the input predictions to make a better output prediction.

In our method, we have trained and tested the processed dataset on different machine learning algorithms namely LR, SVM, KNN, GNB, BNB, DT, RF, XGB, AB, GBC, HGBC and LGBM classifier. Initially, all these models were trained without using any hyper-parameter tuning. After that some of these models were trained by applying hyper-parameter tuning in order to achieve better results. All the non-parameterised and parameterized model results were noted in Tables 6 and 7, respectively. For stacking, we have used stacking classifier *api* from *sklearn.ensemble* library. In total, we have selected nine models for stacking, where we choose XGB, RF, SVC, KNN, DT, AB from Table 2 (tuned model table) and HGBC, LGBM classifier from Table 6 (normal non-tuned table). GBC was chosen as the meta learner and rest eight models for base learner. After building the stacked model, we again analysed test data of balanced dataset on this newly created stacked model and we achieved an accuracy of 98.85% with precision, recall, F1-score, Cohen-Kappa score, ROC-AUC score as 1.00, 0.98, 0.99, 0.97 and 0.99, respectively, as mentioned in Table 8.

Table 6 Performance metric results with respect to twelve machine learning algorithms

Normal model	Accuracy	Precision	Recall	F1-score	Cohen-Kappa score	RoC-AuC score
RF	97.36	0.99	0.95	0.97	0.94	0.97
HGBC	97.31	0.99	0.95	0.97	0.94	0.97
LGBM	97.26	0.99	0.95	0.97	0.94	0.97
XBG	96.95	0.99	0.94	0.96	0.93	0.96
GBC	96.95	0.99	0.94	0.96	0.93	0.96
AB	95.93	0.98	0.92	0.95	0.91	0.95
DT	94.39	0.94	0.94	0.94	0.88	0.94
SVM	93.14	0.95	0.90	0.92	0.86	0.93
KNN	92.98	0.88	0.99	0.93	0.85	0.92
LR	78.23	0.76	0.81	0.78	0.56	0.78
BNB	77.40	0.75	0.79	0.77	0.53	0.76
GNB	61.92	0.56	0.98	0.72	0.23	0.61

Table 7 Performance metric results with respect to best eight tuned machine learning algorithms

Tuned model	Accuracy	Precision	Recall	F1-score	Cohen-Kappa score	RoC-AuC score
GBC	97.73	0.99	0.96	0.97	0.95	0.97
XGB	97.47	0.99	0.95	0.97	0.94	0.97
RF	97.47	0.99	0.95	0.97	0.94	0.97
SVM	96.75	0.95	0.98	0.96	0.93	0.96
KNN	96.59	0.94	0.99	0.96	0.93	0.96
DT	95.51	0.95	0.95	0.95	0.91	0.95
AB	96.23	0.99	0.92	0.96	0.92	0.96
LR	78.44	0.76	0.82	0.79	0.56	0.78

Table 8 Performance metric results with respect to stacked model

Model	Accuracy	Precision	Recall	F1-score	Cohen-Kappa score	RoC-AuC score
Stacked	98.85	1.00	0.98	0.99	0.97	0.99

The ROC-AUC curve for the stacked model is presented in Figs. 2 and 3 presents the confusion matrix for the stacked model.

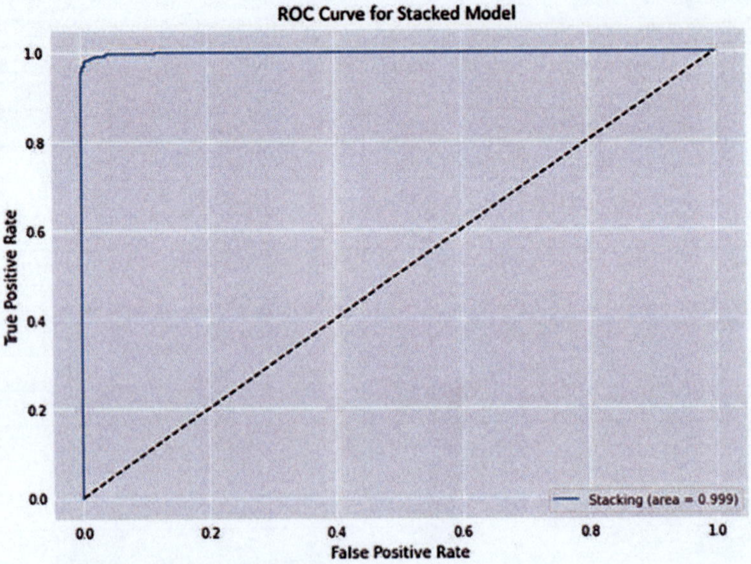

Fig. 2 ROC-AUC curve for the stacked model

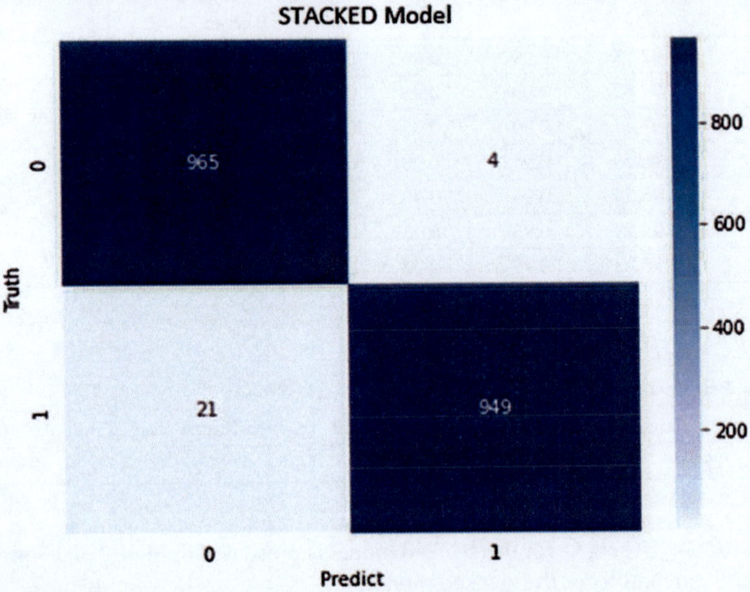

Fig. 3 Confusion matrix for the stacked model

4 Comparative Analysis

This section presents the comparative analysis with existing literature in Table 9. From Table 9, it can be observed that certain proposals fare better than some of the performance metrics individually, but when the complete set of parameters are taken into account, our proposed stacked model excels over the existing counterparts. Barring [13], our proposal fares better than all the other literary proposals presented in Table 9. In contrast to [13], we have implemented 12 machine learning algorithms whereas [13] has implemented only 12. We have implemented the normal as well as hyper-parameter tuned modes for all the 12 machine learning algorithms followed by a stacked model which exhibits the best performance in our analysis.

5 Conclusion

In this study, we have performed classification of stroke using twelve machine learning algorithms. The classification was done in two modes. The first mode used the machine learning models as a base study. In the second mode, the hyper-parameters were tuned in all the twelve models and the best performing eight models were listed. These eight models formed the base model for the stacked model, which was further designed to fetch a better performance. The meta model for the stacked model was the gradient boost classifier. We have observed that the stacked model outperformed most of the proposals in the literature taking into account all the performance metrics. The study can be further extended using deep learning frameworks using artificial neural networks.

Table 9 Comparative analysis with existing literature

Refs #	Algorithms used	Accuracy	Precision	Recall/sensitivity	F1-score	Specificity	RoC-AuC score
[4]	Linear SVC, RF, AB, multinomial NB, Shapiro-Wilk	69					
[5]	RF, random K-label sets		85				
[6]	LR, RF, XGB	99.07	99				
[8]	SVM, margin-based censored regression						77
[9]	LR, DT, KNN, SVM, NB	82	79	82.7	82.3		
[11]	ANN, SVM, RF, boosting and bagging	95	95.9	99.2		99.2	
[12]	DT, two-class boosted DT	96.8					
[14]	KNN, LR, RF, SVC	99.35					
[13]	ANN, SVM, RF, NB	99.8	99.8	99.8	99.8		
[20]	LR, XGB, GBM, RF, SVM, DT	90				100	
[24]	LR, DT, SVM, XGB	93.6					
[23]	SVM	91	84.7	100	91.7	78.75	
[22]	Glow-worm swarm optimization (GSO), SVM	82.58					89
[21]	LR, GNB, KNN, BNB, LR	93					
[19]	SVM, ANN, DT, multilayer perceptron, NB, Dempster-Shafer using gradient descent classifier (DSGD)	85					87

(continued)

Table 9 (continued)

Refs #	Algorithms used	Accuracy	Precision	Recall/sensitivity	F1-score	Specificity	RoC-AuC score
[18]	AB, KNN, GBC, stochastic gradient descent, weighted voting method	97	93	100	97		93
[16]	SVM	70					
[10]	SVM, RF, AB, multinomial Naïve Bayes	98	95				
[15]	SVM, deep learning (DL), KNN, ANN, LR, RF				45.4	83.4	90
[17]	RF, deep neural network and LR						88
Proposed stacked model		98.85	100	98	99		99

References

1. Centers for disease control and prevention. Stroke Facts
2. Prevention C, Know the facts about stroke
3. MedicineNet: cost of treating strokes in U.S. Could Soar to $180B Annually by 2030
4. Fang G, Wang L, Liu W (2020) A machine learning approach to select features important to stroke prognosis. Comput Biol Chem 88
5. Kashi S, Polak RF, Lerner B, Rokach L, Levy-Tzedek S (2020) A machine-learning model for automatic detection of movement compensations in stroke patients. IEEE Trans Emerg Top Comput 9(3):1234–1247
6. Islam F, Ghosh M (2021) An enhanced stroke prediction scheme using SMOTE and machine learning techniques. In: International conference on computing communication and networking technologies (ICCCNT), Kharagpur, India
7. Pedregosa F, Varoquaux G, Gramfort A, Michel V, Thirion B, Grisel O, Blondel M, Prettenhofer P, Weiss R, Dubourg V, Vanderplas J, Passos A, Cournapeau D, Brucher M, Perrot M, Duchesnay E (2011) Scikit-learn: machine learning in python, pp 2825–2830
8. Khosla A, Cao Y, Lin C, Lee H, Hu J, Chiu (2010) An integrated machine learning approach to stroke prediction. In: Proceedings of the 16th ACM SIGKDD international conference on knowledge discovery and data mining, New York, NY, United States, pp 183–192
9. Sailasya G, Kumari GL (2021) Analysing the performance of stroke prediction using ML classification algorithms. Int J Adv Comput Sci Appl (IJACSA), 12(6)
10. Fang G, Xu P, Liu W (2020) Automated ischemic stroke subtyping based on machine learning approach. Feature representation and learning methods with applications in large-scale biological sequence analysis 8(0):118426–118432
11. Govindarajan P, Soundarapandian RK, Gandomi AH, Patan R, Jayaraman P, Manikandan R (2018) Classification of stroke disease using machine learning algorithms. In: Intelligent biomedical data analysis and processing, London, England
12. Ray S, Alshouiliy K, Roy A, AlGhamdi A, Agrawal DP (2020) Chi-squared based feature selection for stroke prediction using AzureML. In: Intermountain engineering, technology and computing (IETC), Orem, UT, USA

13. Shoily T, Islam T, Jannat S, Tanna S, Ali T, Ema R (2019) Detection of stroke disease using machine learning algorithms. In: 10th International conference on computing, communication and networking technologies (ICCCNT), Kanpur, India
14. Krishna V, Kiran JS, Rao PP, Babu GC, Babu GJ (2021) Early detection of brain stroke using machine learning techniques. In: 2nd International conference on smart electronics and communication (ICOSEC), Trichy, India
15. Sirsat M, Ferme E, Camara J (2020) Machine learning for brain stroke: a review. J Stroke Cerebrovasc Dis 29(10):1051–1062
16. Kamal H, Lopez V, Sheth SA (2018) Machine learning in acute ischemic stroke neuroimaging. Front Neurol 9(0):945
17. Heo J, Yoon JG, Park H, Kim Y, Nam H, Heo J (2019) Machine learning–based model for prediction of outcomes in acute stroke. Natl Technol Biotechnol Inf 50(5):1263–1265
18. Emon M, Keya M, Meghla T, Rahman M, Al Mamun MS (2020) Performance analysis of machine learning approaches in stroke prediction. In: 4th International conference on electronics, communication and aerospace technology (ICECA), Coimbatore, India
19. Penafiel S, Baloian N, Sanson H, Pino J (2021) Predicting stroke risk with an interpretable classifier. IEEE Access 9:1154–1166
20. Abedi V, Avula V, Chaudhary D, Shahjouei S, Khan A, Griessenauer CJ, Li J, Zand R (2021) Prediction of long-term stroke recurrence using machine learning models. J Clin Med 10(6)
21. Hossain S, Biswas P, Ahmed P, Sourov MR, Keya M, Khushbu SA (2021) Prognostic the risk of stroke using integrated supervised machine learning techniques. In: 12th International conference on computing communication and networking technologies (ICCCNT), Kharagpur, India
22. Zhang Y, Song W, Li S, Fu L, Li S (2018) Risk detection of stroke using a feature selection and classification method. IEEE Access 6:31899–31907
23. Jeena RS, Kumar S (2016) Stroke prediction using SVM. In: International conference on control, instrumentation, communication and computational technologies (ICCICCT), Kumaracoil, India
24. Monteiro M, Fonseca AC, Freitas AT, e Melo TP, Francisco AP, Ferro JM, Oliveira AL (2018) Using machine learning to improve the prediction of functional outcome in ischemic stroke patients. IEEE/ACM Trans Comput Biol Bioinform 15(6):1953 - 1959
25. Stroke prediction dataset. (Accessed 27 Jan 2021) Available at: https://www.kaggle.com/fedesoriano/stroke-prediction-dataset/metadata

Breast Cancer Detection Using Transfer Learning Techniques in Convolutional Neural Networks

Soma Mitra, Mauparna Nandan, and Randrita Sarkar

Abstract Breast cancer is the primary cause of death in women, despite significant efforts to avoid it through screening programmes. Given the situation, the number of mammograms gathered has increased at an exponential rate. The correct detection of the tumour is vital in determining the course of treatment and the severity of the illness. Computer-assisted diagnosis has become considerably more efficient nowadays. The use of automatic image processing in this context is important. Deep learning-based techniques are a viable option in the detection of breast cancer. In this research work, a transfer learning-based strategy for classifying breast tissue images into two broad categories, benign or malignant, is proposed. The breast histology images corresponding to the BreakHis data set are taken as input from which after normalization, patches are extracted and fed into Google's Inception-V3 and ResNet152V2 Convolutional Neural Networks (CNNs) such that they are able to learn domain-specific features necessary for the categorization of histology images into infectious and non-infectious.

Keywords Breast cancer classification · Deep learning · Transfer learning · Convoluted neural network (CNNs)

S. Mitra
Department of Computational Science, Brainware University, Barasat 700125, India

M. Nandan (✉)
Department of Computer Applications, Haldia Institute of Technology, Haldia 721657, India
e-mail: mauparna2011@gmail.com

R. Sarkar
Department of Information Technology, B. P. Poddar Institute of Management and Technology, Kolkata 700052, India

© The Author(s), under exclusive license to Springer Nature Singapore Pte Ltd. 2023

J. K. Mandal and D. De (eds.), *Frontiers of ICT in Healthcare*, Lecture Notes in Networks and Systems 519, https://doi.org/10.1007/978-981-19-5191-6_19

1 Introduction

Breast cancer is the most prevalent disease in women and the leading cause of death due to cancer worldwide, making it a major public health concern. Indeed, approximately one in every seven women will be impacted by this disease at some point in their lives, with the risk growing as they become older. Furthermore, global studies revealed 522,000 breast cancer deaths in 2012, a 14% increase over 2008 [1].

It is expected that by 2030, this figure will have risen to more than 28 million. According to ACS, breast cancer deaths accounts for approx. 14% amongst all cancer fatalities in the USA and hence the second-leading reason for cancer death in women. Breast cancer accounts for 30% amongst newly discovered cancer cases. Breast cancer is now one of the most common cancers amongst women. When it comes to detecting breast cancer, a biopsy followed by microscopic image analysis is the standard procedure [2].

The pathologist examines the microscopic architecture and other components on a microscopic level in breast tissue biopsy so that the pathologist can distinguish between normal tissue, non-malignant (or benign) tissue, and malignant lesions using these histological pictures. The information gathered is then used to make a prognosis determination.

Benign lesions are deviations in the normal tissue of the breast parenchyma that are unrelated to the progression of malignancy. The two types of carcinoma tissue are in situ and invasive carcinomas. The term "in situ tissue" refers to tissue that is contained within the mammary ductal–lobular. Otherwise, invasive carcinoma cells spread outside the breast ductal–lobular framework.

The afflicted region is determined throughout the diagnosing phase using whole-slide tissue imaging. Zooming, concentrating, and scanning each picture in its entirety are all required when analysing photos with varying magnification factors. This technique is time consuming and exhausting, and as a result, the manual process can occasionally result in incorrect breast cancer detection. Because of the progress of digital imaging techniques, various computer vision and ML algorithms have been developed for evaluating pathological images at a microscopic resolution. These methods might aid in the automation of some pathological process operations in a diagnostic system. However, recent advances in deep learning (DL) have already demonstrated tremendous efficiency on a variety of recognition tasks in the fields of image processing.

These methods have been used in a variety of medical imaging modalities, including pathological imaging, with excellent classification, segmentation, and detection results. In other circumstances, DL-based technologies are an integral part of the workflow for pathologists and clinicians in clinical settings [3].

A Convolutional Neural Network (CNN or ConvNet) is a common deep learning approach that teaches a model to do classification tasks directly from pictures, video, text, or sound. CNNs are particularly useful for recognizing objects and faces, by looking for patterns in images. They learn directly from picture data, classifying images using patterns rather than traditional feature extraction. In our proposed work, we have implemented CNN to classify breast cancer images. We have also evaluated the usefulness of transfer learning to achieve image classification on the BreakHis data set and then analyse the classification performance parameters of the pre-trained Inception-V3 [4] and ResNet152V2 [5] networks, respectively.

2 Related Works

During the recent decade, research on breast cancer detection has increased. The detection of malignant tissue in the breast and the classification of tumours have been the focus of a lot of research. This section gives a complete assessment of several methodologies focused on breast cancer analysis in order to comprehend the concerns and difficulties encountered by prior research studies.

Tourassi et al. [6], for example, preferred a tumour detection content search engine that uses expert information contained in the various mammograms that comprise the imagery database. To do so, matching templates are employed to detect photos which are similar to the ROI request submitted by the system's user. They developed a decision method that successfully integrates numerous similar measures based upon the concept of best matches to determine whether the query ROI incorporates tumour or only healthy tissue.

Bayramoglu et al. [7] developed a CNN-based method for automating breast cancer diagnosis in histopathology photos, regardless of magnification. When this method's classification performance was compared to that of prior models that employed manual feature extraction approaches, the CNN model performed better. Arajo et al. [8] developed a CNN model for multi-classification of breast biopsy pictures in another work to address the limitations of traditional feature extraction classification approaches. For the multi-classification of breast biopsies, this model has a classification accuracy of 77.8%.

Alto et al. [9] chose to extract edge attributes such as roughness, shape, and sharpness. Tao et al. [10] integrated those related to pixel intensity, shape, and texture in order to detect tumours comparable to those in the ROI query and classified them as benign or malignant. Nawaz et al. [11] developed a multi-class breast cancer categorization based on CNN. Their proposed technique achieved a high classification accuracy of 95.4% using the DenseNet and BreakHis training data sets. Kasani et al. [12] used an ensemble deep learning-based technique for binary categorization of histopathological biopsy pictures into malignant and benign cases. Zheng et al. [13] propose a technique in which the user is requested to evaluate the type of the spiking tumour in the query image using ML methods.

Comparatively, in recent research papers, the CNN models are mostly used for breast cancer detection [14–17]. CNN models are mainly proposed for other image recognition purpose, but transfer learning enables the researchers to classify the cancerous cells.

3 System Model Architecture

In this section, we will primarily describe the architecture of our proposed system model, which is made up of four modules: data collection, data processing, feature learning, and data classification.The complete system architecture is depicted in Fig. 1.

3.1 Data Collection

The most widely publicly available BreakHis data set comprises of a database of microscopic biopsy images of malignant and benign breast cancer images. BreakHis breast tumour tissue collection encompasses a set of 9,109 images collected from 82 patients with various magnifying factors (40×, 100×, 200×, and 400×). The details of the images data set into four distinct magnification levels is enumerated in Table 1.

3.2 Feature Learning Module

Feature learning (FL) is referred to as a set of approaches in machine learning that allows a system to discover the representations required to serve the purpose of feature

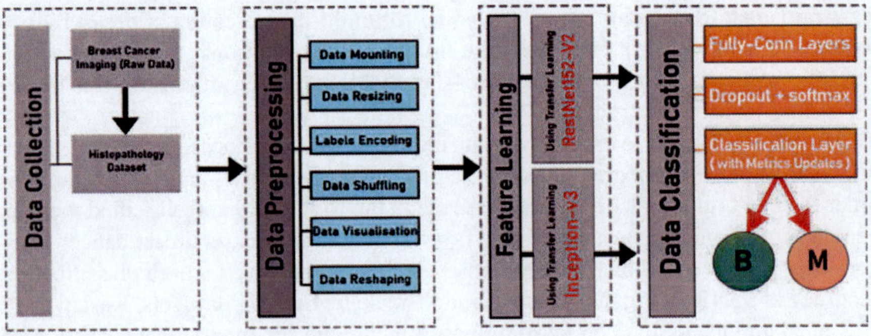

Fig. 1 Schematic diagram of the proposed system architecture

Table 1 Distribution of BreakHis data set

	Magnification level				
Category	40×	100×	200×	400×	Total
Benign	652	644	623	588	2480
Malignant	1370	1437	1390	1232	5429
Total	1995	2081	2013	1820	7909

detection, prediction, or classification from a preprocessed data set automatically [20]. Transfer learning is commonly applied to deep learning (DL) applications which assist us to apply a pre-trained network to perform new prediction/classification tasks. Using this approach, the original network design is preserved and the pre-trained weights are utilized for the initialization of the network. During the fine-tuning phase, the initialization weights are adjusted, thereby allowing the network to learn features with respect to the specific task at hand. In this study, we have employed two CNN architectures, namely Google's Inception-V3 [4] and ResNet152V2 [5]. These models may be used for a variety of tasks, including classification, feature extraction, and prediction. A brief introduction of these two architectures are illustrated below.

- **Inception-V3**: According to a recent study, Google's Inception-V3 network obtained skin cancer classification accuracy that was comparable to that of many dermatologists [21]. Factorized inception modules are implemented in the Inception-V3 network, thereby allowing the network to select appropriate kernel sizes for the convolution layers. This allows the network to learn both low-level and high-level features. By improving earlier Inception designs, Inception-V3 primarily focuses on consuming less processing power. The feature learning module using Inception-V3 is illustrated in Fig. 2.
- **ResNet152V2**: The ResNet model is built on a residual learning architecture in which layers inside a network are reformed to learn a residual mapping between inputs and outputs rather than the desired unknown mapping. As a result, optimization is simpler in such a network which allow training of deeper networks, thereby resulting in enhanced network capacity and performance. ResNet has a large number of layers and is extremely fast [22]. As illustrated in Fig. 3, ResNet152V2 is also employed as a feature extraction model. The input can be learned using the model's pre-trained starting weights. This method shortens the time it takes to train and cover a large area with good precision. The initial model is followed by a reshape step, a flatten step, a dropout layer, two dense layers, and finally an

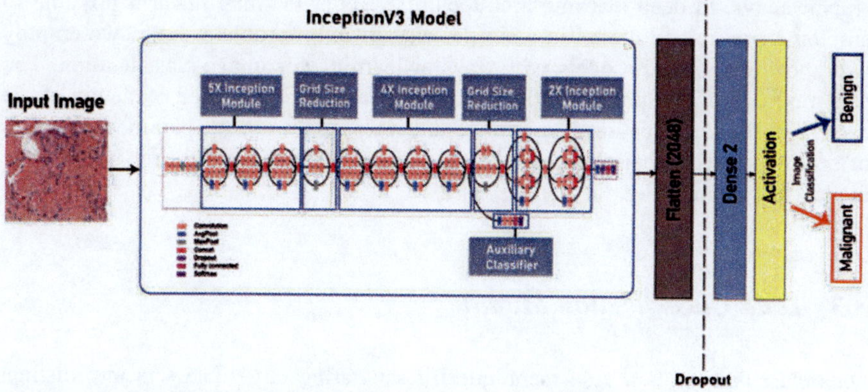

Fig. 2 Feature learning module using Inception-V3 transfer learning

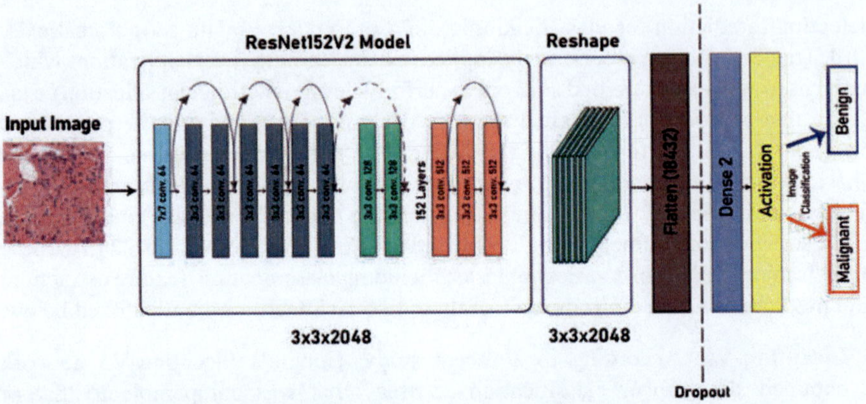

Fig. 3 Feature learning module using ResNet152V2 transfer learning

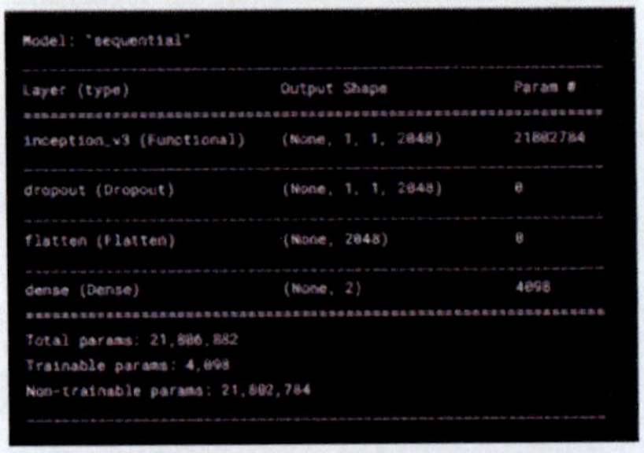

(a) Inception V3 Model Summary

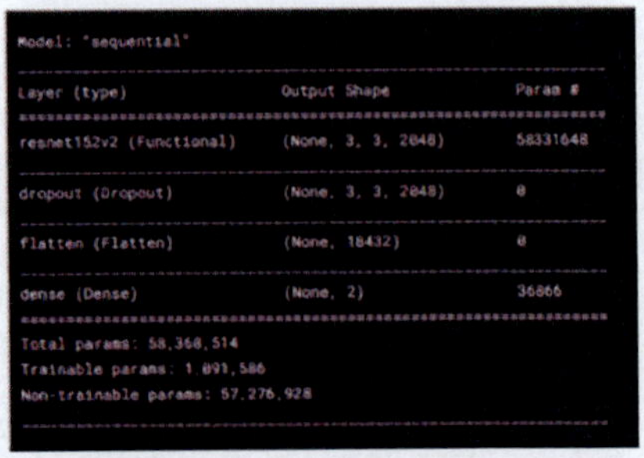

(b) ResNet152V2 Model Summary

Fig. 4 Feature learning models

activation function that classifies the picture as malignant or benign, as seen in the figure. The feature learning module using ResNet152V2 is illustrated in Fig. 3.

Nowadays, in deep learning architecture, transfer learning made it possible to employ a pre-trained model in a similar classification problem. Here, we employ two above-mentioned models with transfer learning for image classification. The said models are incorporated topless and a dense layer is included at the top of the each layer for classification. It minimizes the number of trainable parameters in both of the models. The list of trainable and non-trainable parameters for both of the models are given in Fig. 4.

3.3 *Data Classification Module*

Data classification is a vital technique for separating large data sets into distinct classes for efficient decision-making, pattern recognition, and other purposes. For

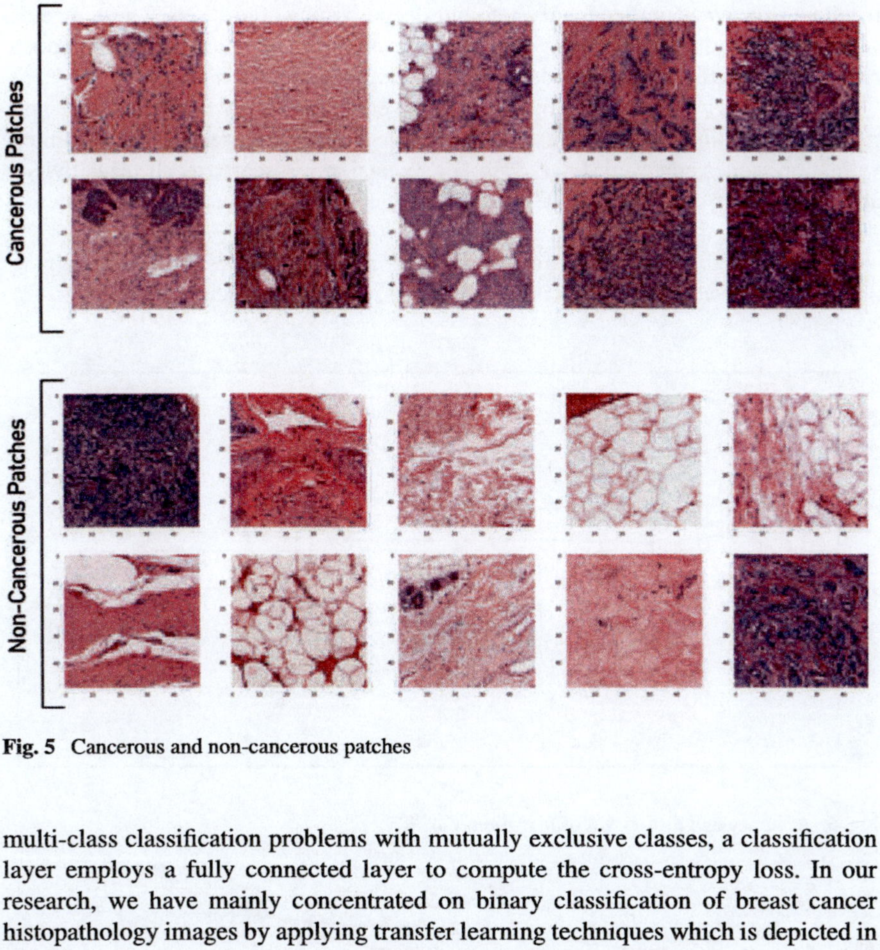

Fig. 5 Cancerous and non-cancerous patches

multi-class classification problems with mutually exclusive classes, a classification layer employs a fully connected layer to compute the cross-entropy loss. In our research, we have mainly concentrated on binary classification of breast cancer histopathology images by applying transfer learning techniques which is depicted in Fig. 5.

4 Experimental Results and Evaluation

In this study, we have used a publicly accessible data set on Breast Histopathology Images in Kaggle, which contains 277,524 images. 162 whole mount slide pictures of breast cancer (BCa) specimens were scanned at 40× in the original data set. 277,524 (50 × 50) patches were retrieved from it (198,738 IDC negative and 78,786 IDC positive).

We have downscaled the photos to 75 by 75 before adding them into the models. The training pictures are allocated as follows in our framework: 70% for training and 30% for validation. Numpy was then used to convert the images into arrays. The resultant images were then loaded into our deep learning algorithms. These models were trained and validated using the optimizer and fit algorithms, with each epoch having 3694 steps and each model running about 10 epochs.

The findings were produced by applying the equations for each performance metric to the validation data outputs, with the recorded results representing the maximum validation values achieved. Loss, accuracy, precision, F_1-score, recall (sensitivity), and Area Under the Curve (AUC) were used to evaluate the deep learning system's performance.

Loss and accuracy curves of training and validation as obtained during the training process of the two models are displayed in Figs. 6 and 7, respectively.

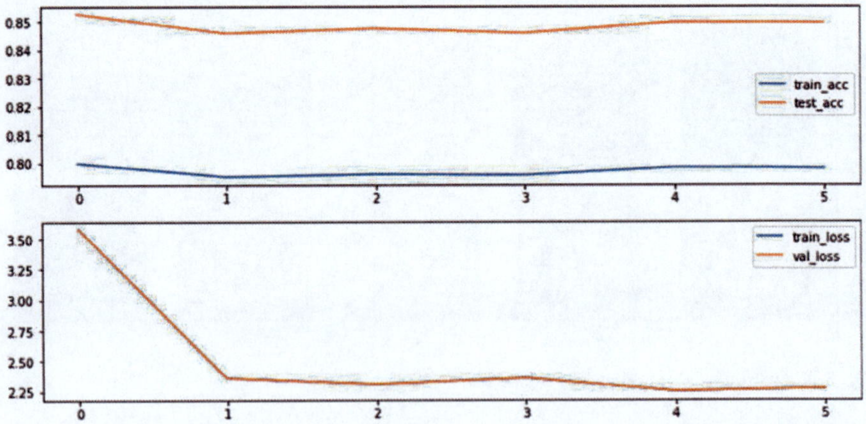

Fig. 6 Accuracy and loss curves of Inception-V3

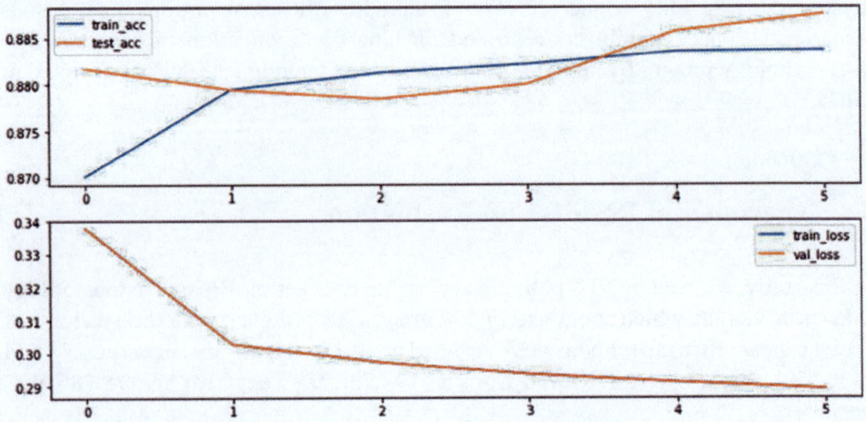

Fig. 7 Accuracy and loss curves of ResNet152V2

Table 2 Inception-V3 performance analysis

Class	Precision	Recall	F_1 score
0	0.86	0.98	0.92
1	0.56	0.11	0.18
Accuracy			0.85
Macro avg.	0.71	0.55	0.55
Weighted avg.	0.81	0.85	0.8

Table 3 ResNet152V2 performance analysis

Class	Precision	Recall	F_1 score
0	0.88	0.99	0.93
1	0.52	0.1	0.16
Accuracy			0.85
Macro avg.	0.7	0.545	0.545
Weighted avg.	0.83	0.86	0.82

It is clearly visible that both the losses start with a large value but systematically diminish as training proceeds with faster threshold. The classification accuracy is measured as the area under the ROC curve (AUC) where an area of 1 indicates perfect classification upon the test set.

And, finally the overall accuracy metrics of the entire architecture after the application of both the models through transfer learning techniques is 86% which is displayed in Tables 2 and 3.

5 Conclusion and Future Work

This paper presents a transfer learning-based strategy for classifying H&E-stained histological breast cancer images. Google's Inception-V3 and residual network (ResNet152V2) designs, which have been pre-trained using ImageNet, are used to teach the network features. Both the networks have been trained with 70% of the data set, and their performance was evaluated on the remaining 30% of images. The proposed transfer learning approach for automatic classification of breast cancer histology images is effortless but fruitful. Despite the lack of training data, the networks directly converted ImageNet knowledge of convolutional features to classify histology images. For the automatic analysis of breast cancer histology images, the given study illustrates the efficiency and effectiveness of transfer learning algorithms.

References

1. Todua F, Gagua R, Maglakelidze M, Maglakelidze D (2013) Estimated cancer incidence, mortality and prevalence worldwide in 2012. In: Globocan 2012, IARC 2013
2. Loukas C, Kostopoulos S, Tanoglidi A, Glotsos D, Sfikas C, Cavouras D (2013) Breast cancer characterization based on image classification of tissue sections visualized under low magnification. In: Computational and mathematical methods in medicine 2013
3. Litjens G, Kooi T, Bejnordi BE, Setio AAA, Ciompi F, Ghafoorian M, Sánchez CI (2017) A survey on deep learning in medical image analysis. Med Image Anal 42:60–88
4. Szegedy C, Vanhoucke V, Ioe S, Shlens J, Wojna Z (2016) Rethinking the inception architecture for computer vision. In: Proceedings of the IEEE conference on computer vision and pattern recognition, pp 2818–2826
5. He K, Zhang X, Ren S, Sun J (2016) Deep residual learning for image recognition. In: Proceedings of the IEEE conference on computer vision and pattern recognition, pp 770–778
6. Tourassi GD, Vargas-Voracek R, Catarious DM Jr, Floyd CE (2003) Computer-assisted detection of mammographic masses: a template matching scheme based on mutual information. Med Phys 30(8):2123–2130
7. Bayramoglu N, Kannala J, Heikkilä J (2016) Deep learning for magnification independent breast cancer histopathology image classification. In: 23rd International conference on pattern recognition (ICPR), Cancun, Mexico, pp 2440–2445
8. Araújo T, Aresta G, Castro E et al (2017) Classification of breast cancer histology images using convolutional neural networks. PloS One 12:e0177544
9. Alto H, Rangayyan RM, Desautels JL (2005) Content-based retrieval and analysis of mammographic masses. J Electron Imaging 14(2):023016–023016
10. Tao Y, Lo S, Freedman MT, Xuan J (2007) A preliminary study of content-based mammographic masses retrieval. In: Medical imaging, 65141Z. International Society for Optics and Photonics
11. Nawaz M, Sewissy AA, Soliman THA (2018) Multi-class breast cancer classification using deep learning convolutional neural network. Int J Adv Comput Sci Appl 9:316–332
12. Kassani SH, Kassani PH, Wesolowski MJ et al (2019) Classification of histopathological biopsy images using ensemble of deep learning networks. In: Proceedings of the 29th international conference on computer science and software engineering, Toronto, Canada, pp 92–99
13. Zheng B, Lu A, Hardesty LA, Sumkin JH, Hakim CM, Ganott MA, Gur DA (2006) A method to improve visual similarity of breast masses for an interactive computer-aided diagnosis environment. Med Phys 33(1):111–117
14. Alanazi SA, Kamruzzaman MM, Islam Sarker MN, Alruwaili M, Alhwaiti Y, Alshammari N, Siddiqi MH (2021) Boosting breast cancer detection using convolutional neural network. J Healthc Eng
15. Meenalochini G, Ramkumar S (2021) Survey of machine learning algorithms for breast cancer detection using mammogram images. Mater Today Proc 37:2738–2743
16. Sinha N, Sharma P, Arora D (2021) Prediction model for breast cancer detection using machine learning algorithms. In: Computational methods and data engineering. Springer, Singapore, pp 431–440
17. Assegie TA (2021) An optimized K-nearest neighbor based breast cancer detection. J Robot Control (JRC) 2(3):115–118
18. Spanhol F, Oliveira LS, Petitjean C, Heutte L (2016) A dataset for breast cancer histopathological image classification. IEEE Trans Biomed Eng (TBME) 63(7):1455–1462. https://doi.org/10.1109/TBME.2015.2496264
19. Dataset. https://www.kaggle.com/paultimothymooney/breast-histopathology-images
20. Bengio Y, Courville A, Vincent P (2013) Representation learning: a review and new perspectives. IEEE Trans Pattern Anal Mach Intell 35(8):1798–1828. PMID 23787338. arXiv:1206.5538; https://doi.org/10.1109/tpami.2013.50
21. Esteva A, Kuprel B, Novoa RA, Ko J, Swetter SM, Blau HM, Thrun S (2017) Dermatologist-level classification of skin cancer with deep neural networks. Nature 542(7639):115
22. Gulli A, Pal S (2017) Deep learning with Keras. Packt Publishing Ltd., Birmingham, UK

A Machine Learning-Based Prediction Model for Fetal Health Assessment

Hirdesh Varshney and Avtar Singh

Abstract Even with multi-fold growth in medical diagnostics, continuous and error-free monitoring of pregnant women during the gestational stage has attracted many eye-catching concerns, globally. These diagnostics play a vital role in the overall assessment of fetal and expecting women's health. Cardiotocography is one such technique that acquires sophisticated information of fetal heart to access the fetus's health status. However, because of human interventions, it is also prone to errors. Therefore, the present work proposes a machine learning-based prognosis tool that will assist the medical practitioners for the early and critical assessment of fetal health. For this purpose, Random Forest, *k*-Nearest Neighbor, Logistic Regression, Gradient Boost, and Extreme Gradient Boost techniques are employed. Also, the grid search cross-validation is utilized to estimate the optimum hyperparameters of these models. The results reveal that the Extreme Gradient Boost algorithm performs remarkably and achieved an accuracy of greater than 94% that is significantly better than all other models.

Keywords Fetal cardiotocography · Fetal health assessment · Machine learning · Maternal mortality ratio

1 Introduction

Proper monitoring of fetal growth during pregnancy is of utmost importance. However, this growth may be affected by various hormonal changes that occurred during the gestation stages of expecting women and her medical history. Further, the

H. Varshney (✉) · A. Singh
Department of Computer Science and Engineering, Dr B R Ambedkar National Institute of Technology, Jalandhar, India
e-mail: hrideshvarshney@gmail.com

A. Singh
e-mail: avtars@nitj.ac.in

H. Varshney
Department of Computer Science and Engineering, Babu Banarasi Das University, Lucknow, India

© The Author(s), under exclusive license to Springer Nature Singapore Pte Ltd. 2023
J. K. Mandal and D. De (eds.), *Frontiers of ICT in Healthcare*, Lecture Notes in Networks and Systems 519, https://doi.org/10.1007/978-981-19-5191-6_20

maternal and paternal attributes also affect significantly in the overall growth of the fetus because of which, keeping an eye on fetal development has been considered as one of the most challenging tasks [1]. Also, it has been found that around 20% of pregnant women experience various levels of complications such as premature birth, intrauterine growth restriction, and birth hypoxia which may lead to fetal/maternal morbidity, or sometimes mortality [2]. This resulted in the death of more than 800 pregnant women per day even with various preventive measures [3]. The associated maternal mortality ratio (MMR) has been found as comparatively very small in developed countries than in developing countries. Similar trends have been witnessed in India where this ratio is quite lesser in states like Kerala and Maharashtra, however, much higher in Assam [4].

To prevent these irreversible damages, medical practitioners widely prefer the assessment of fetal health via cardiotocography (CTG). The main aim of the CTG is to track fetal distress and other common fetal risks including fetal heart rate (FHR), acceleration or deceleration of FHR, etc. [5]. However, even with the international guidelines and experienced clinicians, the assessment of these CTG has not been consistent. Furthermore, the reported literature reveals that the inability to recognize abnormal FHR trends along with the lack of associated preventive actions resulted in more than 50% of fetal deaths [6]. Therefore, in order to lower the fetal mortality and MMR, the errors due to human intervention and unwanted practice variation must be reduced which may be achieved by integrating computer-based patient records and clinical decision support.

Under the umbrella of above discussion, this work employs machine learning (ML) algorithms to develop a prognosis tool for the accurate classification of the CTG dataset. For this purpose, the open source fetal health dataset from Kaggle has been utilized [7]. Also, since there exist no single ML algorithm that can perform sufficiently well for all tasks; therefore, in this work, five most popular ML (Random Forest (RF), K-Nearest Neighbor (k-NN), Logistic Regression (LR), Gradient Boost (GB), and Extreme Gradient Boost (XGB)) techniques have been employed and their effectiveness has been compared on the basis of various key performance parameters.

The rest of the proposed work is organized as follows: Sect. 2 presents the related work done in this field. The brief description of dataset being employed is mentioned in Sect. 3. The methodology used for this work is depicted in Sect. 4. In Sect. 5, the experimental results are presented and discussed. And finally, Sect. 6 gives the concluding remarks of the present work.

2 Related Work

With the amount of data being available, it has become a new oil, and therefore, ML techniques can become very fruitful assistive tool for the medical practitioners in order to predict the various complications during pregnancy so that the MMR and fetal mortality rate (FMR) can be effectively reduced. Being inspired by this, many researchers have employed ML techniques for the classification of fetal health. In

[8], the employability of various ML algorithms has been assessed on CTG data and it has been found that RF performs sufficiently well. In [9], the fetal heart rate has been monitored by employing Artificial Neural Network (ANN). In [10], the CART-based Decision Tree (DT) has been employed for multiclass classification on CTG data with an accuracy of 88.88%. Similarly, Support Vector Machine (SVM) and Naïve Bayes (NB) have been employed to classify CTG data [11, 12]. Though, generally, the classification has been done in the third trimester but monitoring of fetal health even in second trimester can effectively reduce the prenatal mortality with a mean accuracy of 91.10% [13]. Also, a recent rush of ensemble ML techniques has been witnessed for effective interpretation of FHR [14].

Although, these spectra of works reveal that there is an intrinsically interesting association which may assist medical practitioners in lowering the MMR and FMR but most of these studies have utilized balanced dataset only. However, in real world, it is not always the case; therefore, there is an urgent need for the development of ML-based prognosis tool that may predict the fetal health for both balanced and unbalanced dataset with acceptable accuracy.

3 Dataset Description and Preprocessing

There is a close correlation between fetal and maternal health, and the device used to monitor FHR has been referred as cardiotocogram or electronic fetal monitor. The CTG is preferably done in the third trimester of the pregnancy, in which two transducers have been placed onto the abdomen of the pregnant women to estimate the health of both mother and fetal. One transducer records FHR, whereas other uterine contraction (UC). The CTG measures and records the tensions created in the abdominal wall by a time-scaled printed running paper and therefore, provides an indirect indication of intrauterine pressure. In this work, the open source UCI dataset for fetal health classification has been employed. This dataset is a numerical representation of the original CTG measurement and has been subdivided into 21 attributes and 1 target. It contains 2126 samples of fetal carditocograms which has been classified into three classes (N-Normal, S-Suspect, and P-Pathologic) by three obstetricians based on the measurement of FHR and UC. Further, various international agencies have issued several guidelines for interpreting these CTG patterns [15]. These guidelines have been briefly presented in Table 1 and the features of obtained CTG data have been depicted in Table 2.

In any ML driven study, exploratory data analysis (EDA) and preprocessing play a very crucial role. It not only helps in visualizing the dataset but also provides better insight of the dataset. Therefore, by analyzing the dataset, it has been revealed that the utilized dataset does not have any missing or null values; however, 13 samples with duplicate entries have been identified. Further, it has been found that the share of Normal, Suspect, and Pathologic class in the dataset is 57%, 23%, and 20%, respectively (Fig. 1). Therefore, the dataset is highly imbalanced toward Normal class. However, considering all these mentioned pitfalls as the natural part of the

Table 1 Fetal health assessment criteria

Baseline heart beat (bpm)	Variability (bpm)	Decelerations	Accelerations	Health state of fetal
110–160	≥5	None	Present or absent (other parameters in normal state)	Healthy
100–109 or 161–180	<5 for 40–90 min	Early, typical (>90 min) and single (<3 min)	None	Require further investigation
<100 or >180 or sinusoidal ≥10 min	<5 for 90 min	Either typical or late (>30 min) and single (>3 min)	None	Abnormal

Table 2 Data description

S. no	Features	Description	Range	Variable type
1.	FHR_B	FHR baseline	(106–160)	Numeric
2.	AC	Accelerations	(0–0.019)	Numeric
3.	FM	Fetal movements	(0–0.481)	Numeric
4.	UC	Uterine contractions	(0–0.015)	Numeric
5.	D_L	Deceleration (Light)	(0–0.015)	Numeric
6.	D_S	Deceleration (Severe)	(0–0.001)	Boolean
7.	D_P	Deceleration (Prolonged)	(0–0.005)	Numeric
8.	STV_A	Percentage of time with abnormal short term variability (STV)	(12–87)	Numeric
9.	STV_M	Mean value of STV	(0.2–7)	Numeric
10.	LTV_A	Percentage of time with abnormal long term variability (LTV)	(0–91)	Numeric
11.	LTV_M	Mean value of LTV	(0–50.7)	Numeric
12.	H_W	Width of FHR histogram	(3–180)	Numeric
13.	H_{Min}	Minimum of FHR histogram	(50–159)	Numeric
14.	H_{Max}	Maximum of FHR histogram	(122–238)	Numeric
15.	N_{HP}	Histogram peaks count	(0–18)	Numeric
16.	N_{HZ}	Histogram zeros count	(0–10)	Numeric
17.	H_{Mode}	Histogram mode	(60–187)	Numeric
18.	H_{Mean}	Histogram mean	(73–182)	Numeric
19.	H_{Med}	Histogram median	(77–186)	Numeric
20.	H_{Var}	Histogram variance	(0–269)	Numeric
21.	H_{Tend}	Histogram tendency	(−1 to 1)	Categorical
22.	FS	Fetal status	(1-Normal, 2-Suspect, and 3-Pathologic)	Categorical

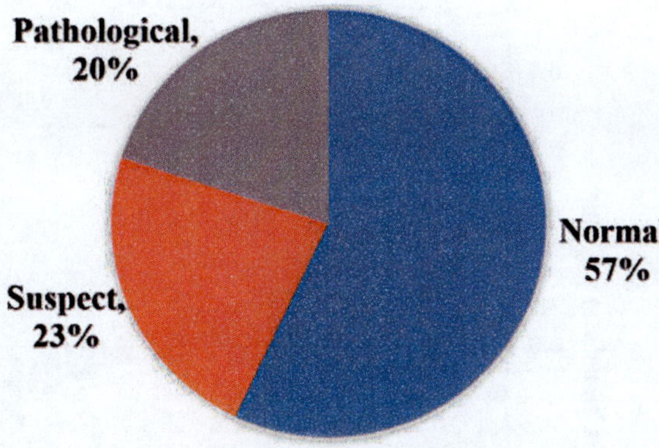

Fig. 1 Fetal health distribution

studied population, no preprocessing technique has been employed in the present study.

Further, correlation between attributes and target has been estimated to find the relation between the available attributes in the dataset with the target. From this analysis, it has been witnessed that the features like DP, STVA, and LTVA have a greater impact on the fetal health as compared to others. This distribution has been depicted in Fig. 2 for more clarity. However, considering other features as the essential part of the CTG dataset, this study employs all the available features for the predicting the health status of fetal. Therefore, the obtained dataset has been randomly distributed in the training and testing subset by employing the open source train-test split from scikit learn library with a policy of 70:30. This policy is mostly preferred in smaller sized datasets (less than 10,000 samples) to avoid high variance.

4 Methodology

Generally, the competency of ML algorithms greatly depends upon the quality of the dataset being employed. For this purpose, most of the reported literature utilizes cleaned and polished dataset [16]. However, the results achieved using these polished datasets loses the practical applicability of the work. Therefore, considering the various levels of irregularities in the obtained dataset as a natural one, this work explores the efficiency of ML algorithms for fetal health assessment in real world. To achieve this goal, five most popular ML (RF, k-NN, LR, GB, and XGB) techniques have been employed.

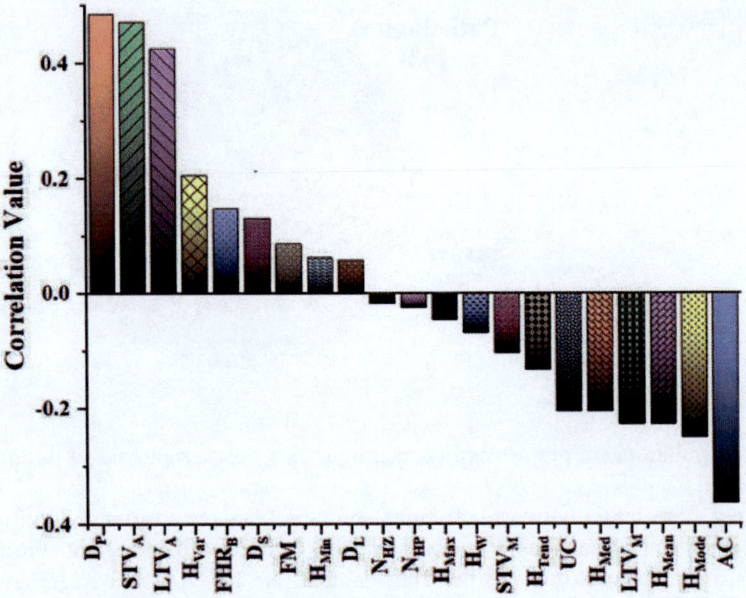

Fig. 2 Correlation of fetal health with other attributes

4.1 *Random Forest (RF)*

RF combines the output of many uncorrelated decision trees, and the most likely classification has been projected as the model prediction. RF predicts the class in two phases: model initialization and residual computation as represented by Eqs. 1 and 2 [17].

$$M_0 = \underset{\varphi}{\arg\min} \sum K(y, \varphi) \tag{1}$$

$$\vartheta = \left[\frac{\delta K(y, M_{\mathrm{RF}}(x))}{\delta M_{\mathrm{RF}}(x)} \right] \tag{2}$$

where (x, y), ϑ, φ, and K represents the attributes of training dataset, regularization, residuals, and differentiable loss function, respectively. Also, $M_{\mathrm{RF}}(x)$ and M_0 depict the model and its initial values, respectively.

4.2 K-Nearest Neighbor (k-NN)

It is an unsupervised learning algorithm which classifies the dataset into k number of classes based on the similarity in the dataset. It memorizes the training data, and therefore, does not require parameter adjustments during training. However, because of this feature, for each prediction, it searches from scratch. It requires comparatively larger time for prediction, and therefore, also called as lazy learner.

4.3 Logistic Regression (LR)

Because of the simplicity with effectiveness, LR remains one of the most popular ML algorithms. It employs logistic function to assess the inherent relationship between the target and available attributes in the dataset. Then, the target has been categorized depending upon the maximum likelihood estimation. Mathematically, it has been expressed by Eq. 3 [8].

$$F(y) = \frac{1}{1 + \mathrm{e}^{-x}} \tag{3}$$

4.4 Gradient Boost (GB)

GB combines fixed size decision trees (weak learners) yet achieved remarkable performance by allowing optimization of a differentiable loss function. It employs back-fitting to limit the loss function $L(y, F(x))$ as mentioned in Eq. 4 [18].

$$F^* = \underset{F}{\arg\min}\, E_{y,x} L(y, F(x)) \tag{4}$$

where $F(x)$ is the objective function. Further, if $\gamma(x; a)$ represents the base learners parameters, then the predicted model is a weighted sum of the base learners and can be mathematically represented as in Eq. 5 [18].

$$F\left(x; \{B_k, a_k\}_1^K\right) = \sum_{k=1}^{K} B_k \gamma(x : a) \tag{5}$$

4.5 *Extreme Gradient Boost (XGB)*

XBG also employs gradient boost methodologies that combines the outcome of many weak learners (Decision Tree). It is a scalable system which provides an end-to-end tree boosting. Further, the execution speed and model performance especially for low to middle level structured data puts it into among the top rated and promising ML algorithms.

The performance of these developed predictive models has also been compared against various crucial parameters such as precision, sensitivity, specificity, accuracy, and F1 score. These parameters can be mathematically calculated using Eq. 6–10 [19].

$$\text{Precision} = \frac{N_{\text{GP}}}{N_{\text{GP}} + N_{\text{FP}}} \tag{6}$$

$$\text{Sensitivity} = \frac{N_{\text{GP}}}{N_{\text{GP}} + N_{\text{FN}}} \tag{7}$$

$$\text{Specificity} = \frac{N_{\text{GN}}}{N_{\text{GN}} + N_{\text{FP}}} \tag{8}$$

$$\text{Accuracy} = \frac{N_{\text{GP}} + N_{\text{GN}}}{N_{\text{GP}} + N_{\text{GN}} + N_{\text{FP}} + N_{\text{FN}}} \times 100 \tag{9}$$

$$F_1 \text{ score} = \frac{2 \times \text{Precision} \times \text{Recall}}{\text{Precision} + \text{Recall}} \tag{10}$$

where NGP, NFP, NGN, and NFN represent the number of gold positives, false positives, gold negatives, and false negatives, respectively. Further, the best parameters for all the mentioned algorithms have been selected by employing fivefold grid search cross-validation, and the impact of cross-validation on the overall model performance has been analyzed using the coefficient of determination of the prediction (R^2). Also, the developed and cross-validated models have been compared against mean square error (MSE), root mean square error (RMSE), training R^2 (R^2_{train}), and test R^2 (R^2_{test}). Summarizing, the step-by-step methodology of the present proposed work can be sketched as in Fig. 3.

5 Result and Discussion

As discussed earlier, this study employs fetal health classification dataset which contains a total of 2126 samples with 21 attributes and 1 target. The target is further classified into 3 classes (Normal, Pathologic, and Suspect). The obtained dataset has been splitted into train and test by employing a policy of 70:30; therefore, 1488 and 638 samples have been used for training and testing, respectively. Further, all

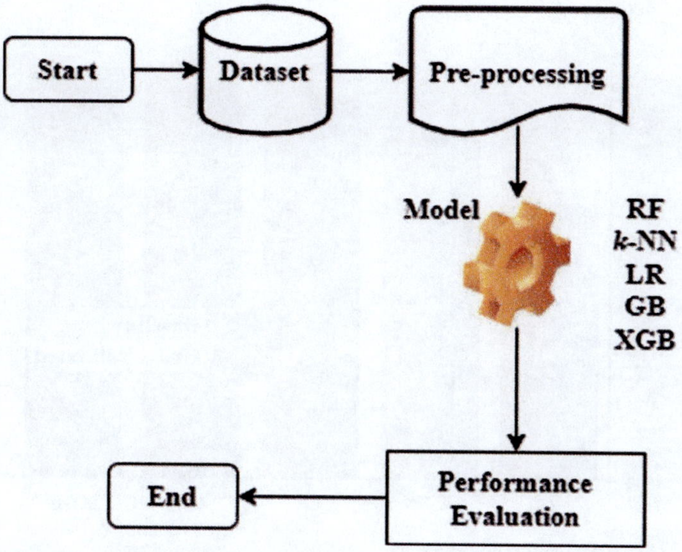

Fig. 3 Flowchart of proposed methodology

the above-mentioned models have been trained to predict the outcome and it has been found that the models when trained with default hyperparameters does not produce acceptable results; therefore, grid search cross-validation with fivefold has been employed to estimate the best hyperparameters. It has been found that the cross-validation improves the models prediction capability by a minimum margin of 0.45% for *k*-NN and maximum margin of 2.84% for RF. This boost in model capability has been estimated on the basis of R^2 and depicted in Fig. 4.

The performance of these boosted models has been compared on the basis of mentioned parameters (Table 3) and it has been found that in terms of MSE, XGB classifier outclasses RF, *k*-NN, LR, and GB classifiers by a margin of 15.24%, 21.93%, 42.21%, and 43.67%, respectively. Similar trends have been witnessed for RMSE where XGB overshadowed other models by 8.02%, 11.83%, 23.98%, and 25.13%, respectively. Though, while training the value of R^2 has been found as approximately same for most of the developed models, a significant improvement with the minimum margin of 1.73% has been estimated while testing. Further, the developed XGB classifier achieved the optimum values of precision, sensitivity, and specificity as 0.916, 0.884, and 0.969, respectively. Therefore, it outperforms RF, *k*-NN, LR, and GB classifiers by a margin of 3.41%, 7.06%, 13.75%, and 13.75% for precision, 4.76%, 8.64%, 29.41%, and 17.33% for sensitivity, and 0.83%, 1.57%, 4.87%, and 2.11% for specificity, respectively. Similarly, it dominates other models by a significant margin of 3.49% and 2.17% for F_1 score and accuracy, respectively. Therefore, it has been perceived that the developed XGB classifier performs outstandingly, and hence, may be used as a prognosis tool for early and accurate assessment of fetal heath.

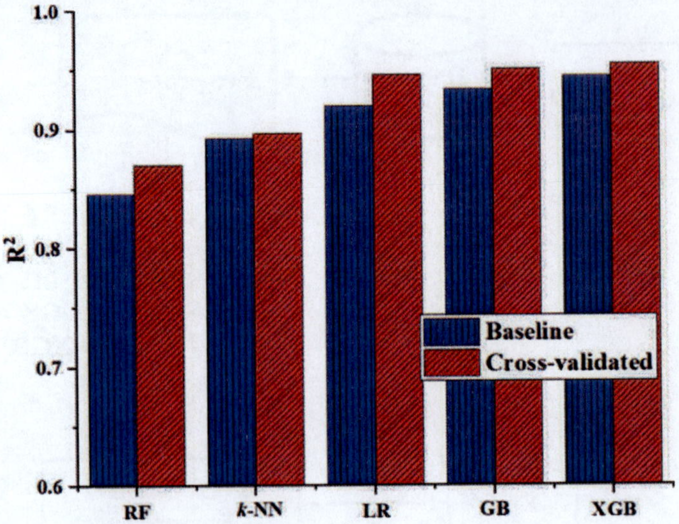

Fig. 4 Boost in model prediction capability

Table 3 Performance comparison of developed classifiers

Model	MSE	RMSE	R^2 train	R^2 test	Precision	Sensitivity	Specificity	Accuracy	F_1 score
RF	0.105	0.324	0.992	0.923	0.883	0.845	0.961	0.922	0.864
k-NN	0.114	0.338	0.999	0.909	0.852	0.817	0.954	0.914	0.836
LR	0.154	0.392	0.886	0.861	0.804	0.683	0.924	0.863	0.734
GB	0.158	0.398	0.978	0.898	0.804	0.756	0.949	0.902	0.777
XGB	0.089	0.298	0.999	0.939	0.916	0.884	0.969	0.941	0.893

Further, to validate the effectiveness of the present proposed work, its results have also been compared with other reported work on the basis of accuracy and given in Table 4. It has been estimated that the proposed methodology performs significantly better than the compared models and outclasses them by an encouraging margin of 9.57% (maximum) and 0.38% (minimum). Therefore, as compared to these techniques, the proposed technique should be preferred.

Table 4 Performance comparison with reported work

S. no	Author's name	Technique	Accuracy (%)
1.	Ramla et al. [10]	DT	88.88
2.	Prasetyo et al. [20]	RF	93.74
3.	Agrawal et al. [11]	SVM	92.39
4.	Afridi et al. [12]	NB	85.88
5.	Ours	XGB	94.10

6 Conclusion

In the present work, fetal health prediction model has been developed by employing various ML algorithms. It has been observed that the utilized raw dataset has lots of variations and should be polished before applying it, for any analysis. However, considering all these as of natural in real-world scenario, it has been employed as obtained. Further, the grid search cross-validation has been used to uplift the model performance by estimating the optimum hyperparameters for all the developed models. The results revealed that XGB classifier performs outstandingly and therefore can be employed as a predictive tool for the early and accurate assessment of fetal health. In the future, the developed classification model will be examined on other fetal health datasets.

References

1. Akbulut A, Ertugrul E, Topcu V (2018) Fetal health status prediction based on maternal clinical history using machine learning techniques. Comput Methods Programs Biomed 163:87–100
2. Vullings R, van Laar JOEH (2020) Non-invasive fetal electrocardiography for intrapartum cardiotocography. Front Pediatr 8:854
3. Mehbodniya A, Lazar AJP, Webber J, et al (2021) Fetal health classification from cardiotocographic data using machine learning. Expert Syst, pp 1–13
4. Meh C, Sharma A, Ram U, et al (2021) Trends in maternal mortality in India over two decades in nationally representative surveys. BJOG
5. Huang M-L, Hsu Y-Y (2012) Fetal distress prediction using discriminant analysis, decision tree, and artificial neural network. J Biomed Sci Eng 2012:526–533
6. Chandra S, Nandipati R, Xinying C (2020) Classification and feature selection approaches for cardiotocography by machine learning techniques. J Telecommun Electron Comput Eng 12:7–14
7. Ayres-de-Campos D, Bernardes J, Garrido A et al (2000) Sisporto 2.0: a program for automated analysis of cardiotocograms. J Matern Fetal Med 9:311–318
8. Sahin H, Subasi A (2015) Classification of the cardiotocogram data for anticipation of fetal risks using machine learning techniques. Appl Soft Comput 33:231–238
9. Mazumdar S, Choudhary R, Swetapadma A (2017) An innovative method for fetal health monitoring based on artificial neural network using cardiotocography measurements. In: Proceedings—2017 3rd IEEE international conference on research in computational intelligence and communication networks, ICRCICN 2017, Dec 2017, pp 265–268
10. Ramla M, Sangeetha S, Nickolas S (2019) Fetal health state monitoring using decision tree classifier from cardiotocography measurements. In: Proceedings of 2nd international conference on intelligent computing and control systems ICICCS 2018, pp 1799–1803
11. Agrawal K, Mohan H (2019) Cardiotocography analysis for fetal state classification using machine learning algorithms. In: 2019 International conference on computer communication and informatics, ICCCI 2019
12. Afridi R, Iqbal Z, Khan M et al (2019) Fetal heart rate classification and comparative analysis using cardiotocography data and known classifiers. Int J Grid Distrib Comput 12:31–42
13. Signorini MG, Pini N, Malovini A et al (2020) Integrating machine learning techniques and physiology based heart rate features for antepartum fetal monitoring. Comput Methods Programs Biomed 185:105015

14. Bhowmik P, Bhowmik PC, Ali UAME, Sohrawordi M (2021) Cardiotocography data analysis to predict fetal health risks with tree-based ensemble learning. Int J Inf Technol Comput Sci 13:30–40
15. Viswanatha RK, Talaulikar VS, Arulkumaran S (2017) Intrapartum fetal surveillance. Obstet Gynaecol Reprod Med 27:363–372
16. Gupta H, Varshney H, Sharma TK et al (2021) (2021) Comparative performance analysis of quantum machine learning with deep learning for diabetes prediction. Complex Intell Syst 1:1–15
17. Kannan E, Ravikumar S, Anitha A et al (2021) Analyzing uncertainty in cardiotocogram data for the prediction of fetal risks based on machine learning techniques using rough set. J Ambient Intell Humaniz Comput 1:1–13
18. Biau G, Cadre B, Rouvière L (2019) Accelerated gradient boosting. Mach Learn 108:971–992
19. Pullagura L, Rao Dontha M, Kakumanu S (2021) Recognition of fetal heart diseases through machine learning techniques. Ann Rom Soc Cell Biol 25:2601–2615
20. Prasetyo SE, Prastyo PH, Arti S (2021) A cardiotocographic classification using feature selection: a comparative study. JITCE J Inf Technol Comput Eng 5:25–32

A Smart System for Assessment of Mental Health Using Explainable AI Approach

Sirshendu Hore, Sinjini Banerjee, and Tanmay Bhattacharya

Abstract Speech emotion recognition (SER) is a popular area of research, and its presence has been observed in various sectors including the smart healthcare system. An SER-enabled smart health system may facilitate the medical practitioners to improve the diagnosis process, by incorporating patient mental health. This is particularly vital in a pandemic/adverse situation when people especially elders are being forced to take psychological counseling/medical advice online. It has been observed that during the counseling stage, patients normally preferred the mother language for communication as they can communicate their problems more easily. However, it has been observed that most of the researchers tried to perceive patient mental health by employing non-regional language audio datasets such as English. Very little work has been done to perceive patient mental health from regional languages such as 'Bangla'. Thus, in the proposed work, an attempt has been made to facilitate the diagnosis process by incorporating patient mental health ('angry', 'fear', 'happy', 'sad', and 'neutral') using widely used ML algorithms. To achieve the objective, important mel-frequency cepstral coefficients (MFCCs) are selected using the explainable AI approach. Here, the random forest (RF) algorithm has been used for the said purpose. SUST Bangla Emotional Speech Corpus (SUBESCO) is used as the training dataset. Experimental result shows the use of important MFCCs gives better accuracy compared to the conventional approach where the first 26 or 13 MFCCs are mostly employed. Comparative results analysis also shows that among the employed ML algorithms 1D CNN has shown better performance. Thus, in the proposed work, 1D CNN-based smart health system has been adopted.

Keywords Bangla · Speech emotion recognition · Psychological state · MFCCs · Feature importance · Explainable AI · Smart health

---

S. Hore (✉) · S. Banerjee
Department of CSE, Hooghly Engineering & Technology College, Pipulpati, Hooghly, West Bengal, India
e-mail: shirshendu.hore@hetc.ac.in

T. Bhattacharya
Department of IT, Techno Main, Salt Lake, Kolkata, India

© The Author(s), under exclusive license to Springer Nature Singapore Pte Ltd. 2023

J. K. Mandal and D. De (eds.), *Frontiers of ICT in Healthcare*, Lecture Notes in Networks and Systems 519, https://doi.org/10.1007/978-981-19-5191-6_21

1 Introduction

The outbreak of the COVID-19 pandemic, lockdown, lack of transportation services, and other restrictions has forced many citizens, especially the elderly and the vulnerable groups, to seek medical advice and care online [1]. These processes have multiplied over time. Understanding their psychological state from these conversations may facilitate the diagnosis process. Speech emotion recognition (SER) has emerged as the front runner to solve various problems in our daily life [2–4]. Consequently, it is being used as an effective tool for understanding the human mental state in the smart healthcare system [5]. During the counseling stage, people prefer regional language as they are more comfortable in doing so. However, most of the research works done so far to determine human mental state have used the RAVDESS, an English corpus [6–8]. Discrete or static label-based systems are used mostly in SER since it is easy to implement. In this process, MFCC coefficients have been used by most researchers [9–11]. Off late both traditional algorithms such as MLP, kNN, RF, XGBoost, and support vector machine and non-traditional algorithms such as CNN, RNN, and AlexNet have been used to determine human mental state using SER [12]. Explainable AI is one of the hot topics in research. One of the fundamental pillars of explainable AI is feature importance [13, 14]. Thus, in the proposed work, we have tried to find MFCCs that have a major impact on the classification process.

Motivation: People prefer to communicate in their mother language or in their native language during psychological counseling be it in person or online. This is more relevant when people are in need. However, there are very few models available in the literature, which is based on regional language. Thus, there is a clear research gap. This motivates the authors to persuade this study.

Objective: The purpose of the study is to develop one smart health system using important MFCCs. *Gini importance or mean decrease in impurity (MDI) model-based random forest algorithm has been employed to find the important features.* SUBESCO, a regional dataset in Bangla, has been used to train the employed ML models. Figure 1 shows the abstracted view of the proposed system.

Takeaways:

- Successfully able to develop one smart health system to determine five mental states of humans using regional language, i.e., 'Bangla'
- Successfully able to find MFCC coefficient having more impact in making the classification decision using feature importance approach.

In section two, some prevailing and relevant works have been discussed. The methodology adopted in this study has been discussed in Sect. 3, which is followed by the result and discussion. Finally, limitations are reported in the conclusion.

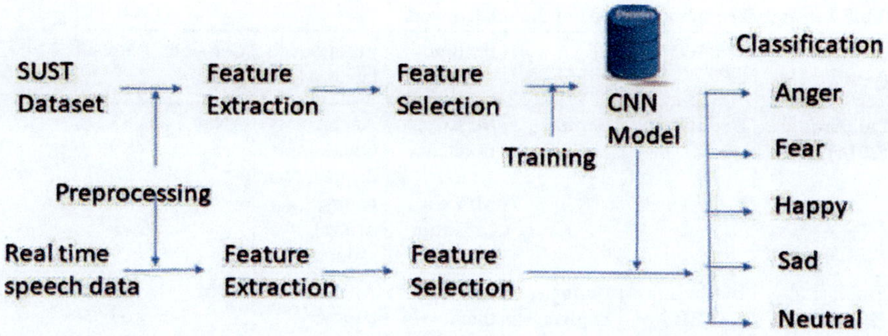

Fig. 1 Block diagram of the proposed smart health system

2 Background

Human emotions can be perceived either in a verbal way or through a non-verbal way [2]. Among the verbal way of emotion recognition, SER has drawn the attention of several researchers since it contains a rich piece of emotional information [3, 4]. The presence of SER is also being observed in the healthcare system. Low et al. [5] tried to find depression a kind of mental health issue among adolescents while they were interacting with their dear and nears. In their research work, author(s) employed SER as a tool. It has been observed that MFCCs have been used widely in SER [6–10]. Pinto et al. [6] developed one 1D CNN model to determine the human emotional state using MFCCs as a feature set. The model has achieved satisfactory accuracy. Yang et al. [7] developed smart home assistance using scaled MFCC as features to get the consumer's psychological state. In their work, author(s) have employed traditional ML models such as SVM, BPNN, and ELM. The proposed model has achieved 92.4% accuracy. In the year 2021, Chatterjee et al. [8] proposed one smart assistant system using 1D CNN. The proposed system used MFCC as an input into the CNN model to obtain higher accuracy. Lalitha et al. [9] and Iqbal et al. [10] applied SER to determine human psychology in real time, using both forms of the ML model. In both works, they have employed MFCCs as a feature vector. Research works of [11, 12] suggested in detail the psychological models, dataset, classifier, preprocessing, and feature to be used in the SER system. Explainable AI has emerged as a hot topic among researchers. Feature importance is one of the major parts of explainable AI. Feature importance can be local or global, or it can be linear or nonlinear. Among the nonlinear approach, random forest is used popularly [13, 14]. RAVDESS [16], EMO-DB [17], and SUBESCO [18] are some of the datasets that are used widely in SER by the researchers. Some of the works found in the literature have been given in Table 1.

Table 1 Brief description of some of the related work

Ref. no. (year)	Dataset		Feature	Emotions labels used	Classifier used	Results
	Name	Language				
Lalitha et al. (2014) [9]	Berlin Emo	German	MFCCs, frequency scaled MFCCs, cepstrum	Anger, boredom, disgust, fear, happy, neutral, sadness (7)	ANN	85.7%
Sinith et al. (2016) [18]	Berlin Emo SAVEE	German English	MFCCs, pitch, intensity	Anger, happy, neutral, sadness (4)	SVM	Males: 67.5%, Females: 70%, Both: 75%,
Iqbal et al. (2019) [10]	RAVDESS SAVEE	English	MFCCs, energy, spectral entropy, etc.	Anger, disgust, fear, happy, neutral, sadness, surprise (7)	Gradient boosting, SVM, KNN	Satisfactory
Yang et al. (2020) [7]	Berlin Emo	German	Scaled MFCCs	Anger, happy, sad, and neutral(4)	SVM, BPNN, ELM, PNN	92.4,77.8, 7881%
Pinto et al. (2020) [6]	RAVDESS	English	MFCCs	Anger, disgust, fear, happy, neutral, sadness, surprise (7)	1D CNN	91%
R.Chatterjee et al. (2021) [8]	RAVDESS, TESS	English	MFCCs	Anger, calm, disgust, fear, happy, neutral, sadness, surprise (8)	1D CNN	90.48, 95.79%

3 Methodology Adopted

3.1 Emotion Dataset

SUST Bangla Emotional Speech Corpus (SUBESCO) is the largest emotional speech corpus available to date on the Bangla language [19]. This emotional speech corpus is made of 7000 sentence-level utterances. The number of target emotions is seven: anger, disgust, fear, happiness, sad, surprise, and neutral. This acted-based audio

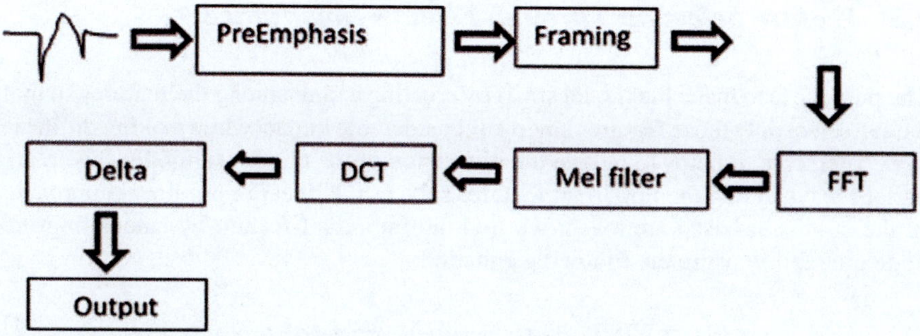

Fig. 2 Process of extraction of MFCCs features from the audio signal

dataset was created by 20 professionals. Ten males and 20 females have participated in this process.

3.2 *Preprocessing*

It is used to improve the quality of speech data for better and more robust classification [15]. Some of the popularly used preprocessing techniques are normalization, pre-emphasis, noise removal, trimming, etc.

3.3 *Mel-Frequency Cepstral Coefficients (MFCC)*

It has been used widely as a feature in the speech processing and machine learning domain. To obtain the MFCCs feature, acquired audio signal is passed through a series of steps as shown in Fig. 2.

3.4 *Feature Extraction*

In the proposed work, MFCC features have been extracted from each waveform. Initially, forty (40) such MFCCs have been extracted and stored. Later, from these 40 features important 26 and 13, having the major impact, have been selected. The selection approach has been described in Sect. 3.5.

3.5 Feature Selection Through Feature Importance

The purpose is to make the model smart by creating a rank among the features so that we can select only those features having a considerable impact while making the decision. Therefore, it helps to reduce the dimension of the employed model. There are various ways to find the important features such as the linear or nonlinear approach. In the nonlinear-based approach, we find the important feature by calculating the node probability using the following equation:

$$ni_j = w_j C_j - w_{left(j)} C_{left(j)} - w_{right(j)} C_{right(j)} \quad (1)$$

Here, the importance of node *j* is represented using $ni_{j,}$ w_j is the weighted number of samples reaching node *j*, the impurity value of node *j is expressed using* C_j, *left(j)*, and *right(j)* is the child node of left and right node of *j, respectively. Then, importance can be derived using*

$$fi_i = \frac{\sum j : \text{node } j \text{ split on feature } i^{ni_j}}{\sum j \in \text{all nodes}^{ni_j}} \quad (2)$$

3.6 ML Models

In the proposed apart from the traditional ML model, CNN is also employed.

3.6.1 MLP

It is a type of biologically inspired neural network, having multiple layers of nodes. The three distinct layers of a typical MLP model are input, hidden, and output layers. In an MLP model, back propagation technique has been employed to train the dataset.

3.6.2 Random Forest (RF)

One of the popularly used ensembles learning approaches, based on the bagging algorithm. In this approach, the most important feature is obtained by searching for the best feature from a random subset of features. This turns out an extensive variety which results in a better model.

3.6.3 K-Nearest Neighbor (kNN)

A similarity-based predicting model that follows the principle of the supervised machine learning algorithm. It makes use of Euclidean distance to reclaim, each new observation. The training dataset is used to make new observations. The final result is then inferred from the outputs of selected observations.

3.6.4 XGBoost

A gradient boosting algorithm, a type of decision tree-based algorithm. It is based on a gradient-boosted tree algorithm and is used widely by the researchers to meet their purpose.

3.6.5 Support Vector Machine (SVM)

A widely used and effective supervised ML algorithm used for classification purposes. The effectiveness of SVM lies in its kernel. This enables researchers to use SVM in high-dimensional spaces.

3.6.6 Convolutional Neural Network (CNN)

It has been applied by several researchers to solve the problem related to real life. It is a type of DNN algorithm that takes the features as input and recognizes features from the rest of the features. The recognition is being made based on weight and bias values obtained during the learning process. The main principle behind the CNN architecture is the 'convolutional layer'. In CNN models, each input goes through a sequence of convolutional layers

$$y = \max\left[\left(\sum_i w_i x_i + a\right), 0\right] \tag{3}$$

3.7 Benchmark Metric Used

- Accuracy is referred to the ratio of the sum of data instances classified properly to the total instances' number, which is given by

$$\text{Accuracy} = \frac{\text{tp} + \text{tn}}{\text{tp} + \text{fp} + \text{fn} + \text{tn}} \tag{4}$$

- Recall (tp-rate) is the ratio of the true positive (tp) to the total number of data instances classified under positive class, given by

$$\text{Recall} = \frac{\text{tp}}{\text{tp} + \text{fn}} \quad (5)$$

- Precision is the ratio of correctly classified data instances in positive class to the total number of data instances classified to be in positive class, given by

$$\text{Precision} = \frac{\text{tp}}{\text{tp} + \text{fp}} \quad (6)$$

where tp (true positive) is the number of data which are positive and fall in the category of positive class, fp (false positive) is the number of data which are 'negative' data but recognized as 'positive', fn (false negative) is the number of data which are positive but categorized as 'negative', and tn (true negative) is the number which are 'negative' but categorized as 'negative'.

4 Results and Discussion

This section has implemented the approach stated in Sect. 3. *In the proposed work, mental health states considered are 'anger', 'fear', 'happiness', 'sad', and 'neutral'. The total sample size (5000) has been divided into training and validation (70%), as well as testing (30%) parts. Gini importance or mean decrease in impurity (MDI) model-based random forest algorithm approach has been employed to obtain the important features.* Figure 3a shows the 40 extracted MFCC mean coefficients, while selected top 26 and top 13 MFCC mean coefficients according to their importance have been shown in Fig. 3b and c. Parameter table of employed XAI-based approach has been depicted using Table 2. Popularly used Python libraries are employed for the stated purpose. Table 3 depicted the competence of our employed ML models. Table 4 demonstrated the classification outcomes of the adopted 1D CNN in terms of benchmark scores. Model accuracy and loss function have been shown in Figs. 4 and 5. The architecture of the MLP model and adopted CNN model has been depicted using Figs. 6 and 7, respectively.

Discussion: Figure 3a shows the 40 important MFCCs according to their importance. Figure 3b shows 22, 23, and 24 MFCCs, based on their importance. It also shows that these three have failed to secure the top 26 positions in the feature space, while 26, 31, and 32 MFCCs took the top place. Again 14, 16, and 18 MFCCs secure the top 13 places, see Fig. 3c. Figure 3c shows the 13 important MFCCs. Result analysis of Table 3 gives that among the traditional ML models, and random forest shows its supremacy over the rest. It has achieved 84.28% and 81.23% accuracy for the top 26 and top

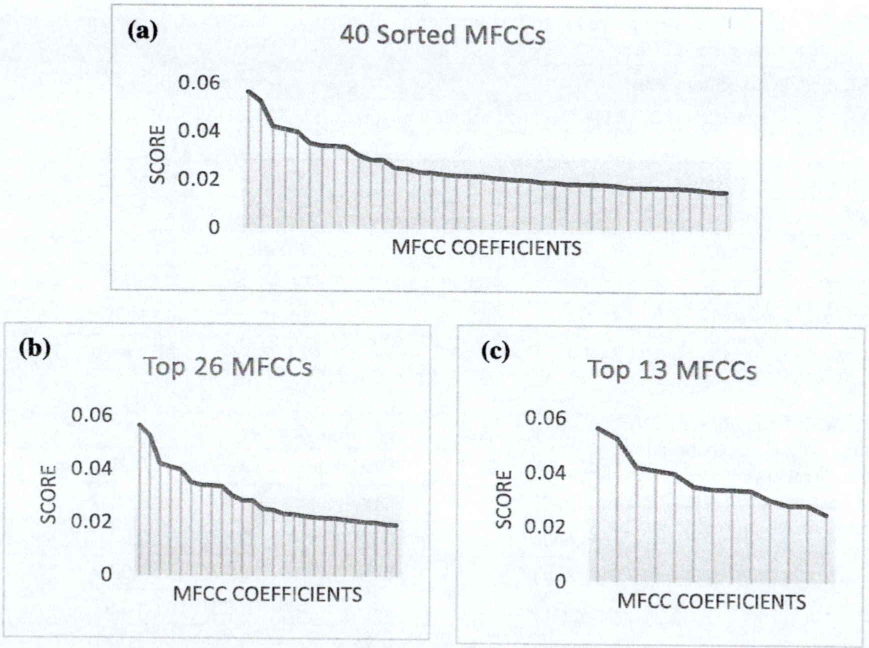

Fig. 3 **a** Sorted 40 MFCCs according to their importance **b** Sorted 26 MFCCs according to their importance **c** Sorted 13 MFCCs according to their importance

Table 2 Parameter table of employed XAI (mean decreases impurity-based random forest algorithm

Parameter name	Value	Parameter name	Value
bootstrap	True	*class_weight*	None
criterion	Gini	*max_depth*	None
max_features	Auto	*max_leaf_nodes*	None
min_impurity_decrease	0.0	*min_impurity_split*	None
min_samples_leaf	1	*min_samples_split*	2
min_weight_fraction_leaf	0.0	*n_estimators*	100
n_jobs	None	*oob_score*	False
random_state	0	*Warm_start*	False

13, respectively, which is marginally more than usually employed MFCCs (40, 26, and 13). Employed 1D CNN is the most suitable model among all the employed models for the study. It has achieved 84.59 and 81.45% accuracy, respectively, using important 26 and 13 MFCCs. Table 4 gives that the recognition rate for mental state happiness is poor compared to the other four mental states. The recognition rate for the other four, namely anger, fear, sad, and neutral is satisfactory. Figures 4 and

Table 3 Evaluation of employed algorithms in terms of accuracy. 40, 26, 13, important 26, and important 13 are the MFCCs

Ml models	Accuracy (%)				
	MFCCs (40)	MFCCs (26)	MFCCs important (26)	MFCCs (13)	MFCCs important (13)
MLP	79.53	72.97	76.96	67.48	67.58
RF	84.04	83.58	84.28	81.03	81.23
kNN	83.67	83.67	83.90	78.96	79.76
SVM	68.50	68.05	68.45	60.06	62.56
XGBoost	68.40	67.19	67.59	62.13	62.58
CNN	85.02	84.23	84.59	81.23	81.45

Table 4 Evaluation of employed 1D CNN based on three benchmark scores against five mental health states using important 26 MFCCs

Mental state	Benchmark score		
	Precision	Recall	F1-score
Angry	0.84	0.87	0.86
Fear	0.88	0.85	0.86
Happy	0.81	0.77	0.79
Neutral	0.87	0.98	0.92
Sad	0.83	0.78	0.81
Accuracy			0.85
Macro avg	0.85	0.85	0.85
Weighted avg	0.84	0.85	0.84

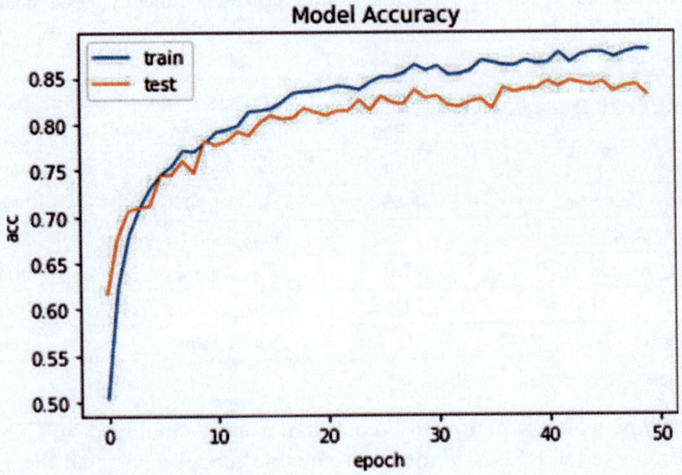

Fig. 4 Model accuracy validated the performance of the adopted 1D CNN model using 26 important MFCCs

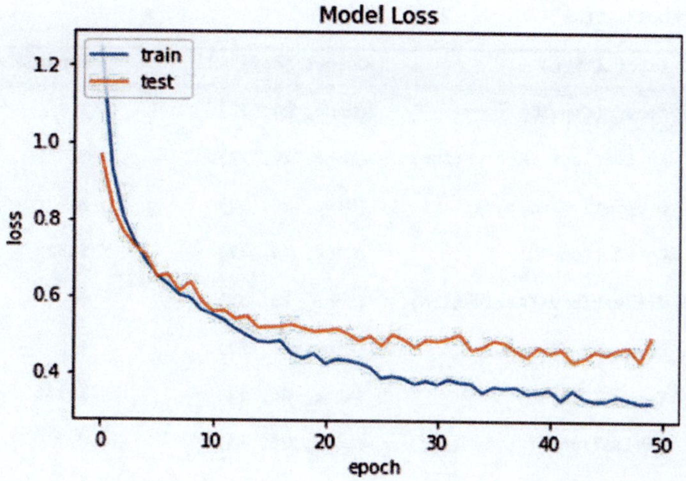

Fig. 5 Model loss measures the stability of the adopted 1D CNN model using 26 important MFCCs

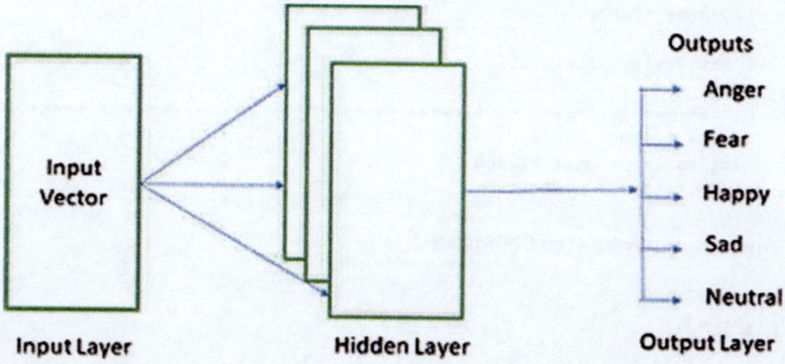

Fig. 6 MLP architecture employed

5 show that the employed CNN model achieved reasonable performance with low iteration having no overfitting issue. Based on Table 4, it may be concluded that during the pandemic/adverse situation or for the elders having a health issue, the proposed system can assist the medical practitioners in the diagnosis process, by incorporating their mental health states from online conversion.

```
Model: "CNN"
_________________________________________________________________
Layer (type)                 Output Shape              Param #
=================================================================
Conv1 (Conv1D)               (None, 26, 32)            192

Activation1 (Activation)     (None, 26, 32)            0

Dropout1 (Dropout)           (None, 26, 32)            0

Conv2 (Conv1D)               (None, 26, 32)            5152

Activation2 (Activation)     (None, 26, 32)            0

Dropout2 (Dropout)           (None, 26, 32)            0

Conv3 (Conv1D)               (None, 26, 64)            10304

Activation3 (Activation)     (None, 26, 64)            0

Dropout3 (Dropout)           (None, 26, 64)            0

Flat1 (Flatten)              (None, 1664)              0

Dense1 (Dense)               (None, 4)                 6660

Activation4 (Activation)     (None, 4)                 0

=================================================================
Total params: 22,308
Trainable params: 22,308
Non-trainable params: 0
```

Fig. 7 Architecture of employed CNN model

5 Conclusion

The proposed work shows the power of the explainable AI approach. Here, instead of considering conventional MFCC coefficients sequence (40, 26, or 13), only important MFCC coefficients have been considered. As a result, better accuracy has been achieved. In addition to this, the use of the regional (Bangla) dataset in the training phase is another unique attempt of its kind.

Limitation: Firstly, in the submitted work, we tried to determine human mental state from their telephonic conversation using 'Bangla' audio corpus. Thus to make the system more robust, so that it can determine the mental state in real time. Other regional datasets such as Tamil and Nepalese can also be used. Secondly, in this study, we make use of MFCCs, a discrete form of speech features. So to make the system strong, other forms of features such as dimensional could be clubbed.

References

1. Socio-economic impact of COVID-19. https://www.undp.org/content/undp/en/home/coronavirus/socio-economic-impact-of-covid-19.html
2. Basharirad B, Moradhaseli M (2017) Speech emotion recognition methods: a literature review. In: AIP conference proceedings, vol 1891, p 020105. https://doi.org/10.1063/1.5005438
3. Ayadia EM, Kamel MS, Karray F (2011) Survey on speech emotion recognition: features, classification schemes, and databases. Pattern Recognit 44:572–587. https://doi.org/10.1016/j.patcog.2010.09.020
4. Poria S, Cambria E, Bajpai R, Hussain A (2017) A review of affective computing: from unimodal analysis to multimodal fusion. Inf Fusion 37:98–125. https://doi.org/10.1016/j.inffus.2017.02.003
5. Low LA, Maddage NC, Lech M, Sheeber LB, Allen NB (2011) Detection of clinical depression in adolescents' speech during family interactions. IEEE Trans Biomed Eng 58(3):574–586. https://doi.org/10.1109/TBME.2010.2091640
6. Pinto MGD, Polignano M, Lops P, Semeraro G (2020) Emotions understanding model from spoken language using deep neural networks and Mel-frequency Cepstral coefficients. In: EAIS. IEEE. 978-1-7281-4384-22020
7. Yang N, Dey N, Sherratt S, Shi F (2019) Emotional state recognition for AI smart home assistants using Mel-frequency Cepstral coefficient features. J Intell Fuzzy Syst
8. Chatterjee R, Majumder S, Sherratt RS, Halder R, Maitra T, Giri D (2021) Real-time speech emotion analysis for smart home assistants. IEEE Trans Consum Electron 67(1):68–76. https://doi.org/10.1109/TCE.2021.3056421
9. Lalitha S, Madhavan A, Bhushan B, Saketh S (2015) Speech emotion recognition. In: Proceedings of the International conference on advances in electronics, computers and communications, ICAECC 2014. IEEE, pp 1–4. https://doi.org/10.1109/ICAECC.2014.7002390
10. Iqbal A, Barua K (2019) A real-time emotion recognition from speech using gradient boosting. In: 2019 International conference on electrical, computer and communication engineering (ECCE). IEEE, pp 1–5
11. Akçay MB, Oguz K (2020) Speech emotion recognition: emotional models, databases, features, preprocessing methods, supporting modalities, and classifiers. Speech Commun 116:56–76. https://doi.org/10.1016/j.specom.2019.12.001
12. Koolagudi SG, Murthy YV, Bhaskar SP (2018) Choice of a classifier, based on properties of a dataset: case study-speech emotion recognition. Int J Speech Technol. https://doi.org/10.1007/s10772-018-9495-8
13. Saarela M, Jauhiainen S (2021) Comparison of feature importance measures as explanations for classification models. SN Appl Sci 3:272. https://doi.org/10.1007/s42452-021-04148-9
14. Fisher A, Rudin C, Dominici F (2019) All models are wrong, but many are useful: learning a variable's importance by studying an entire class of prediction models simultaneously. J Mach Learn Res 20(177):1–81
15. Das N, Chakraborty S, Chaki J, Padhy N, Dey N (2020) Fundamentals, present and future perspectives of speech enhancement. Int J Speech Technol IJST, pp 1–19
16. Livingstone SR, Thompson WF, Wanderley MM, Palmer C (2018) Common cues to emotion in the dynamic facial expressions of speech and song. Q J Exp Psychol, pp 1–19
17. EMO-DB, Berlin database of emotional speech [Online]. 671 Available: http://emodb.bilderbar.info/start.html
18. Sinith MS, Aswathi E, Deepa TM, Shameema CP, Rajan S (2016) Emotion recognition from audio signals using support vector machine. In: Proceedings of the IEEE recent advances in intelligent computational systems, RAICS 2015. IEEE, pp 139–144. https://doi.org/10.1109/RAICS.2015.7488403
19. Sultana S, Rahman MS, Selim MR, Iqbal MZ (2021) SUST Bangla Emotional Speech Corpus (SUBESCO): an audio-only emotional speech corpus for Bangla. PLoS ONE 16(4):e0250173. https://doi.org/10.1371/journal.pone.0250173

Binary Classification of Thyroid Using Comprehensive Set of Machine Learning Algorithms

Diganta Sengupta, Subhash Mondal, Aman Raj, and Ankit Anand

Abstract Binary classification of Thyroid has been observed in several manuscripts in literature. This study also classifies the disease using twelve machine learning algorithms. The results are compared with existing proposals and found to exhibit better performance in terms of the standard machine learning algorithm evaluation parameters. The result improvements are due to the data preprocessing techniques that have been applied in the study. The results that are presented in this paper are void of any tuned machine learning model. Only the basic implementations have been done on the preprocessed data. Random Forest presented the best results amongst all the participants, including literary counterparts with an accuracy of 99.14%, coupled with an F1-Score of 0.991. We have implemented the machine learning models on a resource constraint dataset containing only 3772 instances, and an initial feature vector containing 29 features. Data preprocessing minimized the initial feature vector to a reduced feature vector containing 15 features. We claim this study can form a benchmark for binary classification of thyroid using machine learning models, as our results exhibit implementation on twelve machine learning models as well as improvements in the performances.

Keywords Thyroid · Machine learning · Binary classification · Data preprocessing · Random Forest · Benchmark

D. Sengupta (✉) · S. Mondal · A. Raj · A. Anand
Department of Computer Science and Engineering, Meghnad Saha Institute of Technology, Kolkata 700150, India
e-mail: sg.diganta@ieee.org

S. Mondal
e-mail: subhash@msit.edu.in

A. Raj
e-mail: aman_r.cse2019@msit.edu.in

A. Anand
e-mail: ankit_a.cse2019@msit.edu.in

D. Sengupta
Department of Computer Science and Business Systems, Meghnad Saha Institute of Technology, Kolkata 700150, India

© The Author(s), under exclusive license to Springer Nature Singapore Pte Ltd. 2023

J. K. Mandal and D. De (eds.), *Frontiers of ICT in Healthcare*, Lecture Notes in Networks and Systems 519, https://doi.org/10.1007/978-981-19-5191-6_22

1 Introduction

One of the major hormones involved in development, growth and metabolism in a human body is the thyroid hormone. A steady secretion of metered quantity in the bloodstream in human blood vessels keeps the major functions alive in the human anatomy. This hormone is secreted by the gland known as the thyroid gland. This gland has two lobes (hence, sometimes called butterfly shaped) placed in the lower neck in front of the windpipe. Inflammation of the gland results in enhanced (hyperthyroidism) or reduced (hypothyroidism) amount of hormone secretion to a number of conditions in the human body, including near fatality in certain cases. Thyroid controls our metabolism by producing few specific hormones T4 (thyroxine, contains four iodide atoms) and T3 (triiodothyronine, contains three iodide atoms) which generates right amount proteins and direct the body cells how much energy to use in the ordnance of body temperature [1]. This study focuses on classification of the disease based on historical dataset using traditional machine learning (ML) models. United States accounts for an estimated count of 20 million of the population suffering from either type of thyroids [2]. Also it has been observed that females are more prone to the disease in the order of 5–8 times than the opposite gender.

Twelve ML models have been implemented on a dataset containing 3772 instances [3]. The ML algorithms used in this study are presented in Table 1. It is to be noted that prior to deployment of the ML algorithms, a series of data preprocessing has been done on the initial dataset.

Timely diagnosis and cure of a disease in general is of huge concern for healthcare professionals. In this regard, machine learning algorithms have aided in efficient diagnosis of thyroid throughout the different stages of the disease. The algorithms detect with higher accuracy thereby aiding the healthcare professional in better decision making and minimizing fatality risks [4]. This study classifies the disease

Table 1 Machine learning algorithms used and their acronyms

Machine learning algorithms	Acronym
Random Forest	RF
XGB Classifier	XBG
Gradient Boosting Classifier	GBC
Ada Boost Classifier	AB
Histogram Gradient Boosting Classifier	HGBC
LGBM Classifier	LGBM
Decision Tree	DT
K-Nearest Neighbour	KNN
Support Vector Machine	SVM
Logistic Regression	LR
Bernoulli NB	BNB
Gaussian NB	GNB

and provides a benchmark for future classification of the disease using ML models presented in Table 1.

The paper is organized by having Related Work section after the Introduction followed by our proposal in Sect. 3. Section 4 provides the result and comparative analysis with Sect. 5 concluding the study.

2 Related Work

This section presents the literature in thyroid disease classification using mainly ML models, and some examples of prior art concerning implementations using deep learning (DL) models. Authors in [5–7], and [8] have used machine learning models to classify thyroid.

In [9] the authors presented a comprehensive analysis of different machine learning algorithms by considering the different performance parameters to diagnosis of thyroid disease. The authors in [10] had used three feature selection techniques along with different ML classification algorithms to predict hypothyroid particularly amongst females in early stage. The authors claimed that amongst the others feature selection techniques; RFE obtained the best accuracy of 99.35% amongst all the classification algorithms.

Yadav et al. [11] proposed an ensemble-based method to predict early stages of thyroid disease. To extract the hidden pattern of the dataset they were used decision tree algorithm. Initially the disease was examined by using three algorithms namely Decision Tree, Random Forest and Classification and Regression Tree (CART) with an accuracy of 98%, 99% and 93%, respectively, on the basis of different num-fold and seed values. To achieve the better accuracy, the bagging ensemble combined the three basic tree classifications and obtained 100% accurate result with seed value 35 and num-fold 10. Tyagi et al. [12] proposed a model for diagnosis of the thyroid disease prevention by using different classical machine learning algorithms. They were used the open-source dataset from UCI machine learning repository. The algorithms were evaluated in term of accuracy and obtained results in support vector machine (99.63%), KNN (98.62%), Decision Trees (75.76%) and ANN (97.50%), respectively. The authors claimed that the chances of thyroid disease prediction risk amongst patients.

In [13] the authors proposed a classification model to detect the thyroid disease by using Random Forest algorithm. They were taken different dataset collected from open-source and used PCA approaches to preserve the visibility of the dataset. Their claimed average accuracy of their method reached to 95.63% on the open-source dataset. To verify the result, the authors compare their proposed method with the clinical medical dataset and obtained accuracy of 96.16%. In [14], the authors analysed the effect of thyroid disease detection by using the two feature selection approaches namely Filter-based and Wrapper-based. They were also used the PCA technique to reduce the dimensionality of the dataset. Four different machine learning classification algorithms namely MLP, BPNN, SVM and Extreme Linear Machine (ELM) were used to evaluate the performances by using three matrices like accuracy, sensitivity and specificity. Their claimed results showed that both F-Score and Recursive Feature Elimination perform the best with accuracy 96.60% and 98.14%, respectively. In [15], the authors proposed a model that predicts the thyroid disease after that by using binary classification algorithms namely Decision Tree ID3 and Naïve Bayes to classify the disease stage later. For this purpose, thyroid disease patient dataset was used with all attributes to predict by using Decision Tree and lately to classify by using Naïve Bayes.

The authors in [16] proposed a predictive model of disease detection by using Filter-based feature selection algorithm with two-class-based Neural Network (NN) classifier on Azure Machine Learning tool. The proposed model obtained result with an accuracy of 98.1%, precision 0.968, recall 0.995 and F1 score 0.982, respectively, amongst others classification algorithms. Shahid et al. in [17] compared the results of three machine learning algorithm namely Random Forest, SVM and KNN for the detection of disease on a dataset collected from open-source database. The best accuracy obtained through RF rather than SVM and KNN of 98.50%, 97.02% and 95.81%, respectively.

3 Proposed Work

As discussed earlier, the dataset [3] comprised of 3772 instances for 29 feature vectors. We preprocessed the data and reduced the feature vector having a feature count of 14. The proposed model is presented in Fig. 1. The final features in the feature vector are presented in Table 2. The target label has been denoted by the term Label.

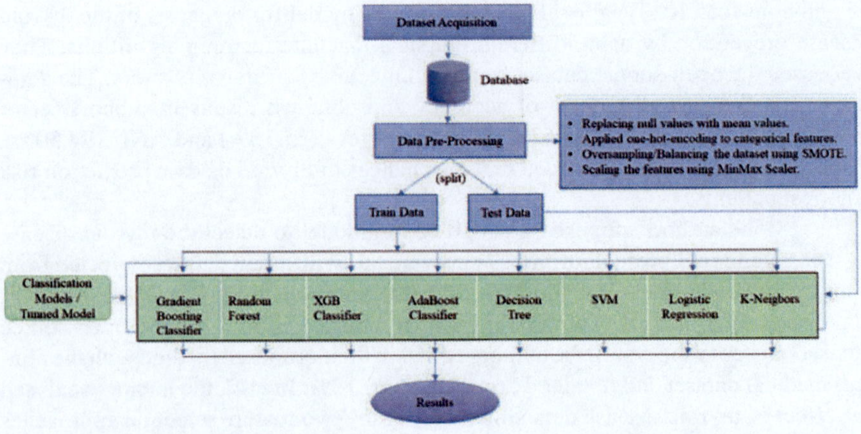

Fig. 1 High level diagram for the proposed model

Table 2 Features in the final feature vector with the target as label

Index	Attributes	Data type
1	Age	Object
2	Sex	Object
3	Sick	Object
4	Pregnant	Object
5	Thyroid surgery	Object
6	I131 treatment	Object
7	Lithium	Object
8	Goitre	Object
9	Tumour	Object
10	TSH	Object
11	T3	Object
12	TT4	Object
13	T4U	Object
14	FTI	Object
15	Label	Object

We renamed the Target feature from Binary class to Label. The Label variable class is divided into two types: positive (True) and negative (False) denoted by 1 and 0, respectively. The missing values in the dataset were replaced by using the average method (Mean), so that the dataset does not contain any missing values. All features in this dataset were having categorical values. To convert these categorical values to numerical values Label Encoding method was used. In our observation this dataset was imbalanced so to balance our dataset we have used most useful SMOTE method to balance the target class Label. Before using SMOTE method, this data has (3481:291) instances 3620 instances. And after using smote it changed to 5344 instances. The values are presented in Table 3.

Feature scaling using min–max scalar technique has been used on the dataset as the dataset contained huge disproportions. After performing all the above-mentioned data preprocessing, we have split the data into training and testing sets into the ratio of 0.80:0.20 of total data, respectively. The values are presented in Table 4.

Table 3 Imbalance data balancing

	Before SMOTE	After SMOTE
Label 1 count	3481	3481
Label 0 count	291	3481

Table 4 Split data

	Dataset split after SMOTE
Count of Training instances	5569
Count of Test instances	1393

3.1 Model Training

To train the model we have applied 12 ML algorithms on the dataset for predicting thyroid disease precisely. Different parameters were calculated like accuracy, Cohen-Kappa Score, precision, F1 score, Recall, Std. Deviation and ROC-AUC for both default hyper-parameters. In case of default hyper-parameter Random Forest came up with best accuracy of 99.14%. The results thus obtained are furnished in Table 5. It can be observed that RF presents the best results in terms of the performance metrics. It is to be noted that the performance metrics used in this study are the standard evaluation parameters for ML models. Figure 2 presents the ROC-AUC scores followed by the confusion matrices in Fig. 3 for all the ML models.

Figure 3 presents the confusion matrices for all the 12 ML algorithms that have been used in this study. Instead of different figures, all the 12 confusion matrices have been clubbed in a single figure.

Table 5 Performance results of the 12 ML algorithms on the thyroid dataset

ML model	Accuracy	K-fold mean accuracy	Standard deviation	RoC-AuC score	Precision	Recall	F1-score	Cohen-Kappa score
RF	99.14	99.10	0.253	0.991	0.998	0.984	0.991	0.982
XBG	99.07	99.07	0.298	0.990	0.997	0.984	0.990	0.981
GBC	99.07	99.03	0.268	0.990	0.997	0.984	0.990	0.981
AB	98.92	98.92	0.300	0.989	0.995	0.982	0.989	0.978
HGBC	98.85	98.99	0.312	0.988	0.994	0.982	0.988	0.977
LGBM	98.85	98.97	0.254	0.988	0.995	0.981	0.988	0.977
DT	98.27	98.56	0.300	0.982	0.981	0.984	0.982	0.965
KNN	89.87	89.96	1.501	0.898	0.952	0.839	0.892	0.797
SVM	85.14	85.65	1.500	0.851	0.841	0.866	0.854	0.702
LR	81.33	81.59	1.378	0.813	0.819	0.805	0.812	0.626
BNB	65.25	65.93	1.192	0.653	0.788	0.420	0.548	0.306
GNB	56.06	55.05	0.933	0.562	0.906	0.138	0.240	0.123

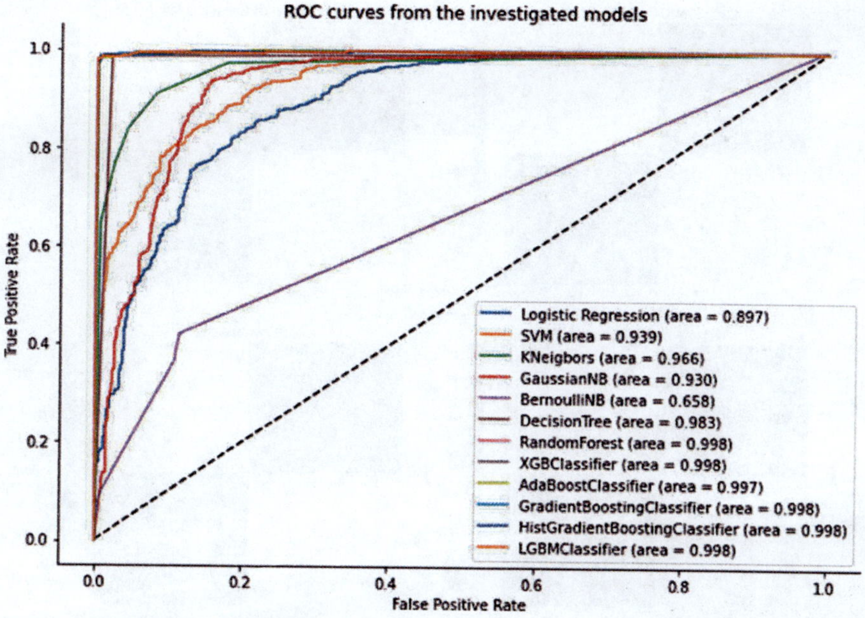

Fig. 2 ROC-AUC Score

4 Comparative Analysis

This section presents the comparative analysis with respect to existing proposals in literature. Table 6 presents the occurrences of ML algorithms in prior art for classification of thyroid disease. Table 7 presents results from the published literature. Figure 4 presents the heatmap.

From Table 7, it can be observed that the results from our model excel over prior art. Conclusion.

5 Conclusion

In this study, we classify thyroid based on a publicly available dataset. In our approach, we conduct data preprocessing resulting in feature reduction, thereby generating better results in comparison to existing literature. The results fare better in terms of traditional machine learning model evaluation parameters. We believe this study can form a benchmark for future proposals in binary classification of thyroid using machine learning models. Future extension of this study can be done in terms of use of deep learning models for binary classification of the disease. Moreover,

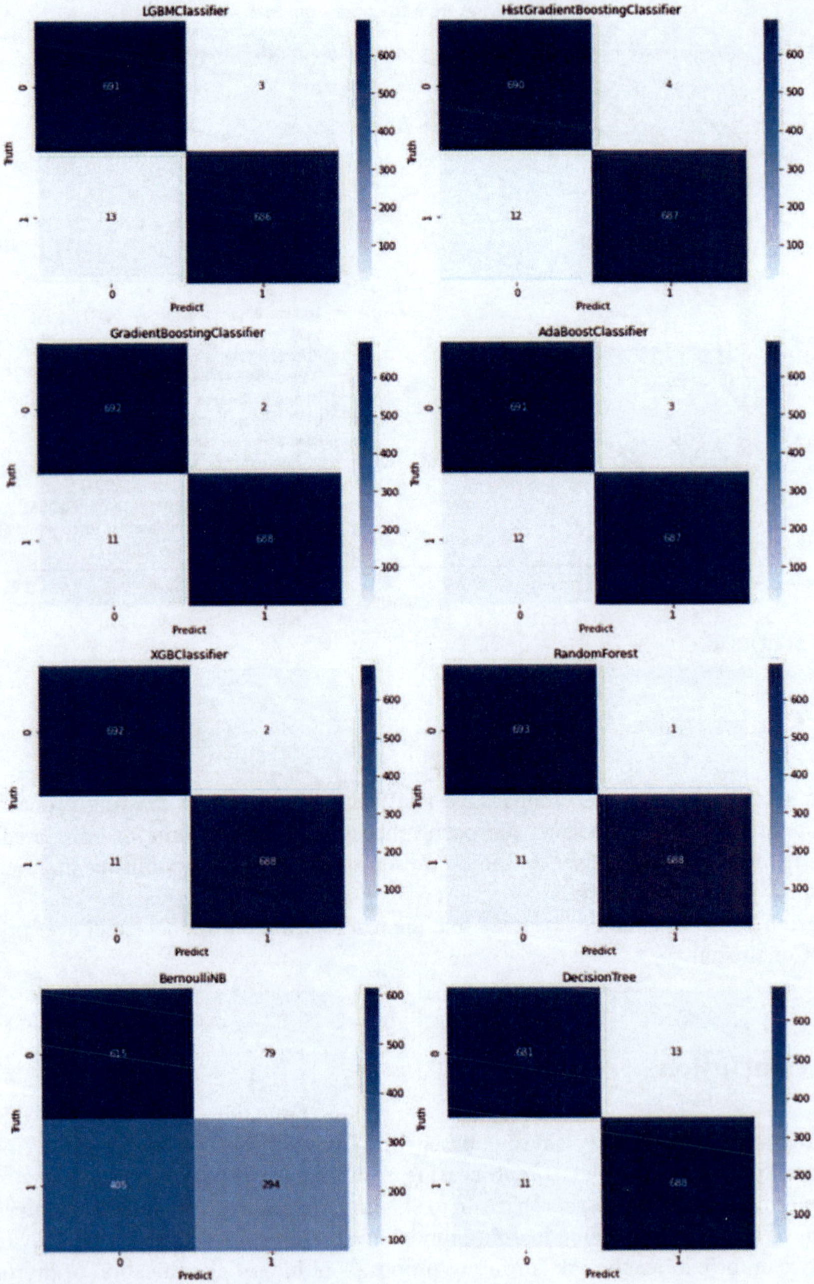

Fig. 3 Confusion matrices for all the 12 ML algorithms

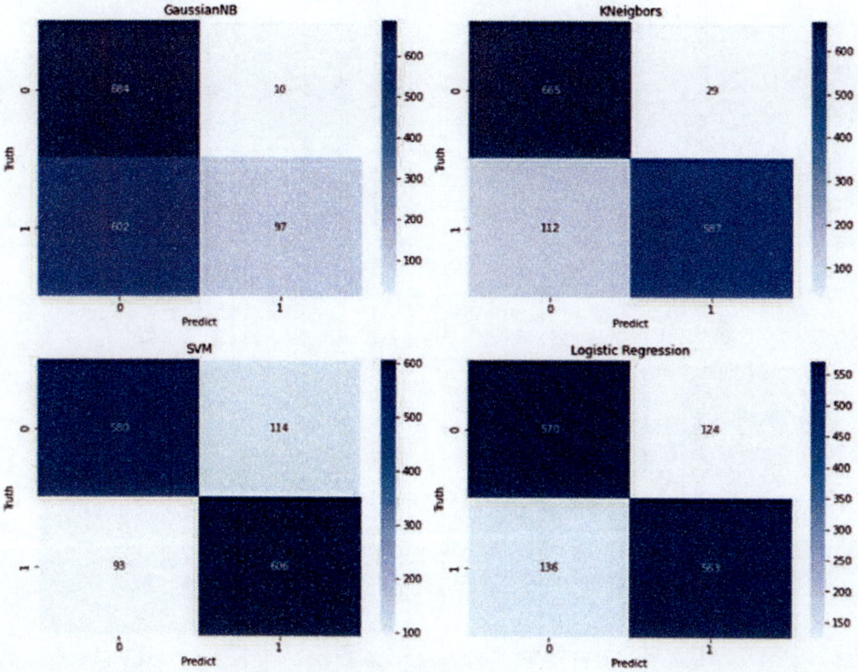

Fig. 3 (continued)

Table 6 ML algorithm occurrences in prior art

Model name	No of occurrence
SVM	10
RF	7
DT	7
LR	4
KNN	7
NB	5
ANN/NN/BPNN	5
MLP	5
XGB	2
GBC	2
ABC	2
MLPC	2

Table 7 Comparative analysis of published literature

Refs #	Algorithm(s) used	Accuracy	Precision	Recall/sensitivity	F1-score	Specificity	RoC-AuC score
[5]	Multi Class SVM	83.37	85.00	69	74		
[6]	KNN, SVM, LR, NN	99.08	98.82	97.5	98.15	99.61	
[9]	KNN, SVM, AdBC, XGB, GPC, GBC, MLPC	99.70	98.78	98.78	98.78	99.82	95.7
[8]	DT, NB, KNN, RF, EXTC, MLPC, XGB, CBC, AdBC, GBC	82.00	84	82	82		
[7]	DT, SVM, RF, NB, LR, LDA, KNN, MLP	98.93					
[10]	SVM, DT, RF, LR, NB, Feature Selection Technique—UFS, REF, PCA	99.35					
[11]	DT, RF, ET, Ensemble Method	100					
[12]	ANN, KNN, SVM, DT	99.63					
[13]	SVM, C4.5, NN, RF	96.16					
[14]	MLP, BPNN, SVM, ELM	98.14					
[15]	DT, NB	95.00					
[16]	Two-class-based NN	98.1	96.8	99.5	98.2		
[17]	RF, SVM, KNN	98.5	98.54	98.57	98.52	94.69	
[18]	SVM, RF, DT, NB, LR, KNN, MLP, LDA	98.93		98.6		100	
Proposed	RF with data preprocessing	99.10	0.998	0.984	0.991		0.991

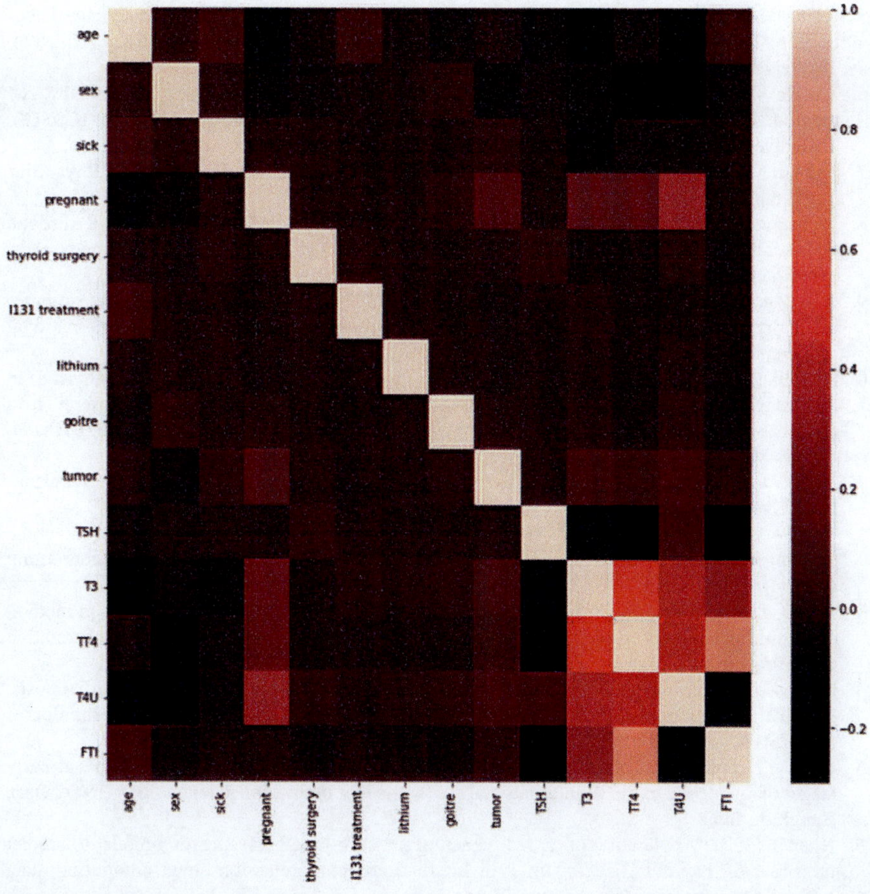

Fig. 4 Heatmap

hyper-parameter tuned models in both the domains of machine learning as well deep learning can be used to further observe the results.

References

1. Temurtas F (2009) A comparative study on thyroid disease diagnosis using neural networks. Expert Syst Appl 36(1):944–949
2. General information/press room. Available at: https://www.thyroid.org/media-main/press-room/
3. Shakir YH (2020) Thyroid disease data set. (Accessed 10 Dec 2020) Available at: https://www.kaggle.com/yasserhessein/thyroid-disease-data-set
4. IoniŃă I, IoniŃă L (2016) Prediction of thyroid disease using data mining techniques. Broad Res Artif Intell Neurosci 7(3)

5. Kumar HH (2020) A novel approach of SVM based classification on thyroid disease stage detection. In: Third international conference on smart systems and inventive technology (ICSSIT), Tirunelveli, India
6. Vairale V, Shukla DS (2019) Classification of hypothyroid disorder using optimized SVM method. In: International conference on smart systems and inventive technology (ICSSIT), Tirunelveli, India
7. Salman K, Sonuç E (2021) Thyroid disease classification using machine learning. J Phys Conf Ser 1963(1):1–12
8. Aversano L, Bernardi M, Cimitile M, Iammarino M, Aversano P, Macchia P, Nettore I, Verdone C, Macchia E (2021) Thyroid disease treatment prediction with machine learning approaches. Procedia Comput Sci 192:1031–1040
9. Asif MA, Nishat MM, Faisal F, Shikder MF, Udoy MH, Dip RR, Ahsan R (2020) Computer aided diagnosis of thyroid disease using machine learning algorithms. In: 11th International conference on electrical and computer engineering (ICECE), Dhaka, Bangladesh
10. Riajuliislam M, Rahim KZ, Mahmud A (2021) Prediction of thyroid disease (hypothyroid) in early stage using feature selection and classification techniques. In: International conference on information and communication technology for sustainable development (ICICT4SD), Dhaka, Bangladesh
11. Yadav D, Pal S (2020) Prediction of thyroid disease using decision tree ensemble method. Hum Intell Syst Integr 2(10)
12. Tyagi A, Mehra R, Saxena A (2018) Interactive thyroid disease prediction system using machine learning technique. In: Fifth international conference on parallel, distributed and grid computing (PDGC), Solan, India
13. Pan Q, Zhang Y, Zuo M, Xiang L, Chen D (2016) Improved ensemble classification method of thyroid disease based on Random Forest. In: 8th International conference on information technology in medicine and education (ITME), Fuzhou, China
14. Pavya K, Srinivasan B (2017) Feature selection algorithms to improve thyroid disease diagnosis. In: IEEE International conference on innovations in green energy and healthcare technologies (ICIGEHT'17), Coimbatore, India
15. Rao A, Renuka B (2020) A machine learning approach to predict thyroid disease at early stages of diagnosis. In: IEEE International conference for innovation in technology (INOCON), Bangluru, India
16. Khan T (2021) Application of two-class neural network-based classification model to predict the onset of Thyroid Disease. In: 11th International conference on cloud computing, data science & engineering (confluence), Noida, India
17. Shahid AH, Singh MP, Raj RK, Suman R (2019) A study on label TSH, T3, T4U, TT4, FTI in hyperthyroidism and hypothyroidism using machine learning techniques. In: International conference on communication and electronics systems (ICCES), Coimbatore, India
18. Salman KA (2021) The efficiency of classification techniques in predicting thyroid disease. Karabuk University

Interpretability Approaches of Explainable AI in Analyzing Features for Lung Cancer Detection

Mahua Pal, Sujoy Mistry, and Debashis De

Abstract The XAI mechanism unboxes the AI model by providing proper explanation for why the important features are taken by AI/ML algorithms. Many AI models are used to detect lung cancer using certain biomarkers detected in CT scan of pulmonary nodules. It is expected that if these models brings out the prediction along with explanation by highlighting the correct features responsible for the prediction, then the automated model would act as augmented doctor; henceforth the model becomes trustworthy and can win the faith of the experienced professional human decision makers of high-stake decision system. The main objective of this research work is to develop an interpretable (XAI-based) machine learning model (AI CAD model) with high performance that can be implemented for lung cancer detection with complete trust. To achieve this goal, six standard ML models were built with biomarkers values identified in CT scan reports as input features. The models were built using SVM, KNN, GBM, XGBoost, RFC and feed forward neural network, respectively. The differences in their performances were analyzed by using an XAI mechanism, SHAP which was used to assess the reasons behind the better and poor performances of the models. XAI outputs revealed that the models with better performances accentuated the similar set of input features with higher weightage. Finally, a trustable XAI model was reconstructed with the classifier (GBM) which made best possible correct selections of input features for lung cancer detection and with the help of the most important biomarkers as input features sorted out from the XAI outputs.

Keywords CAD model · Lung cancer · Pulmonary nodules · SHAP · XAI

M. Pal (✉)
Department of Sciences and Commerce, J. D. Birla Institute, Kolkata, India
e-mail: mahuag@jdbikolkata.in

S. Mistry · D. De
Department of Computer Science and Engineering, Maulana Abul Kalam Azad University of Technology, Kolkata, India
e-mail: debashis.de@makautwb.ac.in

© The Author(s), under exclusive license to Springer Nature Singapore Pte Ltd. 2023
J. K. Mandal and D. De (eds.), *Frontiers of ICT in Healthcare*, Lecture Notes in Networks and Systems 519, https://doi.org/10.1007/978-981-19-5191-6_23

1 Introduction

Explainable Artificial Intelligence (XAI) mechanisms bring the transparency in Machine Learning (ML) models which are now being used quite often in building Computer Aided Diagnostic (CAD) AI models to assist the healthcare systems in producing automated accurate prediction or decision. In the last decade, many models were built to support medical system in detection of diseases based on some input features. But due to the lack transparency of these models, since they did not produce the reasons of the decision taken, there was always a trust issue in accepting them as a tool of decision support systems in healthcare industries. Recent developments of Explainable Artificial Intelligence (XAI) can overcome the black-box problem of ML architectures by providing after the fact explanations. XAI output can be used for validating the prediction, and also can be used to recommend some correction in the prediction model. XAI can be used to explore some new risk factors of a disease, potential biomarkers or some unknown relationships between them, as well. XAI tools produce local, global, post-hoc, ante-hoc, visual and textual explanations. In the last decade some CAD AI models [3] were developed to predict lung cancer using different ML algorithms. The initial detection of lung cancer is made from the CT scan reports of pulmonary nodules which are the abnormal growths in one or both lungs. Intelligent CAD models could act as an Augmented Doctors by reducing the work load of the clinical practitioners by assisting them while taking some decision or making any prediction.

With this perspective, our research work attempted a novel approach by using one state of the art XAI tool, SHapley Additive explanations (SHAP) [1] tool by highlighting the important features selection carried out by six different ML models and thus was investigated and was revealed the reasons behind their performance differences. It is important to find out whether a ML model is making prediction based on the correct feature selection or not. To achieve this goal, six different XAI models were built by using well-known standard ML algorithms and a post-hoc XAI tool, SHAP. The models were support vector machine (SVM) [4], k-nearest neighbors (KNN) [5], gradient boosting algorithm (GBM) [6], eXtreme gradient boosting (XGBoost) [7], random forest classifier (RFC) [8] and feed forward neural network [9] with 5 neurons. All those models were fed with same input biomarkers after oversampling the input dataset with ADASYN [10] algorithm, since the dataset had an imbalance dataset problem with less benign cases and more malignant cases. After executing the ML algorithm separately for classifying the benign and malignant cases, the models' metrics were determined. The SHAP tool was next applied on the top of each model for digging out the interpretations behind each model's prediction, separately. The visual heat maps produced in SHAP method brought a clear picture of the reason behind the better performance of some models. It was observed that the models with high accuracy had set more weightage to few important input features for prediction, whereas the model with low accuracy emphasized on other input features with higher weightage. Finally, GBM was chosen for rebuilding the lung cancer detection XAI CAD model. XGBoost also performed well, whereas KNN and

SVM performed not-so-well due to putting low priorities to some important features. Our experiment highlighted the fact that the XAI tools bring the interpretability in the machine model that can help to construct trustworthy reliable decision support AI system. We have arranged this research paper in the next few sections with the background motivation in Sect. 2, methodology in Sect. 3, result discussions in Sect. 4 and finally the conclusion with future work in Sect. 5.

2 Background

The main motivation of this research work is to enforce trust and reliability to the AI-based CAD model to detect lung cancer from the CT scan reports. Once this target could be achieved, the model could be put into practice with minimum AI implementation risk. To achieve this goal, our research work evaluated the highs and lows of six XAI models' performances on lung cancer prediction by applying SHAP XAI tool and finally the best XAI model was suggested. SHAP produces visual heat maps for local and global explanations. It is a game theoretic approach which is probably the state of the art in ML explainability. The Shapley value for a certain feature i out of n total features (there is a set N with n features) with the given prediction p is

$$\phi i(p) = \sum_{S \subset N/i} \frac{|S|!(n - |S| - 1)!}{n!}(p(S \cup i) - p(S))$$

ϕ is the Shapley value of feature i predates machine learning. S is the coalition of features to obtain a certain gain or a result. At a very high level, this equation calculates the prediction of the model without feature i, and the prediction of the model with feature i, and then calculate the difference:

$$\text{Importance of } i = p(\text{with } i) - p(\text{without } i)$$

The model's prediction changes by adding features, as it sees new features. The change in the model's prediction is basically the effect of the features. Here, all the input features act like players playing their respective roles in winning a match. Their cumulative contributions would be counted to win or lose the match. If any player or input feature has no contribution in winning the match or game, that feature's contribution would be excluded. Local explanations are useful for explaining a single data sample at a time, whereas global-level explanations are useful for understanding the model performance as a whole.

Lung cancer is by far the leading cause of cancer death making up almost 25% of all cancer deaths. This research work was conducted on lung cancer screening thoracic CT scan data to predict the malignancy of pulmonary nodules which are abnormal growths in a lung, but not necessarily would be cancerous. The literature review of some previous works on lung cancer related XAI models are mentioned in this section. Potie et al. [11] developed interpretable AI models using evolutionary fuzzy systems (EFS) for lung cancer prediction with liquid biopsy. Ahmed et al. [12] applied XAI techniques in stack ensemble ML framework and visualized the risk factors of lung and bronchus cancer (LBC) mortality from the stack ensemble model's output in global and local scales after considering the input features such as air-pollution, socio-economic status. Pino et al. [13] developed interpretable deep learning model to automate lesion segmentation and to predict whether non-small-cell lung cancer in CT scans were gene-addicted or not by using adversarial training (PGD) on 3D CNN. Siddhartha et al. [14] proposed an XAI model to predict the postoperative life expectancy in the lung cancer patients after surgery by using SHAP and LIME techniques on the top of ML model. Bartczak et al. [15] proposed another XAI model to predict the postoperative life expectancy in the lung cancer patients after surgery by using SHAP and Ceteris Paribus methods. Venugopal et al. [16] had developed a model with CNN and applied occlusion technique on a nodule for interpretation of model's decision. It is observed that very insignificant amount of work has been accomplished on XAI-based CAD models to detect lung cancer so far and in this work a hybrid approach was adopted by using different well-known ML algorithms and one XAI technique. Henceforth this work suggested a novel idea of selecting important input features which could fine-tune the model to a best diagnostic model.

3 Methodology and Data Preparation

In this research work, we brought into play six XAI ML models using well-known standard ML algorithms and a post-hoc XAI tool, SHAP. Then the best ML algorithm for this work was marked based on the performance metrics. Each model's predictions were interpreted using SHAP tool and finally, the important input features of the better performed models were selected. Thus, we propose a hybrid approach to construct a final trustworthy XAI CAD model. The flow of work of this study is shown in Fig. 1.

The dataset was collected from the LIDC-IDRI (Lung Image Database Consortium image available at wiki.cancerimagingarchive.net/display/Public/LIDC-IDRI) collection which provides diagnostic data and lung cancer screening thoracic computed tomography (CT) scans with marked-up annotated lesions. In this study, 1307 data was investigated. This dataset contained images from a clinical thoracic CT scan and an associated XML file that recorded the results of a two-phase image annotation process. In each CT scan, the marked lesions belong to one of the three categories.

- nodule > or = 3 mm may be Malignant
- nodule < 3 mm could not be annotated and not Malignant
- non-nodule > or = 3 mm is not Malignant

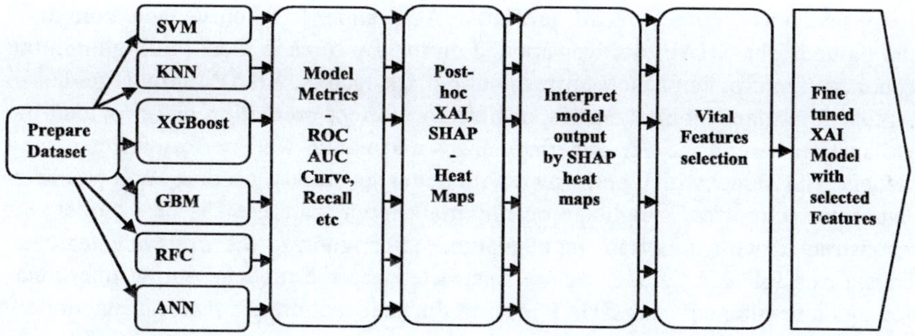

Fig. 1 Work flow

The dataset from XML file which is shown in Fig. 2, was collected after referring to the pylidc document [2]. Our dataset which is shown in Table 1, comprised of categorical values which ultimately were required for labeling the features during interpretation by SHAP.

The dataset used for this research work comprised of eleven attributes with ten input biomarkers with categorical values, shown in Table 1. Malignancy was detected using supervised classification models.

We classified Malignancy into two states—Malignant (High-Risk) and Benign (Low-Risk). The pylidc document was referred and the annotated grading 1 and 2 under Malignancy heading were considered as **Benign** class (493 data) and the grading 3, 4 and 5 were considered as **Malignant** class (814 data). The categorical data were converted to numerical and the problem related to the imbalance classes was handled by the ADASYN method to balance the dataset. The 80% data were used for training the model and 20% data were used for testing. After oversampling, these ten different features or biomarkers were fed into the SVM, KNN, GBM, XGBoost, RFC and feed forward neural network models, separately. Each model's performance

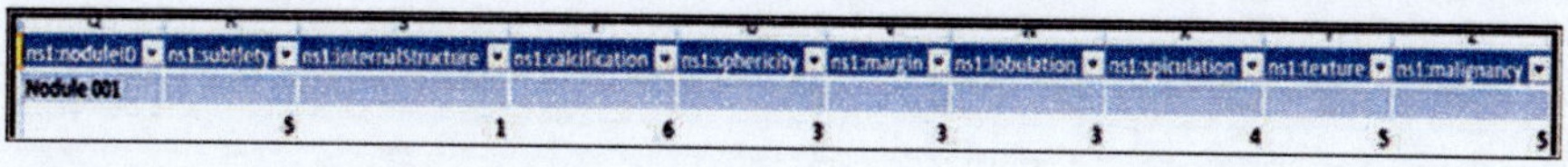

ns1:noduleID	ns1:subtlety	ns1:internalStructure	ns1:calcification	ns1:sphericity	ns1:margin	ns1:lobulation	ns1:spiculation	ns1:texture	ns1:malignancy
Nodule 001	5	1	6	3	3	3	4	5	5

Fig. 2 One sample data in XML file before preprocessing

Table 1 One sample data after collection

Calcification	Absent	Subtlety	Obvious
Internal Structure	Soft Tissue	Texture	Solid
Lobulation	Medium Lobulation	Number_of_Nodules	1
Margin	Medium Margin	Nodule_Size_More_Than_3 mm	1
Sphericity	Ovoid	Malignancy	1
Spiculation	Near marked		

metrics such as accuracy, recall, precision, AUC under ROC curve were computed and plotted. The SHAP tool was applied on the top of each model to highlight the important features with their corresponding risk factors. SHAP outputs guided to explore important biomarkers responsible for correct prediction and provided the explanation behind the better performances and not-so-well performances of any models. The model which performed with better specificity, accuracy and precision values has set correct weightage on important input features. The best model was reconstructed with important input features after ignoring the irrelevant features. Thus a trustable XAI model was reconstructed and the model's output interpretation again revaluated using SHAP tool. In the next section, the result is elaborately discussed.

4 Results and Discussion

Google Colaboratory platform which provides high-end supports was utilized for this research experiments. The imbalance dataset problem was resolved by using an oversampling algorithm ADASYN (Adaptive Synthetic) that generated synthetic data. The dataset fed in six machine learning models separately with fivefold cross validation and the model's performances was observed based on the different metrics such as AUC value, accuracy, precision and specificity, shown in Table 2. It was observed that GBM performed best compared to other models while making the binary classification of the malignancy of pulmonary nodules for lung cancer detection. XGBoost also performed quite well compared with the performance of other models.

After observing the values of important metrics, each model's explainer was fed in SHAP tool to find Shapley values of input features. The SHAP Summary plots with feature contributions were plotted based on the result of Shapely values of the input features or biomarkers that contributed in classifying the benign (0) and malignant (1) classes. The SHAP summary plots of all models are shown in Fig. 3. The feature contribution summary plots of all the models were considered and few observations were noted to infer the reasons behind the better performance of some models and under performance of some other models. There were differences in setting the

Table 2 Models' performance metrics

ML algorithm	Accuracy	Precision	Recall (TPR)	Specificity (TNR)	AUC under ROC curve
GBM	0.942	0.943	0.959	0.918	0.939
XGBoost	0.939	0.918	0.983	0.877	0.930
KNN	0.895	0.881	0.948	0.820	0.884
RFC	0.884	0.835	1.000	0.721	0.970
ANN	0.847	0.793	1.000	0.631	0.863
SVM	0.830	0.780	0.988	0.607	0.797

weights of input features in different models. Here it was observed that GBM and XGBoost focused more on the features called Calcification, Subtlety, Number_of _Nodules, Texture, Margin, Sphericity, Nodule_Size_More_ than_3mm. But SVM, KNN had set low weightage to those features such as Calcification, Margin and by putting low priorities to those features were the reasons of low accuracy and specificity. It was also observed that even after almost similar selections of input features like GBM and XGBoost, the performance of ANN, RFC models were quite low. Our experiment showed that there may be serious contrariety to give proper explanation in how different machine learning models give the same prediction. The experimental results of AI models may be uncertain for highlighting on unrelated data features to detect pulmonary nodules besides providing the correct prediction. This research work focused that XAI tool can reveal the facts of AI system through its prominent predictability and understandability. These valuable facts can be used for explanation of a model, reconstruct an old model to new model and so on.

Finally GBM and SHAP tool were chosen to reconstruct a trustworthy XAI CAD AI model for lung cancer detection using few biomarkers. This model was fed with seven important features which are shown in Fig. 4.

The AUC curves which are shown in Fig. 5 and the models' performance metrics which are displayed in Table 3, depicted the performance of the reconstructed model was better than that of the first model, although the influence of biomarkers remained the same to predict the malignancy of pulmonary nodules that is shown in Fig. 6.

The Force Plot which is shown in Fig. 7 was used for local prediction and it was formed based on any single record of an individual patient by calculating the SHAP values of the biomarkers. The 10th record which was malignant was verified. Here, all of the feature values led to the prediction value 1 (Malignant Class). SHAP plotted the top most influential features for the sample under study. Features in red color influenced positively, features in blue color influenced the opposite.

5 Conclusion with Future Work

In this research work, the predictions of AI binary classification models were interpreted by a post-hoc XAI tool, SHAP and the interpretations achieved by using SHAP were used to interpret, explain, evaluate and analyze six different model's performances. This approach assisted to focus in the rebuilding a best model for lung cancer detection by emphasizing on the important input biomarkers. It was observed that the final model performed best among all the previous models with AUC value 94.6%. It was also observed that through experimental results, many times AI approaches look indecisive for irrelevant oversampling data features to detect pulmonary nodes besides it may correctly predicted. Sometime there may be serious contrariety to give proper explanation in how different models predict the same result. By analyzing all the facts, the final XAI model could be fine-tuned for better performance and interpretability. Our study mainly focused on to reduce AI implementation risk and build the trust while implementing the AI model in real life decision support system in

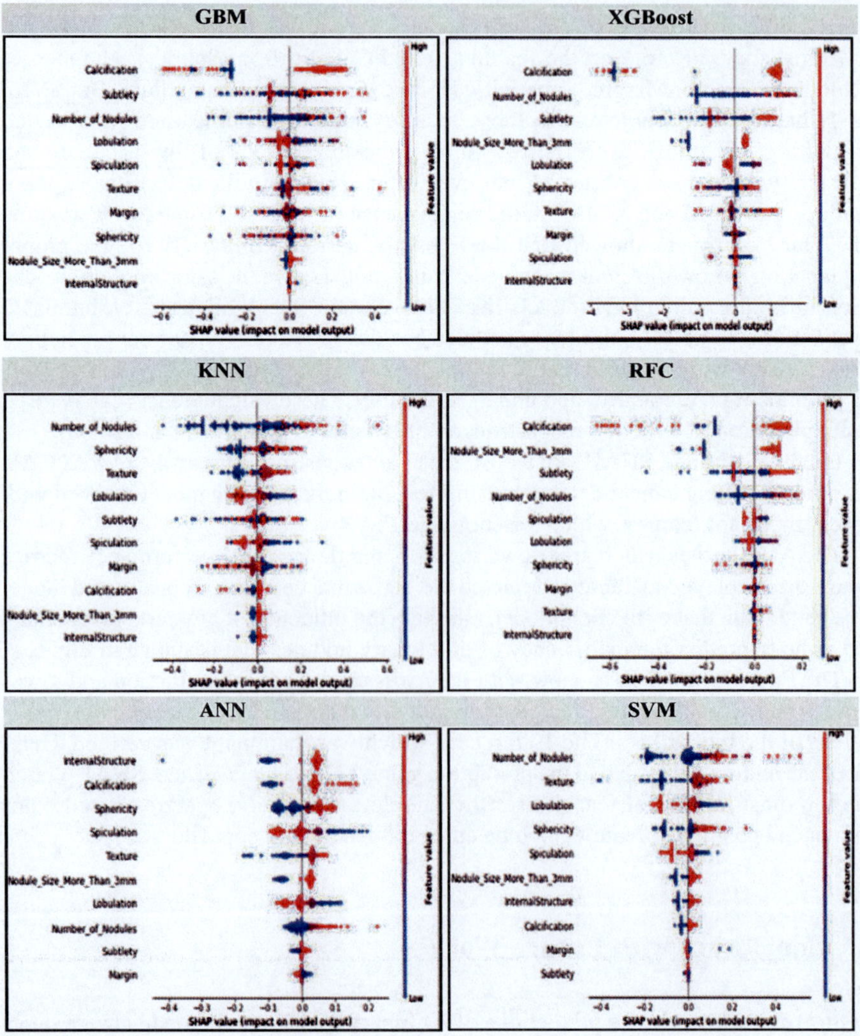

Fig. 3 Summary plots of machine learning models

healthcare domain. Similar approach can be used to build XAI models to diagnose other cancer diseases like prostate cancer, breast cancer etc., as well. In future, we would investigate other new XAI methods and different statistical approaches on hybrid AI models including deep learning models for guaranteed predictions with explanations and the work could be extended to solve multi-class problem to grade cancer stages.

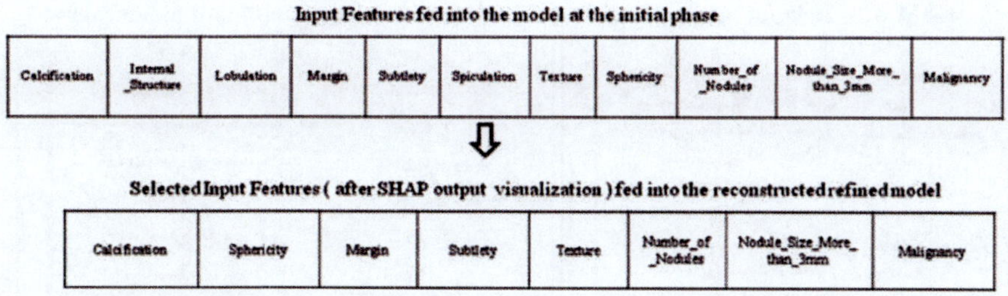

Fig. 4 Important features selection

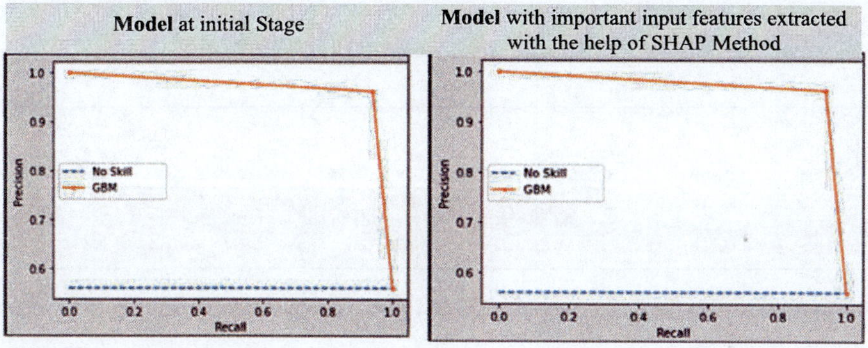

Fig. 5 AUC curve of the models

Table 3 Model's performance metrics

Accuracy	Precision	Recall	Specificity	AUC
Model performance with important input features extracted with the help of SHAP method				
0.945	0.963	0.939	0.953	0.946
Model performance at initial stage				
0.942	0.943	0.959	0.918	0.939

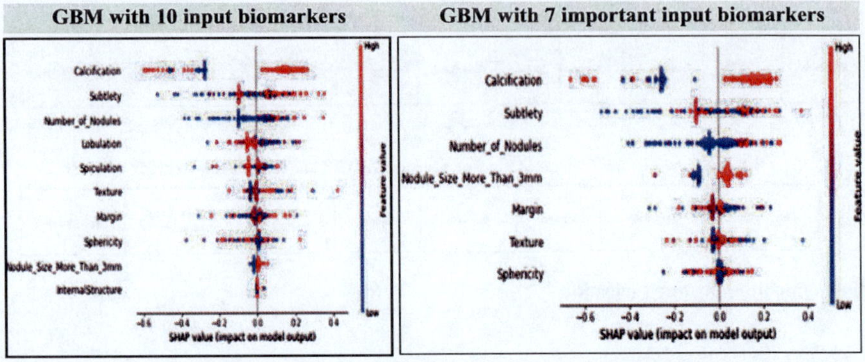

Fig. 6 Feature contribution summary plots of previous and reconstructed models

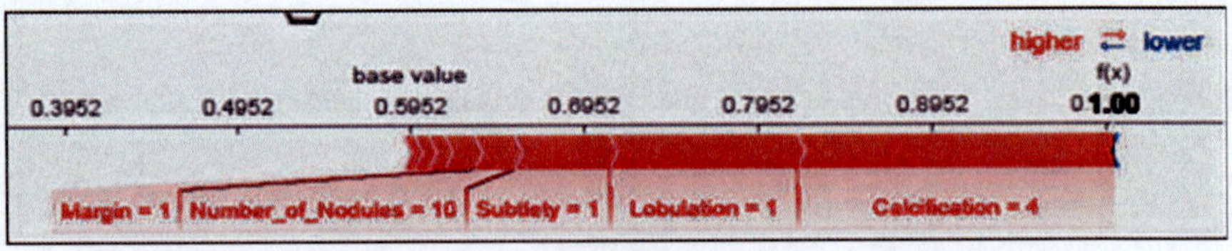

Fig. 7 Force plot for local prediction of single data in reconstructed model

References

1. An introduction to explainable AI with Shapley values. https://shap.readthedocs.io/en/latest/overviews.html. Last accessed 19 Dec 2020
2. Hancock M, Pylidc, MIT. https://pylidc.github.io/tuts/annotation.html
3. Zhu P, Ogino M (2019) Guideline-based additive explanation for computer-aided diagnosis of lung nodules. In Interpretability of machine intelligence in medical image computing and multimodal learning for clinical decision support. Springer, Cham, pp 39–47
4. Escalera S, Baró X, Guyon I, Escalante HJ (2018) Guest editorial: apparent personality analysis. IEEE Trans Affect Comput 9(3):299–302
5. Zhang S, Li X, Zong M, Zhu X, Cheng D (2017) Learning k for kNN classification. ACM Trans Intell Syst Technol (TIST) 8(3):1–19
6. Sahab AR, Zarif MH (2009) Improve backstepping method to GBM. World Appl Sci J 6(10):1399–1403
7. Chen T, Guestrin C (2016) Xgboost: a scalable tree boosting system. In: Proceedings of the 22nd ACM SIGKDD international conference on knowledge discovery and data mining, Aug 2016, pp 785–794
8. Breiman L (2001) Random forests. Mach Learn 45(1):5–32
9. Svozil D, Kvasnicka V, Pospichal J (1997) Introduction to multi-layer feed-forward neural networks. Chemom Intell Lab Syst 39(1):43–62
10. He H, Bai Y, Garcia EA, Li S (2008) ADASYN: adaptive synthetic sampling approach for imbalanced learning. In: 2008 IEEE international joint conference on neural networks (IEEE world congress on computational intelligence). IEEE, June 2008, pp 1322–1328
11. Potie N, Giannoukakos S, Hackenberg M, Fernandez A (2019) On the need of interpretability for biomedical applications: using fuzzy models for lung cancer prediction with liquid biopsy.

In: 2019 IEEE international conference on fuzzy systems (FUZZ-IEEE). IEEE, June 2019, pp 1–6
12. Ahmed ZU, Sun K, Shelly M, Mu L (2021) Explainable artificial intelligence (XAI) for exploring spatial variability of lung and bronchus cancer (LBC) mortality rates in the contiguous USA. Sci Rep 11(1):1–15
13. Pino C, Palazzo S, Trenta F, Cordero F, Bagci U, Rundo F, Battiato S, Giordano D, Aldinucci M, Spampinato C (2021) Interpretable deep model for predicting gene-addicted non-small-cell lung cancer in CT scans. In: 2021 IEEE 18th international symposium on biomedical imaging (ISBI). IEEE, pp 891–894, Apr 2021
14. Siddhartha M, Maity P, Nath R (2020) Explanatory artificial intelligence (XAI) in the prediction of post-operative life expectancy in lung cancer patients. Int J Sci Res, vol 8
15. Bartczak M, Partyka M, Chapter 8 Story Lungs: eXplainable predictions for post operational risks. Available at: https://pbiecek.github.io/xai_stories/story-lungs.html
16. Venugopal VK, Vaidhya K, Murugavel M, Chunduru A, Mahajan V, Vaidya S, Mahra D, Rangasai A, Mahajan H (2020) Unboxing AI-radiological insights into a deep neural network for lung nodule characterization. Acad Radiol 27(1):88–95

Healthcare Security and Blockchain

Impregnable Healthcare Ecosystem Using Blockchain and Artificial Intelligence Approaches

Anto Rahul Mahiban, Pritish Gupta, Aditya Raj, and Sumaiya Thaseen Ikram

Abstract Blockchain holds the potential to revolutionize health care. The ledger technology facilitates secure access and storage of electronic health records (EHRs). The proposed blockchain architecture coalesced with artificial intelligence (AI) and data obtained from the Internet of Things (IoT) provides a significant platform that can benefit the medical industry exceptionally. The data in blockchain can be viewed in a folder-file structure by the branched blockchain approach. Moreover, analytics dashboards are built on the prediction results of the AI models and the providers can envision the data interpreted in a comprehensive manner. Multiple attack predictions are computed after analyzing the EHR data stored in the blockchain. Hyperglycemia live prediction is implemented using a time-series model and random forest. Pulmonary infection classification is determined using visual geometry group-16 (VGG), convolutional neural network (CNN) model and heart attack prediction using K-nearest neighbor (KNN) binary classification. An accuracy of 93, 84 and 88 are obtained for the prediction of hyperglycemia, pulmonary and heart attack, respectively.

Keywords Blockchain · Electronic health records · Random forest · Smart health care · U-Net and VGG-16

A. R. Mahiban · P. Gupta · A. Raj · S. T. Ikram (✉)
School of Information Technology and Engineering, Vellore Institute Technology, Vellore, Tamil Nadu 632014, India
e-mail: sumaiyathaseen@gmail.com

A. R. Mahiban
e-mail: rahulm.a2019@vitstudent.ac.in

P. Gupta
e-mail: pritish.gupta2019@vitstudent.ac.in

A. Raj
e-mail: aditya.raj2019@vitstudent.ac.in

© The Author(s), under exclusive license to Springer Nature Singapore Pte Ltd. 2023

J. K. Mandal and D. De (eds.), *Frontiers of ICT in Healthcare*, Lecture Notes in Networks and Systems 519, https://doi.org/10.1007/978-981-19-5191-6_24

1 Introduction

The healthcare industry has grown into one of the largest sectors in India in terms of revenue and employment according to the Indian Brand and Equity Foundation report [1]. With the increasing surge in health care, it is crucial to address optimal solutions to handle the spiraling domain. Being decentralized and transparent in nature, blockchain drives the most encashed sector toward its intense features. Blockchain facilitates the worldwide interoperability of EHRs, which would allow authorized providers, access patients' medical histories. The decentralized approach of blockchain eliminates data corruption by removing the dependency on a centralized admin database. Thereby, the EHRs stored in the blockchain are free from corruption, unlike the traditional applications where it is still a possibility due to limitations in the physical memory. Data loss could be prevented by forming a common agreement between multiple nodes by implementing the consensus algorithm since the loss of EHRs can have severe consequences. The immutability of blockchain ensures that the EHRs are free from data tampering because modified reports can cause serious tension in the healthcare industry. Between 2005 and 2019, around 249.09 million individuals were afflicted in healthcare data breaches [2] and the sensitive data collected is then used for frauds and financial forgery. Blockchain can serve as an efficient solution to tackle the growing concern of data exposure by following coherent cryptographic techniques and appropriate cybersecurity practices. Furthermore, the integration of blockchain with AI and IoT will be the future of healthcare applications. Advancement in AI has reduced human effort by a significant margin in almost every field. Health care is one the biggest as well as an important field where AI models' assistance is highly appreciable. Drug discovery, disease prediction, emergency alert, administrative work and many more can result in high accuracy using machine learning (ML) and deep learning (DL) models. The integration of AI with IoT forms a robust smart ecosystem. Such as wristwatches to radiology devices, IoT has a huge range of gadgets that helps the healthcare industries collect medical data with ease.

The research work aims to provide a smart healthcare management system (SHMS) as a combination of blockchain, AI and IoT. Figure 1 contains the high-level design of the SHMS framework. Figure 2 specifies the use case diagram which depicts the authorized user actions of healthcare professionals and patients. The SHMS framework comprises three different layers, a blockchain layer that allows data storage and retrieval, the interface layer which allows the end-users to access the stored data using authentication credentials and a separate application programming interface (API) endpoint for IoT devices inputs. Blockchain is developed as a self-contained structure that communicates with the other two layers. Due to the independent nature of the blockchain with respect to the other two layers, multiple custom interfaces can be fabricated, on-demand for the healthcare centers. Data visualization is enhanced by introducing the branched blockchain approach into the decentralized structure thereby the EHRs can be envisioned in a folder-file structure through the interface. The IoT API endpoint encompasses self-trained AI models which will be

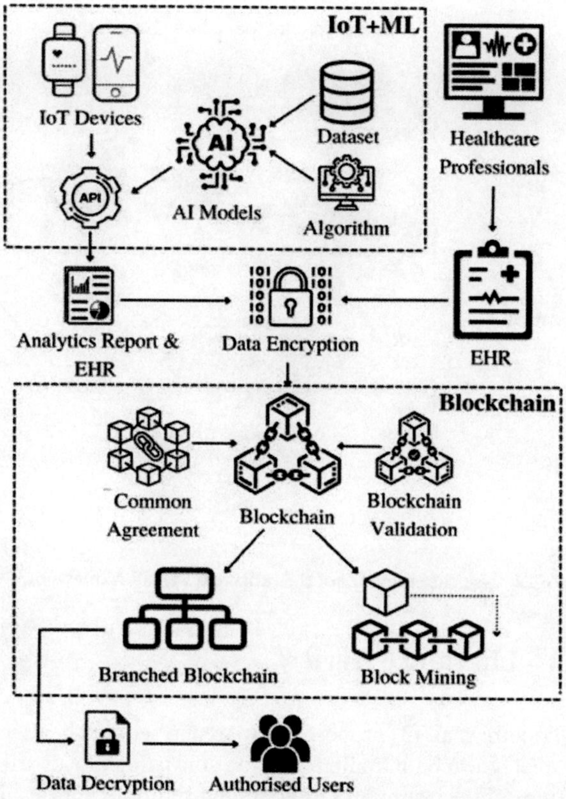

Fig. 1 High-level architecture of the proposed SHMS framework

triggered on the inputs provided by the smart devices to compute predictions and generate subsequent EHRs comprising of both IoT inputs and the predicted results, which are stored in the blockchain.

The remainder of this paper is organized as follows: Sect. 2 presents a literature survey on various blockchain-oriented approaches in health care integrated with AI, ML and DL models. Section 3 elaborates on the proposed SHMS framework. Section 4 presents a discussion of the results obtained with a bibliographic overview. Finally, Sect. 5 gives conclusive remarks along with the future scope and areas of development. Section 6 presents the current limitations and addresses the future revisal, which could enhance the research work.

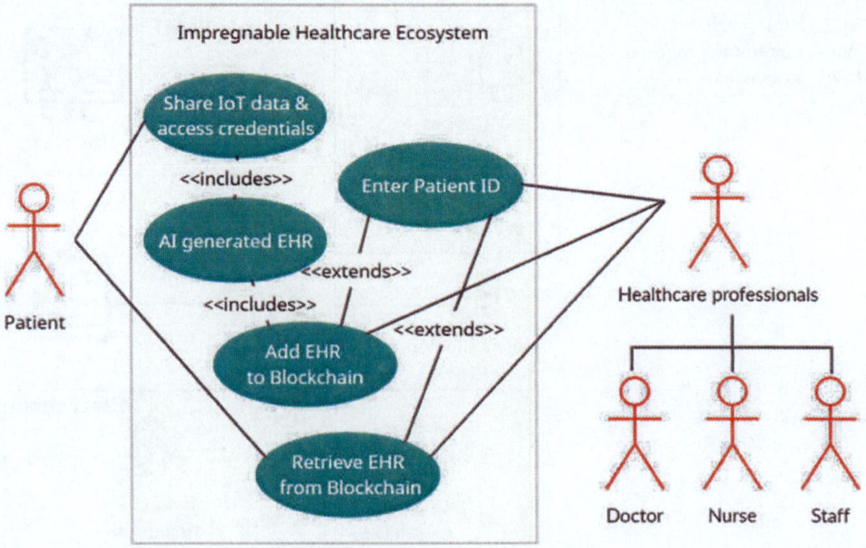

Fig. 2 Use case diagram of the proposed SHMS framework

2 Literature Review

Tripathi et al. [3] proposed a smart and secured healthcare system, which uses a two-level blockchain implementation consisting of a distributed and centralized architecture. This ensures isolation among multiple entities thereby providing a consistent and transparent workflow in a secure manner. Nagasubramanian et al. [4] suggest the keyless signature infrastructure with blockchain for ensuring the secrecy of digital signatures and other aspects of authentication. The proposed system is efficient in terms of multiple aspects including response time, which is 50% faster and cost, which is 20% lower than the conventional techniques. Cirstea et al. [5] introduce MedBlocks, a web application in which the data is encrypted through diverse encryption techniques like SHA-2, SHA-3. However, the technique is 20–30% slower than MD5 or SHA-1, it ensures data integrity which has a higher priority rank in the case of blockchain. Esposito et al. [6] propose off-chain storage, where the data is stored in a conventional database and the hashes are stored in the blockchain. The immutable hashes ensure authenticity and accuracy. The idea is efficient in terms of data portability, analytics and accessibility but may have serious concerns about cost efficiency and data processing. Ismail et al. [7] presented a lightweight blockchain architecture for health care which reduces the computational and communicational overheads over the bitcoin network. It introduces the canal method for confidential data transfer and is also free from forking. The proposed structure generates eleven times low network traffic as the number of nodes increases, the ledger update time is 1.13 times faster than the bitcoin network. Tandon et al. [8] review the idea of blockchain as a means to store medical data in order to ensure the safe distribution of individual health monitoring reports so that it is compliant with all the privacy laws. This work uses a meta-ethnography approach to study a pool of 42 studies to identify the challenges faced by the traditional EHRs such as data loss, delay in communication, memory efficiency and so on thereby stressing the importance of blockchain in health care. Hence, Singh et al. [9] propose a novel patient-centric architectural framework for blockchain enabled applications. It provides a basic data distribution interface for dis-joint parties of this application. Su et al. [10] propose a revocable attribute-based signature for blockchain-based healthcare systems to ensure users' privacy. The implementation mainly involves the use of KUNodes algorithm for identity-based encryption. Signature key is independently calculated by the user on the basis of a super and updated key in order to avoid any loss. Wilber et al. [11] review the advantages of blockchain in this field, where the features such as immutability, patient-centric architecture, interoperability and more are detailed as a viable long-term approach for health industry issues. Ahmed et al. [12] proposed discrete wavelet transform to enhance the security of the system and a genetic algorithm technique to optimize the processing. The work also introduces a cryptographic hash generator, MD5 that enhances the insusceptibility and access control. Shynu et al. [13] came up with a blockchain-based healthcare system for disease identification using AI models. Various types of ML clustering algorithm are primarily applied to the patient's medical records, and then, diabetic and cardiac diseases are predicted using feature selection-based self-learning neural networks. Aujla et al. [14] presented a decoupled blockchain-based approach in the AI applied edge nodes ecosystem. It also reduces data redundancy. Shaheen et al. [15] analyzed the application of AI in the field of health care. It is observed that medicine discovery, clinical trials, patient care, robotics and equipment as well as in administrative work, AI is capable of advancing the health system.

3 Proposed Work

Blockchain combined with IoT and AI is the future of the healthcare industry. This paper proposes the SHMS framework as a front-runner for modern healthcare applications. The blockchain is developed as a standalone entity to accept and return API calls from interfaces and other APIs registered under the cross-origin resource sharing policy of the network, for authorized users. Each block consists of five parameters: timestamp, version, nonce, previous_hash and data. The timestamp records the block creation timestamp, the version allows to track changes in blockchain functionalities, the nonce is the proof generated by the proof of work algorithm, and the previous_hash contains the hash of the previous block in hexadecimal format encrypted by SHA-256 algorithm. The data attribute contains key-value pairs of information regarding the EHRs stored across the block. The consensus algorithm checks for the longest chain across the blockchain network and replaces the chain with a shorter length. A common agreement is achieved between the multiple nodes on the blockchain network, and it is executed every time before any operation is performed on the blockchain. In addition, the blockchain is also validated every time before invoking any blockchain functionalities. For successful validation, the previous_hash parameter in every block, except for the elemental block, should contain a block associated with it and the nonce value of every block must comply with the proof of work algorithm.

The agile interface is built with the best user interface/user experience practices for increased productivity. The authentication process is carried out using JavaScript Object Notation Web Token, and all blockchain endpoints are secured and only authorized users can access and interact with the blockchain. The providers must request access, in the name of the hospital, to add/retrieve the EHRs of the particular patient before exercising the privilege of block addition for the individual. Once the patient approves the request, all the staff working in the hospital gain add/retrieve access to the patient's EHRs. After gaining one time access, the hospital staff can insert the EHRs of the particular individual into the blockchain and the files get uploaded to the simple storage service (S3) of Amazon Web Services and the respective keys are stored in the blockchain. The documents are uploaded to S3 to maintain high scalability and minimize production costs.

The IoT devices send data along with the patient credentials to a separate API endpoint. Further, pre-trained AI models are deployed such that the raw data from the smart devices are coupled with the corresponding self-learning AI model predictions to generate EHRs. These EHRs find their place in the blockchain under smart_entry. Furthermore, the EHRs under the smart_entry are classified and the staff members are presented with a comprehensive statistical analytics dashboard. The ecosystem comprehends three AI models namely hyperglycemia live prediction model, pulmonary infection classification model and heart attack prediction model.

In the hyperglycemia live prediction model, the data such as heart rate, skin temperature, posture are collected from the smartwatches in the.csv format. The input from the devices is sent to the API where the AI model is pre-trained with over 15,000 data, can return calls with the prediction results and notify the patients spontaneously. Due to the interdependency of data, the direct split can be unyielding. So, time-series split is applied with quantile transform for uniform distribution and frequent values, reducing the outliers. The data is then sent to an ensemble learning method, random forest with parameters, number of estimators = 500, criterion = 'entropy', number of jobs = 6. The result of the model is presented in Table 1. In the case of the hyperglycemia live prediction model, the analytics dashboard consists of the number of patients who are type-1 diabetic and the number of patients who are not type-1 diabetic, in a graphical format. The pulmonary infection classification model categorizes the patients based on the chest X-ray images shared by the smart devices. A total of 4500 chest X-ray images were resized, augmented and rescaled to train the CNN model. The model uses VGG-16, and VGG is a very deep CNN model with a 3×3 convolution filter. There are around 16–19 layers which help the architecture classify 1000 images into 1000 classifications, and the error in classification of the model is only 7.2%. The parameters used to compile the model are categorical cross-entropy loss, Adam optimizer, accuracy as metrics and sigmoid activation

Table 1 Hyperglycemia live prediction model results

Metrics	Values
Accuracy:	93.94%
Precision:	96.62%
Recall:	93.06%
F1-score:	94.81%
Confusion matrix:	[[13204 462] [984 9209]]

function. The X-ray images are processed through this model, to give a spontaneous result. Table 2 illustrates the results associated with the CNN model. The heart attack prediction model utilizes the KNN for the accurate classification of data points based on similarity trends. The optimum nearest neighbor value of K is determined to be eight. The training data is of size 305 rows × 14 columns, which are separated based on the categorical and continuous data and the continuous model is divided by time-series split, and finally, the KNN model is built. The results of the KNN model are illustrated in Table 3.

Table 2 Pulmonary infection classification model results

Metrics	Values			
Accuracy:	84.33%			
Average Precision:	85.42%			
Average recall:	82.29%			
F1-score:	83.97%			
Confusion matrix:		Pneumonia	Normal	COVID-19
	Pneumonia	2648	385	0
	Normal	250	779	0
	COVID-19	32	18	260

Table 3 Heart attack prediction model results

Metrics	Values
Accuracy:	88.53%
Precision:	91.17%
Recall:	0.837838
F1-score:	0.873239
Confusion matrix:	[[21 3] [6 31]]

3.1 Coupling Method

The immutable healthcare data generated by healthcare professionals and IoT devices are added to the blockchain ensuring it is free from data tampering and highly reduces the risk of medical error through proper documentation. However, the personal details that are subjected to change, which includes password, email address, personal address and so on are stored off-chain in a centralized database, protected by cybersecurity practices, due to the immutability of the blockchain. Thus, the coupling method involves the combination of blockchain and the centralized database to provide an efficient way for data storage across the blockchain applications.

3.2 Branched Blockchain Approach

The EHRs are stored in the blockchain in a linear format. The branched blockchain approach is introduced for enhanced data visualization by introducing two parameters namely collection and document, into the data dictionary. This is derived from the non-structured query language approach of the centralized database. The parameters introduced allows the data to be visualized in a tree structure, where the values containing key as collection form the parent nodes and the subsequent document values are the children nodes. The tree structure allows the data to be displayed as a folder-file structure through the interface. The unique collection names are listed as folders, and the documents under each collection can be viewed as files under the respective folders.

4 Result

4.1 Blockchain EHRs Addition

On gaining access, providers can add EHRs of patients into the blockchain. Figure 3 contains the interface for the addition of documents into the blockchain. On successful execution, the data dictionary records the paitent_id in the primary key and the staff_id along with the hospital_id which is stored in the secondary key. The folder name is stored in the collection parameter, the files get uploaded to S3, and the subsequent keys are stored in the document key. Additionally, the nonce, previous_hash and the timestamp are calculated along with the version and the block gets added into the blockchain.

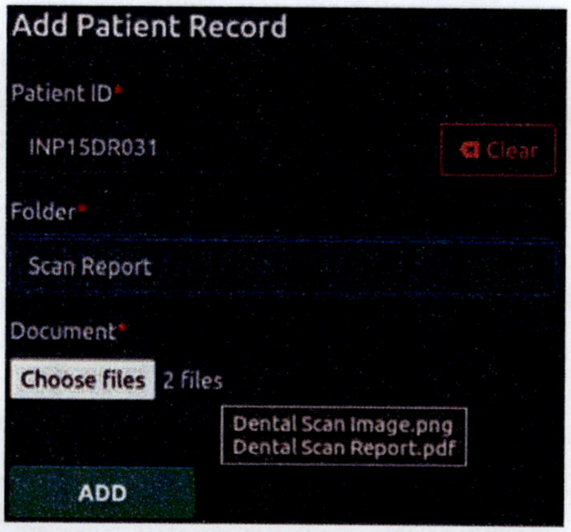

Fig. 3 Interface allows the addition of documents into the blockchain

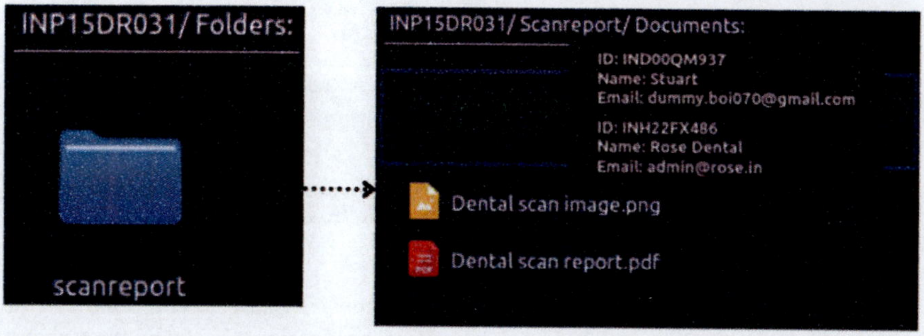

Fig. 4 On tapping the folder icon the list of blocks present under the collection is displayed

4.2 Blockchain EHRs Retrieval

The data in blockchain can be viewed in a folder-file structure by the branched blockchain approach. The folder represents the collection, and after selecting the particular folder, the blocks are listed along with the documents present inside the respective collection. Figure 4 represents the flow after clicking on the particular folder which displays the list of added documents.

4.3 IoT Endpoint + AI

The smart devices send the healthcare data, collected from the patients, as mentioned in Fig. 5. The AI model predicts and generates a subsequent report encompassing the results along with the IoT inputs. The created EHR is stored in the blockchain. Figure 5 shows a sample report generated by the hyperglycemia live prediction model.

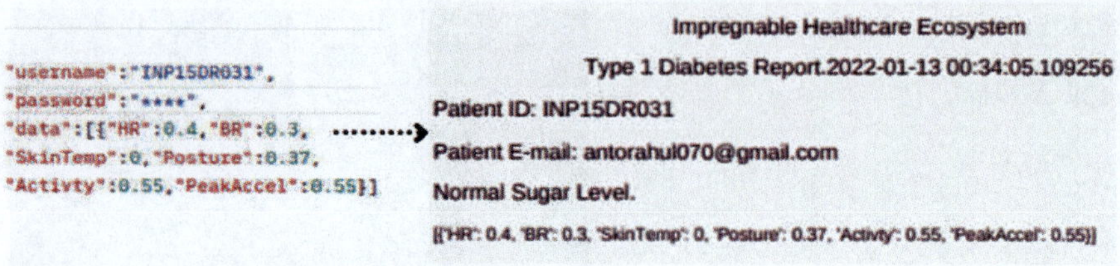

Fig. 5 Healthcare data shared from IoT devices along with the generated EHR containing the hyperglycemia live prediction model results

Fig. 6 Statistical analytics dashboard for the hyperglycemia live prediction model

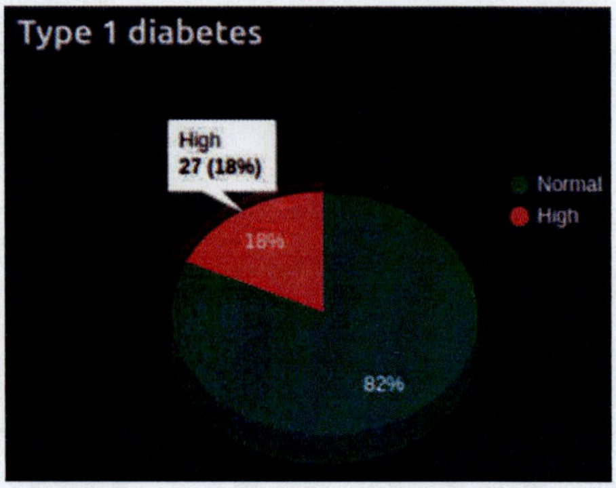

The analytics dashboard developed on top of the AI model predictions can be accessed from the staff login. The graph classifies their patients based on their health attributes predicted by the AI models as represented in Fig. 6.

4.4 AI Models Metrics

5 Conclusion

The challenges during the adoption of blockchain in health care such as unfeasible variable storage due to the immutability of blockchain and the difficulties in data visualization due to the linear structure of the blockchain are addressed and resolved by introducing new approaches such as the coupling method and the branched blockchain approach, respectively, in the proposed approach. The coupling method facilitates the management system with a combination of conventional and decentralized storage, and the branched blockchain approach provides a logical tree structure to enhance data visualization. The SHMS framework can prospectively replace the conventional medical management systems to a far extent. Moreover, the integration of AI and IoT along with blockchain provides a significant leap for the enhancement of existing applications. Pulmonary infection classification is determined using visual geometry group-16 (VGG) convolutional neural network (CNN) model and heart attack prediction using K-nearest neighbor (KNN) binary classification. An accuracy of 93, 84 and 88 is obtained for the prediction of hyperglycemia, pulmonary and heart attack, respectively. The AI models deployed yielded promising results. An accuracy of 93, 84 and 88 is obtained for the prediction of hyperglycemia, pulmonary and heart attack, respectively. In the future, more and more models can be deployed in the API to accept IoT inputs and compute subsequent predictions. Therefore, the designed SHMS framework is agile and can also support the introduction of imminent technologies, due to the lack of interdependency among the layers.

6 Future Work

The SHMS framework applies blockchain for healthcare application. In addition, AI models and IoT devices are integrated to provide a sustainable and secure ecosystem. The proposed framework, being a front-runner of blockchain in health care, is one of the very few potential architectures present in this domain. Therefore, extensive comparative analysis has been limited in our research work, which could possibly be performed in the future studies.

A pipeline developed using ML will ease the burden on doctors by minimizing the diagnosing time and effort. As a prototype, chest X-rays (CXR) are utilized for COVID-19—infection segmentation model which is built using U-Net architecture with VGG-16 and CNN as its backbone. There are 20,000 images containing CXR, lung masks and infection masks of both COVID-19 and non-COVID-19 patients which could be used for segmenting purposes. In parallel to this, another ML pipeline for COVID-19 classification using clinical data can be integrated for comparison with the segmentation model. This hybrid will assist in obtaining double assurance and, chances of false positives and negatives will reduce. If in any case, the ML models produce a contradicting result, it will be transferred to the doctor for verification. If not, an EHR will be generated and sent to the patient with the model's output.

References

1. Indian Brand Equity Foundation. https://www.ibef.org/industry/healthcare-india.aspx
2. Privacy Rights Clearinghouse. https://privacyrights.org/data-breaches
3. Tripathi G, Ahad MA, Paiva S (2020) S2HS-A blockchain based approach for smart healthcare system. Healthcare 8(1):100391
4. Nagasubramanian G, Kumar Sakthivel R, Patan R, Gandomi AH, Sankayya M, Balusamy B (2020) Securing e-health records using keyless signature infrastructure blockchain technology in the cloud. Neural Comput Appl 32(3):639–647

5. Cirstea A, Enescu FM, Bizon N, Stirbu C, Ionescu VM (2018) Blockchain technology applied in health the study of blockchain application in the health system (II). In: 2018 10th international conference on electronics, computers and artificial intelligence (ECAI). IEEE, pp 1–4
6. Esposito, C, De Santis A, Tortora G, Chang H, Raymond Choo K-K (2018) Blockchain: a panacea for healthcare cloud-based data security and privacy? IEEE Cloud Comput 5(1):31–37
7. Ismail L, Materwala H, Zeadally S (2019) Lightweight blockchain for healthcare. IEEE Access 7:149935–149951
8. Tandon A, Dhir A, Islam N, Mäntymäki M (2020) Blockchain in healthcare: a systematic literature review, synthesizing framework and future research agenda. Comput Ind 122:103290
9. Singh, AP, Pradhan NR, Luhach AK, Agnihotri S, Jhanjhi NZ, Verma S, Ghosh U, Sinha Roy D (2020) A novel patient-centric architectural framework for blockchain-enabled healthcare applications. IEEE Trans Ind Inf 17(8):5779–5789 (2020)
10. Su Q, Zhang R, Xue R, Li P (2020) Revocable attribute-based signature for blockchain-based healthcare system. IEEE Access 8:127884–127896
11. Wilber K, Vayansky S, Costello N, Berdik D, Jararweh Y (2020) A survey on blockchain for healthcare informatics and applications. In: 2020 7th international conference on internet of things: systems, management and security (IOTSMS). IEEE, pp 1–9
12. Hussein, AF, ArunKumar N, Ramirez-Gonzalez G, Abdulhay E, Manuel J, Tavares RS, de Albuquerque VHC (2018) A medical records managing and securing blockchain based system supported by a genetic algorithm and discrete wavelet transform. Cognit Syst Res 52:1–11 (2018)
13. Shynu PG, Menon VG, Lakshmana Kumar R, Kadry S, Nam Y (2021) Blockchain-based secure healthcare application for diabetic-cardio disease prediction in fog computing. IEEE Access 9:45706–45720
14. Aujla GS, Jindal A (2020) A decoupled blockchain approach for edge-envisioned IoT-based healthcare monitoring. IEEE J Select Areas Commun 39(2):491–499
15. Shaheen MY (2021) Applications of artificial intelligence (AI) in healthcare: a review. Sci Open Preprints

RIWT Generative Feedback Residual Network for Secure Clinical Data Communication in Healthcare Unit

Prabhash Kumar Singh, Biswapati Jana, Kakali Datta, Partha Chowdhuri, and Pabitra Pal

Abstract At present, data hiding has moved from a traditional approach to deep learning models. Deep learning has the potential to strengthen the security and privacy of sensitive information in medical images. In this paper, a novel RIWT-based generative feedback residual CNN model has been designed for hiding and recovery of secret information. Feedback system helps to re-learn and refine the deep features, while the residual system maintains the integrity and quality of the cover image. The model is trained simultaneously both on data hiding and recovery network with a learning rate of 0.001 and epoch of 1200. The model demonstrates an average PSNR of 42.73 dB and SSIM value of 0.99 for the stego images. Also, in comparison with state-of-the-art learning schemes, the proposed model performs superior for stego images, while its limitations are seen for a recovered secret images.

Keywords Data hiding · Deep learning · Wavelet transform · Residual network · Feedback system

1 Introduction

The advancement of communication technologies and their acceptance by communities across the globe has led to the progress of the use of multimedia technology in numerous real-life fields. In the healthcare sector, clinical information is shared as reports over insecure public networks via video, text and images. Digital multimedia technology allows for multiple copies of the reports to be made and gives the flexibility of simple adjustments using specialist software. The security of the med-

P. K. Singh · B. Jana (✉) · P. Chowdhuri
Department of Computer Science, Vidyasagar University, Midnapore, West Bengal, India
e-mail: biswapatijana@gmail.com

P. K. Singh · K. Datta
Department of Computer and System Sciences, Visva-Bharati University, Santiniketan, West Bengal, India

P. Pal
BSTTM, IIT Delhi, New Delhi, India

© The Author(s), under exclusive license to Springer Nature Singapore Pte Ltd. 2023
J. K. Mandal and D. De (eds.), *Frontiers of ICT in Healthcare*, Lecture Notes in Networks and Systems 519, https://doi.org/10.1007/978-981-19-5191-6_25

ical record is jeopardised by such flexibility. Medical data is particularly sensitive, making it prone to serious dangers including data manipulation and eavesdropping.

Digital watermarking and image information masking technology, as essential technologies in the realm of information security, could effectively protect network participants' privacy and information security [1]. The robust image steganography should make it more difficult to suspect hidden information along with the recovery of the secret data. A piece of secret information is converted into its binary equivalent for embedding the bits in the cover image. With the increase in the embedding of bits per pixel (bpp), the visual quality of the stego image degrades. A consistent trade-off has to be maintained among image quality and effective embedding capacity for better results.

It is seen in the literature that traditional algorithms do not meet the escalated security and capacity demands. However, recent research interest has concentrated on exploring neural networks [2] and augmentation reality [3]. Although most previous watermarking approaches incorporated binary data in greyscale or colour images, neural networks did not. The idea was to combine a greyscale and a colour image, or even a colour image with another colour image. Simultaneously, the use of neural networks for data hiding proved to be resilient, surviving traditional geometric attacks [4]. Deep steganography, a deep learning-based steganography system, was proposed by Baluja [5]. Authors used three different networks, preparation network, hidden network and expose network to embed and extract secret data. A year later, Rehman et al. [6] involved CNN with encoder and decoder for training. Another big development came with the introduction of adversial network for data hiding [7, 8].

In this paper, a model has been designed on the backbone of the residual and feedback CNN network system. A novel Redundant Integer Wavelet Transform (RIWT) has been incorporated for enhancing the security and convenience of recovering the secret data at the recovery network. The secret image was converted into wavelet components for hiding the information through convolutional layers. The efficiency and potential of the designed model get clearly visible by the results obtained in the experimental section.

2 Related Work

According to prior research, a 2D-DWT can be divided into four sub-bands: approximation (A), horizontal (H), vertical (V) and diagonal (D), which correspond to the LL, HL, LH and HH sub-bands, respectively. Approximation sub-bands hold maximum information, while diagonal sub-bands have less information [9]. The data embedding at HH sub-bands improves the imperceptibility. Furthermore, embedding at LL sub-bands contributes to resist attacks. Wang et al. [10] presented a method for reducing the possibility of a stego image being classified as a stego image by burying confidential clinical information in the camouflage zones. Since DWT technique does not guarantee complete reversibility, IWT is preferred. But, it has also its limitation in terms of embedding capabilities. The RDWT-based hiding methodology outperformed the DWT- and IWT-based embedding approaches in terms of capacity and resilience, according to [11]. The Redundant Integer Wavelet Transform (RIWT) is an unique approach that combines the benefits of both RDWT and IWT to produce better reversibility, high embedding capacity and good robustness [12].

It is true that deep learning has been around, but its recent advancement has been eye catching due to multi-layered deep neural networks. The present configuration of computer system has expedited its execution. Some outstanding deep learning solutions have been applied in the field of data hiding in recent years of research, including models like image generation, segmentation and target identification. Goodfellow et al. [13] introduced a Generative Adversarial Network (GAN) for an image in 2014. Zhang et al. [14] employed GAN to hide information. The GAN network produced good aesthetic effects while producing images carrying secret information since it performed well in the realm of image generation.

Researchers have recently become interested in steganography, which is a technique for hiding images within images. Duan et al. [15] employed a U-Net structure to create an image steganography model in which complex texture objects were used to hide hidden images. The quality of the retrieved secret image was pretty poor because this method compressed the secret image information. In the same year, Baluja [16] proposed a new neural network-based steganography model that successfully concealed a secret image within a similar-sized image. These algorithms produced a good hiding result for colour photos, but there is still room to improve image hiding capability.

3 Preliminaries

4 RIWT

When doing inverse transformation, the DWT enhances imperceptibility and durability, but also generates an inaccuracy. However, IWT perpetuates for exact reversibility of values. IWT embodies Haar lifting transform to obtain minimal loss transform error. The forward and inverse transformations are computed as follows:

$$d_{1,n} = s_{0,2n+1} - s_{0,2n} \tag{1}$$

$$s_{1,n} = s_{0,2n} + \lfloor d_{1,n/2} \rfloor \tag{2}$$

$$s_{0,2n+1} = d_{1,n} + s_{0,2n} \tag{3}$$

$$s_{0,2n} = s_{1,n} - \lfloor d_{1,n/2} \rfloor \tag{4}$$

where $s_{i,n}$ indicates nth low-frequency coefficient and $d_{i,n}$ indicates nth high-frequency coefficient of the ith level wavelet. RDWT divides a single image into

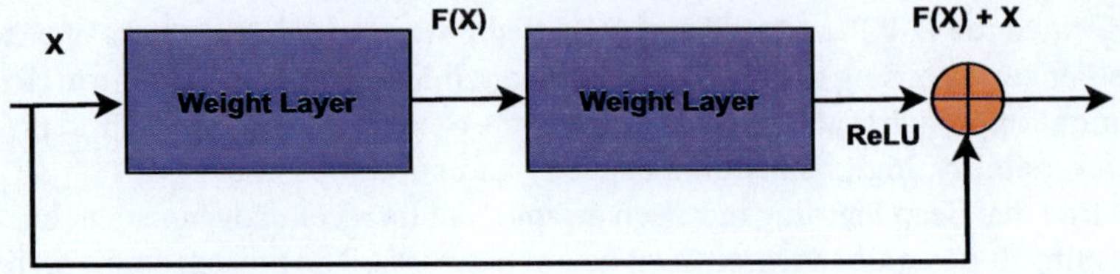

Fig. 1 Basic residual network

four coefficient matrices and repeats the procedure till the level of decomposition is satisfactory. The Redundant Integer Wavelet Transform (RIWT) [12] is a new hybrid transformation that improves reversibility, robustness, imperceptibility and embedding capacity by combining both RDWT and IWT.

5 Residual Network

Classical linked networks and convolutional neural networks may result in the loss of important information, gradient disappearance and explosion while hiding or extracting information. The concept of residual learning was invented by Kaiming and four other Chinese, and ResNet largely solved the problem [17]. The CNN feature reveal network, which is presently the most widely used, not only simplifies learning objectives and barriers, but also preserves the integrity of the data by learning the difference between input and output. Several $y = x$ congruent mapping layers are added if the shallow network gets saturated. As a result of the deeper network, there will be no more errors in the training set. The use of equality mapping to pass the previous output directly to the latter influenced ResNet. The learning goal is $F(x) = H(x) - x$ if the network's input is x and the expected output is $H(x)$. The leftover block is depicted in Fig. 1.

6 Proposed Scheme

The proposed method involves RIWT, Generative Feedback and Residual network to construct a data hiding scheme for secure data communication and resilience to attacks encountered over the unreliable media. The proposed novel Generative Feedback Residual Network (GFRN) works in two phases through two different networks: data hiding network and data recovery network. Multiple cover images ($256 \times 256 \times 3$) along with the secret image ($256 \times 256 \times 1$) of same dimensions but of different channels are fed into the network for feature extraction, convolution and concatenation. Both the networks are trained simultaneously. The recovery network trained to recover the secret image from the container (stego image), while the hiding network learned to hide the secret information in the least obvious areas of the carrier image (cover image). The embedding approach ensures reversibility and enhanced imperceptibility, making it impossible for any unauthorised user to suspect the presence of a concealed secret data. The secret data is accurately recovered from the stego image by reversing the embedding process.

6.1 Hiding Network

The 29 convolutional layers, 2 deconvolutional layers, 4 concat operations, one feedback and one residual block make up the hidden network. Network inputs took into account an RGB carrier image holding a size of $256 \times 256 \times 3$, as well as a greyscale secret image possessing a size of 256×256, while an RGB image owning a size of 256×256 served as a network output. Prior to actual embedding, the secret image passes through first level of RIWT to produce the four sub-bands A, H, V and D. Convolution features are extracted from these components and concatenated to different network layers. Because of the modelled linking approach, the hidden image's attributes were kept, and the influence on the carrier image was limited.

Batchnormalization and ReLU are used as an activation function for the designed model. The feature map of the A sub-band was concatenated with the feature map of the cover image seven convolution layers including two downsampling as well. This combined feature map passes through another three convolution layers where the concatenated feature maps of the sub-bands A, H and V are concated. To re-learn and refine the features a feedback system in employed to transfer the deep features to the shallow layers. The advantage of using the feedback mechanism is that the loss output can be predicted in advance in parallel to transmitting deep carrier image features back to the low-level network for learning.

In the residual network, multiple layer skip connections can be used to retain the cover image properties to the greatest extent possible while also improving the aesthetic effect of the final stego image through optimization. The 11th convolution layer of the cover image is mixed with the outputs of the 14th convolution layer of the specified model.

Figure 2 clearly illustrates the proposed data hiding network. Two convolution functions of filter size 3×3 and 4×4 with stride 1 and 2 were used respectively. A deconvolution function of filter size 4×4 was processed with stride 2 and one layer padding. Throughout the model, three different channels of size 4, 12 and 24 were used at the convolutional layers.

6.2 Recovery Network

The recovery network has been tasked with extracting the secret data present in the stego image. For learning to extract the secret information, it uses 24 convolution

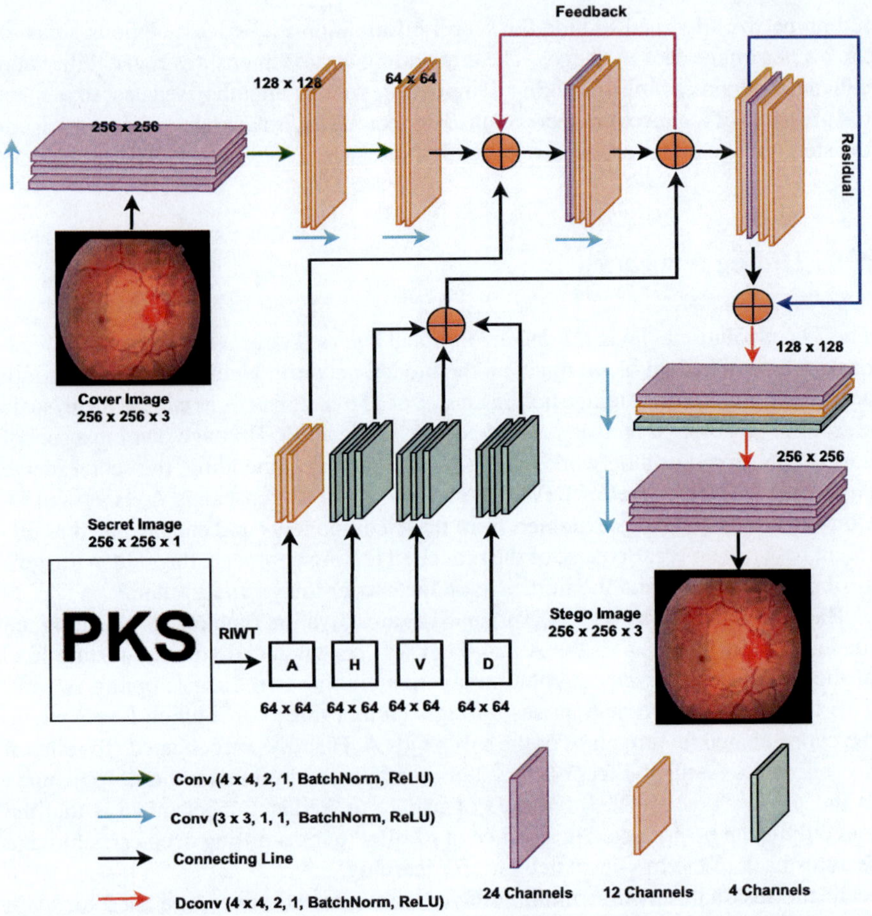

Fig. 2 Proposed hiding network

layers, one deconvolution layer, 2 feedback operations, 4 concat operations and one residual operation. At first, the received colour image of size $256 \times 256 \times 3$ is provided to the system which passes through three convolutions layers of 24 channels. Four concat operations were carried out after 3rd, 6th, 14th and 16th convolution layers. Two feedback systems have been enrolled for better learning within short interval. One supplies feedback from the 10th convolution layer to the concat operation used after 3rd layer, while another was used from 16th layer to concat operation present after 6th layer. Finally, at the end of the network the features were separated into four wavelet components. Thereafter, the inverse Redundant Integer wavelet Transform (iIRWT) was applied to obtain the secret image. The details of the recovery network are shown in Fig. 3.

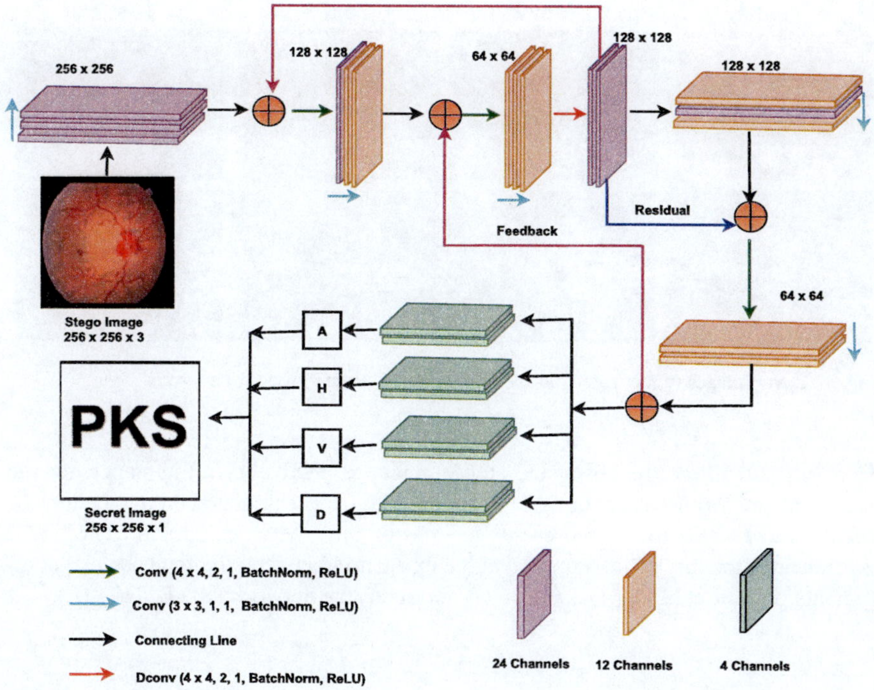

Fig. 3 Proposed recovery network

6.3 Loss Function

The mean square error (MSE) was utilised to calculate the loss function for the proposed networks. The low difference indicates lower MSE value which implies high quality of derived images. The loss function needed to contain both information concealing and information extraction loss functions in order to assure high quality data hiding and recovery at the same time. MSE was calculated in the following way.

$$\text{MSE}(I^1, I^2) = \frac{1}{M \times N} \sum_{i=1}^{M} \sum_{j=1}^{N} (I^1_{i,j} - I^2_{i,j})^2 \tag{5}$$

$$L = L_1 + L_2 \tag{6}$$

$$L_1 = \text{MSE}(\text{CI}, \text{SI}) \tag{7}$$

$$L_2 = \text{MSE}(A, A') + \text{MSE}(H, H') + \text{MSE}(V, V') + \text{MSE}(D, D') \tag{8}$$

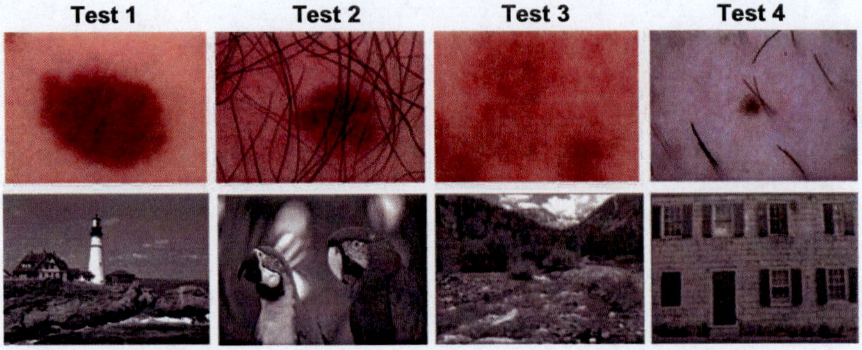

Fig. 4 Cover images (upper row) and secret images (lower row) used for analysis

Here, CI and SI are the cover and stego image, respectively. In this paper, for the proposed network loss function (L) as shown in Eq. 6 is calculated on two factors L_1 (Eq. 7) and L_2 (Eq. 8). L_1 represents the loss of MSE between CI and SI, whereas L_2 indicates the loss of information at the extraction between the four wavelet components present at hiding (A, H, V, D) and recovery network (A', H', V', D').

7 Experimental Analysis

The proposed model was trained on the HAM10000 data set, which contains 5000 medical colour images [18]. However, a total of 3000 images with a size of $256 \times 256 \times 3$ were employed in this study, with 2400 and 600 images used for training and testing, respectively. The experiments were conducted on a workstation having Intel Xeon processor, 8 GB RAM and 4 GB Nivdia graphics under the IDE python 3.6 and pytorch. Each images were restricted to size $256 \times 256 \times 3$. For an optimization of the loss function, Adam optimizer was called upon with default starting learning rate of 0.001 and finally iterated (epoch) upto 1200.

To measure the performance of the designed model, study on visual effects, imperceptibility, payload and robustness analysis was conducted. As shown in Fig. 4, a set of four images were selected randomly from test set to act as cover image along with four other secret images for hiding as information.

7.1 Visual Analysis

Figure 5 shows the image obtained as an output of the hiding network (stego image) and extracted secret image as an output of the recovery network. The comparison was made using histogram analysis of the image used in the model. Analysis reveals that

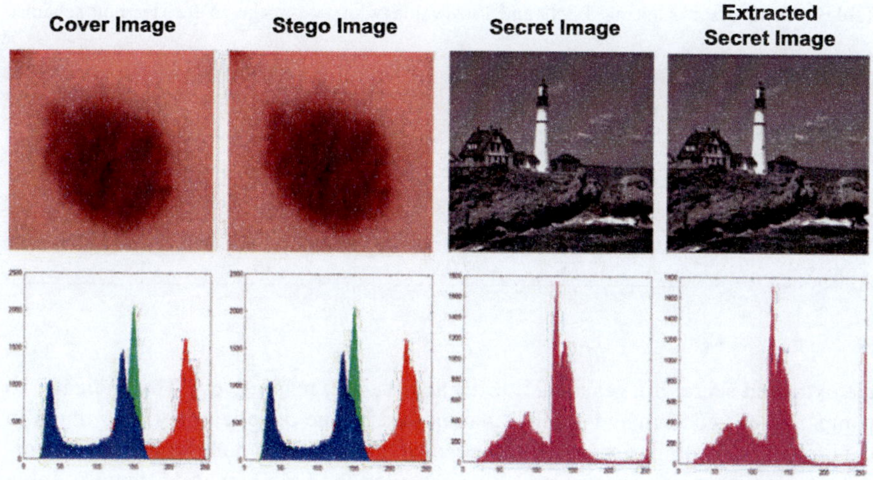

Fig. 5 Comparison of histogram for visual analysis

the pixel distribution in both the cover and stego image almost remains the same. It is visually not possible to identify any trace of noise directly looking into the histogram. As a result, the hiding and extracting procedures proposed in this work have good aesthetic effects.

7.2 *Image Quality and Comparison*

The quality of the image was measured by PSNR and SSIM. PSNR represents the difference between the two images based on MSE. Higher PSNR indicates to good quality of the image. Moreover, SSIM is the similarity index calculated on three factors: luminance, contrast and structure. Its value ranges between −1 and 1.

Table 1 clearly points that the average PSNR and SSIM values for the stego images are 42.73 dB and 0.9860, respectively. Also, the average PSNR and SSIM values for

Table 1 PSNR and SSIM values of the selected cover images

Cover images	Stego image		Extracted secret image	
	PSNR (dB)	SSIM	PSNR (dB)	SSIM
Test 1	43.95	0.9864	20.38	0.8234
Test 2	40.87	0.9889	20.33	0.8416
Test 3	42.44	0.9853	23.63	0.8754
Test 4	43.67	0.9834	23.51	0.8562
Average	42.73	0.9860	21.96	0.8492

Table 2 Comparison of average PSNR and SSIM values with state-of-the-art deep learning schemes

Cover images	Stego image		Extracted secret image	
	PSNR (dB)	SSIM	PSNR (dB)	SSIM
Baluja [16]	36.49	0.96	30.54	0.90
Rahim and Nadeem [6]	32.50	0.93	34.75	0.93
Zhang et al. [14]	34.89	0.96	39.90	0.96
Duan et al. [15]	40.47	0.97	40.66	0.98
Proposed	42.73	0.99	21.96	0.85

the extracted secret images are 21.96 dB and 0.8492, respectively. This indicates to comparatively good image quality as indicated by the deep learning algorithms in the literature. A comparison of the proposed model has been done with four state-of-the-art deep learning schemes as demonstrated in the literature. Additionally, Table 2 indicates that the proposed method performed better in terms of quality for stego image; however, the quality of the extracted secret image was not upto mark in comparison with the standard techniques.

8 Conclusion

Nowadays, health care is playing a pivotal role in everyday life. The security and privacy of clinical information are of paramount importance. Thus, a deep learning generative model has been proposed involving feedback and a residual network system. The secret image is first transformed into RIWT coefficients for the embedding information through various convolutional layers of the hidden network. Essentially, the recovery of the information is done at the recovery network. The experimental results advocate the superiority of the designed model over the stego image; however, some refinement needs to be done on the recovery network for better extraction of secret information and resilience to adversaries.

References

1. Ma K, Zhang W, Zhao X, Yu N, Li F (2013) Reversible data hiding in encrypted images by reserving room before encryption. IEEE Trans Inf Forensics Secur 8(3):553–562
2. Lee JE, Seo YH, Kim DW (2020) Convolutional neural network-based digital image watermarking adaptive to the resolution of image and watermark. Appl Sci 10(19):6854
3. Li C, Sun X, Li Y (2019) Information hiding based on augmented reality. Math Biosci Eng 16(5):4777–4787
4. Jiao S, Zhou C, Shi Y, Zou W, Li X (2019) Review on optical image hiding and watermarking techniques. Opt Laser Technol 109:370–380

5. Baluja S (2017) Hiding images in plain sight: deep steganography. In: Advances in neural information processing systems, vol 30, pp 2069–2079
6. Rahim R, Nadeem S (2018) End-to-end trained CNN encoder-decoder networks for image steganography. In: Proceedings of the European conference on computer vision (ECCV) workshops
7. Li Q, Wang X, Wang X, Ma B, Wang C, Xian Y, Shi Y (2020) A novel grayscale image steganography scheme based on chaos encryption and generative adversarial networks. IEEE Access 8:168166–168176
8. Chen B, Wang J, Chen Y, Jin Z, Shim HJ, Shi YQ (2020) High-capacity robust image steganography via adversarial network. KSII Trans Internet Inf Syst (TIIS) 14(1):366–381
9. Baby D, Thomas J, Augustine G, George E, Michael NR (2015) A novel DWT based image securing method using steganography. Procedia Comput Sci 46:612–618
10. Wang J, Wu J, Wu Z, Anisetti M, Jeon G (2018) Bayesian method application for color demosaicking. Opt Eng 57(5):053102
11. Makbol NM, Khoo BE (2013) Robust blind image watermarking scheme based on redundant discrete wavelet transform and singular value decomposition. AEU-Int J Electron Commun 67(2):102–112
12. Sukumar A, Subramaniyaswamy V, Ravi L, Vijayakumar V, Indragandhi V (2021) Robust image steganography approach based on RIWT-Laplacian pyramid and histogram shifting using deep learning. Multimedia Syst 27(4):651–666
13. Goodfellow I, Pouget-Abadie J, Mirza M, Xu B, Warde-Farley D, Ozair S et al (2014) Generative adversarial nets. In: Advances in neural information processing systems, vol 27
14. Zhang R, Dong S, Liu J (2019) Invisible steganography via generative adversarial networks. Multimedia Tools Appl 78(7):8559–8575
15. Duan X, Jia K, Li B, Guo D, Zhang E, Qin C (2019) Reversible image steganography scheme based on a U-Net structure. IEEE Access 7:9314–9323
16. Baluja S (2019) Hiding images within images. IEEE Trans Pattern Anal Mach Intell 42(7):1685–1697
17. He K, Zhang X, Ren S, Sun J (2016) Deep residual learning for image recognition. In: Proceedings of the IEEE conference on computer vision and pattern recognition, pp 770–778
18. Tschandl P (2018) The HAM10000 dataset, a large collection of multi-source dermatoscopic images of common pigmented skin lesions. Harvard Dataverse, V3, UNF:6:/APKSsDGVDhwPBWzsStU5A==. https://doi.org/10.7910/DVN/DBW86T

Blockchain-Based Smart Integrated Healthcare System

Deepa Parasar, Preet Viradiya, Aryaa Singh, Sumit Chahar, Vivek Prasad, and Varun Iyengar

Abstract The goal of this research is to implement a smart healthcare application based upon blockchain technology, to construct a theoretical model that is hierarchical for smart healthcare, and to build a smart healthcare development software system based on stakeholder theory. Currently, electronic health records allow for just the automatic updating and exchange of medical data on a single patient inside a single organization or network of organizations. This could be extended if the data was organized in a way such that the blockchain's uppermost layer only contained non-PHI or personally identifiable data (PII). Decentralization, anonymity, tamper resistance, and auditability are all properties of blockchain. It is a key fourth industrial revolution technology. The combination of blockchain and smart healthcare can help to alleviate traditional smart healthcare's pain points in information sharing, data protection, and privacy preservation, as well as optimize user-centered smart healthcare systems and establish a multiparty medical cooperation chain involving government, businesses, and individuals, all of which can imperialize smart healthcare.

Keywords Blockchain · Healthcare system · PII · Medical information · Smart records · Decentralization · Consensus

1 Introduction

Going digital has a plethora of potential benefits for both patients and professionals. Digital care may speed up procedures, improve clinical decision-making, and eliminate errors by connecting caregivers and exchanging clinical data, all with the goal of improving patient outcomes and increasing care efficiency. The all-in-one healthcare solution.

D. Parasar (✉) · P. Viradiya · A. Singh · S. Chahar · V. Prasad · V. Iyengar
Amity School of Engineering and Technology, Amity University Maharashtra, Mumbai, India
e-mail: dparasar@mum.amity.edu

V. Prasad
e-mail: vivek.prasad1@s.amity.edu

© The Author(s), under exclusive license to Springer Nature Singapore Pte Ltd. 2023
J. K. Mandal and D. De (eds.), *Frontiers of ICT in Healthcare*, Lecture Notes in Networks and Systems 519, https://doi.org/10.1007/978-981-19-5191-6_26

The process of converting information into a digital (i.e., computer-readable) format is known as digitization. The end result is digital representation, or more precisely, a digital picture of the object and a digital form of the signal. Digitization is critical for data processing, storage, and transmission because "information of all kinds in all forms can be transported with the same efficiency and also mixed." Though analog data is typically more durable, digital data is easier to exchange and retrieve, and it can theoretically be transmitted indefinitely without generation loss if converted to new, stable forms as needed. This is why many organizations all over the world prefer it as their preferred method of data preservation. Healthcare consumes a sizable portion of developed countries' gross domestic product (GDP). However, hospital expense is continued to rise, as do inefficient practices, and health data breaches are on the rise. This is an area where technology based on blockchain can be beneficial. It can perform a variety of activities, including secure encryption of medical information and epidemic control. Currently, electronic health records allow for just the automatic updating and exchange of medical data on a single patient inside a single organization or network of organizations. This might be extended if the data was organized in such a way that the blockchain's top layer only contained non-PHI or personally identifiable information (PII).

Decentralization, confidentiality, auditability, and tamper-resistant are all properties of blockchain, which is the fourth industrial revolution's key technology [1, 2]. The approach of combining blockchain and smart healthcare can address traditional smart healthcare's pain points in information sharing, digital security, and data preservation, optimize user-centered smart health systems, and create a multi-party medical alliance chain involving government, businesses, and individuals, all of which will help to promote smart healthcare industrialization. A "blockchain" is a shared, immutable record of a series of events, each of which is made up of a single block and linked by cryptographic keys. These signatures or keys are stored in a network of nodes or processes that are linked together. Each node has a replica chain, which is regularly synchronized and updated.

2 Literature Review

A Blockchain-based health information exchange might uncover the true value of interoperability. With blockchain-based systems, current middleman friction and expenditures might be minimized or eliminated. Furthermore, in terms of reproducibility, data sharing, personal data privacy, and patient participation in clinical trials, Blockchain technology poses severe medical concerns [3]. The blockchain is pushing the Internet closer to its ultimate aim of decentralization in the realm of the Internet. It is predicted that the blockchain's health would suffer serious implications. This is an exciting period in health care and information technology. Health care is seeing a new approach to sickness prevention as a result of developments in genetic research and clinical research.

2.1 Motivation and Contribution

Contribution and inspiration blockchain-based medical systems are still in the developmental stages. The following are some disadvantages of existing schemes: (1) The majority of the plans are simply outlined and do not include particular implementation specifics [4, 5]. (2) Despite the fact that some plans include specifics, the cost of calculation and communication is significant [6]. The idea is to create a blockchain-based system for sharing medical data. It facilitates the storage, management, and dissemination of medical data. In this system, the security standards for plans of medical data to be exchanged must be met. In terms of computing and connectivity, it should also be low-cost.

The following is a list of the paper's main contributions: (1) A lightweight medical data sharing and security model based on blockchain is proposed. The model can communicate data across doctors from other hospitals using proxy re-encryption technology. Because medical data is recorded on the blockchain, it is extremely secure and cannot be readily tampered with [7]. (2) By building on the usual delegated proof, a better consensus procedure is presented. It is secure, dependable, and effective. (3) For patients who register at various hospitals but exhibit symptoms of the same condition, we develop a symptom-matching algorithm. When mutual authentication is complete, the patients can exchange a session key. Patients can use the system to get disease-related information [8].

2.1.1 Blockchain

Blockchain is a digital ledger of distributed databases that combines data blocks in chronological sequence, and it primarily handles transactional trust and security challenges. The private, consortium, and public blockchains are the three types of blockchains [9, 10]. Each blockchain is made up of several blocks, each of which has a block header and a block body. The block header provides a variety of meta-data about the current block. For example, the timestamp, the blockchain body's hash value, and the prior block's hash value. The genuine data of current transactions is generally recorded in the block body.

2.1.2 Basic Requirements for Sharing of Medical Data and Protection Plan

Basic requirements for an optimal sharing of medical data and protection strategy include consistent standards, privacy and security protection, data access, patient management (user engagement), and security and privacy protection [5, 11]. Medical data would be secure and private, and no one will be in a position to utilize it in an unauthorized way. The system should be able to withstand harmful assaults and track illicit activity. Patients may access all of their medical records after being approved, and doctors can access previous medical information with patients' permission. Patient control: the patient had control over his or her medical records in the past, which meant that no one could access the data without the patient's permission. All players in the model should utilize a single data standards and management scheme, which is effective in implementing data sharing and improving system stability.

2.1.3 Proof-of-Stake with Delegated Ownership

In blockchain, the consensus process ensures that all legitimate nodes maintain the same global record. Delegated Proof-of-Stake (DPOS) is a secure and rapid consensus method [12, 13]. Coin holders elect select nodes to vote on behalf of all DPOS participants, similar to how the board votes. It has the ability to shorten the time it takes to achieve an agreement. Everyone who has coins must vote and create 101 delegates first, according to the DPOS system. The delegates can be compared to supernodes who have the same rights as each other. These supernodes are then in charge of generating a new block. If delegates fail to fulfill their obligations, the network will require new supernodes, and the existing nodes will be fined.

3 Proposed System

This proposed system will house various data layers, comprising the storage layer, data management layer, and data usage layer, which will all work together to assure data security and functionality. Furthermore, improving blockchain-based smart contracts may aid in the secure operation of monitoring devices. The blockchain activity will be verified and monitored by smart contracts. Smart contracts will also allow for real-time patient monitoring by securely providing critical notifications to patients and healthcare providers. Patients may handle their own care while a healthcare practitioner is always available with real-time updates, which is crucial for safe home care. While offering hospitals quick access, our system safeguards and allows patients to retain ownership of their own documents. The actual medical records will not be stored on a decentralized cloud storage system, but rather a unique identifier for each document will be added to the blockchain. The root chunk will be formed by combining the swarm hash with the decryption key from each medical record. The content is only accessible to individuals who know the root chunk's reference. As a result, the root chunks are securely stored in smart contracts on the blockchain and only released under certain conditions.

The presentation logical, view, and physical layer architecture are shown in Fig. 1. The presentation layer is the interface between humans and computers, as well as the means through which a user interacts with a program or a website.

The logical layer works between the user and the real database, the GraphQL server works as a mediator. When a client application has to specify which fields in a long query format are required, this might be utilized. When adding functionality

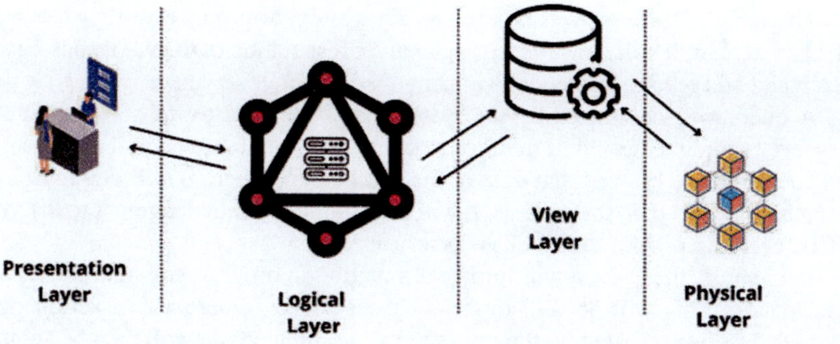

Fig. 1 4-Tier architecture

to old or current APIs, it may be fully utilized. An abstraction over an existing API for defining a response structure based on user requirements.

The view layer represents the database, which is where the logical layer's activities are processed. The same data should be accessible to every user, but they should be able to see a personalized representation of it. The user is not required to deal directly with the physical layer specifics. Changes to the display layer in terms of storage should have no effect on the database's fundamental structure.

The physical layer represents the core of a blockchain-based system provides a balance of medical privacy and system-wide access to healthcare records. Users have more faith in their practitioners when they have more control. Furthermore, providing medical personnel with tools to keep track of the patient's whole medical history.

The backend architecture of GraphQL and database is shown in Fig. 2 and explained below.

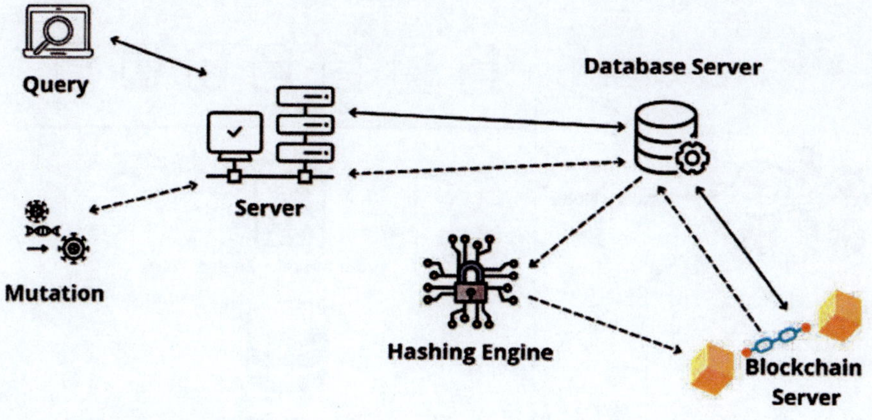

Fig. 2 Backend architecture

The GraphQL server will be used by the system to produce and read data from the blockchain. It will construct a graphical representation of the whole database and fetch and add records as nodes to it using the GraphQL server.

A query will be created by the system and submitted to the server in order to retrieve records. Query will then try to search the data in the stored database, then try to search the hash of that data in the blockchain, where it will employ indexed searching to speed up the process. It will transmit the acknowledgment to the system after receiving it from the blockchain server.

In contrast, the system will initiate a mutation in order to add new entries to the blockchain. This will be sent to the database server, where a transaction will be started. The hash created by the transaction's hashing engine will then be submitted to the blockchain server. Now, the blockchain server will attempt to store the records, and if the records are successfully saved, the database transaction will be committed; otherwise, the transaction will be rolled back. Finally, it will send the system the identical acknowledgment it received from the blockchain server.

The blockchain architecture of the proposed system is shown in Fig. 3. A private blockchain is mapped over a database by the blockchain server. To reach consensus across the nodes, this bespoke blockchain employs the proof of stake mechanism.

The blockchain's nodes will only be staked by the blockchain's administrators. Records will be indexed in the blockchain in order to shorten the time it takes to find a certain record from the current list. Smart contracts will be used to add these entries, which will be initiated by the blockchain server. Furthermore, in order to preserve the density of records, if a node's capability for producing new transaction blocks hits its limit, it will no longer be able to do so.

It will employ multi-signature contracts to address the issue of data ownership and control. To be authenticated, a transaction must be signed by multiple users, in this case, the patient and the hospital, using their private keys. The patient can't update the record without the hospital's permission, but he may choose who has access to it.

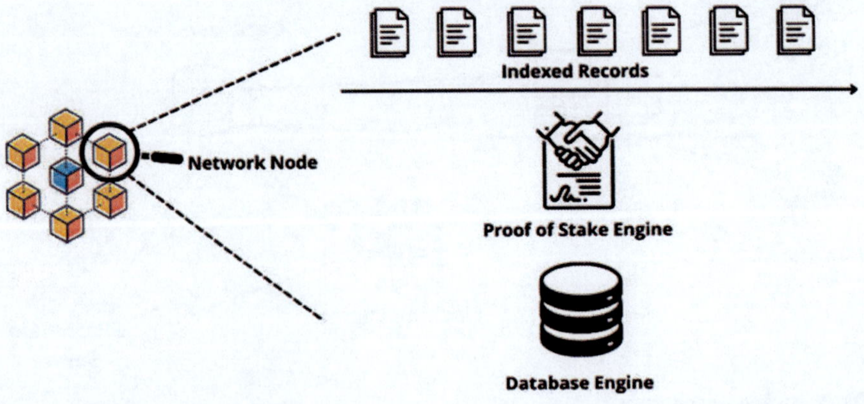

Fig. 3 Blockchain architecture

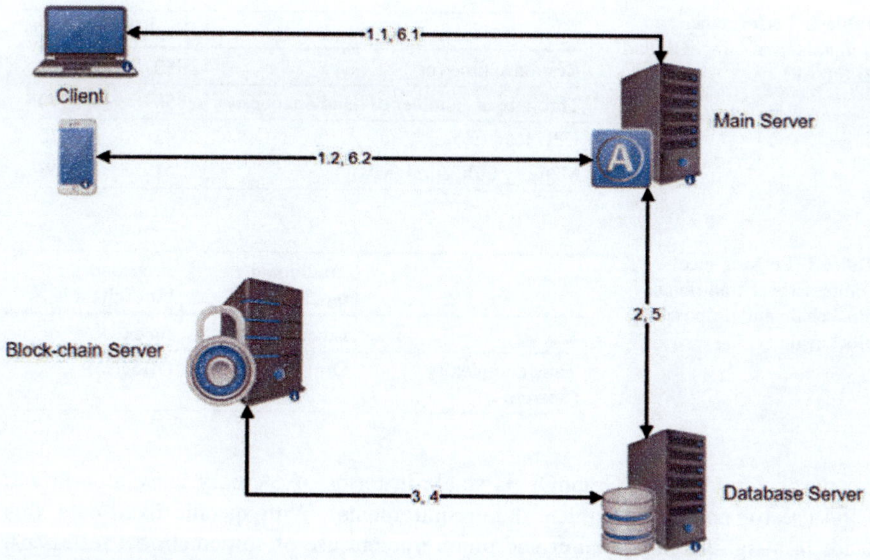

Fig. 4 Dataflow between layers

Because the previous swarm hash is now known, a new swarm hash must be created each time the data is collected, thus a "last accessed" timestamp will be supplied.

As the data changes, the swarm hash will be immediately updated, allowing it to be protected until it has the necessary access rights. This paradigm not only delivers blockchain's immutability and security but also a multi-signature solution to data ownership and accessibility.

The data flow diagram is depicted in Fig. 4. The user requests data from the main server via a web application or a mobile application, which is processed. The main server then asks the database server for the same information. The database server examines the request and attempts to locate it in both the database and the blockchain server. Only if both answers are identical will the client receive the required response.

4 Experimental Results

This method makes it possible to view one's medical records from anywhere in the globe, with data security and access speed not being a concern. As big data issues might strike REST APIs with increased demand, GraphQL was used to effectively do this.

The GraphQL service pattern is more reliable and normal than REST, as seen in Table 1. In terms of resource usage and utilization, GraphQL outperforms REST. GraphQL is 28% more efficient and consistent in utilizing processing resources while under demand. Because the query includes specified data fields or attributes

Table 1 Performance comparison of GraphQL and REST API

	GraphQL	REST
Response time (ms)	1850	920
Throughput (number of handle request)	2850	4570
CPU load (%)	47	75
Memory utilization (MB)	41	68

Table 2 Performance comparison of traditional blockchain and proposed blockchain

	Traditional blockchain	Proposed blockchain
Search	Linear	Indexed
Time complexity (Search)	O(n)	O(log(n))

for particular requests, GraphQL is stable in terms of memory consumption and CPU use (or contains complete data requirements). With specific fixed data, this leads in a significantly smaller and more efficient use of computational resources. Furthermore, the client can provide flexible answer formats to avoid excessively massive data transfers (over fetching) or sparse data responses (under fetching), which might occur with the REST API service.

The long-term danger to a traditional blockchain may be readily addressed with the private, indexed blockchain, which is the time it takes to add and get any record on the blockchain, which is done using linear search in the traditional one but indexed in this one and comparison of traditional blockchain and proposed blockchain is shown in Table 2.

5 Conclusion

Usage of blockchain in healthcare management systems is still in the development phase and need in today's evolving healthcare system. To summarise, the elements that influence the usage of blockchain in the long-term growth of innovative healthcare are several. Because of the mode of influence, the process of impact, a system integration framework for establishing a sustainable intelligent healthcare system on the blockchain, as well as a scientific application framework, has been established, and the degree of action varies based on the conditions.

Single information technologies, like the Internet of Things in healthcare, are the focus of current smart healthcare research. Data of patients cannot be securely transmitted across institutions, in today's smart health business, privacy protection has become a barrier. Although there are a few studies that combine blockchain and smart medical care, the great majority of them focus on the use of a single blockchain feature in the field of smart medical care, with patients and medical institutions as the research subjects. Few research takes multiagent cooperative development into account, and there is no blockchain application system for smart healthcare development. Blockchain TeleHealth Services aims to establish a secure and safe platform to store data and managing information all of the data in the healthcare system. Cloud computing technology has been employed in the proposed system to securely store data on the cloud, making data storage and access for the necessary stakeholders much easier and faster.

References

1. Yue X, Wang H, Jin D, Li M, Jiang W (2016) Healthcare data gateways, found healthcare intelligence on the blockchain with novel privacy risk control. J Med Syst 40(10):218
2. Gong T, Huang H, Li P, Zhang K, Jiang H (2015) A medical healthcare system for privacy protection based on IoT. In: Proceedings of the 2015 seventh ınternational symposium on parallel architectures, algorithms and programming (PAAP). IEEE, Nanjing, China , pp 217–222
3. Linn LA, Koo MB (2016) Blockchain for health data and ıts potential use in health ıt and health care related research. In: ONC/NIST use of blockchain for healthcare and research workshop. ONC/NIST, pp 1–10
4. Xia Q, Sifah EB, Asamoah KO, Gao J, Du XJ, Guizani M (2017) MeDShare: trust-less medical data sharing among cloud service providers via blockchain. IEEE Access 5:14757–14767
5. Xia Q, Sifah EB, Smahi A, Amofa S, Zhang XS (2017) BBDS: Blockchain-based data sharing for electronic medical records in cloud environments. Information 8(44):1–16
6. Zhang AQ, Lin XD (2018) Towards secure and privacy-preserving data sharing in e-health systems via consortium blockchain. J Med Syst 42:140
7. Liu X: A blockchain-based medical data sharing and protection scheme. IEEE Access PP(99)
8. Wang Z, Jin C (2019) A blockchain-based medical data sharing and protection scheme. IEEE Access PP(99):1–1
9. Mettler M (2016) Blockchain technology in healthcare: the revolution startshere. In: 2016 IEEE 18th ınternational conference on e-health networking, applications and services (Healthcom), Munich, Germany, pp 1–3
10. Zheng ZB, Xie SA, Dai HN, Chen XP, Wang HM (2017) An overview of blockchain technology: architecture, consensus, and future trends. In: 2017IEEE ınternational congress on big data, Honolulu, USA, pp 557–564
11. Xue TF, Fu QC, Wang C, Wang XY (2017) A medical data sharing modelvia blockchain. Acta Automat. Sinica 43(9):1555–1562
12. Bentov I, Lee C, Mizrahi A, Rosenfeld M (2014) Proof of activity: extending bitcoin's proof of work via proof of stake [extended abstract]y. ACM Sigmetrics Perform Eval Rev 42(3):34–37
13. Yuan Y, Wang FY (2016) Blockchain: the state of the art and future trends. Acta Automat. Sinica 42(4):481–549

Designing a Secure Robust Medical Image Authentication Based on Watermarking Using the ED-DWT and Encryption

Chandan Kumar and Sadaf Hussaini

Abstract The COVID-19 scenario, there was a massive increase of medical imaging data. Designing an authentication technique for safeguarding medical photographs is a difficult task. This research intended to create a hybrid authentication system that combines image encryption with a durable watermarking mechanism. The invisibility of the watermark and its resistance to attacks are the two most important requirements for watermarking. The sensitivity of encryption algorithms in the presence of noise is also discussed in the paper. For watermark embedding, the paper presented edge detection (ED) of the discrete wavelet transform (DWT) coefficient. The first-level DWT coefficients are deconstructed from the enlarged medical image. To maintain invisibility, the edge coefficients are calculated over the high-frequency DWT sub-band. Objective of this paper is to safeguard the watermark image with quick and simple image encryption. For image encryption, a random key is created. The efficiency of encryption is also tested over noisy attack for the PSNR and NC.

Keywords Image security · Watermarking · Edge detection · DWT · Random key encryption · Watermark attacks

1 Introduction

The invisible watermark was once a popular way to protect medical imaging for protecting the patient data from copyright infringement. The goal of this research is to create a groundbreaking blend of invisible watermarking of medical images along with a random key-based secure encryption algorithm [1]. The watermarking algorithms can be designed to claim the authentication of the patients imaging data. This could be done by hiding the watermark info within the imaging data. The major design challenge is the selection of the watermark and scaling it to be invisible.

C. Kumar (✉)
SAGE University, Bhopal, India
e-mail: mckv.chandan@gmail.com

S. Hussaini
Truba College of Science and Technology, Bhopal, India

© The Author(s), under exclusive license to Springer Nature Singapore Pte Ltd. 2023

J. K. Mandal and D. De (eds.), *Frontiers of ICT in Healthcare*, Lecture Notes in Networks and Systems 519, https://doi.org/10.1007/978-981-19-5191-6_27

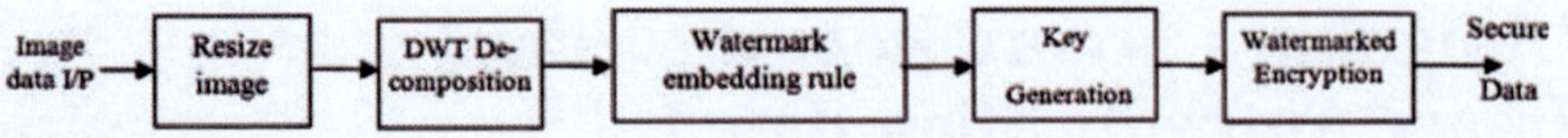

Fig. 1 Basic building block of the secure watermarking process

The proposed watermarking algorithm is expected to be utilized for improving the authentication and security of medical images [2]. The basic flow of the proposed watermarking methodology is shown in Fig. 1. It is clear that the proposed approach is a combination of the watermarking and the secure encryption. Additional security in existing watermarking method is the prime contribution of this work.

Other than watermarking, there are various types of data security or hiding techniques that are used for copyright protection. These techniques include cryptography, which can either be public or private. Steganography [3], which is a secret communication technique, and digital signatures, which are used to verify data. Finally, watermarking is a commonly used data concealment method.

The key contribution of this study is to accomplish the secure watermarking via ED component over the DWT coefficient and encryption. To generate multi-resolution coefficients, the medical image is deconstructed using the second-level DWT transform. Using edge detection on the HH wavelet band, the edge coefficients are computed. Watermark embedding takes advantage of the difference among dilation and edges intensity to provide further robustness. A random key shuffling cipher technique is used to encrypt a watermark image on medical images. The image is recreated just after decryption on receiver side. For both stages, the statistics are presented for the PSNR results and compared to those obtained at a greater level of security.

An example of the various applications of the medical image watermarking is presented and shown in Fig. 2. As the watermarking is three stage processes, thus many variants of method are available. Therefore, watermarking can be used in a variety of applications as in [4–6], and the most widely being opted applications of the medical watermarking are given in Fig. 2. These applications are used for data authentication and protection purpose for medical imaging data.

Fig. 2 Usual applications of medical image watermarking

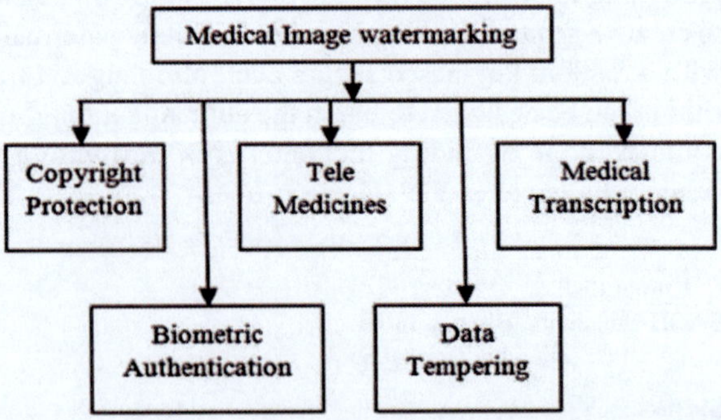

1.1 Contribution of Work

The security is major motivation behind the image storage for protecting them from copyright. The main contribution of the paper is to design the secure image encryption-based robust digital medical image watermarking method. The paper evaluated the performance of fast AES encryption method for making the ED based watermarking techniques.

2 Literature Review of Secure Watermarking

Basic classification of the various encryption standards opted for image watermarking is represented in Fig. 3.

The basic encryption methods in Fig. 3a are classified as advanced encryption standard (AES), and data encryption standards (DES). These methods can be implemented for the images as 2D methods. Generally, the concept varies based on the key generation process. In this paper, we prefer the method of the random binary key generation. The basic classification of ED based watermarking methods is given in Fig. 3b. In past, ED-based watermarking methods were widely being used and most widely classified as the methods of ED-based method using the contrast sensitivity function (CSF) for the watermark embedding as suggested by the Ellinas et al. [7, 8] They have used the CSF in 2007 and then replaced it by image dilation in the 2008. The ED is used for the invisibility and in the DWT domain.

Fig. 3 Classification of Image Watermarking and Encryption methods

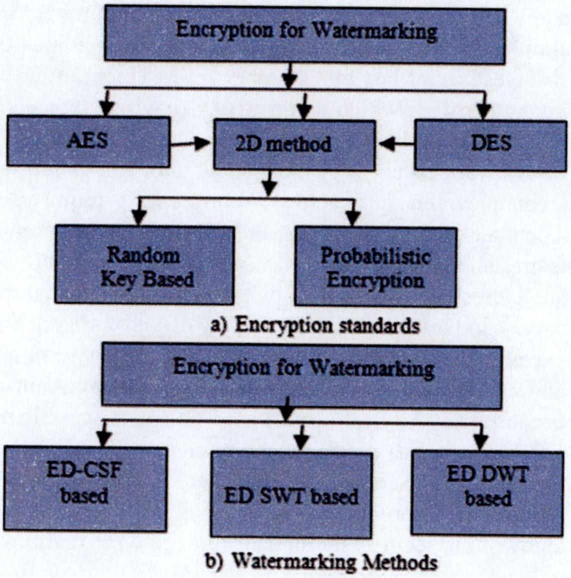

Using the 2 × 2 dilation masks, Ramanand Singh et al. [9] increased the performance of invisible watermarking in the edge detection domain. For watermark embedding, they opted the high-frequency sub-band coefficient. Using watermark embedding in Region of interest (ROI) blocks of medical pictures, Xiao et al. in [10] developed a robust multipurpose watermarking technique. Singh et al. [11] proposed employing the ED coefficients to design a watermarking approach for medical photos using the stationary wavelet transform (2D-SWT). In this paper, the approach is shortened as ED-SWT-based watermarking as shown in Fig. 3b. However, it was discovered that this method is only suitable for single-level SWT because extending the SWT levels may cause the integer values to be lost.

2.1 Review of Encryption Methods

The updated technique was proposed by Kawle et al. [12] to increase the performance of AES-based encryption standards. They did, however, demonstrate the strategy for a 1D data set. Although it is asserted that the AES-based encryption approach is more efficient and uses symmetric key. Mehdi-Laurent et al. [13] have designed the algorithm for comparing the performance of the AES and DES-based encryptions methods under the influence of certain image attacks and it is found the AES works efficiently.

Kamal et al. [14] proposed novel encryption technique, which works equally for color and gray medical images. They have also given introduction of a novel image-splitting technology based on image blocks. The image blocks were then scrambled in a zigzag pattern, rotated, and randomly permuted. Then, using a chaotic logistic map, a key is generated to diffuse the previously jumbled image. It is required to design simple and fast image encryption methods. Sandipan Basu [15] proposed one of the strongest secret-key block cipher IDEA (International Data Encryption Algorithm) in another way, which is too strong (having taken care for weak keys) for medical image encryption.

Wazirali et al. [16] compared and contrasted various digital watermarking techniques and approaches. Watermarking requirements and obstacles were also discussed in depth. In addition, common architecture of the watermarking system is presented. The major concern is on the Internet of Things (IoT) and its problems are addressed. For medical picture security and watermarking systems, a number of survey and review publications [17–19] are offered. Sadkhan et al. [20] provided an excellent overview of many lightweight encryption methods. A multilevel security and encryption system has been presented by Amna Shifa et al. [21]. They have proposed security solutions based on smart surveillance security. Mannepalli et al. [22] have recently presented the extension of the ED-DWT-based watermarking using the block chain-based security. Method seems to be complex, and it is required to reduce the complexity of security algorithm. Overall, this paper provides a good study of the security methods for image watermarking applications.

3 ED Coefficients Determination

In this research work, it is proposed to use Sobel edge detector mask for the determination of ED coefficients. The Sobel mask is a smallest difference filter with an odd number of coefficients.

That averages the image in the perpendicular direction to the differentiation as suggested by R. O. Duda and P. E. Hart in 1973. The Sobel averaging operator is more Gaussian-like, which makes it better at reducing white noise and so improves ED's performance. Furthermore, using finite differences, it is possible to estimate the x and y gradient.

$$\frac{\delta f}{\delta x} = \lim_{h \to 0} \frac{f(x+h, y) - f(x, y)}{h} \tag{1}$$

$$\frac{\delta f}{\delta y} = \lim_{h \to 0} \frac{f(x, y+h) - f(x, y)}{h} \tag{2}$$

The Sobel ED is a differentiating mask determined using gradients mask as

$$S = \begin{bmatrix} -1 & -2 & -1 \\ 0 & 0 & 0 \\ 1 & 2 & 1 \end{bmatrix} t = \begin{bmatrix} -1\,0\,1 \\ -2\,0\,2 \\ -1\,0\,1 \end{bmatrix} \tag{3}$$

An example of the detected edge coefficients in proposed work is given in Fig. 4 for the CT-scan image using the Sobel mask.

It is suggested that the DWT transform should be used first, followed by the ED over coefficients, because the wavelet transform increases the watermark's robustness and makes it more invisible.

The wavelet transform quantifies the local regularity of signals by dissecting them into simple building blocks that are well localized both in space and frequency. An example of DWT decomposition is given in Fig. 5.

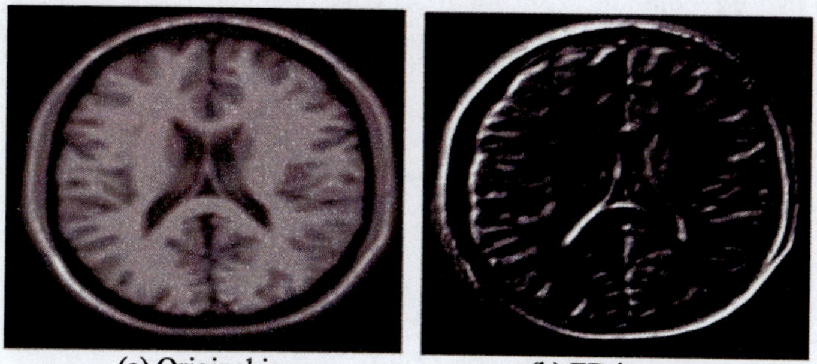

(a) Original image (b) ED image

Fig. 4 Edge detections using the Sobel ED mask an example for CT scan image

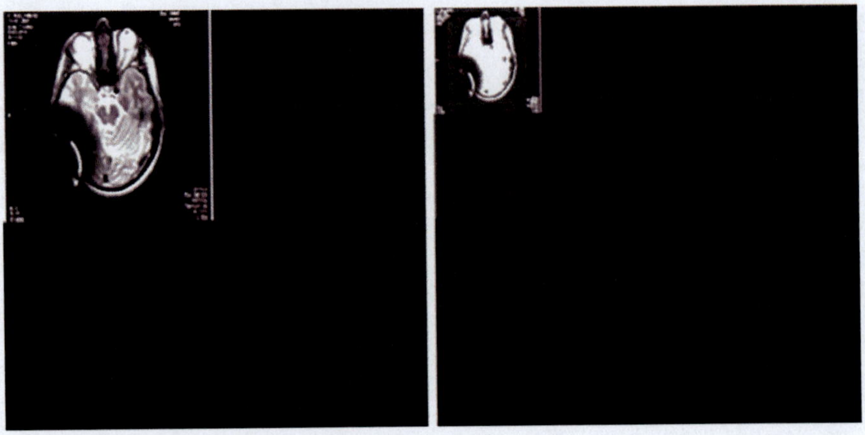

Fig. 5 An example of the DWT decomposition

4 Proposed Watermark Embedding

This study develops an encrypted watermarking technique that is both durable and secure. Figure 6 depicts the ED and DWT-based watermarking technology's basic block diagram. This procedure refers Mannepalli et al. [22] and their suggested watermarking method is implemented in three phases.

The first step is to use a watermark embedding based on ED coefficients. The watermark is embedded using the deconstructed DWT domain. As referred by the method of [6], the watermark is made up of the difference between the edge component of the LL wavelet coefficient and the dilation component.

The cover or host medical image is read and transformed to 512×512 image sizes before being embedded. There is no need for an external watermark logo. The ED coefficients of the cover medical image are used as the watermark in the proposed method. Paper proposed to take the 2nd level DWT decompositions of cover medical image, then extract the low and high pass DWT coefficients. The edge coefficient is computed over LL components using Sobel edge operator. The watermark insertion rule is used to produce the watermark using the edge coefficients.

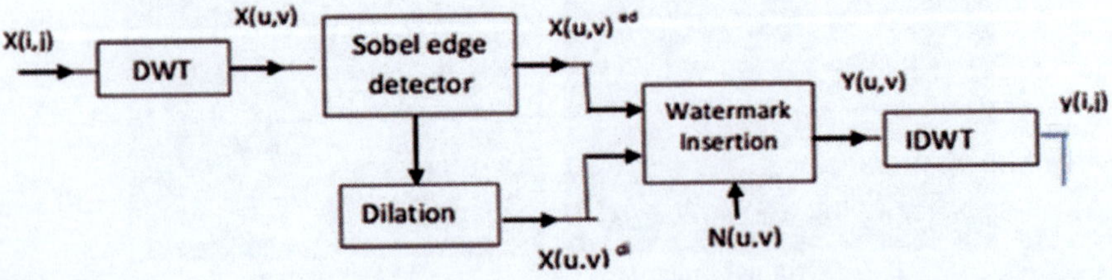

Fig. 6 Process of ED-based watermark insertion Ref. [6]

4.1 Watermark Insertion Rule

Following existing watermark rule is used for the watermarking in this research.

$$Y(u, v) = X(u, v)^{\mathrm{di}} - X(u, v)^{\mathrm{ed}} \tag{4}$$

where $X(u, v)^{\mathrm{di}}$ is the dilated edge coefficient, and $X(u, v)^{\mathrm{ed}}$ is the ED coefficient of LL sub-band of DWT. To improve the invisibility, use the scaling factor to implement the watermark features. Changing the scale factor is an effective way to increase invisibility. The watermark looks like this;

$$W = (1 - \alpha)*(Y) + \alpha N_{x,y} \tag{5}$$

where $N_{x,y} is AWGN$ noise. It is proposed to hide the watermark to LL sub-band of DWT of cover image the watermarked image is IDWT image of

$$W_E = LL^L_{x,y} + W(x, y) \tag{6}$$

5 Secure and Fast Encryption

The major contributing factor to the research is to design the random key generation-based crypto cipher encryption method which is implemented over the watermarked image. The sequential methodology for the random key-based AES encryption is as follows:

1. The watermarked image based on ED-DWT algorithm is considered as the input for encrypting using cipher text random key.
2. The process of the key generation is initialized by scanning the size of the input image.

$$n = r * c * 8 \tag{7}$$

   This assumes the image to be 8 bit image.
3. Generate the random key in binary form as.

$$x_N = 1 - 2 * (\mathrm{bin}(x_N) - 1)^2 \tag{8}$$

4. Encode the image using the bit wise XOR of the key data and row wise generated image data.
5. The noise assaults are applied to the encrypted image that has been transmitted.
6. The image is reconstructed by decrypting the data with and without assaults.
7. The watermark extraction procedure is exactly the same as the extraction process.

6 Experimental Results and Analysis

In this part, the findings of the suggested ED-DWT watermarking approach are presented in order. The four separate medical images are taken into account while evaluating the outcomes. As illustrated in Fig. 7, these images are CT scan image, MRI_T2, brain tumor image, and MRI_T1 image. All of these images were commonly used to validate results in papers. Medical images have lower color brightness values than other types of images. The proposed method is resilient, and it is projected to improve the watermarking technique's efficiency.

Initially, the sequential ED-DWT-based results for watermarking methods by Mannepalli et al. [22] are validated for the brain Tumor image in Fig. 8.

It can be observed that using ED, the watermark is invisible in image. But, the proper scaling needs to improve invisibility further. The watermarking method of [22] is opted, but the encryption is implemented using the proposed fast binary key-based encryption.

The results of the image security using the encryption for the MRI_T1 image are shown in Fig. 9. Figure represents the comparison of the cipher weights in terms of histograms. Histogram is representation of frequency of gray levels and shows cipher weights as referred in Kama et al. [14]. It can be observed from Fig. 9 that the encryption and decrypti8on weights are in close proximity to each other without noise.

Sequential results of our proposed secure encrypted Watermarking using random binary key generation process are shown in Fig. 10 for two MRI images and offers the

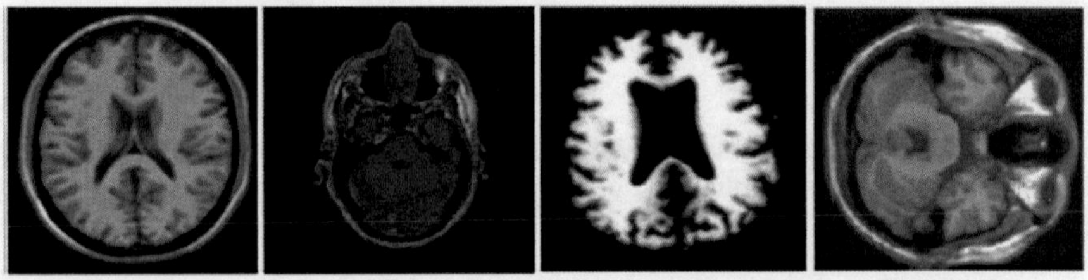

(a), CT-Scan_1, (b) MRI_T2 (c) Brain Tumor MRI Image (d) MRI_T1

Fig. 7 Input medical images used for study

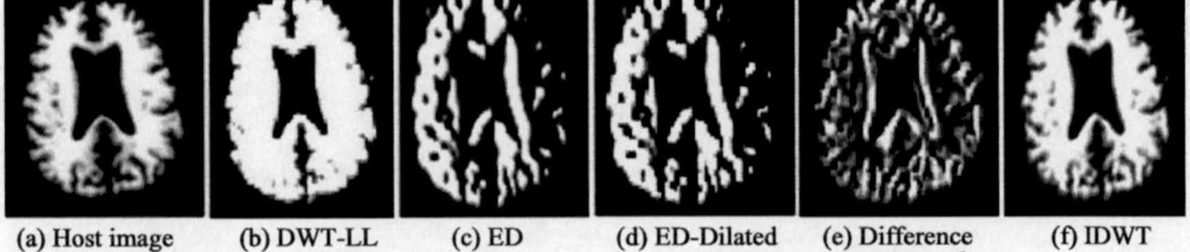

(a) Host image (b) DWT-LL (c) ED (d) ED-Dilated (e) Difference watermark (f) IDWT

Fig. 8 Validation of ED-DWT results [22]

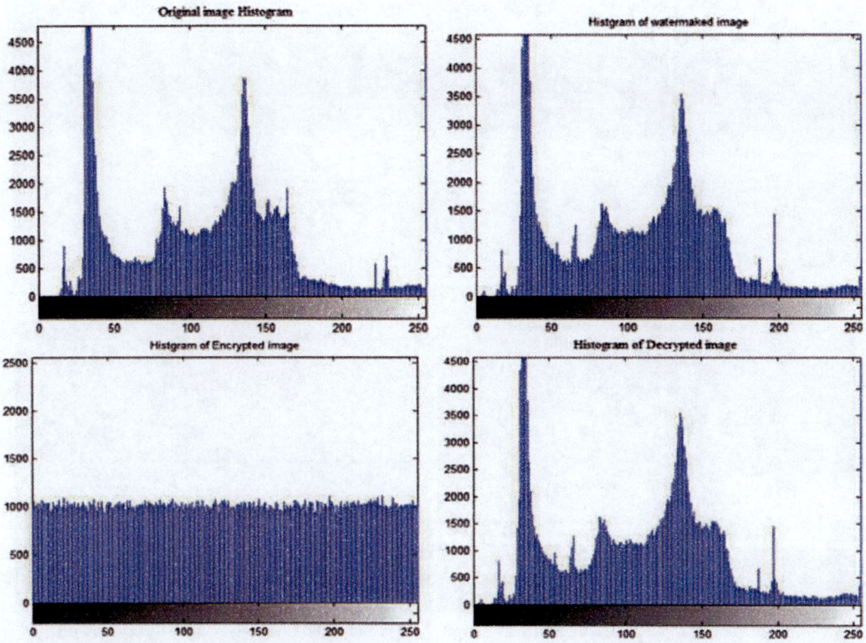

Fig. 9 Comparison of the cipher weights during the watermarking and the encryption process for MRI_T1 image

good encryption quality. The decrypted data also have good enough visual quality. The qualitative comparison of performance of our encryption method and block chain-based encryption method [22] is presented in Fig. 11. It can be observed that the proposed method is simpler than the method of Mannepalli et al. [22].

7 Comparison of Results

This section presents evaluation of our method under the presence of noisy attack. The Gaussian noise is added to the watermarked image and decryption performance is evaluated. The PSNR and the NC are evaluated for the parametric evaluation as shown in Tables 1 and 2, respectively. Our proposed method performs well enough. The NC without noise is nearly equal to 1, which justifies the invisibility as in Table 2. Although there is reduction in NC with noise attack watermarks are recoverable.

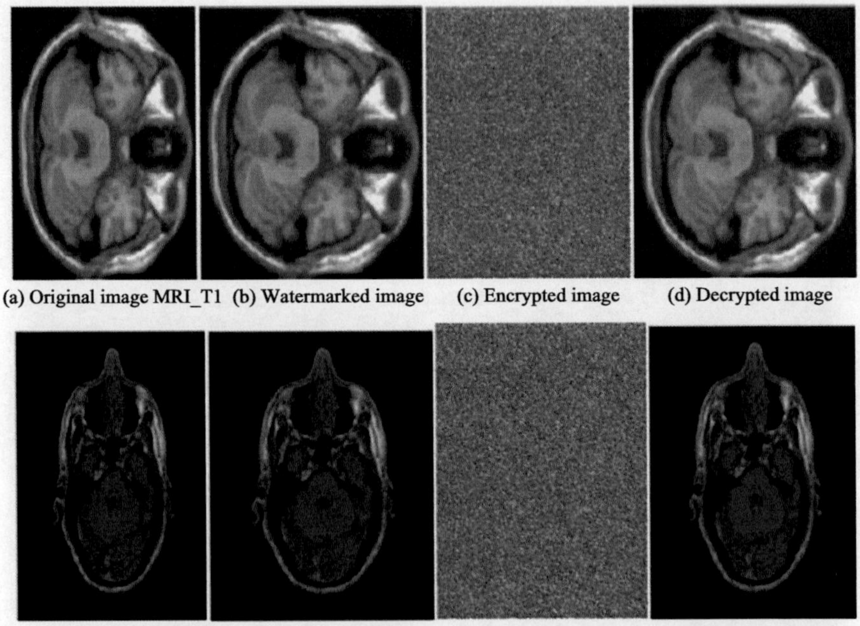

(a) Original image MRI_T1 (b) Watermarked image (c) Encrypted image (d) Decrypted image

(e) Original image MRI_T2 (f) Watermarked image (g) Encrypted image (h) Decrypted image

Fig. 10 Sequential results of proposed secure watermarking using random binary keys for Two MRI images

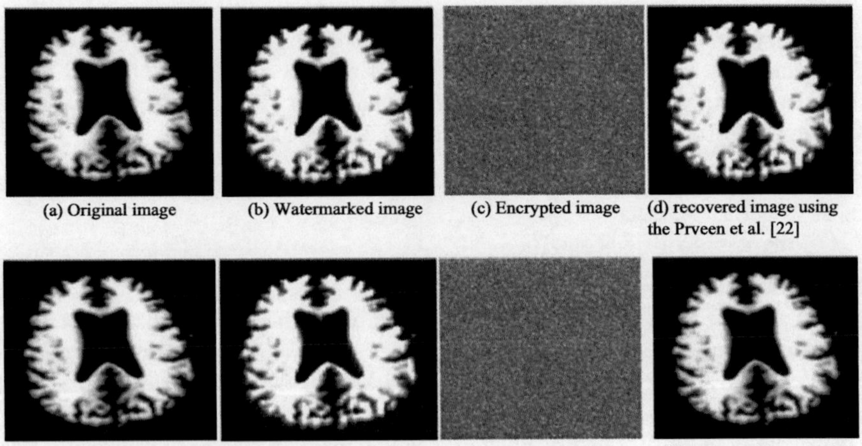

(a) Original image (b) Watermarked image (c) Encrypted image (d) recovered image using the Prveen et al. [22]

(e) Original image (f) Watermarked image (g) Encrypted image (h) recovered image using proposed method

Fig. 11 Comparison of Encryption performances for two methods

Table 1 Comparison of PSNR for the Watermarking without attacks

Images	Watermarked	Decrypted
MRI_T1	16.6350	15.9782
MRI_T2	6.5209	15.9587
Brain Tumor	18.1007	15.9687

Table 2 Comparison of NC for the watermarking Gaussian noise attacks

Images	Without noise	With noise
MRI_T1	0.9982	0.8716
MRI_T2	0.9893	0.7947
Brain tumor	0.9985	0.8250

8 Conclusions and Future Scope

The secure watermarking is important for protecting the images. Considering these issues, this paper has designed a fast and simple encryption method for the medical images. Paper is designed in two pass; initially, in the first pass, the ED-DWT-based watermarking method is validated. Then in the second pass, the random key-based binary encryption methods using XOR operator are implemented. The qualitative comparison of performance of our encryption method and block chain-based encryption method [22] are presented. Maximum value of the NC without noise clearly states the invisibility of watermark.

The performance is evaluated under the Gaussian noise, and it is found that the NC is relatively in the range of above 80% for all images even under the highly noisy attacks. Overall, it is concluded that our proposed method is simple and fast encryption standard, which is also used efficiently for securing the Watermarking applications. It is an open field of problems to improve the performance in future onwards.

8.1 Future Scope and Drawbacks

But in the future, it is required to improve the performance of the encryption method under the various attacks like image sharpening, Gaussian noise, rotation, cropping, and motion. As it is observed that encryption in the edge domain-based watermarking is sensitive to the presence of the noise, and the performance significantly decreases. Thus, in the future, noise investigation problem for encrypted watermark is an open issue.

References

1. Zhang X, Seo S-H, Wangm C (2019) A lightweight encryption method for privacy protection in surveillance videos. J IEEE Access 4
2. Shukla A, Singh C (2014) Medical image authentication through watermarking. Int J Adv Res Comput Sci Technol (IJARCST 2014), 2(2), Ver. 2
3. Bala BK, Kumar AB (2017) The combination of steganography and cryptography for medical image applications. Biomed Pharmacol J 10(4)
4. Jogendra Kumar M, Raghavendra Sai N, Vijaya Kumar Reddy R, Ravi Kumar T, Pavan Kumar A (2021) Using DWT-DCT-SVD watermarking for securing medical images. In: 2021 2nd international conference on smart electronics and communication (ICOSEC), pp 1127–1138
5. Shankar, Kannammal A (2021) A hybrid of watermark scheme with encryption to improve security of medical images. In: 2021 third international conference on intelligent communication technologies and virtual mobile networks (ICICV), pp 226–233
6. Singh AK, Dutta MK (2020) DWT, DCT and PBFO based approach for biometric image security. In: 2020 International conference on contemporary computing and applications (IC3A), pp 298–303
7. Ellinas JN, Kenterlis P (2007) A wavelet-based watermarking method exploiting the contrast sensitivity function. World Acad Sci Eng Technol 31
8. Ellinas JN (2008) A robust wavelet-based watermarking algorithm using edge detection. J Image Proc 197–208
9. Ramanand Singh P, Shukla RP, Shukla PK (2019) Invisible medical image watermarking using edge detection and discrete wavelet transform coefficients. Int J Innovat Technol Expl Eng (IJITEE) 9(1)
10. Xiao S, Zhang Z, Zhang Y, Yu C (2020) Multipurpose watermarking algorithm for medical images. J Hindawi Sci Programm
11. Singh R, Rawat P, Shukla P (2017) Robust medical image authentication using 2-D stationary wavelet transform and edge detection. In: 2nd IET international conference on biomedical image and signal processing (ICBISP 2017), pp 1–8
12. Kawle P, Hiwase A, Bagde G, Tekam E, Kalbande R (2014) Modified advanced encryption standard. Int J Soft Comput Eng 1–3
13. Akkar M-L, Giraud C (2001) An implementation of DES and AES, secure against some attacks. Springer, pp 309–318
14. Kamal ST, Hosny KM, Elgindy TM, Darwish MM, Fouda MM (2021) A new image encryption algorithm for grey and color medical images. IEEE Access 9:37855–37865
15. Basu S (2011) International data encryption algorithm (Idea), a typical illustration. J Glob Res Comput Sci, 116–118
16. Wazirali R, Ahmad R, Al-Amayreh A, Al-Madi M, Khalifeh A (2021) Secure watermarking schemes and their approaches in the IoT technology: an overview. MDPI J Electron 10:1744
17. Mancy L, Maria Celestin Vigila S (2015) A survey on protection of medical images. In: 2015 International conference on control, instrumentation, communication and computational technologies (ICCICCT), pp 503–506
18. Singh G (2017) A review of secure medical image watermarking. In: 2017 IEEE international conference on power, control, signals and instrumentation engineering (ICPCSI), pp 3105–3109
19. Rana P, Mittal U, Chawla P (2020) Medical images security using watermarking, hashing and RGB displacement. In: 2020 8th international conference on reliability, Infocom technologies and optimization (Trends and Future Directions) (ICRITO), pp 532–536
20. Sadkhan SB, Salman AO (2018) A survey on lightweight-cryptography status and future challenges. In: 2018 International conference on advance of sustainable engineering and its application (ICASEA), Wasit, pp 105–108

21. Shifa A, Asghar MN, Fleury M, Kanwal N, Ansari MS, Lee B, Herbst M, Qiao Y (2020) MuLViS: multi-level encryption based security system for surveillance videos, vol 8. IEEE Access
22. Mannepalli PK, Richhariya V, Gupta SK, Shukla PK, Dutta PK (2021) Block chain based robust image watermarking using edge detection and wavelet transform. Research Square

IoT-Based Secure Blockchain Framework for Patient Record Management Using MPRESENT Lightweight Block Cipher

Rajdeep Chakraborty and Runa Chatterjee

Abstract This paper deals with the patient record management framework and its security by our novel lightweight block cipher MPRESENT. Blockchain is a distributed data repository and used nowadays in various use cases, and one of them is Patient Record Management. Blockchain also provides a trusted distributed network. Internet of things (IoT) is the one mostly used network to record patient data in various units of a hospital. A Blockchain framework for storing patient records and its management from IoT devices installed at various units in a hospital and the security established by lightweight block cipher is proposed in this paper. Further, we also provided a second layer of security in the IoT sensor layer through MPRESENT.

Keywords IoT · Lightweight cryptography · Blockchain · Patient Record Management

1 Introduction

This section gives a brief introduction of Internet of things (IoT) and lightweight cryptography (LWC). Section 1.1 discusses the basics of Internet of things (IoT), and Sect. 1.2 and Sect. 1.3 discuss lightweight cryptography and the Blockchain, respectively.

1.1 Internet of Things (IoT)

Many advanced devices are currently being used in the progressive world which are highly constrained. To accomplish some tasks, these devices are interconnected and communicated by transferring information to one another. The Internet of things (IoT) is one of the important areas where we use these advanced devices. The IoT

R. Chakraborty (✉) · R. Chatterjee
Department of CSE, Netaji Subhash Engineering College, Kolkata, India
e-mail: rajdeep_chak@yahoo.co.in

© The Author(s), under exclusive license to Springer Nature Singapore Pte Ltd. 2023

J. K. Mandal and D. De (eds.), *Frontiers of ICT in Healthcare*, Lecture Notes in Networks and Systems 519, https://doi.org/10.1007/978-981-19-5191-6_28

can be defined as a system of interlinked computing appliances, digital as well as mechanical machines, objects, animals or people. All are recognized by a specific identifier and that has the ability for transferring data through a network having no interaction between human–human or human–computer. Although a wide range of IoT-enabled applications are there, the application in the medical field plays a significant role in various aspects. For example, the admission procedure of the patients to the hospital can be made faster and accurate.

Some important features of IoT are described below.

- Connectivity: It is the key feature of IoT. The devices are connected via Wi-Fi, radio waves, Bluetooth, etc.
- Sensing: People choose appropriate sensing paradigm based on their needs.
- Active Engagements: To establish active engagements among various IoT products, services, and platforms, cloud computing in Blockchain is generally used.
- Scale: On demand, scaling should be applicable to IoT devices.
- Dynamic Nature: To fulfill certain demand, IoT components should change their state (i.e., collection and converting procedure of data) dynamically.
- Intelligence: Knowledge extraction from generated data is very important to make data useful.
- Energy: IoT components should be designed in such a way so that it consumes minimal energy.
- Safety: To keep our data secure, a proper safety mechanism is needed.
- Integration: Proper integration over various cross-domain models ensures proper trade-off between cost and infrastructure.

1.2 Lightweight Cryptography (LWC)

The growing use of massive devices that are in the field of electronics raised security concerns. Within this environment, some fields are present where conventional cryptographic algorithms are not applicable due to constraints like power dissipation, area, and cost. Here a challenging term "lightweight cryptography" (LWC) is used which secures the information in an efficient way. It utilizes very low resources and power, provides high throughput, and maintains conservativeness.

The word "lightweight" within LWC is measured in terms of heaviness of an algorithm and has target platform-based description. The heaviness is measured in hardware by counting the number of logic gates (gate equivalent or GE) required to implement the cipher. In software, it is measured in terms of time complexity. The ISO/IEC organization standardized the number of allowable GE for designing ultra-lightweight cryptography is up to 1000, whereas for low-cost implementation, it is up to 2000, and for lightweight it is extensible up to 3000.

1.3 The Blockchain (BC)

Blockchain consists of a system of recording to keep the information in such a way that changing data, hacking the data, or cheating the system is quite impossible. So, a Blockchain is defined as a ledger, digital, with transactions that are kept and distributed across the network nodes.

Figure 1 typically depicts a Blockchain framework. The primary component of a Blockchain is the block. A block is composed of hash values of the current block as well as previous block; this ensures the immutability of data. Timestamp is another important record stored to keep the time of the transaction. Other information is kept thereafter, and finally, the data are kept. The decentralized and distributed nature and various structure of Blockchain is discussed in Harshini et al. [1].

Section 2 gives the literature and motivation, Sect. 3 gives the IoT security with MPRESENT [2], Sect. 4 gives the proposed framework and implementation, Sect. 5 gives the discussion, and finally, Sect. 6 draws the conclusion. References are given at last.

2 Literature Survey and Motivation

Of late, one of the common, famous, and highly demanding applications of the Internet of things (IoT) is medical sector management. Parallelly, the rising Blockchain technology helps in data and resource sharing among nodes in the IoT network. This technology is radically changing medical research and industry. The use of smart devices in the IoT domain enhanced the grade of self-health monitoring

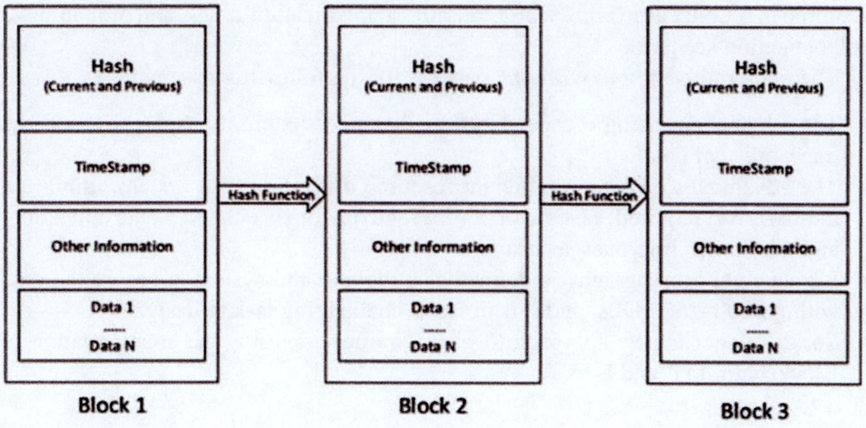

Fig. 1 Nodes of a Blockchain

as well as providing fast and accurate data for proper diagnosis and treatment. This rising demand is motivating more and more researchers to work in this field.

This section reviews some earlier paper works done by different researchers on the same domains. In this work [3], the researchers Veeramakali et al. developed ODLSB, it is an optimal deep learning and secure Blockchain that enabled intelligent IoT and healthcare diagnosis model [4]. Secured transaction which are hashed valued encryption with medical diagnosis consist of three processes that are used for transferring medical data in a secure manner and also used for diagnosis purposes. The ODLSB technique is to secretly share medical images. The hashed valued encryption is used for encryption purposes. At last, the optimal deep neural network (ODNN) is used for diagnosing diseases.

In another paper [5], the researchers proposed a Blockchain-based patient health monitoring platform which tracks vital signs using smart contracts. For this Blockchain-based application, the researchers used Hyperledger fabric, enterprise, and distributed ledger framework for designing and developing purposes. The patients benefited from this approach by generating extensive, immutable history log. Not only that the patients were also capable of accessing remote data from anywhere at any time. The Hyperledger Caliper, a standard benchmark tool, is used for measuring the performance of the designed and developed system. They demanded that for patient data monitoring, the proposed system goes beyond the traditional healthcare system.

In the next paper [4], the researchers mainly focused on the security issues that arise in IoT devices during personal and sensitive data storage or transferring data from one place to another. To prevent such issues in real-time conditions, they used Blockchain technology for secrecy and protection purposes. They secured information by generating a hash of each data to ensure that any alteration or breaching of medicines conveys all Blockchain network users. Using Blockchain technology, they got 86% success in data analysis against conventional approaches. The success acquired in product drop ratio, wormhole attack, falsification attack, and probabilistic authentication scenario.

The main motivation to write the paper is for the following reasons:

- The Blockchain being a trusted system, secured system, transparency, and the traceability of data.
- The advantages of IoT are efficient resource utilization of a system, minimum human effort required, saves a lot of time, and obviously enhances data collection, and with much improves security.
- Lightweight cryptography is defined as a method and system to secure the data within 2000–2500 GEs, and it is in fact a challenging task to design.
- So, this paper is new approach to give a framework using the amalgamation of Blockchain, IoT, and LWC.

3 MPRESENT and IoT Security

This section describes the lightweight block cipher Modified-PRESENT (MPRESENT) details which give better response than so-called PRESENT [6]. Section 3.1 illustrates the said algorithm, Sect. 3.2 gives IoT security with MPRESENT, and Sect. 3.3 gives the mathematics behind PRESENT LWC block cipher.

3.1 MPRESENT Algorithm

The MPRESENT block cipher is lightweight and less complex and has greater efficiency than the existing PRESENT. The efficiency is comparable with some parameters like non-homogeneity, *N*-gram, frequency distribution, and floating frequency. The original PRESENT takes 64-bit plaintext and considers either of the key variants 80 or 128-bit. But the MPRESENT requires 64-bit plaintext with 80-bit key. The block diagram of MPRESENT cipher is shown in Fig. 2. Section 3.1.1 gives the details of the key register updating method, and Sect. 3.1.2 discusses how extra layer is being stuffed (Figs. 3 and 4).

The modified version MPRESENT possesses two steps. The first one is key register updating technique, and the second one is extra layer stuffing. These two parts are described in the below mentioned Sect. 3.1.1 and Sect. 3.1.2.

3.1.1 Key Register Updating Method

Unlike PRESENT, the MPRESENT divides the 64-bit key registers contents into two parts. Each part has a length of 32-bit. The right part uses the delta value addition technique of tiny encryption algorithm for encryption purposes. The encryption starts from the MSB position of the right part key. The XOR operation is performed between the original left part and the encrypted right part key. The original 32-bit left part key is now updated by the resultant value of XOR operation. Again, the updated left part and right part perform the same operation. This process will repeat for 10 times. Finally, the 64-bit key is generated by combining two parts which will be used as a key input for the next iteration. This entire process is depicted in Fig. 5.

3.1.2 Stuffing the Extra Layer

The MPRESENT algorithm stuffs an extra layer in between the S-box layer and the permutation layer of the original PRESENT. Within the new layer, first the output of the S-box breaks into two 32 bits parts. After that, the left and right parts perform XOR operation between them. The output is treated as the new left part. This process exhibits 32 times. The right part is updated by performing 5-bit right rotation. At

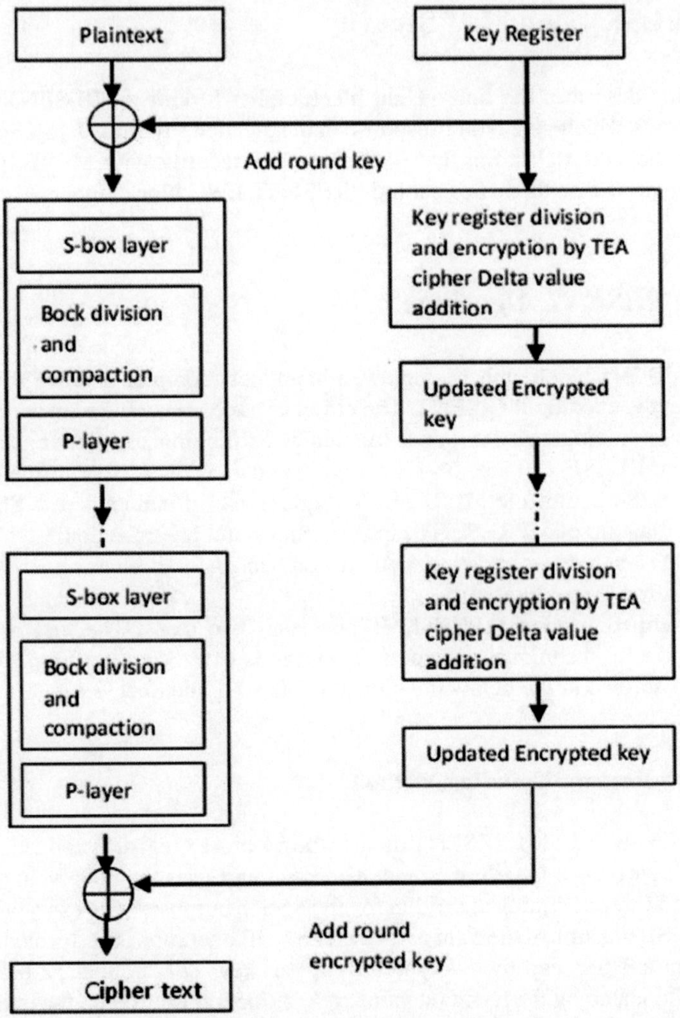

Fig. 2 Block diagram of MPRESENT cipher

last, two parts merge to generate 64-bit resultant new combination. This is fed to the permutation layer as an input. The decryption process is similar to encryption process except that is rotation done left which was done right before. Figure 4 displays the detailed procedure of stuffing the extra layer using a block diagram method.

The MPRESENT has reduced the PRESENT's 31 rounds to 25 rounds. It shows better performance with respect to efficiency measuring parameters like *N*-gram analysis, non-homogeneity or chi^2 test, histogram, and floating frequency. It is an efficient lightweight block cipher which is suitable in the IoT environment for encryption purposes.

Fig. 3 Pseudocode of MPRESENT

```
/* 1.Pseudo code of Key Register
Updating by Encrypting S-Box output
with TEA Cipher Delta Value
Addition*/

Function_KEY_Updating (KEY)
{
Repeat steps 1 to 5 10 times
1. Key_Left= Left_Half_Key[KEY];
2. Key_Right= Right_Half_Key[KEY];
3.Encrypt_right_key_TEA.Delta(Key_Ri
ght, TEAKey);
4. Key_Left ^ = Key_Right;
5. KEY =Merge (Key_Left, Key_Right);
}
/*Updated KEY is now taken as an
input to the next step*/
```

```
/*2.Pseudo code of Stuffing Extra
Layer In Between S-Box Layer and
Player of PRESENT Encryption */

Function _stuffing_layer(SBOX)
{
1. S_box_new[0] = LEFT[SBOX];
2. S_box_new[1] = RIGHT[SBOX];
3. Repeat step 4 32 times
4. S_box_new[0] ^ = S_box_new[1];
5. Rotation_right (S_box_new[1],
NO_of_Bits);
6. SBOX=
Merge(S_box_new[0],S_box_new[1]);
}
/*SBOX now feed to the permutation
Layer*/
```

3.2 *MPRESENT in IoT Security*

At present, our emerging world is continuously adopting new technologies and services. IoT is one of the highly demanded fields where a huge number of nodes participating in the IoT domain are a major constraint. As devices have limited computational power, low memory, and work in different operating environments, it is not possible to fulfill the security challenge in all aspects. Security requirements in IoT are very much crucial due to three characteristics of IoT such as heterogeneity, dynamic environment, and resource constraint.

There are different cryptographic primitives present in the security domain. The block cipher is one of the main primitives that is treated as a workhorse of the encryption process. Block cipher is comparatively better than stream cipher in terms

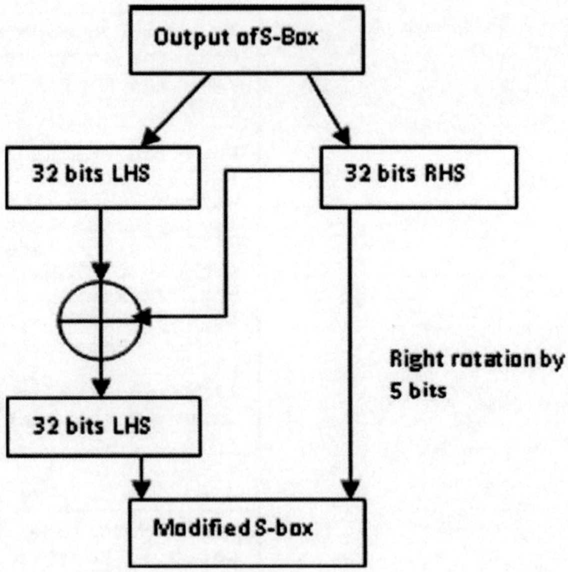

Fig. 4 Detailed block diagram of stuffing (extra layer)

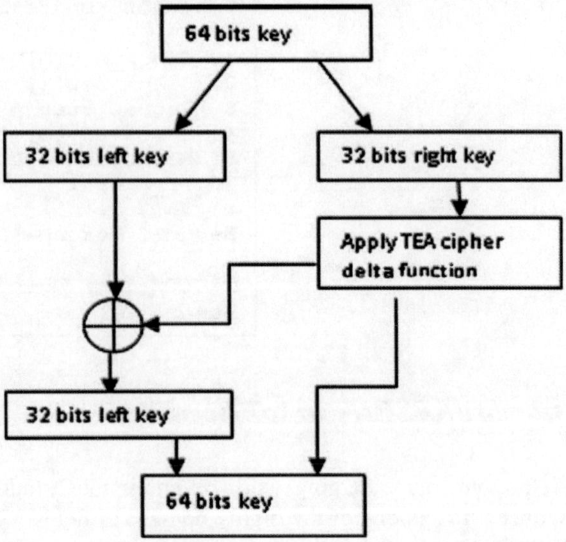

Fig. 5 Block diagram of key register (updating method)

of implementation complexity and efficiency. It also has a higher diffusion and error propagation rate than stream ciphers. Some of the specific designed block ciphers served as a purpose of security in terms of authentication or integrity protection. Here, MPRESENT is a highly efficient and lightweight block cipher which enables it to maintain security in the IoT domain.

3.3 Mathematics Behind PRESENT Algorithm

We define here addRoundKey, *S*-box, *p*-layer, and the key scheduling.

addRoundKey: For a particular round key, $K_i = K_i^{63}\ K_i^{62}$ to ... K_i^0 where $1 \le i \le 32$ with the current state b^{63} ... b^0, the operation is $0 \le j \le 63$, and Eq. (1) represents the particular output.

$$b^j \to b^j \oplus K_i^j \quad (1)$$

S-box: The *S*-box used in PRESENT is one 4-bit to 4-bit *S*-box *S*: ${F^4}_2 \to {F^4}_2$; thus, the input–output mapping of this box in HEX format is given in Table 1.

For *S*-BoxLayer, the current state $b^{63}\ b^{62}$ to ... b^0 is considered of and as 16 4-bit words, w_{15} ... w_0, where

$$w_i = b_{4*i+3}||b_{4*i+2}||b_{4*i+1}||b_{4*i} \text{ for } 0 \le i \le 15 \quad (2)$$

and it is calculated as output nibble $S[w_i]$ that provides with the updated state values in the given way.

p-layer: It is a bit permutation technique used in PRESENT as given in Table 2. Bit *i*th of a state is to move to bit position *P*(*i*).

The key schedule: PRESENT algorithm takes keys of either 80 or 128 bits which is continuned in MPRESENT also. But the focus is on 80-bit keys. The session key is stored in a key register *K* and that are represented by $k_{79}\ k_{78}$ ... k_0. During *i*th round, 64-bit key $K_i = K_{63}\ K_{62}$ ... K_0 consists of the 64 LSB of current content of register *K*. Thus, Eq. (3) gives the value of K_i at *i*th round.

$$K_i = K_{63}K_{62}\ldots K_0 = K_{79}K_{78}\ldots K_{16} \quad (3)$$

Table 1 Input (*x*) to output *S*[*x*] mapping

x	*S*[*x*]	*x*	*S*[*x*]	*x*	*S*[*x*]	*x*	*S*[*x*]
0	*C*	1	5	2	6	3	*B*
x	*S*[*x*]	*x*	*S*[*x*]	*x*	*S*[*x*]	*x*	*S*[*x*]
4	9	5	0	6	*A*	7	*D*
x	*S*[*x*]	*x*	*S*[*x*]	*x*	*S*[*x*]	*x*	*S*[*x*]
8	3	9	*E*	*A*	*F*	*B*	8
x	*S*[*x*]	*x*	*S*[*x*]	*x*	*S*[*x*]	*x*	*S*[*x*]
C	4	*D*	7	*E*	1	*F*	2

Table 2 Input to output bit mapping in *p*-layer bit

İ	P(i)	i	P(i)	i	P(i)	i	P(i)
0	0	16	4	32	8	48	12
İ	P(i)	i	P(i)	i	P(i)	i	P(i)
1	16	17	20	33	24	49	28
İ	P(i)	i	P(i)	i	P(i)	i	P(i)
2	32	18	36	34	40	50	44
İ	P(i)	i	P(i)	i	P(i)	i	P(i)
3	46	19	52	35	56	51	60
İ	P(i)	i	P(i)	i	P(i)	i	P(i)
4	1	20	5	36	9	52	13
İ	P(i)	i	P(i)	i	P(i)	i	P(i)
5	7	21	21	37	25	53	29
İ	P(i)	i	P(i)	i	P(i)	i	P(i)
6	33	22	37	36	41	54	45
İ	P(i)	i	P(i)	i	P(i)	i	P(i)
7	49	23	53	39	57	55	61
İ	P(i)	i	P(i)	i	P(i)	i	P(i)
8	2	24	6	40	10	56	14
İ	P(i)	i	P(i)	i	P(i)	i	P(i)
9	8	25	22	41	26	57	30
İ	P(i)	i	P(i)	i	P(i)	i	P(i)
10	34	26	38	42	42	58	46
İ	P(i)	i	P(i)	i	P(i)	i	P(i)
11	50	27	54	43	58	59	62
İ	P(i)	i	P(i)	i	P(i)	i	P(i)
12	3	28	7	44	11	60	15
İ	P(i)	i	P(i)	i	P(i)	i	P(i)
13	19	29	23	45	27	61	31
İ	P(i)	i	P(i)	i	P(i)	i	P(i)
14	35	30	39	46	43	62	47
İ	P(i)	i	P(i)	i	P(i)	i	P(i)
15	51	31	55	47	59	63	63

4 The Blockchain Framework

We use the Ethereum [7] for this framework, Sect. 4.1 gives some mathematical concepts behind the implementation platform, Ethereum, and Sect. 4.2 gives the proposed framework.

4.1 Mathematics Behind Ethereum

Section 4.1.1 defines a cryptographic hash function, Sect. 4.1.2 defines the Elliptic Curve Cryptography (ECC) and Digital Signature with the Elliptic Curve Digital Signature Algorithm (ECDSA), Sect. 4.1.3 mathematically formalizes the Ethereum, and Sect. 4.1.4 defines proof of work.

4.1.1 Cryptographic Hash Function

Definition 1 One-way function

$$f : \{0, 1\}^* \rightarrow \{0, 1\}^* \tag{4}$$

Equation 4 is the computable function where * represents arbitrary finite length message, it is the probability of finding x by providing random value, and $y = f(x)$ is negligible in polynomial time.

Definition 2 $H(x)$ is hash function, and in there, x has an arbitrary finite length of bits that produces output Y with fixed length. Hash output is a random bit string. This definition is represented by Eq. (5).

$$\{\{0, 1\}^* \rightarrow \{0, 1\}^n \text{ and } Y = H(x) \tag{5}$$

4.1.2 The Elliptic Curve Cryptography (ECC) and Digital Signature

The elliptic curve is a simplified form of Weierstrass equation over algebraic field K as a form of Eq. (6)

$$\begin{aligned} &Y^2 = x^3 + aX + b \,(\text{mod } p) \\ &4a^3 + 27b^2 \neq 0 \text{ nonsingular condition} \end{aligned} \tag{6}$$

In cryptography, the coefficients and the variables must belong to field K which can be prime number finite fields or prime number binary fields. All points must lie on the equation that are added with abstract notation ∞ in the form of an Abelian algebraic group with additive operation.

The Elliptic Curve Digital Signature Algorithm (ECDSA) is defined by the Algorithm 1, Algorithm 2, and Algorithm 3.

Algorithm 1 Key generation in ECC

Input: $Y^2 = x^3 + aX + b$, where a, b are prime numbers in Z_p and the base point is G, The order of this subgroup is n, and cofactor is h

Output: private and public key

1. *Privatekey* $\leftarrow$ *Choosearandomnumberamong* $\{1, 2, 3, \ldots, n-1\}$
2. *Publickey* $\leftarrow$ *Computeprivatekey* $\times$ *G* (*notethatthepublickeyispointoncurve*)
3. *Return* private key and public key.

Algorithm 2 Signing ECDSA

Input: $Y^2 = x^3 + aX + b$, where a, b are prime numbers over Z_P and the base point is G. The order of this subgroup $= n$, private key, message $= M$
Output: M, signature 1, signature 2

1. $r \leftarrow$ *Chooserandomintegerr*, $r \in [1, n-1]$
2. $e\,(x_e, y_e) \leftarrow$ *Computer* $\times$ *G*
3. $S_0 \leftarrow$ *Compute* (*xemodn*)
4. *If* $S_0 == 0$ *then* Go to 1

Else $S \leftarrow$ *Compute* $[r^{-1}\,(M + S_0 \times privatekey)]$ *modn* ($r - 1$ *ismultiplicationinverse*)

5. *Return* (S_0, S)

Algorithm 3 Verifying ECDSA

Input: S, S_0, *Publickey*, *Message* $= M$, *orderofsubgroup* $= n$, *basepoint G*
Output: True, False

1. $V_1 \leftarrow$ *Compute* $(S^{-1} \times M)$ *modn*
2. $V_2 \leftarrow$ *Compute* $(S^{-1} \times S_0)$ *modn*
3. $P \leftarrow$ *Compute*$V_2 \times G + (V_2 \times Publickey)$
4. *If* $xp == S_0$ (*modn*) *thenReturnTrue*

Else *ReturnFalse*

4.1.3 Mathematical Formalization of Ethereum

Definition 3 A transition system is defined as a mathematical object which consists of two parts: first set of configurations that defines the various states and second with having binary relation among the states.

The abstraction of this mathematical modeling of these systems with a memory being carried out by state machines in turn helps us to understand the underlying structuring of systems. So, this model is having various finite/infinite states also having input/output sets giving output to function and transition function. This model is further denoted by tuple (S_0, S, I, O, T, F), where $S_0 =$ genesis state, $S =$ non-empty set of states, $I =$ input set, and $O =$ output set. The transition function and output function are defined by Eqs. (7) and (8).

$$T = \text{transition function which } T(x \in I, y \in S) \rightarrow z \in S$$

$$(T \text{ takes inputs at time } t \text{ and outputs at time } (t+1)). \quad (7)$$

$$F = \text{output function which } F(x \in I, y \in S) \rightarrow o \in O \text{ (regard to the time so that } F \text{ takes inputs at time } t \text{ and outputs at } t + \epsilon \text{ such that we can neglect } \epsilon). \quad (8)$$

4.1.4 The Proof of Work

In short, the proof-of-work mechanism for mutual consensus was first introduced, implemented, and coined in bitcoin by Satoshi Nakamoto that provide a valid mining process for all nodes. This protocol, proof of work, is also known as Nakamoto protocol that is based mainly as a non-interactive cryptographic puzzle that can be solved, and it is also that each node is verified independently. The goal is finding a hash of some inputs which starts with a specific number of zeros called leading zeros and less or equal that target value. The proof of work can be summarized in Eq. (9).

$$\text{SHA} - 256(A_1||A_2||A_3||A_4||A_5||A_6) \leq \text{CurrentTarge} \quad (9)$$

where A_1 is previous hash, A_2 is Merkle root of transactions, A_3 is nonce, A_4 is target difficulty, A_5 is timestamp, and A_6 is bitcoin protocol version.

4.2 The Framework and Implementation

In the proposed framework, the IoT devices collect the patient record and which is then encrypted by our own designed, MPRESENT. The data are then fed to each of the Blockchain nodes over the Internet which is decrypted by MPRESENT. Then the proof of work is used to validate the data to store it permanently in each of the Blockchain (Fig. 6).

In this pseudocode as given in Fig. 7, the first IoT nodes collect the patient data and make a block as illustrated in Fig. 1. This data block is small in size as it is made in sensor/physical layer of IoT. The data structure of this medical record has only Medical Data Type [array *n*] (MRI images, X-ray images, blood report values, value ranges, etc.), Corresponding Medical Records [array *n*], and Sensor/Device_ID. Now the first communication is between sensor layer/physical layer and edge layer. This security is provided by MPRESENT, and we use CBC mode for encryption and decryption. In the edge layer more information is added to this data. So, now the data in the block may contain Patient_ID, Doctor_ID, IoT_ID, Medical Data Type [array *n*] (MRI images, X-ray images, blood report values, value ranges, etc.), Corresponding Medical Records [array *n*], Sensor/Device_ID, and Collector_ID. This block is encrypted with TDES in CBC mode and propagated to various nodes

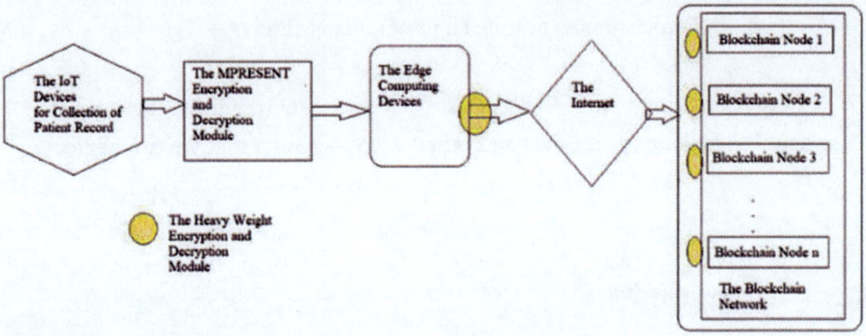

Fig. 6 Proposed framework

of the Ethereum Blockchain [8] through internetwork, and in the receiver side, this block is decrypted. Here we use TDES in CBC as LWC not provides security in internetwork.

Then proof of work is called in each of the node with this block and if the result is success with our framework then this block is committed to each Blockchain node by adding timestamp. The cryptographic hash with Merkle tree of previous hash and current hash with other information if required then an alarm is raised.

```
Framework (){
InputData_IoT(Data Block);
Encrypt(Data Block, MPRESENT_CBC, ESData);
FTP(ESData, Edge_Device);
Decrypt(ESData, MPRESENT_CBC, Data Block);
Edge_Computing(DataBlock, Add_ID[n], Add_Other_Data[n], ResultDataBlock);
Encrypt(ResultDataBlock, TDES_CBC, EData)
FTP1(EData, BN1);
FTP2(EData, BN2);
………..
FTPn(EData, BNn);
Decrypt1(EData, TDES_CBC, DataBlock1);
Decrypt2(EData, TDES_CBC, DataBlock2);
…………
Decryptn(EData, TDES_CBC, DataBlockn);
Call Proof-of-Work (Node [Bn1, Bn2 ….. BNn] , Block[DataBlock1, DataBlock2 ….. DataBlock3])
{ If (Success)
Commit (Node [Bn1, Bn2 ….. BNn] , Block[DataBlock1, DataBlock2 ….. DataBlock3]);
Else
Alarm ("The data block is wrong or consensus not matching for any wrong ID");}
Return;}
```

Fig. 7 Pseudocode of the framework

5 Discussion

The first is the security of the lightweight cryptography. Here we use MPRESENT [2], which is well established, and already published LWC and the security features of PRESENT are already discussed in Sect. 3. The use of IoT sensor layer or physical layer is highlighted in this paper. Since IoT devices and amalgamated medical devices are used everywhere nowadays in IoMT, the security is provided with the LWC. The Blockchain-based record framework is also highlighted in this paper. We use Ethereum which is already discussed in Sect. 4, and the consensus is well established with the equations and algorithms in the same section.

Thus, this framework is an amalgamation of IoT, LWC, and Blockchain to keep medical records and can be effectively used in IoMT.

A comparative discussion against the work on "Health Record Management through Blockchain Technology" [1] is as follows:

a. Our proposed framework is given a second layer of security through MPRESENT.
b. Our work is based and focused on IoT and IoMT.
c. We have given the detailed discussion and implementation as pseudocode in this paper.
d. Since Blockchain is platform dependent or depends on developer network, a direct comparison cannot be given.
e. We also defined the related theories with mathematical equations in our paper.

6 Conclusion

In this paper, we started with the introduction of IoT, lightweight cryptography, Blockchain, and Internet of Medical Things, IoMT. Then we give a detailed discussion of lightweight cryptography, PRESENT, and MPRESENT. Thereafter, we give the Blockchain framework and Ethereum followed by proposed model and implementation.

Therefore, we successfully delivered IoT-based secure Blockchain framework for Patient Record Management using MPRESENT.

The future scope is to develop an IoT protocol itself that should be lightweight in nature as compared to MQTT, XMPP, and CoAP. The application of this LWP will be in diverse fields using Blockchain.

References

1. Harshini VM, Danai S, Usha HR, Kounte MR (2019) Health record management through blockchain technology. In: 2019 3rd International conference on trends in electronics and informatics (ICOEI), pp 1411–1415. https://doi.org/10.1109/ICOEI.2019.8862594

2. Chatterjee R, Chakraborty R (2020) A modified lightweight PRESENT cipher for IoT security. In: 2020 International conference on computer science, engineering and applications (ICCSEA), pp 1–6. https://doi.org/10.1109/ICCSEA49143.2020.9132950
3. Veeramakali R, Siva R, Sivakumar B, Senthil Mahesh PC, Krishnarajl N (2021) An intelligent internet of things-based secure healthcare framework using blockchain technology with an optimal deep learning model. J Supercomput 77:9576–9596. https://doi.org/10.1007/s11227-021-03637-3
4. Rathee G, Sharma A, Saini H et al (2020) A hybrid framework for multimedia data processing in IoT-healthcare using blockchain technology. Multimedia Tools Appl 79:9711–9733. https://doi.org/10.1007/s11042-019-07835-3
5. Jamil F, Ahmad S, Iqbal N, Kim D-H (2020) Towards a remote monitoring of patient vital signs based on IoT-based blockchain integrity management platforms in smart hospitals. Sensors 20(8):2195. https://doi.org/10.3390/s20082195
6. Mahantesh RS, Mohapatra S (2018)Design of secured block ciphers PRESENT and HIGHT algorithms and its FPGA implementation. In: 2018 Second international conference on intelligent computing and control systems (ICICCS), pp 1113–1118. https://doi.org/10.1109/ICCONS.2018.8663165
7. Rouhani S, Deters R (2017) Performance analysis of Ethereum transactions in private blockchain. In: 2017 8th IEEE International conference on software engineering and service science (ICSESS), pp 70–74. https://doi.org/10.1109/ICSESS.2017.8342866
8. Dagher GG, Mohler J, Milojkovic M, Marella PB (2018) Ancile: privacy-preserving framework for access control and interoperability of electronic health records using block chain technology. Sustain Cities Soc 39:283–297. ISSN 2210-6707

A Secure Electronic Health Record Storage System Based on Hyperledger Fabric, IPFS, and Secret Sharing Scheme

Puja Sarkar, Lopamudra Pathak, Rohan Molia, Sima Boro, and Amitava Nag

Abstract Electronic health records (EHR) systems are now becoming widely used as a system for storing and managing patients' health records. Patients should be able to access their health records as and when required. Traditional EHR systems have challenges with data security, integrity, interoperability, and management. The typical client–server system is vulnerable to single-point-of-failure since it is centralised. Medical data that is dispersed across different EHR systems is frequently difficult to access. Due to its positive features such as security, privacy, secrecy, and decentralized, blockchain technology has the potential to significantly enhance the healthcare sector, despite all of the existing problems. In this paper, we present a health data storage system based on the permissioned Hyperledger blockchain, an InterPlanetary File System (IPFS), and a multi-image secret sharing approach. Hyperledger Fabric is a peer-to-peer tamper-proof private-permissioned blockchain network that allows an organisation to simultaneously participate in multiple, separate blockchain networks via channels. And further, multi-image secret sharing is applied to provide security to sensitive medical image data during transmission against illegal access or alteration. Our system is integrated with IPFS for EHR storage. The proposed framework provides a secure, decentralised, and distributed model of EHR management system. Hyperledger Fabric is a tamper-proof private-permissioned blockchain network that allows an organisation to participate in many blockchain networks at the same time using channels. Furthermore, multi-image secret sharing is used to protect sensitive medical picture data from unauthorised access or manipulation during transmission. Using which our system is free from single-point-of-failure. For EHR storage, our system is connected with IPFS. The proposed framework provides an EHR administration system that is secure, decentralised, and distributed.

Keywords Blockchain-based EHR system · Hyperledger Fabric · InterPlanetary File System · Image secret sharing

P. Sarkar (✉) · L. Pathak · R. Molia · S. Boro · A. Nag
Central Institute of Technology, Kokrajhar, India
e-mail: p.sarkar@cit.ac.in

A. Nag
e-mail: amitava.nag@cit.ac.in

© The Author(s), under exclusive license to Springer Nature Singapore Pte Ltd. 2023

J. K. Mandal and D. De (eds.), *Frontiers of ICT in Healthcare*, Lecture Notes in Networks and Systems 519, https://doi.org/10.1007/978-981-19-5191-6_29

1 Introduction

An electronic health record is a health-related, extremely sensitive record used to diagnose and treat patients with care. The amount of patient data is increasing at a breakneck speed. The access, sharing, and sensible distribution of EHR among numerous healthcare stakeholders such as hospitals, clinicians, and patient families is one of the most essential and critical difficulties the healthcare industry is now experiencing. The electronic health record system has a variety of flaws, including the following:

Interoperability: The capacity of multiple information systems to communicate with one another is referred to as interoperability. The information should be able to be shared and put to various uses.

Information Asymmetry: According to opponents, today's biggest concern in the healthcare sector is information asymmetry, which refers to one side having better access to information than the other. This difficulty emerges in the case of EHR systems or the wider healthcare sector since doctors or hospitals have access to the patient's information, making them central. A patient must go through a lengthy and rigorous process in order to view his medical records. The data, which is centralised at a single healthcare organisation, is only accessible to hospitals or organisations.

Data Breach: Without the knowledge or authority of the system owner, information is stolen or taken from the system, requiring the need for a better platform in the healthcare industry [1, 2].

To overcome all of the aforementioned concerns, we devised a system based on blockchain technology. Blockchain is a distributed, decentralised ledger that records transactions in an ever-growing chain of unchangeable blocks linked by cryptographic hashes. Due to their transparency, blockchains can instantly detect fraudulent information, and smart contracts on the blockchain can operate as security measures [3, 4]. These smart contracts can record evaluations and provide data that can be utilised to design new and more effective treatments.

For patient privacy and confidentiality, such as health-related personal information, a private-permissioned blockchain is appropriate. It focuses on specific security and interoperability weaknesses and issues, as well as present EHR system roadblocks. With all of the advantages of blockchain technology, there are also some disadvantages.

Using a blockchain network to store massive volumes of data makes it slow and computationally expensive. So, in our system, we kept our data files separate in off-chain storage, and we employed an InterPlanetary File System (IPFS) to do so. Our objectives can be described as follows: A decentralised platform that would store a patient's medical records and allow physicians and other interested parties, such as the patient and the patient's trusted party (PTP), to access them. A patient- centric paradigm is one in which the patient determines who has access to their data and how it is used. In the event of an emergency, data can be easily shared with other organisations. Before uploading important EHRs to off-chain storage, make sure they are secure. This paper is organised as follows: Sect. 2 discusses comparable efforts by others. The preliminary knowledge of the technologies involved is covered in Sect. 3. In Sect. 4, the proposed system and workflow are discussed. Section 5 looks at the conclusion and security analysis.

2 Related Works

Shahnaz et al. [1] established a strategy for adopting blockchain technology in the healthcare sector for EHR to address issues including data leaks, information asymmetry, and scalability. The purpose of their suggested framework is to first embrace blockchain technology for EHR and then to provide secure electronic record storage by creating granular access controls for users of the proposed framework, as well as off-chain record storage, thereby addressing the scalability issue.

Tith et al. cite [2] presented a distributed system based on the Hyperledger Fabric that combines existing EHR. To protect a patient's privacy, they use a proxy re-encryption process when transferring data. Doctors can use the system to find patient records and check that the patient has given their consent to data access. The hospital has easy access to the patient's information. The access log is transparently and immutably maintained in the ledger for auditing purposes.

In Zhang et al. [5], Shamir's Secret Sharing was used to suggest a cloud storage solution for EHRs that fully secures data privacy by splitting the system into several components and distributing them across various cloud servers. Because reconstruction of a shared EHR might be time consuming during recovery, they propose a feasible cloud storage system that outsources it to a cloud computing service provider.

Kumar et al. [6] proposed a blockchain-based consortium structure for storing medical report details. They also describe a system for patient diagnostic reports that employs off-chain storage.

Sultana et al. [7] proposed a technique for dealing with vulnerabilities in medical/health data. The approach leverages blockchain's immutability, zero-trust principles' additional security, and the scalability of off-chain data storage via IPFS.

In paper Tanwar et al. [8], a blockchain-based approach for sharing electronic health records was presented. Many methods and configurations for block transactions are utilised on the network. A shared symmetric key and private key can be used to distribute the EHR to other users of the blockchain network.

3 Preliminary Knowledge

3.1 Blockchain

It is a decentralised digital ledger that records transactions without the need for a central authority in a public or private peer-to-peer network. It allows community members to record transactions in a shared ledger. Every transaction is recorded with a hash, which is a cryptographic signature that cannot be changed. Since the blockchain's inception, each blockchain node has a comprehensive record of all data recorded on it. In most cases, once a transaction has been published, it cannot be changed. Blockchain has a number of advantages, including no central administration, built-in transparency, distributed record-keeping, and immutability [9, 10].

3.1.1 Categorisation

Blockchain can be categorised into four categories: public, private, hybrid or consortium blockchain network.

1. **Public blockchain**: This has no restrictions as to who can use it. Anyone who wants to transmit, view, or modify to the database can do so. Anyone can send transactions to it and become a validator, hence anyone can use it.
2. **Private blockchain**: A private blockchain necessitates permissions. Only those who have been invited by the network's administrator are allowed to access it.
3. **Hybrid blockchain**: It is a hybrid of centralised and decentralised characteristics.
4. **Consortium blockchain**: A permissioned blockchain that allows many organisations to participate in decision-making, allowing for real decentralisation.

3.2 Hyperledger Fabric

Hyperledger Fabric is a private blockchain that allows organisations to collaborate in the formation of the blockchain network. It aims to advance blockchain technology. It is an open source framework implementation for private chain in which membership and roles are known to other members. Some of its features are [3, 4] (Table 1).

1. In a peer-to-peer blockchain network, it provides a private and adaptable framework for completing multiple transactions.
2. The adaptable, pluggable endorsement model aids in the realisation and attainment of consensus among network stakeholders.
3. It allows us to construct communication channels between different member organisations, allowing us to meet the privacy and security goals.
4. It uses channels to create a method that ensures transaction privacy and integrity.

Table 1 Distinction between permission-less blockchain and permissioned blockchain

	Permission-less	Permissioned
Access	Access to the database is enabled for both read and write operations	Database access with read/write permissions
Scale	Scale to a high number of nodes, but not at the expense of transaction throughput	Scale transaction throughput but not to a huge number of nodes
Consensus	Proof of work/proof of state	Algorithms for closed membership consensus
Identity	Anonymous/pseudonymous	Although node identities are known, transaction identities might be private, anonymous, or pseudonymous
Asset	Indigenous	Any data/state

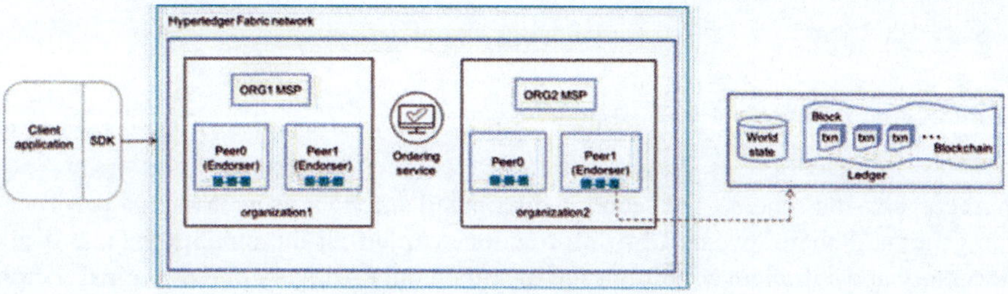

Fig. 1 Flow of operations/compositions in our proposed framework

The components and composition of HLF is shown in Fig. 1.

3.3 *InterPlanetary File System*

The InterPlanetary File System (IPFS) is a distributed file system protocol and peer-to-peer network. Content-addressing is used by IPFS to uniquely identify each file in a global namespace that connects all computing devices. In a similar way to BitTorrent, IPFS allows users to host and receive content. Rather than relying on a single server, IPFS is based on a decentralised system of user-operators who each hold a fraction of the overall data, resulting in a robust file storage and sharing system.

IPFS aims to establish a distributed and permanent web. This is accomplished by employing a content-addressed approach rather than HTTP's location-based mechanism. Instead of employing a physical address, IPFS addresses the content using a representation of the content itself. A file is broken into smaller bits, cryptographically hashed, and given a unique fingerprint called a content identifier (CID) when it is added to IPFS. This CID serves as a permanent record of the file at the moment it was created. A user can obtain this "beginning point" of data instead of talking to a server. When other nodes search up your file, they inquire as to which of their peer nodes is storing the content indicated by the CID.

IPFS uses a distributed hash table, or DHT, to store data. Data is transmitted between nodes in the network using BitTorrent-like processes. On the IPFS web, a user looking for material discovers neighbours who have access to that content. They then download little portions of the content from individuals who are close by. IPFS utilises a Merkle tree in addition to DHT and BitTorrent protocols. This is a data format that is akin to Git's version management system and the bitcoin blockchain technology. It is used to maintain source code versions in Git, but it is also used to track material across the Internet in IPFS.

IPFS and blockchains can operate well together due to their structural similarities. In fact, IPFS creator Juan Benet describes this as a "wonderful marriage." IPFS is one of a few initiatives that are part of Protocol Labs, an organisation that was formed by Benet as well [11, 12].

3.4 Secret Sharing Scheme

In secret sharing scheme, the secret is distributed among n users in such a way that, the generated share reveals zero information without all the random values. If all necessary and sufficient conditions are met, then only recovery of the original secret is possible [13–16].

4 Proposed System

4.1 System Conceptual Design

A user would be the one interacting with the system. Users could be patients, doctors, or an administrator. An administrator would be the one assigning roles to the other users and performing the backend operations. The basic tasks of the users would be to perform operations like create, update, query, and delete medical records. All the users would interact with the system with the help of a GUI (Fig. 2).

4.2 Workflow

4.2.1 Proposed Application

All the users of the system would be registered in the system by the admin and their respective IDs would be generated. Every user would also have their respective

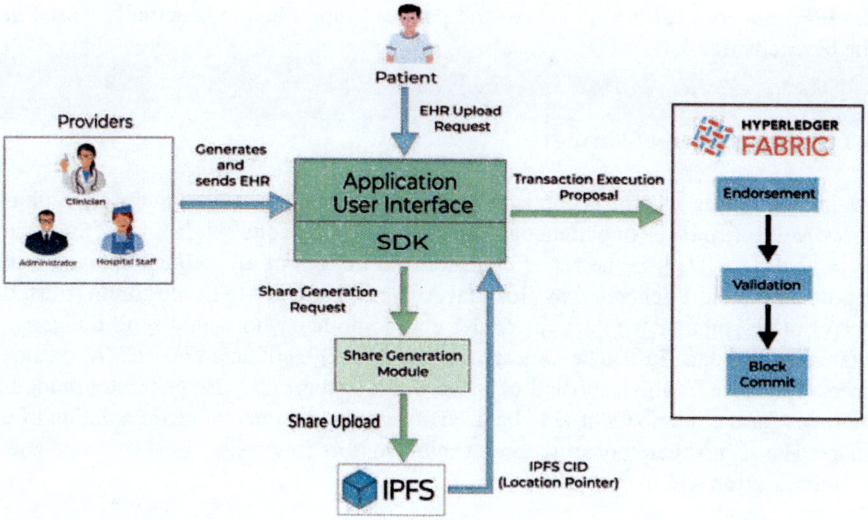

Fig. 2 System design

profiles which they would access through their login credentials. This login module would provide the outermost layer of security.

After successful login, a user can perform any CRUD operation to the network through the web UI. Let us say, a patient wants to view his details. He/she would make a request through the web page. This transaction would invoke the respective smart contract and make a transaction proposal to the fabric network. The Fabric SDK provides various APIs to interact with the network. The SDK will try to establish a connection to the network using the respective client identity. The client identity must be registered and enrolled in the network and recognised as a valid identity. After successful connection and invoking the respective smart contract, the network will return the response back to the SDK. The SDK will then parse the response accordingly and display it to the client through the webpage. In our proposed system, the large files like medical scan reports (image files) are not directly stored in the ledger, stored outside the blockchain network, known as off-chain storage. Here, we used another decentralised technology, the InterPlanetary File System or IPFS.

IPFS is a distributed file system protocol and peer-to-peer network. In a global namespace that connects all computing devices, IPFS uses content-addressing to uniquely identify each file. Along with the medical data fields available for the patient, the doctor can also upload/update the medical image files associated with the medical examination of the concerned patient. Before uploading the file needs to be encrypted in some sort. So in our proposed system, we are using the concept of secret sharing to hide the raw information of the EHR. The system would send a request to the share generation module. A secret share of the EHR would be generated and the system would then upload it to IPFS. After successfully adding the file to the IPFS network, a content identifier or CID (hash string) of the file is returned by the IPFS network. This CID acts as the pointer to the file and is actually stored in the blockchain.

4.2.2 Image Secret Sharing

An image sharing scheme is applied on the patient data to be stored in the IPFS platform. Multiple images of patient data are concatenated in one single image. Suppose $I_C = I_1||I_2 \dots ||I_K||$ is the set of concatenated images of all medical examination reports of Patient 1 generated by Hospital A. We consider 'A' to be the admin (trusted party) of Hospital A who acts as dealer and combiner who would send the secret share generated to IPFS. The concatenated images I_C is of size $W \times H$. 'A' creates access structure G which consists of authorised members and also generates random matrices for the members of G to be used during generation and reconstruction of a share. The secret share construction mechanism is as follows:

Initialisation and user verification:

1. 'A' generates I_C.
2. 'A' constructs the access structures G, which is the authorised subset of members $G = P_i|3$ 'P_i' k, $k =$ maximum number of members.
3. For each I_C, 'A' generates random matrices for each of the members in G.
4. First, 'A' encrypts the random matrices with his private key, then sends them to the concerned members after encrypting it with their public keys.

Algorithm 1: Share Generation

1. 'A' computes the secret share using random matrices of members by XORing it with I_C.

$$I_{\text{Secret Share}} = I_C \oplus R_1 \oplus R_2 \oplus \cdots \oplus R_K.$$

2. 'A' uploads the secret share, $I_{\text{Secret Share}}$ on the IPFS network.

Example Let $I_C = I_1||I_2 \dots ||I_K||$ be the set of concatenated images and we are considering two access structures G_1 and G_2.

$G_1 = \text{P1, D1, PTP}$

$G_2 = \text{PTP, D1, D2,}$ (To be used as backup if patient is not in the state to share its random matrix)

$\text{D1} = \text{Doctor 1}, \text{D2} = \text{Doctor 2}, \text{P1} = \text{Patient 1}, \text{PTP} = \text{Patient Trusted Party}$

'A' generates random number matrices R_{D1}, R_{D2}, R_{P1}, R_{PTP} for G_1 and G_2 using random functions. Secret share is generated $I_{\text{Secret Share}}$ by XORing I_C with the random matrices.

$$I_{\text{Secret Share}} = I_{\text{C}} \oplus R_{\text{P1}} \oplus R_{\text{D1}} \oplus R_{\text{PTP}} \text{ (using } G_1\text{)}$$
$$I_{\text{Secret Share}} = I_{\text{C}} \oplus R_{\text{D1}} \oplus R_{\text{D2}} \oplus R_{\text{PTP}} \text{ (using } G_2\text{)}$$

Algorithm 2: Image Recovery
Considering that all the participants agrees on recovering of data I_{C} by any member from the access structure, the mechanism of reconstruction is as follows:

1. Combiner will download the secret share, $I_{\text{Secret Share}}$ from the IPFS public network.
2. Each member will share their random matrices (R_1, R_2, ..., R_K) to reconstruct the image I_{C}.

$$I_{\text{C}} = I_{\text{Secret Share}} \oplus R_1 \oplus R_2 \cdots \oplus R_K$$

Example

$$G_1 = \text{P1, D1, PTP}$$
$$R = R_{\text{P1}}, R_{\text{D1}}, \text{RPTP}$$
$$I_{\text{C}} = I_{\text{Secret Share}} \oplus R_{\text{P1}} \oplus R_{\text{D1}} \oplus R_{\text{PTP}}$$
$$G_2 = \text{PTP, D1, D2}$$
$$R = \text{RPTP}, R_{\text{D1}}, R_{\text{D2}}$$
$$I_{\text{C}} = I_{\text{Secret Share}} \oplus R_{\text{PTP}} \oplus R_{\text{D1}} \oplus R_{\text{D2}}$$

5 Discussion and Security Analysis

We discuss some of the features that our present framework proposes. For this, we have discussed some security measures with respect to the parameters (Figs. 3, 4 and 5):

- **Scalability**: The storing of large amounts of data on blockchain is a problem that demands a long-term solution. For storing patient's huge image files, our proposed model uses an off-chain storage mechanism. As a result, our methodology resolves the scalability issue.
- **Confidentiality**: In our architecture, we use a permissioned blockchain powered by the HLF network, which prevents access from any unauthorised third-party outside the network.
- **Integrity**: As we are leveraging tempar-proof blockchain technology, it is built specifically to protect data integrity.
- **Access Control**: Our suggested paradigm is patient-centric, which means that individuals have the power to grant access to their data to whoever they wish. Authorised parties are also permitted to see only a portion of the data, i.e. they are permitted to know only what they require.

(a) Patient Random Matrix (b) Doctor Random Matrix (c) PTP Random Matrix

Fig. 3 Random matrices

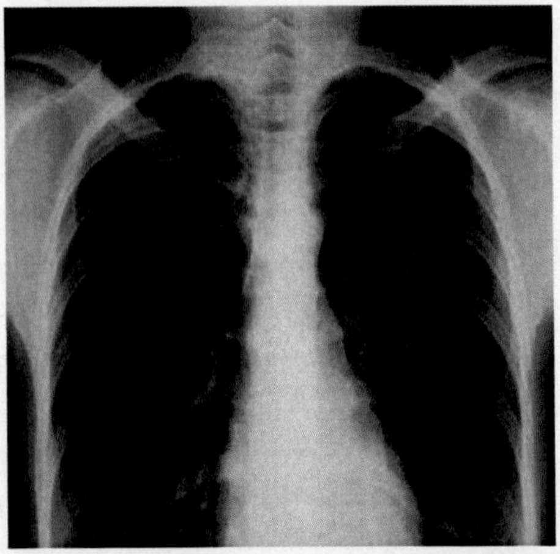

Fig. 4 I_C

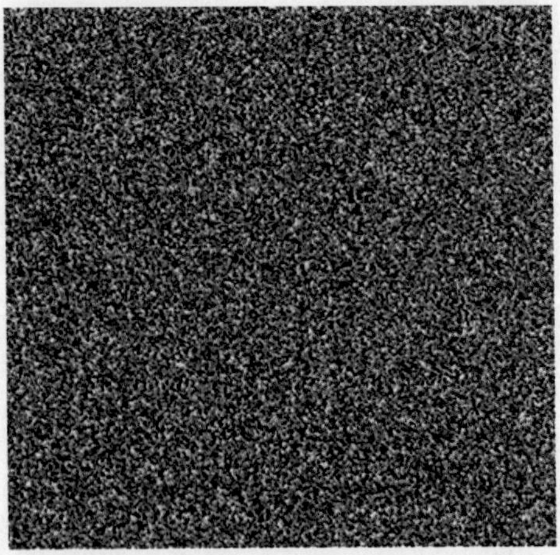

Fig. 5 $I_{\text{Secret Share}}$

6 Conclusions and Future Scope

Our proposed architecture is a patient-centric framework that provides a secure, decentralised, and distributed EHR administration system that employs the IPFS method for off-chain data storage. The IPFS network ensures that a hash named CID is generated. As a result, the cryptographic hash generated for each file stored in IPFS protects its security. We intend to update the system in future by adding features such as verifiability to secret sharing method.

References

1. Shahnaz A, Qamar U, Khalid A (2019) Using blockchain for electronic health records. IEEE Access 7:147782–147795. https://doi.org/10.1109/ACCESS.2019.2946373
2. Tith D et al (2020) Application of blockchain to maintaining patient records in electronic health record for enhanced privacy, scalability, and availability. Healthc Inf Res 26(1)
3. Biswas S et al (2020) Blockchain for E-health-care systems: easier said than done. Computer 53(7):57–67
4. Aswin AV, Basil KY, Viswan VP, Reji B, Kuriakose B (2020) Design of AYUSH: a blockchain-based health record management system. In: Ranganathan G, Chen J, Rocha Á (eds) Inventive communication and computational technologies. Lecture notes in networks and systems, vol 89. Springer, Singapore. https://doi.org/10.1007/978-981-15-0146-3_62
5. Zhang H et al (2018) Cloud storage for electronic health records based on secret sharing with verifiable reconstruction outsourcing. IEEE Access 6:40713–40722
6. Kumar R, Marchang N, Tripathi R (2020) Distributed off-chain storage of patient diagnostic reports in healthcare system using IPFS and blockchain. In: 2020 International conference on communication systems networks (COMSNETS). IEEE
7. Sultana M et al (2020) Towards developing a secure medical image sharing system based on zero trust principles and blockchain technology. BMC Med Inf Decis Making 20(1):1–10
8. Tanwar S, Parekh K, Evans R (2020) Blockchain-based electronic healthcare record system for healthcare 4.0 applications. J Inf Secur Appl 50:102407
9. Aswin AV et al (2020) Design of AYUSH: a blockchain-based health record management system. In: Inventive communication and computational technologies. Springer, Singapore, pp 665–672
10. Choi Y-J, Kim K-J (2020) Secure healthcare data management and sharing platform based on hyperledger fabric. J Internet Comput Serv 21(1):95–102
11. Jeong J et al (2020) Design and implementation of a digital evidence management model based on hyperledger fabric. J Inf Process Syst 16(4)
12. Mukne H et al (2019) Land record management using hyperledger fabric and IPFS. In: 2019 10th International conference on computing, communication and networking technologies (ICCCNT). IEEE
13. Shamir A. How to share a secret. http://web.mit.edu/6.857/OldStuff/Fall03/ref/Shamir-HowToShareASecret.pdf
14. Ulutas M, Ulutas G, Nabiyev VV. Medical image security and EPR hiding using Shamir's secret sharing scheme. https://www.sciencedirect.com/science/article/pii/S0164121210003274
15. Chattopadhyay AK, Nag A, Singh JP et al (2020) A verifiable multi-secret image sharing scheme using XOR operation and hash function. Multimed Tools Appl. https://doi.org/10.1007/s11042-020-09174-0
16. Nag A, Singh JP, Singh AK (2020) An efficient Boolean based multi-secret image sharing scheme. Multimed Tools Appl 79:16219–16243. https://doi.org/10.1007/s11042-019-07807-7

Attribute-Based Personal Health Record Protection Algorithm for Cloud-Based Healthcare Services

F. Sammy and Gadisa Kana

Abstract Today, personalized health records (PHR) have been created as a forum for the processing of patient data. The practical implementation of PHR in cloud-based technologies raises the security and privacy problems that must be addressed. Even then, such as personal health records, there has been large security implications. This could be created for remote server and considered as cloud storage that is not authorized. The huge percentage of PHR customers and data owners could have a high computation and administrative workload on the resources throughout the methodology; this will limit the functionality and availability of PHR records. The attribute-based patient records security (AHRP) method is used to provide security, integrity, and privacy of data access control in order to create a better resolution to above problems. It offers user access to ensure data security and a privileged feature to authenticate a document before discovering the person's medical details. The encode and decode times are used to assess the system's performance. The result clearly shows that the proposed approach requires less encode and decode time for the appropriate medical data.

Keywords Cloud security · Privacy preserving · Health care · Personal health record · Attribute-based encryption (ABE) · Cryptographic algorithms

1 Introduction

Personal health records (PHR) seem to have become prominent as a forum for the processing of healthcare information. It is some kind of medical records which is associated with both the customer's merchandise and ventures or psychiatric information. The method helps a person to profoundly collect, store, maintain, and share opinions about his health condition. Through distinguishing from regurgitated repetitive clinical experiments or complicated documentation preparation, PHR might

F. Sammy (✉) · G. Kana
Department of Information Technology, Dambi Dollo University, Dembi Dolo, Welega, Ethiopia
e-mail: fvr.sammy@gmail.com

© The Author(s), under exclusive license to Springer Nature Singapore Pte Ltd. 2023
J. K. Mandal and D. De (eds.), *Frontiers of ICT in Healthcare*, Lecture Notes in Networks and Systems 519, https://doi.org/10.1007/978-981-19-5191-6_30

even save expense and risks for clinicians. As smart watches are becoming increasingly intensive, at a certain time and everywhere, clinicians can discover something about all of their own medical conditions. Then, they store the details in cloud.

The PHR maintained mostly in cloud provider PHR is accessed by a proactive competitor, even though it is transmitted on the website or Internet. For retaliation, income, seek retribution, or specific functionality, the competitor can leak out all the person's medical information. Such behaviors can pose a significant threat to a patient. Fortunately, physicians inadvertently relinquish direct control of their medical information while keeping PHRs as cloud providers, requiring each client to encode each PHR record before uploading it to cloud servers. A malignant patient can gain unauthorized access to the data and modify the PHR [1] prior to accessing an authorized recipient (e.g., a doctor). This could cause a problem of diagnostic errors, leading to the patient's condition. These behaviors may pose a significant trouble to the health of patients. Sensitive information including an infection can be integrated into the PHR; quality assurance must be maintained simultaneously during delivery of PHRs to different customers. This is a complex job for a framework to share PHR data securely in cloud applications without exposing the sensitive information about patients.

2 Related Work

Duncan and Whittington [2] integrated an acknowledgment and assessment system for organizations employing cloud natural ecosystems by leveraging goat-starting descriptive and organizational structures. This will establish a fair mechanism to increase the efficiency of cloud-based security verification. Also, the data caretaker as the integrator/framework that enhanced the reliability and maintainability of the system by sustaining and extending the existence of its unstated functional scope is described. The clear goal suit, addressed by Duncan et al. [3], may also deprive an experienced specialist the ability to develop an adapted understanding of the situation through being required to focus on the specific branches rather than the woods in general.

The importance of providing evidence to improve confidence in cloud computing circumstances was explored by Chinnasamy and Deepalakshmi [4]. Following the modification of the standard validation protocol to practicable forms of evidence, it was applied and safety measures were investigated. In [5, 6], the population at large cloud system is inward toward organization is discussed, cloud customers may have a particular degree of internal security operations, and an upgrade of encryption use in the customers' side could be carried around in the direction that moves to a cloud. Low and Chen [7] demanded to organize antioxidant effects and must gain the necessary medicinal services also at negligible cost to clinicians at the desired level of quality and on an ongoing basis that could be done by updating a most suitable manufacturer preference outsourcing device to better respond to resource considerations.

The structure presented here has been recognized by Poulymenopoulou et al. [8] to aid in the evaluation of requirements in settings where adversarial access to social resources has been a legitimate problem in the past. Chinnasamy and Deepalakshmi [9] experimented on a cloud-based solution that is less feasible as a massive data transfer to exchange hospitals and healthcare centers information in the cloud. Chinnasamy et al. [10] addressed keeping in mind the data security of the properties of their customers. Any unauthorized party may unjustly access cloud services to preserve the security of the customer's data.

A safe and protected AROcrypt mechanism to ensure the security of outsourced data was demonstrated in [11]. Security as a Service (SEaaS) also is represented within cloud, and ASCII parameters are being used to transform plain text into cypher text. Kumari and Kamal [12] presented CP-ABE (Ciphertext policy-attribute-based encryption) to provide reliable authentication of legitimacy for encrypted information that have to be transmitted in reasonable protection. The incorporated attribute-based cryptographic approach through bilinear modeling is to enhance privacy protection.

3 The Proposed Method

Through suggested strategies and application information, the framework clarified the conceptual framework. The application design discussed is demonstrated in Fig. 1 including data preprocessing phases of the process and specifications of mathematical functions. In the meanwhile, the framework is introduced to include data access control, confidentiality, integrity, and security. The proposed solution fulfills critical security goals including protection of knowledge and protection of customer data.

4 The Proposed PHR Security Algorithm

In a medical records security algorithm, various attributes are intended to provide anonymity, integrity, and privacy throughout the clouds for fine-grained access control. This is a new and justifiable framework for patient-driven reliable transmission under inter-owner configurations of PHR personal data through distributed cloud computing. Each owners of the PHR and the customers of the PHR has personal relationships within the individual domain. In terms of dealing through PHR users and features, the public domain is focused on a false agent trusted authority of attributes (TAA). A disjointed group of elements or attributes is supervised by each TAA distribution of resources. Although there are no specific systems, the security of everything in this system can still be handled. In addition, in increasing circumstances, the approach addresses strategies for motivating efficient removal of PHR users and drop-glass entry. The proposed method contains four phases including setup, key generation, encoding, and decoding.

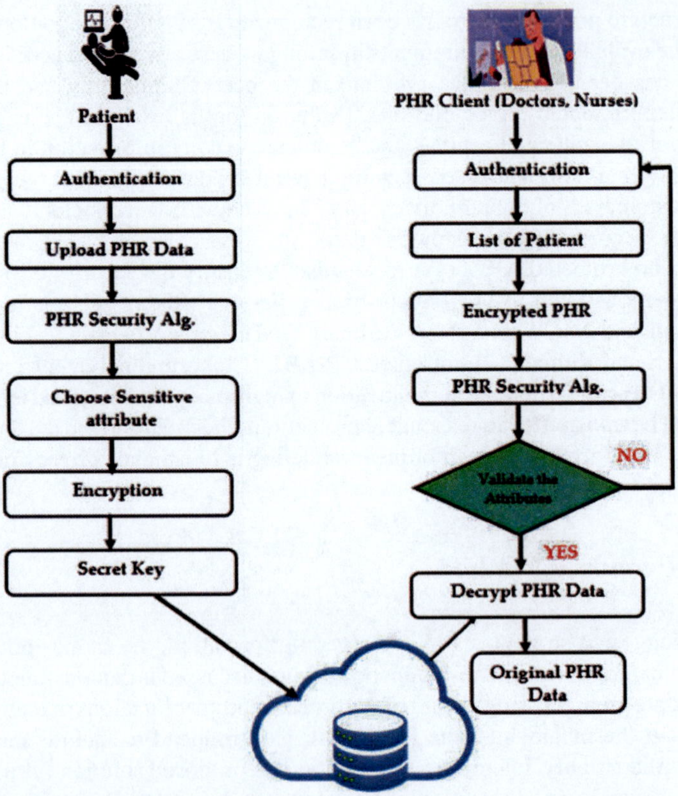

Fig. 1 Process of proposed scheme

4.1 Setup

The initialization phase generates the set of attributes and master secret for our proposed environments as follows:

$$\text{Setup} \rightarrow \text{MSK, SA}$$

4.2 Key Generation

$$\text{KeyGen(MSK, SA)} \rightarrow \text{SK}$$

This procedure runs master secret key (MSK) and set of attributes (SA) as input, producing a secret key for the legitimate user verifying the user attributes (SA_v) and secret key (SK_v).

4.3 Encryption Phase

The encoding stage is performed via a securely encrypted PHR owners or patient who receives the PC's public parameters, a document F together with its subject label, SA_v verification attribute or feature collection, SK_v private key verification, and Y_v (for verification) and Y_e (for encryption) assertion-predicate as outputs. The process will encode F and create a cypher CT text that has collection of parameters and is simply a PHR owner or patient. It satisfies Y_e, which will encrypt and verify the secret key.

$$CT = F, SA_V, SK_V, Y_V Y_e, t$$

4.4 Decryption

A recipient (doctors or nurses) that requires public/open parameters PC, recipient attribute SA_r, an encrypted text CT, and secret key attributes takes as inputs and runs the decoding process. A document F or a declined model is returned by the process.

5 Simulation Settings

The execution function is performed with an Intel i6 Core processor computer, 8 GB of RAM, 1000 GB of storage, and Windows 10. In the creation of PHR-based web applications, we are utilizing NetBeans 8.0.2, JDK 1.8, Apache Tomcat 8.0.15, MYSQL 5.5, and Jelastic cloud environments. In this, Jelastic cloud is being used to launch efficient web applications for PHRs data to protect and accurate data exchange between client, doctor, and insurers provider geographically. Several forms of medical records PHR with distinct formats (document, paper, and PDF) together with previous techniques are anticipated throughout the proposed methodology.

6 Performance Evaluation

For the proposed system, the section represents a computational interpretation to measure the PHR data-sharing performance, protection, and cost-effectiveness. The developed system operates on both the owners or patient of PHR and the user of PHR (doctors or nurses). The system design has data storage server efficiency and operates independently for enhancing secure data sharing and PHRs data retrieving. The performance evaluation of this technique is measured against existing methods in terms of key generation, encoding, and decoding processing time.

Pursuant to Figs. 2 and 3 findings, an algorithm based on attribute medical records security (AMR) is tested via traditional techniques with encryption time and decryption time. The highest accuracy of descriptive statistics forms, including text, document, and multimedia data, would be the proposed attribute-based algorithm. The proposed method is calculated on consideration of an encode and decode time of IKGSR and developed approaches. Also for intention of public-key cryptosystems as well as message authentication, the IKGSR approach is really a traditional encryption paradigm which really recognizes each data file as a numerical. The RSA system, furthermore, used enormous storage and time complexity.

The SHA1 + AES, furthermore, consumes a lot of time for encryption and decryption processing. In [11], technique is being used to encrypt a confidential non-statistical unit documents. If customers upload a combination of confidential info

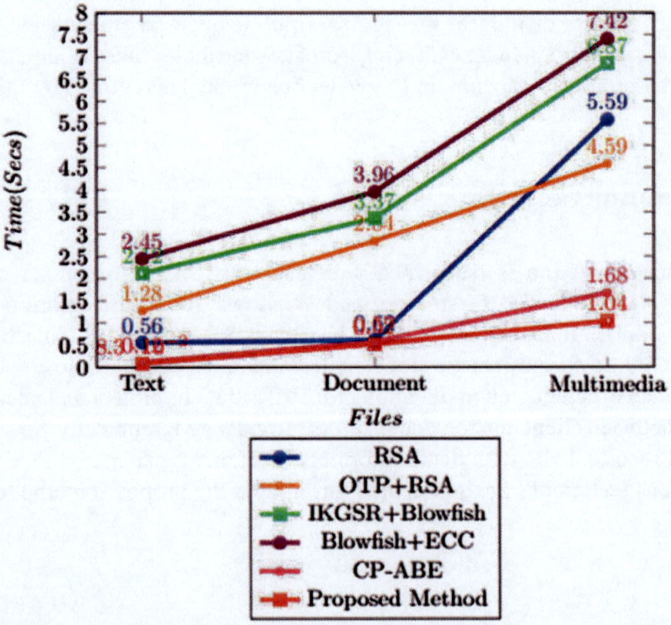

Fig. 2 Comparison of encryption time with different files

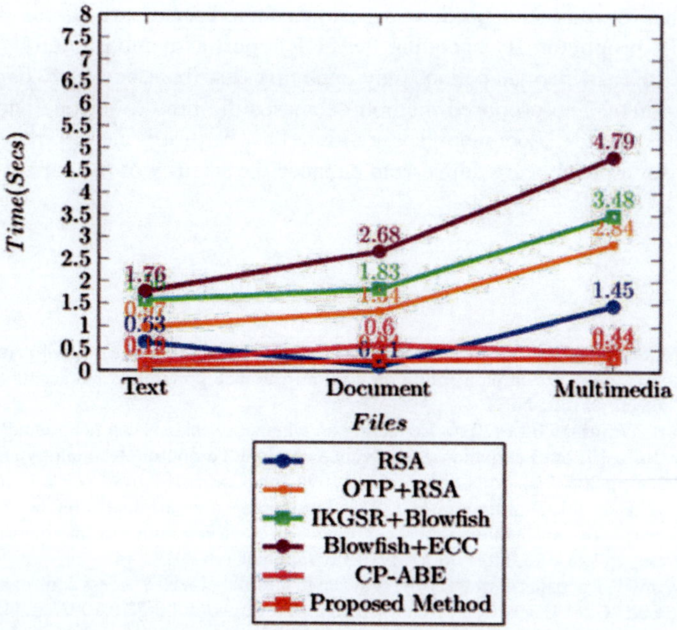

Fig. 3 Comparison of decryption time with different files

files that are numeric and non-numeric data, the AROcrypt, furthermore, encrypts non-numerical data as well as other forms of files of numerically sensitive data. However, highly confidential files are not secured, which would not be a guarantee through a public cloud storage.

The developed system safeguards highly confidential files and provides protection mostly on public cloud provider. CP-ABE on aggregate parameters was its suggested nearest opponent process. To accomplish forward as well as backward security, the CP-ABE [12] methodology has been used. The proposed methodology helps in improving the quality of encryption and decryption efficiency. The medical records security algorithm based on attributes decreases 0.364 in seconds and 0.188 in seconds with respect to encode and decode process.

7 Conclusion

The paper discusses attribute-based medical records cryptographic algorithms to provide confidentiality, integrity, and privacy for data access control. It is also providing secured data access control as well as a secure method toward verifying a text against revealing its personal data. In this, the owner of the PHR ensures complete access to control regarding everyone's PHR results. The proposed method is being used for rudimentary encoding, and its shared secret structure is generated by any PHR proprietor. By encoding the PHR report as demonstrated by a set of features, a PHR owners or patient may explicitly distribute any PHR data with a set of customers. The proposed method decreases the time to encode and decode different files like text, document, and multimedia. The results clearly show that it is applicable for all healthcare domains to enhance the security of the patient data.

References

1. Scholl M, Stine K, Hash J, Bowen P, Johnson A, Smith CD, Steinberg DI (2008) An introductory resource guide for implementing the health insurance portability and accountability act (HIPAA) security rule. NIST
2. Duncan B, Whittington M (2014) Reflecting on whether checklists can tick the box for cloud security. In: IEEE 6th international conference on cloud computing technology and science. IEEE Press, pp 805–810. https://doi.org/10.1109/CloudCom.2014.165
3. Duncan B, Pym DJ, Whittington M (2013) Developing a conceptual framework for cloud security assurance. In: 5th International conference on cloud computing technology and science. IEEE Press, pp 120–125. https://doi.org/10.1109/CloudCom.2013.144
4. Chinnasamy P, Deepalakshmi P (2018) A scalable multilabel-based access control as a service for the cloud. Trans Emerg Telecommun Technol 29. https://doi.org/10.1002/ett.3458
5. Chinnasamy P, Deepalakshmi P, Shankar K (2020) An analysis of security access control on healthcare records in the cloud. In: Intelligent data-centric systems, intelligent data security solutions for e-health applications. Academic Press, pp 113–130. https://doi.org/10.1016/B978-0-12-819511-6.00006-6
6. Chinnasamy P, Ganesan A, Prasathkumar V, Praveena V (2020) A trusted-role based access control model for secure cloud storage. Int J Adv Sci Technol 29(9s):3253–3259
7. Low C, Chen Y (2012) Criteria for the evaluation of a cloud-based hospital information system outsourcing provider. J Med Syst 36:3543–3553. https://doi.org/10.1007/s10916-012-9829-z
8. Poulymenopoulou M, Malamateniou F, Vassilacopoulos G (2011) Emergency healthcare process automation using mobile computing and cloud services. J Med Syst 36:3233–3241. https://doi.org/10.1007/s10916-011-9814-y
9. Chinnasamy P, Deepalakshmi P (2018) Design of secure storage for health-care cloud using hybrid cryptography. In: 2nd International conference on inventive communication and computational technologies. IEEE Press, pp 1717–1720. https://doi.org/10.1109/ICICCT.2018.8473107
10. Chinnasamy P, Padmavathi S, Swathy R, Rakesh S (2020) Efficient data security using hybrid cryptography on cloud computing. In: Lecture notes in networks and systems. Springer, Singapore, pp 537–547. https://doi.org/10.1007/978-981-15-7345-3_46
11. Monikandan S, Arockiam L (2014) A security service algorithm to ensure the confidentiality of data in cloud storage. Int J Eng Res Technol 3:1053–1058
12. Kumari S, Kamal AR (2016) Optimal integrity policy for encrypted data in secure storage using cloud computing. Indian J Sci Technol 9(8):1–10. https://doi.org/10.17485/ijst/2016/v9i11/88453

Pixel Interpolation Followed by Prediction Error Expansion-Based Reversible Information Hiding Algorithm for Securing Healthcare Data

Sakhi Bandyopadhyay, Sunita Sarkar, Subhadip Mukherjee, and Somnath Mukhopadhyay

Abstract Reversible information hiding is a type of data concealing in which the cover picture can be retrieved after the embedded data has been extracted. We presented an information concealing strategy based on linear interpolation and prediction error expansion in this research for securing healthcare-related information. A well-predicted technique for the pixels is required for the supremacy of a prediction error expansion (PEE)-based information hiding system. The picture is recursively decomposed into triangles for forming a B-tree structure for the data embedding. The suggested prediction technique uses the vertices for concealing the private bits. The planar linear interpolation of the vertex pixels is anticipated for every pixel within the triangle or on its sides. By increasing the prediction error, private data bits are inserted in pixels. Furthermore, according to the findings of the experiments, two bits can be hidden within a single pixel. Extensive experiments demonstrate the suggested method's higher performance.

Keywords Reversible data hiding · Linear interpolation · B-tree · PEE · Information security

1 Introduction

Since it has the capability to recover the cover picture without any distortion in any pixel values, information hiding with reversibility is also called lossless information hiding [1, 2]. As a result, it has uses in medicine, the military, and satellites [3]. The literature has a number of information concealment strategies [4]. The DE-based method in [5] is a well-known algorithm for reversible information concealing. By extending the difference between two pixels, it incorporated one-bit data. Several notable research efforts have advanced this topic since the introduction of the first approach in this sector. In [6], a vector of nearby pixels was employed. To hide the

S. Bandyopadhyay (✉) · S. Sarkar · S. Mukherjee · S. Mukhopadhyay
Department of Computer Science and Engineering, Assam University, Silchar, Assam 788011, India
e-mail: banerjeesakhi18@gmail.com

© The Author(s), under exclusive license to Springer Nature Singapore Pte Ltd. 2023
J. K. Mandal and D. De (eds.), *Frontiers of ICT in Healthcare*, Lecture Notes in Networks and Systems 519, https://doi.org/10.1007/978-981-19-5191-6_31

private bits into the enlarged gaps between a referred element in the vector and the items inside the vector, an integer transform has been proposed. The data bits in [6] were inserted using four adjacent pixels of size 2×2 with the help of the differences among a pixel's neighbours. To boost embedding capacity even more, [7] suggests using a companying strategy. The incidence of overflow/underflow is a prevalent concern with these strategies. If after embedding, the altered values of the pixels do not belong to the range 0–255, overflow/underflow occurs. To avoid the aforesaid scenario, a location map is utilized to define the places where hiding must not be performed. This picture must have a location map included in it. When compared to the technique in [6], it has much improved embedding capacity. Furthermore, in a DE-based method, an intelligent pairing of pixels avoids the necessity for the location map on overflow. In a recent technique [8], the gap among the most significant bits of the neighboring pixels was calculated to hide private bits.

The notion of PEE is a development of the DE concept. The change between the pixel value of the cover picture and its expected value is extended to integrate the data in PEE-based algorithms. When compared to standard DE-based methodologies, these strategies perform better in general. The PEE-based RDH method was initially published in [9]. Since then, a great deal of study has been done in this area. They vary in the following aspects: (i) embedding process and (ii) prediction technique. The DT-based technique [10], on the other hand, uses a collection of randomly dispersed pixels to generate triangles according to the DT attribute. This condition assures that no additional vertex is located within a circumcircle of Delaunay triangle. It is not based on the proximity of values between non-vertex and vertex pixels. The following are our contributions: (i) linear interpolation over the pixels in the vertices is anticipated for every pixel within the triangle or on its sides. (ii) Recursive decomposition, using triangular forms, is to determine and anticipate the related pixels. (iii) PE expansion is utilized to add two private bits to a pixel. (iv) The prediction error is minimized by using an iterative technique to revising the prediction value.

The remainder of this paper is organized as follows: Literature review of information hiding strategies are discussed in Sect. 2. In Sect. 3, the proposed scheme is illustrated. Experimental results are analyzed in Sect. 4. In Sect. 5, the conclusion is stated.

2 Literature Review

The picture is partitioned into non-overlapping pieces using a pixel value ordering or PVO-based technique [11]. The values of the pixels are then arranged in ascending order within this chunk. After that, for the highest and lowest values, the second largest and second smallest elements are cast-off to forecast them, respectively. The approaches based on PVO in [12, 13] build on the work in [11]. The limitation of partitions of fixed blocks in PVO-oriented methods has been eliminated in PPVO prediction [14] scheme, which is a version of the aforementioned techniques. A prediction in PPVO depends on the sorting the reference pixels. An obtuse angle is needed to be formed between the boundary lines of the current and context pixels; from the satisfaction of this condition, the context pixels are chosen [15]. In this situation, PPVO-based prediction is used.

In 2007, Thodi and Rodríguez [9] developed a PEE-based information hiding method using a median edge detector (MED) which is a lossless image coding technique [16]. A pixel is projected using top-left neighbors, left, and top based on the existence of a line at either the top or the left of it, according to MED predictor. In [17], right-lower, lower, and right neighbors were used in a modified variant of the MED predictor. Gradient adjusted predictor [18] makes advantage of vertical and horizontal gradients in a pixel's immediate neighbor. Several studies have employed this predictor for RDH, despite the fact that it was initially developed for image coding. The direction (horizontal or vertical) is chosen based on which of these two orientations has the lowest prediction error. Naskar and Chakraborty [19] developed a prediction method depending on a median of neighbour pixel with weightage. For reversible information hiding, least square predictor is used in [20] for localize prediction. Prediction using least square method is performed by centering each pixel in a square-shaped block. As a result, for each block, this prediction's coefficients vary, and it also has the effect of using a unique predictor for every squared block. The proposed study is further motivated by the fact that pixel values for PE expansion-based information hiding may be predicted using an image coding technique. This research proposes a unique reversible information hiding strategy based on the expansion of prediction error and linear interpolation for solving above-mentioned problems.

3 Proposed Method

The picture is divided into triangles in a recursive manner until a given condition is met (see Fig. 1). The flowchart of the proposed method is shown in Fig. 2. The picture plane is split into reasonably smooth smaller sections as a result of this. As a result, the variations in pixel values between a triangle's vertices and adjacent triangle pixels are tiny. In the smoother portions of the picture, larger triangles may be seen, while the rougher regions are divided into tiny triangles. Furthermore, higher threshold values result in larger triangles on average. Unlike [21], which decomposes the picture into two triangles based on prediction errors, the suggested technique decomposes the image using cover image pixel values. The reference pixels are the triangles' vertices. The linear interpolation of the triangle's vertices is used to forecast the intended pixels in a triangle. The enlarged prediction errors of the pixels contain payload bits. As a result, before decomposition, the suggested technique does not need the projected values. Instead, the decomposition is done to get the expected values. The value determined by employing a triangle, which might be visited later on, replaces the prior projected value. During extraction, the sequence of the visited triangles is preserved to provide the similar anticipated values of those pixels. The prediction error is reduced when the threshold is set to a lower value. This is due to the fact that smaller thresholds result in smoother triangles.

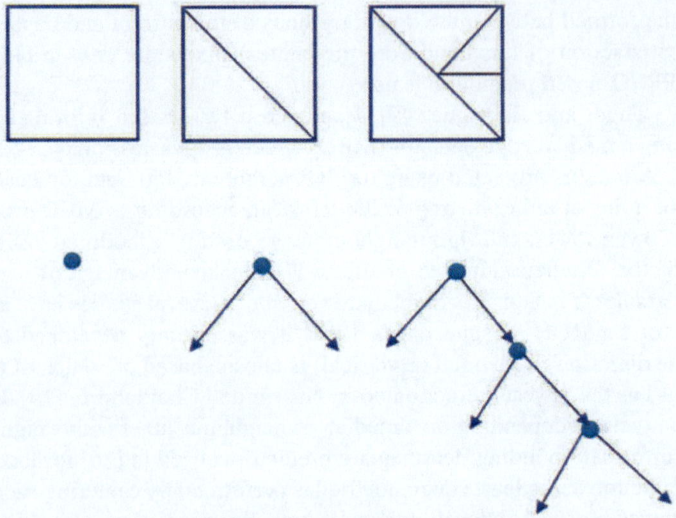

Fig. 1 Image decomposition into triangles and forming a B-tree structure

Fig. 2 Flowchart of the proposed method

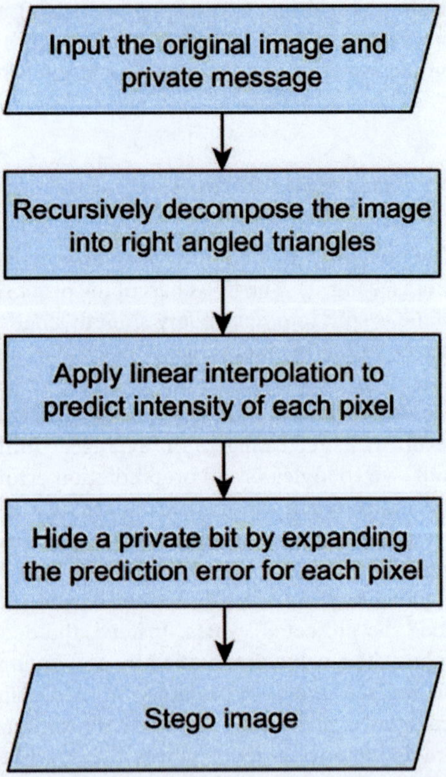

3.1 Data Embedding

Step 1: Input private message and an image.

Step 2: Recursively decompose the image into two triangles having a 90° angle until the pixels in the afresh-generated triangles satisfy any one of the following conditions:

(i) $n_T \leq 5$, where n_T is the number of pixels in a triangle including the pixels on the sides.

(ii) $|P_{v_{max}} - P_{v_{min}}| \leq T$, where T is the threshold, $P_{v_{max}}$ is the maximum pixel value and $P_{v_{min}}$ is the minimum pixel value in a triangle.

Step 3: For the intensity values I_1, I_2 and I_3 of the vertices (x_1, y_1), (x_2, y_2) and (x_3, y_3) of any right-angled triangle, every pixel (x, y) on the sides or on the vertices of the triangle is predicted by performing the linear interpolation over vertices as expressed in Eq. 1:

$$I'(x, y) = I_1 + \alpha * (I_2 - I_1) + \beta * (I_3 - I_1) \tag{1}$$

where α and β are defined by Eqs. 2 and 3, respectively.

$$\alpha = \frac{(y_3 - y_1)(x - x_1) - (x_3 - x_1)(y - y_1)}{(y_3 - y_1)(x_2 - x_1) - (x_3 - x_1)(y_2 - y_1)} \tag{2}$$

$$\beta = \frac{(y - y_1)(x_2 - x_1) - (x - x_1)(y_2 - y_1)}{(y_3 - y_1)(x_2 - x_1) - (x_3 - x_1)(y_2 - y_1)} \tag{3}$$

Step 4: Compute the prediction error by differencing between the predicted pixel $I'(x, y)$ and original pixel $I(x, y)$ using Eq. 4.

$$\text{PE}(x, y) = I(x, y) - I'(x, y) \tag{4}$$

Step 5: Embed two bits $b_1 b_2$ of the private message using the following Eq. 5.

$$Ib = I + 3 * \text{PE} + b \tag{5}$$

where $b = 2 * b_1 + b_2$ and I_b and I are the pixels after and before data hiding, respectively.

Step 6: Repeat Step 5 until all the secret bits are embedded and obtain the marked image.

3.2 Data Extraction

Step 1: Input the marked image.
Step 2: Obtain the prediction error using Eq. 6

$$\mathrm{PE}_b = I_b - I' \tag{6}$$

Step 3: Extract the secret bits using Eq. 7 and reconstruct the original image using Eq. 8, where $b \in 0, 1, 2, 3$.

$$b = \lfloor \mathrm{PE}_b \rfloor - 4\left\lfloor \frac{\mathrm{PE}_b}{4} \right\rfloor \tag{7}$$

$$I = I_b - 3\left| \frac{\mathrm{PE}_b}{4} \right| - b \tag{8}$$

Step 4: Obtain the private message and the original image.

4 Experimental Results and Analyses

For assessing the performance of the proposed data concealing strategy, a set of eight standard test pictures (as shown in Fig. 3) of size 512×512 are used from the

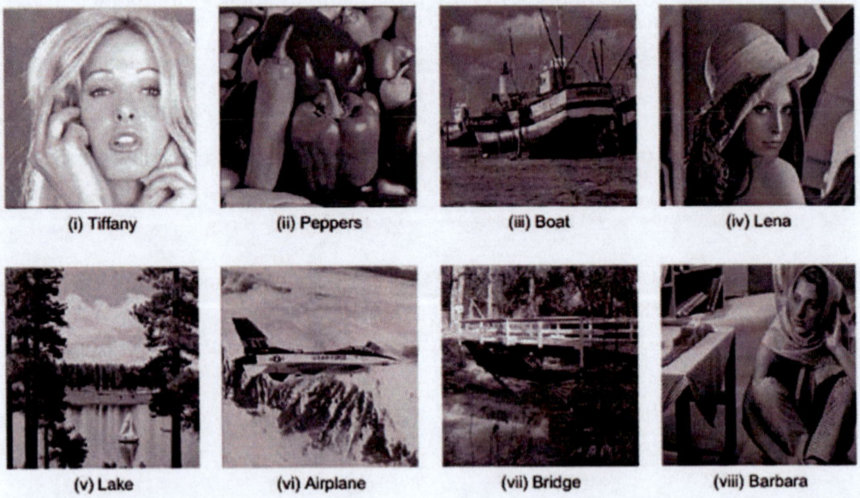

Fig. 3 Test images taken for experiments

Table 1 Different PSNR values for different thresholds from 1 to 10 for 1.7 bpp of EC

Images	Thresholds										Selected (threshold, PSNR)
	1	2	3	4	5	6	7	8	9	10	
Tiffany	55.47	54.80	55.62	54.94	54.72	55.38	54.59	53.98	55.61	54.42	(3, 55.62)
Peppers	54.65	55.81	55.12	54.95	55.88	55.32	56.06	55.96	56.01	55.57	(7, 56.06)
Boat	55.20	55.05	54.75	55.14	55.23	54.84	54.53	54.28	55.17	55.60	(5, 55.23)
Lena	54.49	55.18	53.97	54.85	54.78	54.21	54.54	55.05	53.62	53.55	(2, 55.18)
Lake	56.58	56.21	55.84	56.33	56.01	56.71	56.22	55.52	55.87	56.45	(6, 56.71)
Airplane	55.40	56.39	55.64	56.09	54.89	55.65	55.32	56.15	55.95	55.77	(2, 56.39)
Bridge	55.39	55.38	55.96	55.16	55.96	55.26	55.48	54.67	55.44	55.01	(3, 55.96) and (5, 55.96)
Barbara	55.35	55.48	55.76	55.83	55.53	54.68	54.95	55.25	55.66	54.62	(4, 55.83)

Table 2 Comparison of PSNR and EC

Images	[25]		[17]		[23]		[24]		Proposed	
	PSNR	EC	PSNR	EC	PSNR	EC	PSNR	EC	PSNR	EC
Tiffany	59.58	1.5	40.62	0.29	56.72	1.4	40.31	0.6	55.62	1.7
Peppers	59.69	1.5	41.13	0.29	55.95	1.4	41.68	0.6	56.06	1.7
Boat	60.55	1.5	40.46	0.29	57.36	1.4	42.01	0.6	55.23	1.7
Lena	58.89	1.5	39.87	0.29	58.20	1.4	38.40	0.6	55.18	1.7
Lake	58.64	1.5	41.06	0.29	58.03	1.4	41.77	0.6	56.71	1.7
Airplane	60.81	1.5	40.71	0.29	56.44	1.4	42.10	0.6	56.39	1.7
Idge	58.94	1.5	40.74	0.29	55.30	1.4	39.14	0.6	55.96	1.7
Barbara	59.45	1.5	41.92	0.29	58.47	1.4	42.05	0.6	55.83	1.7

Table 3 Comparison of PSNR and EC

Metric	MPX1008 synpic48839	MPX1013 synpic34889	MPX1022 synpic17321	MPX1024 synpic40272	MPX1026 synpic32821	MPX1033 synpic45449
PSNR	55.71	56.12	56.22	55.75	55.86	56.04
EC	1.7	1.7	1.7	1.7	1.7	1.7

SIPI database [22]. A test picture is recursively decomposed into B-tree structured triangles based on an appropriate decomposition threshold T, and the pixel prediction is associated with linearly interpolated pixels, according to our suggested technique. Because good prediction results in reduced distortion, an appropriate threshold value for each of the test pictures is chosen by evaluating the peak signal-to-noise ratio (PSNR) in the range of 1–10.

In Table 1, different PSNR values are shown for different thresholds ranging from 1 to 10 for 1.7 bpp of embedding capacity. In the last column, the suitable T is selected to get the maximum PSNR value for each test image. For example, the threshold 7 is selected because for $T = 7$ the proposed method gives the maximum PSNR value, i.e., 56.06 dB. For the image Sailboat, it can be observed that there are two threshold values, i.e., 3 and 5, for which it gives same and highest PSNR value, i.e., 55.96 dB.

In Table 2, a comparison of the proposed method with other methods [17, 23–25] is shown. From this table, it can be observed that [23] has achieved, minimum 58.64 dB of PSNR for image Lake and maximum 60.81 dB of PSNR for image Airplane, whereas the proposed method has achieved minimum 55.18 dB of PSNR for the image Lena and maximum 56.71 dB of PSNR for the image Lake. The average PSNRs of [17, 23–25] are 59.57 dB, 40.81 dB, 57.06 dB and 40.93 dB, respectively. The average PSNR of the proposed method is 55.87 dB which is lesser that [23, 25] because the EC of the proposed scheme is higher than [23, 25]. But the schemes [17, 24] both has achieved lesser average PSNR value and lesser EC than the proposed method.

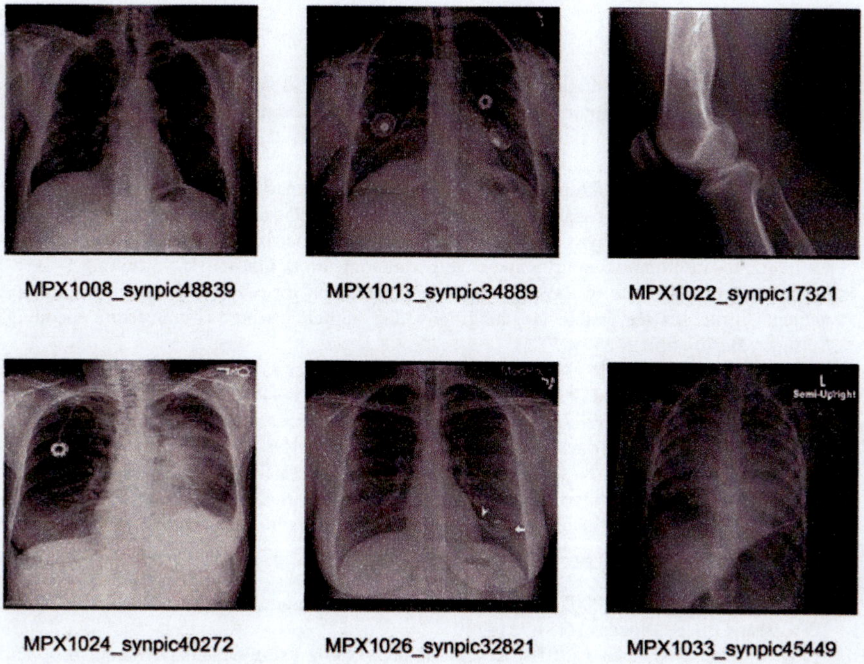

Fig. 4 Medical test images

In Table 3, the outcomes of PSNR and EC of some medical images, taken from the image database [26], are shown in Fig. 4. Like the standard test images, the medical images can also hide 1.7 bpp of healthcare information inside. The qualities of the stego images are also impressive, and human cannot detect whether any information hidden inside the images or not.

5 Conclusion

This paper proposes a novel information hiding scheme based on linear interpolation and expansion of prediction error. The proposed method decomposes the cover image recursively into a B-tree structure. The recursive decomposition process continues until the triangle's pixels are homogenous or the triangle is too tiny to breakdown. Using this B-tree triangular decomposition and planar linear interpolation, the suggested prediction technique beats numerous other known predictors. It is to be noted that the proposed scheme is capable to hide 1.7 bpp with an average 55.87 dB of PSNR to ensure the robustness of the method since it is essential for several security applications such as medical data security and satellite image security.

References

1. Mukherjee S, Sarkar S, Mukhopadhyay S (2021) A LSB substitution-based steganography technique using DNA computing for colour images. In: Proceedings of international conference on innovations in software architecture and computational systems. Springer, Berlin, pp 109–117
2. Mukherjee S, Sarkar S, Mukhopadhyay S (2021) Pencil shell matrix based image steganography with elevated embedding capacity. J Inf Secur Appl 62:102955
3. Mukherjee S, Mukhopadhyay S, Sarkar S (2022) A shell-matrix-based image steganography technique for multimedia security and covert communication. Innov Syst Softw Eng 1–16
4. Mandal JK (2020) State of the art in transform encoding for reversible steganography and authentication. In: Reversible steganography and authentication via transform encoding. Springer, Berlin, pp 19–26
5. Mukherjee S, Jana B (2019) A novel method for high capacity reversible data hiding scheme using difference expansion. Int J Nat Comput Res (IJNCR) 8(4):13–27
6. Alattar AM (2004) Reversible watermark using the difference expansion of a generalized integer transform. IEEE Trans Image Process 13(8):1147–1156
7. Weng S, Zhao Y, Pan JS, Ni R (2007) A novel reversible watermarking based on an integer transform. In: 2007 IEEE International conference on image processing, vol 3. IEEE, pp III–241
8. Lakshmi H, Borra S (2021) Difference expansion based reversible watermarking algorithms for copyright protection of images: state-of-the-art and challenges. Int J Speech Technol 24(4):823–852
9. Thodi DM, Rodríguez JJ (2007) Expansion embedding techniques for reversible watermarking. IEEE Trans Image Process 16(3):721–730
10. Hong W, Chen TS, Chen J (2015) Reversible data hiding using Delaunay triangulation and selective embedment. Inf Sci 308:140–154
11. Li X, Li J, Li B, Yang B (2013) High-fidelity reversible data hiding scheme based on pixel-value-ordering and prediction-error expansion. Signal Process 93(1):198–205
12. Kaur G, Singh S, Rani R (2021) PVO based reversible data hiding technique for roughly textured images. Multidimension Syst Signal Process 32(2):533–558
13. Tang X, Zhou L, Tang G, Wen Y, Cheng Y (2021) Improved fluctuation derived block selection strategy in pixel value ordering based reversible data hiding. In: International workshop on digital watermarking. Springer, Berlin, pp 163–177
14. Qu X, Kim HJ (2015) Pixel-based pixel value ordering predictor for high-fidelity reversible data hiding. Signal Process 111:249–260
15. Xiang H, Liu H (2017) A pixel-based reversible data hiding method based on obtuse angle prediction. In: 2017 2nd International conference on multimedia and image processing (ICMIP). IEEE, pp 191–195
16. Weinberger MJ, Seroussi G, Sapiro G (2000) The LOCO-I lossless image compression algorithm: principles and standardization into JPED-LS. IEEE Trans Image Process 9(8):1309–1324
17. Coltuc D (2011) Improved embedding for prediction-based reversible watermarking. IEEE Trans Inf Forensics Secur 6(3):873–882
18. Wu X, Memon N (1997) Context-based, adaptive, lossless image coding. IEEE Trans Commun 45(4):437–444
19. Naskar R, Chakraborty R (2012) Reversible watermarking utilising weighted median-based prediction. IET Image Process 6(5):507–520
20. Dragoi IC, Coltuc D (2014) Local-prediction-based difference expansion reversible watermarking. IEEE Trans Image Process 23(4):1779–1790
21. Distasi R, Nappi M, Vitulano S (1997) Image compression by b-tree triangular coding. IEEE Trans Commun 45(9):1095–1100
22. USCID Image Database. http://sipi.usc.edu/database/

23. Dragoi IC, Coltuc D (2018) Improved pairwise embedding for high-fidelity reversible data hiding. In: 2018 26th European signal processing conference (EUSIPCO). IEEE, pp 1412–1416
24. Lu TC, Chen CM, Lin MC, Huang YH (2017) Multiple predictors hiding scheme using asymmetric histograms. Multimedia Tools Appl 76(3):3361–3382
25. Wang W, Ye J, Wang T, Wang W (2017) Reversible data hiding scheme based on significant-bit-difference expansion. IET Image Process 11(11):1002–1014
26. National Library of Medicine . https://openi.nlm.nih.gov/

Healthcare in COVID-19 Scenario

Similarity Study of Spike Protein of Coronavirus by PCA Using Physical Properties of Amino Acids

Jayanta Pal, Soumen Ghosh, Bansibadan Maji, and Dilip Kumar Bhattacharya

Abstract The properties of amino acids, some of which are physical or chemical in nature, are found to have a significant role in comparing sequences of proteins of different species. In similarity/dissimilarity study of sequences of proteins, normally, an arbitrary combination of such properties is used. In the present study, all five known physical properties of amino acids are taken into consideration. It may be remarked that comparison of DNA sequences is more frequent than that of protein sequences, as DNA sequence contains four nucleotides, whereas protein sequence contains twenty amino acids. In sequences of protein, the complexity of spatial information is relatively high. The principal component technique, which is based on the numerical values of the aforesaid five properties of amino acids, is used to reduce space complexity. As a result, twenty TP values are obtained corresponding to twenty amino acids. Non-degenerate representations of each protein sequence under comparison are obtained by adding these represented values cumulatively. Now, non-central moments of order j are defined referred to minimum value of each sequence. Finally, three-dimensional descriptors are defined involving such non-central moments of order one, two, and three. Next, to obtain the distance matrix, measure of distance is taken to be Euclidean. Finally, the UPGMA algorithm is used to generate phylogeny using the distance matrix. The proposed approach is tested on sequences of 50 coronavirus spike protein. The current method's result is found to be comparable to those produced earlier for the same species using other methods, and they agree with their biological references as well. Furthermore, the process requires less space.

Keywords Distance matrix · Moment vector · Physical property · Principal component analysis (PCA) · Spike protein · TP value · UPGMA algorithm

---

P. Jayanta (✉) · G. Soumen
Narula Institute of Technology, Kolkata, India
e-mail: jayanta.pal@gmail.com

P. Jayanta · G. Soumen · M. Bansibadan
National Institute of Technology, Durgapur, India

B. Dilip Kumar
Calcutta University, Kolkata, India

© The Author(s), under exclusive license to Springer Nature Singapore Pte Ltd. 2023

J. K. Mandal and D. De (eds.), *Frontiers of ICT in Healthcare*, Lecture Notes in Networks and Systems 519, https://doi.org/10.1007/978-981-19-5191-6_32

1 Introduction

In the field of bioinformatics, comparing DNA and protein sequences remains a difficult task. Two forms of analysis have been discovered in the similarity study of protein sequence: alignment based and alignment free. However, because of some constraints of alignment based methods, alignment free techniques are preferable. There are various approaches for comparing sequences of protein, but references are provided only for those articles that compare sequences of proteins on the basis of properties (either physical or chemical) of the constituent amino acids. For example, using relative weight, a well-known physical property and hydrophobicity, a well-known chemical property of amino acids, a three-dimensional graphical representation is developed in [1]. Unfortunately, it is a degenerate representation, as the whole sequence of an individual protein is represented by twenty distinct three-dimensional points only. It is desirable to check that the representation ceases to be degenerate before the descriptors are calculated. In [2], authors consider amino acid's chemical properties such as pKa NH^{3+} and pKa COOH. In biochemistry, these characteristics are essential because they may be utilised to generate a protein map. These features can also be used to determine enzyme activity. The authors of [3] use isoelectric point and hydrophobicity value, two indices relating to the physical and chemical characteristics, respectively, of 20 amino acids, and applied the same, resulting in a non-degenerate graphical form of representation. The cosine of the correlation angle, as well as the distance between two vectors associated with the two curves previously produced, is then determined. The final descriptor is a ratio of these two. In [4], a model is presented based on position-feature for comparing sequence of proteins by measuring graph energy. The representation's physiochemical attributes include pI and pKa values. A typical B-vector emerges from this representation. The relative entropy, which represents B-vectors, is then used to calculate the similarity or dissimilarity. The results acquired by this method shows significant meaning when compared to those obtained by other methods. In [5], one more physical property side-chain mass and one more chemical property hydrophobicity are considered to obtain two-dimensional representation. As a result, the "2D-MH" curve is generated, with "H" representing hydrophobic quantity and "M" representing mass of the amino acid side-chain. This too comes out as degenerate representation. In [6], 2D mapping is utilised to create two-dimensional representation in graphical form. The coordinates are calculated based on only two chemical properties viz., the pKa NH3 value and pKa COOH value. Alignment of protein can also be shown in this diagram. In [7], only six physiochemical parameters corresponding to all the twenty amino acids are explored in a unique two-dimensional graphical form. This graphical representation is used to compute the distance between 2 sequences that are to be examined. Advantage of the method is that it remains unaffected difference in length of the sequence under examination. In [8], only twelve fundamental physicochemical properties are used to demonstrate a new mapping technique for comparing some sequences of protein. Principal component analysis is used to calculate the proportion of amino acids present on 12 principal axes only. Accordingly, a simplified 2D representation of sequence of proteins is obtained. Finally, a 20-dimensional vector is selected as a descriptor for all of the sequences under comparison. The descriptor is independent of sequence length. This proposed approach is first tested on ND6 proteins dataset, then on haemagglutinin genes from influenza A isolates and on several others sequences of protein. In all cases, the method works well. In [9], authors propose a 2D graphical depiction of sequence of proteins based on another six random physicochemical attributes. The author employs numerical characterisation generated from a two-dimensional graphical representation for the descriptor. It demonstrates its utility in comparing protein sequences as well as encoding native protein structural information. Finally, the proposed approach is tested using eight different species' of ND6 proteins. The author of [10] uses a strong technique for protein sequence categorization based on protein mapping. This approach's unique feature, which distinguishes it from rest of its kind, is that it provides computing efficiency, specially for huge amounts of data. Another crucial point is that it takes into account amino acid phylogeny factors when making mutations. For this, ten distinct amino acid physiochemical properties are used. This is yet another random selection. In [11], author uses indices of only three physicochemical parameters, such as PH, PI, and Hp, to transform a protein sequences into a 23-dimensional vector. Finally, the similarity or dissimilarity of ND5 proteins from nine different species is calculated using Euclidean distance. In [12], a completely new form of IFSis introduced based on four entirely random and arbitrarily chosen physicochemical properties of amino acids, viz., pK1, h, pK2, and pI. This results in a 2D graphical representation. This is applied in the similarity/dissimilarity analysis of 9 ND5 and 8 ND6 sequences of proteins. Method of principal component analysis is also used in comparison of protein sequences in [13]. Although both of [8, 8] use PCA approach for comparison of sequences of protein successfully, still arbitrary and random combination of physical and chemical characteristics of amino acids are taken into account. This remains a haphazard mixture of chemical and physical properties. So it is still debatable what occurs if only chemical or only physical properties are taken into account. In this study, only some physical properties are considered. It would be fascinating to see whether some new descriptors could be discovered and further research be conducted using those new descriptors for comparing sequences of different types of proteins. These are the two motivations of this paper.

2 Methodology

(i) The current technique considers all known five physical properties of amino acids listed in Table 1, out of all of their physical and chemical properties. To lower the dimension, PCA is applied to all of the values of the considered qualities (on a 20×5 matrix) that results in 20 TP values based on the least eigenvalue.

(ii) Now, cumulative sum is taken for all such TP values to obtain a non-degenerate representation of the sequences of protein under comparison.

Table 1 Value of five physical properties of amino acids

Amino acid	Sym.	Relative dis. RD	Side-chain class	Residue volume	Residue Wt	Mole vol
Alanine	S	0.2227	15	43.5	71.08	31
Cysteine	C	1.000	47	60.6	103.14	55
Methionine	M	0.1882	75	77.1	131.191	105
Proline	P	0.2513	41	60.8	97.12	32.5
Valine V	V	0.1119	43	81	99.13	84
Phenylalanine	F	0.2370	91	91.3	147.17	132
Isoleucine	I	0.1569	57	107.5	113.16	111
Leucine	L	0.1872	57	107.5	113.16	111
Tryptophan	W	0.4496	130	105.1	186.21	170
Tyrosine	Y	0.1686	107	121.3	163.18	136
Aspartic acid	D	0.3924	59	123.6	115.09	54
Lysine	K	0.1739	72	144.1	128.17	119
asparagine	N	0.2513	58	78.0	114.10	56
Arginine	R	0.0366	100	90.4	156.19	124
Serine	S	0.2815	31	74.1	87.08	32
Glutamic acid	E	0.1819	73	93.9	129.12	83
Glycine	G	0.3229	1	108.5	57.05	3
Histidine	H	0.0201	81	111.5	137.14	96
Glutamine	Q	0.0366	72	99.3	128.13	85
Threonine	T	0	45	72.5	101.11	61

(iii) Now, non-central moments of order j are defined with respect

(i) To the minimum value of the sequence given as follows:

$$M^j = \frac{1}{N}\sum_{k=1}^{N}(x_i - m)^j, k = 1, 2, \ldots, N$$

where (x_i), $i = 1, 2, \ldots, N$ is the numerically represented sequence of protein and $m =$ minimum of all x_i.

(ii) Descriptors are taken as three component vectors comprising of moments of orders one, two, and three.

(iii) Distance matrix is calculated by taking Euclidean distance as the distance measure.

(iv) Phylogeny are constructed from the distance matrix by applying UPGMA algorithm.

In a nutshell, the process is shown in Fig. 1 in the form of a flowchart.

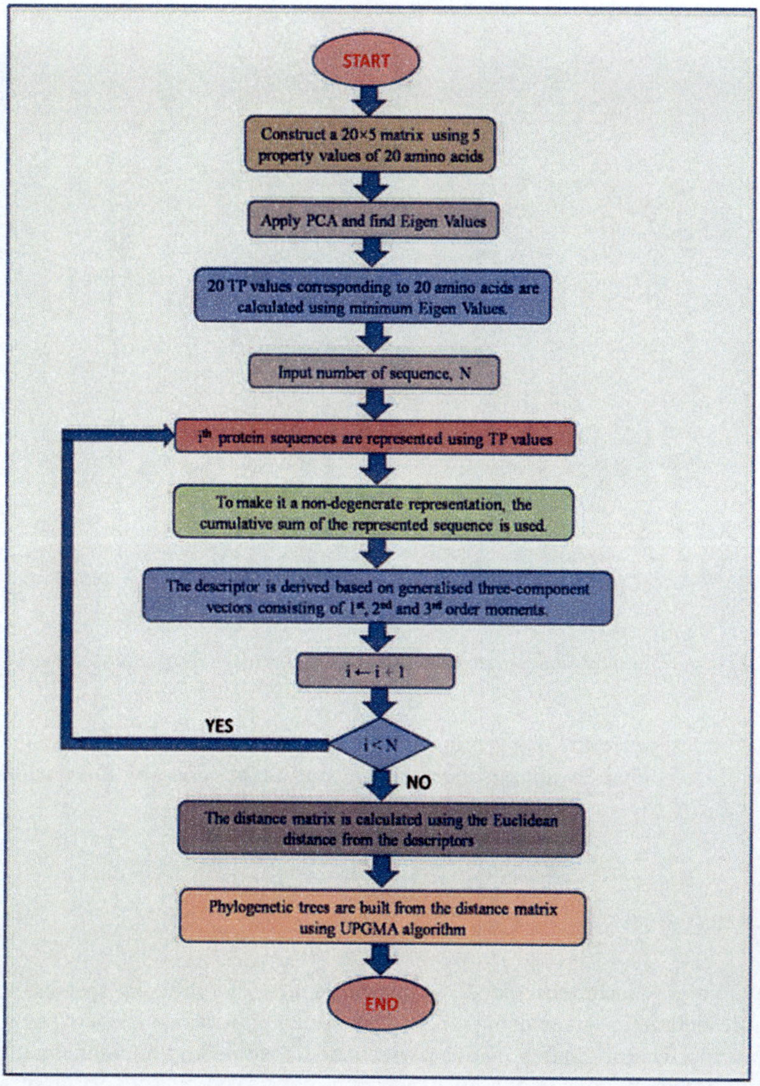

Fig. 1 Flowchart of the proposed method

3 Result and Discussion

Figure 2 shows the results of this method for 50 spike proteins of the coronavirus. The results are found to be identical to the known biological reference. By analysing results to those achieved previously by other authors by other approaches, the method's efficacy is proved. Figure 3 shows phylogenetic trees of 50 coronavirus

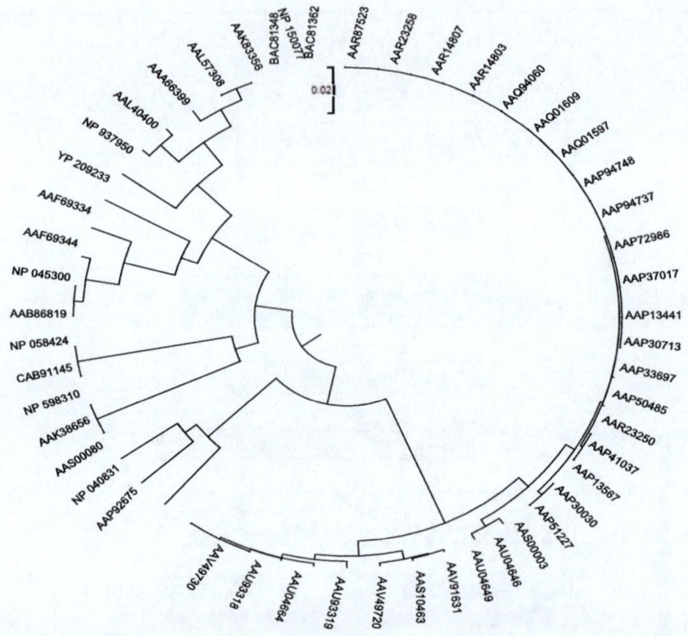

Fig. 2 Result obtained by proposed method 50 spike proteins in the form of phylogenetic tree

spike proteins generated using a unified approach based on classified amino acid groups [14]. For the identical sequences, the results obtained by this method are comparable to those obtained by other methods.

4 Conclusion

In the literature on similarity study of protein sequence of different species, numerical representation is given using randomly selected physiochemical attributes of 20 amino acids. The originality of this paper is demonstrated by the numerical representation given by considering all five known physical property's value of amino acids. This study initially employs PCA to lower the dimension in order to deal with the spatial complexity required in protein sequence analysis due to the need to accommodate 20 amino acids. Although PCA has been utilised in previous works, the current study is unique in that it uses generalised moments of the first, second, and third orders instead of standard ones as descriptors.

The method's efficacy is determined by comparing results that are similar to a recognised biological reference as well as data acquired using other methods. As a result, it is possible to conclude that the current analysis is well-motivated, and the outcome demonstrates that it is sound and correct, using less space. Finally,

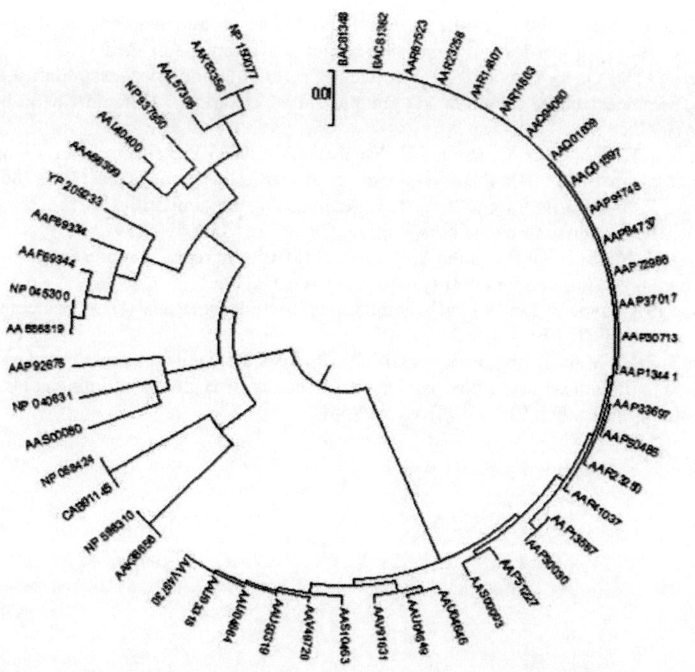

Fig. 3 Result obtained by unified approach for 50 spike proteins as found in [14]

regardless of the length of the protein sequence, it can be applied to both equal and unequal length sequences as the descriptor is derived using a 60-component moment vector using first, second, and third order moment.

References

1. Wenbing H, Qiuhui P, Mingfeng H (2016) A new graphical representation of protein sequences and its applications. Phys A 444:996–1002
2. Jia W, Zhang Y (2009) A 2D graphical representation of protein sequence and its numerical characterization. Chem Phys Lett 476:281–286
3. Yuxin L, Dan L, Kebo L, Yandong J, Ping-An H (2013) P-H curve, a graphical representation of protein sequences for similarities analysis. MATCH Commun Math Comput Chem 70:451–466
4. Lulu Y, Yusen Z, Ivan G, Yongtang S, Matthias D (2017) Protein sequence comparison based on physicochemical properties and the position-feature energy matrix. Sci Rep 7:46237
5. Zhi-Cheng W, Xuan X, Kuo-Chen C (2010) 2D-MH: a web-server for generating graphic representation of protein sequences based on the physicochemical properties of their constituent amino acids. J Theor Biol 267:29–34
6. Milan R (2007) 2-D graphical representation of proteins based on physicochemical properties of amino acids. Chem Phys Lett 444:176–180
7. Dandan S, Chunrui X, Yusen Z (2016) A novel method of 2D graphical representation for proteins and its application. MATCH Commun Math Comput Chem 75:431–446

8. Zhao-Hui Q, Meng-Zhe J, Su-Li L, Jun F (2015) A protein mapping method based on physicochemical properties and dimension reduction. Comput Biol Med 57:1–7
9. Yu-Hua Y, Dai Q, Li L, Nan X, He P, Zhang Y (2010) Similarity/dissimilarity studies of protein sequences based on a new 2D graphical representation. J Comput Chem. https://doi.org/10.1002/jcc.21391
10. Chenglong Y, Shiu-Yuen C, Rong LH, Stephen SY (2011) Protein map: an alignment-free sequence comparison method based on various properties of amino acids. Gene 486:110–118
11. Yan-ping Z, Ji-shuo R, Ping-an H (2013) Analyzes of the similarities of protein sequences based on the pseudo amino acid composition. Chem Phys Lett 590:239–244
12. Tingting M, Yuxin L, Qi D, Yuhua Y, Ping-an H (2014) A graphical representation of protein based on a novel iterated function system. Phys A 403:21–28
13. Pengyao P, Xianyou Z, Lei W (2017) Similarities/dissimilarities analysis of protein sequences based on PCA-FFT. J Biol Syst 25:29–45
14. Ghosh S, Pal J, Maji B, Bhattacharya DK (2018) A sequential development towards a unified approach to protein sequence comparison based on classified groups of amino acids. Int J Eng Technol. https://doi.org/10.14419/ijet.v7i2.9546

Analysis of Spread of COVID-19 Based on Socio-economic Factors: A Comparison of Prediction Models

Seema Patil, Isha Patil, Ravneesh Singh, Aayushi Verma, and Raghav Gaur

Abstract COVID-19 is a rapidly spreading virus, which was encountered first in December 2019 in Wuhan, China. Being a severe virus that dominantly targets the respiratory tract of the human body has taken a toll over nearly 120 million people. The vaccination process around the world against COVID-19 started around January 2021, and the world has seen a steady decrease ever since. However, new variants keep coming into picture, deadlier than the previous making it difficult to overcome this deadly disease. Many factors that range from the availability of hospital beds in particular areas to the GDP Index have been taken into consideration while performing this experiment. Thus, this study aims to model and predict COVID-19 outbreak in Albania, Chile, Georgia, Malaysia, Panama, Sri Lanka, Turkey, Ukraine, and Uruguay. An analysis is performed to see the correlation between various socio-economic factors and the COVID-19 spread. Furthermore, prediction was performed using various algorithms to see which algorithm gives the best result. Data was accumulated from February 2020 to 16 August 2021. The data contained COVID-19 infection spread related statistics and data related to various socio-economic factors. Various machine learning algorithms like XGBoost, Light GBM, Lasso regression, and support vector machine were considered during the study. The central focus of our prediction model was around finding which algorithm gives a better prediction going forward into the pandemic as every country has started vaccination in one form or another. Countries that have extensively used the AstraZeneca vaccine were only considered in this study. Our analysis is focused on the direct correlation between the spread of COVID-19 and socio-economic factors like the availability of hospital beds, handwashing facilities, population density, etc.

Keywords AstraZeneca · Coronavirus · COVID-19 · Machine learning · Socio-economic factors

---

S. Patil (✉) · I. Patil · R. Singh · A. Verma · R. Gaur
Symbiosis University, Symbiosis Institute of Technology, Pune, India
e-mail: seemahpatil2007@gmail.com

© The Author(s), under exclusive license to Springer Nature Singapore Pte Ltd. 2023
J. K. Mandal and D. De (eds.), *Frontiers of ICT in Healthcare*, Lecture Notes in Networks and Systems 519, https://doi.org/10.1007/978-981-19-5191-6_33

1 Introduction

The SARS-COV-2 COVID-19 has spread rapidly, since it was first reported in the Wuhan district of China, towards the end of 2019. COVID-19 is a rapidly spreading severe acute respiratory syndrome that has been wreaking havoc around the world. Originally, it was reported as three people with pneumonia that contracted a cluster of respiratory disease. As time goes on, we are seeing that this disease is getting more and more dangerous with its increasing number of mutations and variants effectively hampering the efforts that are being undertaken to immunize the community. The COVID-19 pandemic has unfolded new obstacles for understanding the factors associated with the spread of contagious viral diseases. This project helps us understand the role that social, economic, and environmental stimuli play in the meteoric spread of the deadly disease. In this study, we explore how socio-economic factors can knowingly and unknowingly play a vital role in the widespread of COVID-19.

There are many variants of the virus that are currently contributing to the new waves that are setting across the world. The delta variant that is likely to cause more infections and spread faster was a major concern until the third week of November 2021, where now new cases of the Omicron variant can be seen in many countries of South Africa.

The offset of the pandemic defined a set of factors that are considered the most important while referring to the spread of the virus. One of which included the reproduction number (R0). The reproduction number generates the mean of child cases (considering the spread of COVID-19 in the shape of a tree), caused by one root case given the population is largely susceptible to infection, can tell us about the number of people that most likely to get infected further [4].

The dataset was procured from ourworldindata.org. It is a research and database centre that provides huge databases for research purposes. The timestamp for the data begins from February 2020 which is just one month after COVID-19 was declared as a public health emergency by the WHO. The dataset had a list of over hundred countries. To convert the data into a data frame that is efficiently computed, countries with excessive missing values were dropped after assessment. To further narrow down the list of countries.

Summarizing, this paper makes the following contributions:

1. XGBoost, support vector machine, Lasso regression, and light GBM are used to predict the further spread of the cases.
2. It aims to understand which algorithm works best with data after the vaccination process began to predict the spread of COVID-19 over various countries.
3. Analysis and understanding the relation of socio-economic factors with the spread of COVID-19.

The rest of the paper consists of Sect. 2 which describes related work that has been done previously to understand such data. Section 3 talks about the methodology, mainly pre-processing of the data, exploratory data analysis, outlier detection and removal, and feature engineering. Section 4 will talk about the algorithms that have been applied, i.e. the prediction methodology. Section 5 will consist of the results and discussions. The final part of the paper which will be Sect. 6 is the conclusion of the entire experiment (Fig. 1).

2 Related Work

A number of authors from different fields have tried to find the reasons behind the consecutive waves of COVID-19 all over the world. There are many factors that have come in the limelight and that are considered to be the possible explanation for the spread of COVID-19 at a tremendous level.

Some works consider demographical factors which mostly include the influence of age structure, population age, etc., that may explain the remarkably visible variation in the number of fatalities across Italy. This work suggests that demographically informed projections will have a better chance at predicting the COVID-19 trends further suggesting that the social distancing measures also might be equally important to the process of flattening the curve [1].

Other work also talks about creating models using cross sectional data of over 184 countries to understand the spread of COVID-19 according to the doctor's population per thousand, population over the age of 65, obesity, etc., further suggesting that per capita income is not positively related to the COVID-19 mortality rates. These experiments that were conducted using quartile regression also suggest that old people are more prone to this respiratory disease than younger people [2]. The direct impact of climatic factors on the spread and waves of the virus. Data for climatic indicators for New York, the capital of New York City was considered from March 2020 to April 2021 to prove this which was mostly done using the Kendal correlation test. This paper further suggested that average air quality played a significant role in the count of the new cases along with average and minimum temperature. It also suggests that features that describe the wind might also cause the spread of COVID-19 to rise and decrease day-wise at times [3].

There are other works that focus on the risk caused to healthcare workers in the hospitals and the disease transmission caused by them. These works suggest that in samples that are fully tested and have provided with a positive result consisted of asymptomatic cases ranging from 51 to 88% of the total cases [5]. Estimating the spread level of the virus of a particular country given a date by assigning each country to a specific level that tells us about the total number of confirmed cases which can be less than 1000, between 1000 and 10,000, between 10,000 and 50,000, and more than 50,000. The results of which suggested that the range of countries having confirmed cases manly lied between less than 1000 and between 1000 and 10,000. This was done using the classification approach, which relied heavily on the socio-economic indicators which were as high as 1429 in number from the fields of science and technology, education, financial sector, social protection, etc. [9].

Considering the work that has been done to understand the spread of the virus in Brazil, it is assumed that it being a country with strong demographic heterogeneity,

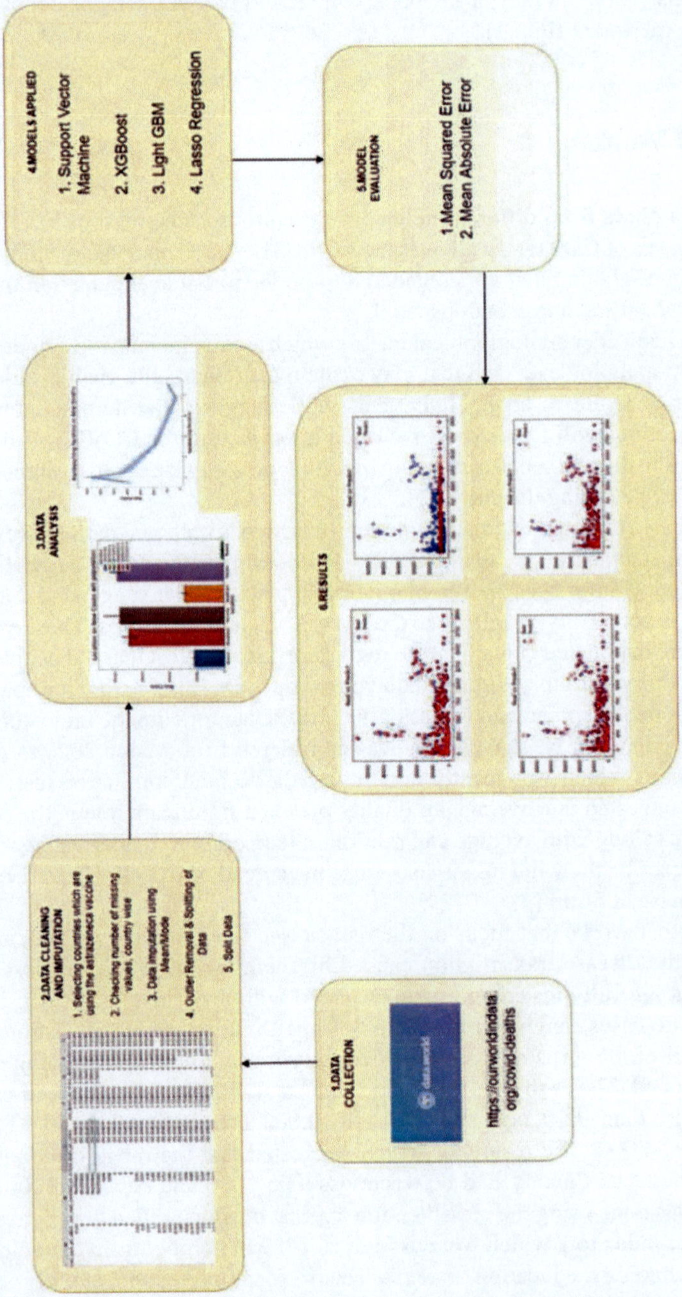

Fig. 1 Architecture diagram for prediction of spread of COVID-19 based on socio-economic factors

might not be able to give access to public health and might tamper the socio-economic indexes. This inequality should impact every section of the population differently. Thus, performing classification on the basis of three main criteria which were population mobility, socio-economic characteristics, and available health benefits to the population with respect to the hospital capacity [10].

Among other works that have been done on Italy, correlation between the rate of infection and family habits have also been considered. Such factors have also been evaluated considering them as a possible trigger of the epidemic [11].

Works that specifically concentrated on the correlation analysis of the spread of COVID-19 and factors such as age and urban population show that a significant positive relationship is seen with the median age of the population of certain countries and the COVID-19 day-to-day cases [16].

Relation between the socio-economic factors and the spread of COVID-19 was done using statistical modelling methods such as Poisson regression modelling (PRM) and negative binomial regression modelling (NBRM) which showed that prevalence of obesity, smoking, and diabetes (Type 1 and Type 2) had effects in the percentages (22.1%, 34.0%, and 6.75%) [14]. Apart from the socio-economic factors, like mentioned in the above points, healthcare workers were affected by a major pandemic due to the proximity they had with the other COVID-19 patients. As testing increased, it also became clear that a huge population of younger persons was infected with the virus in Wuhan, China [15], thus suggesting that age might also play a role in the spread of the infection keeping the health conditions aside.

Apart from the above discussed climatic, geographic, health, and socio-economic factors, social, legal, and political factors also have a significant role to play in the increase of COVID-19 outcomes [17]. Abusing certain social conditions endangering health of the people leading to smuggling of certain health products, lack of people working in the semi-clinical services, lack of use of disinfectants, and the effect of certain persons in the spread of mouth aspect of spreading awareness among people about disinfection, social distancing, etc., all play a major role in the spread of this virus. Despite the vast research that continues to follow trying to understand the behaviour of this virus, this paper tries to predict the inflow of new cases specifically based on the AstraZeneca vaccine which has been used by a large number of countries and understand what socio-economic factors play a specific role in the increase or decrease in the number of new cases. The results of this paper will help researchers to have an existing base on which work can be done and the respective authorities to take action which will help control the spread of this deadly virus.

3 Proposed Work

Figure 2 demonstrates in detail the factors that have been worked with while understanding the study of COVID-19 across the world. We propose four prediction models that are constructed using machine learning to predict the spread of COVID-19 which are XGBoost, support vector machines, Lasso regression, and light GBM using socio-economic factors such as GDP per capita, population, hospital beds per thousand, positivity index, stringency index, age, total cases, and new cases per day. A brief exploratory data analysis over these factors also allows us to understand what factors a major impact on the new cases that have come in per day. Figure 3 gives a brief overview of how the experiment was conducted.

Collection of appropriate data was done which provided the project with the above-mentioned factors that were to be considered. Followed by data was the initial step of cleaning the data, pre-processing the data, selecting appropriate machine learning algorithms to work with, and finally the evaluating the models and making appropriate predictions.

4 Data Source and Collection

The dataset used for this project was taken from ourworldindata.org, a popular website to get datasets from. Various datasets can be published and explored on this platform. The dataset that was used in our project was the one found under coronavirus (COVID-19) deaths. The dataset on the site is updated daily. The main groups of features this dataset covers were as following:

- Country data (i.e. the ISO code of the country, continent name, and location)
- Data of the data record
- Total cases of the day
- New cases of the day
- New deaths of the day
- Reproduction rate
- Hospitalization
- Data related to testing (positive tests and new tests)
- Stringency index
- Population
- Age
- GDP
- Cardiovascular deaths
- Diabetes
- Smokers
- Life expectancy.

5 Data Cleaning and Pre-processing

Data cleaning was done using the traditional method of looking for null values and either removing rows with 90% or more missing values or imputing the values using mean and mode. Data imputation refers to the filling of inconsistent data points

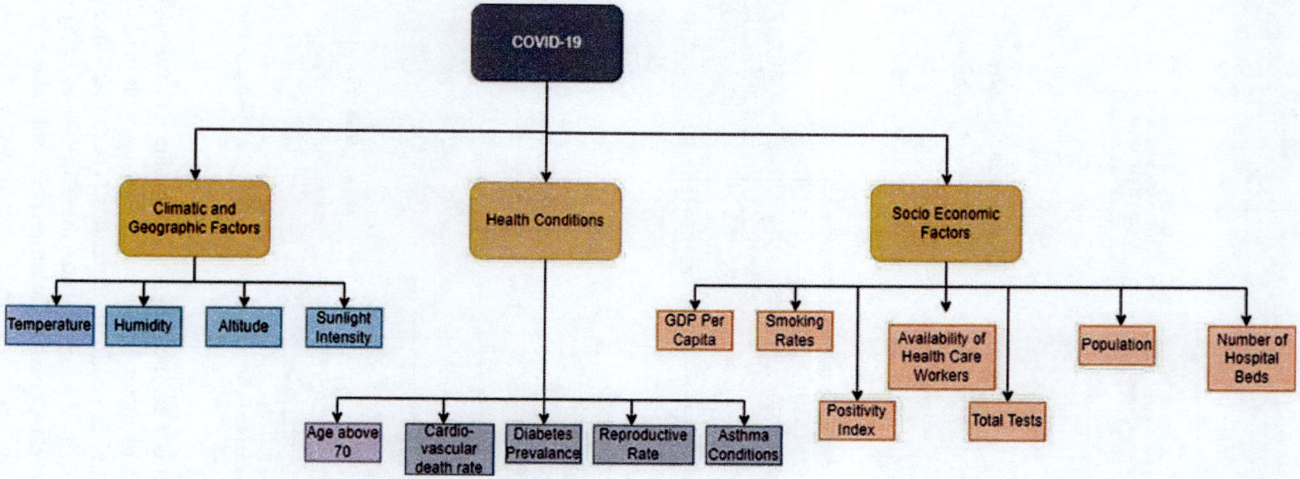

Fig. 2 General factors that were considered in various studies

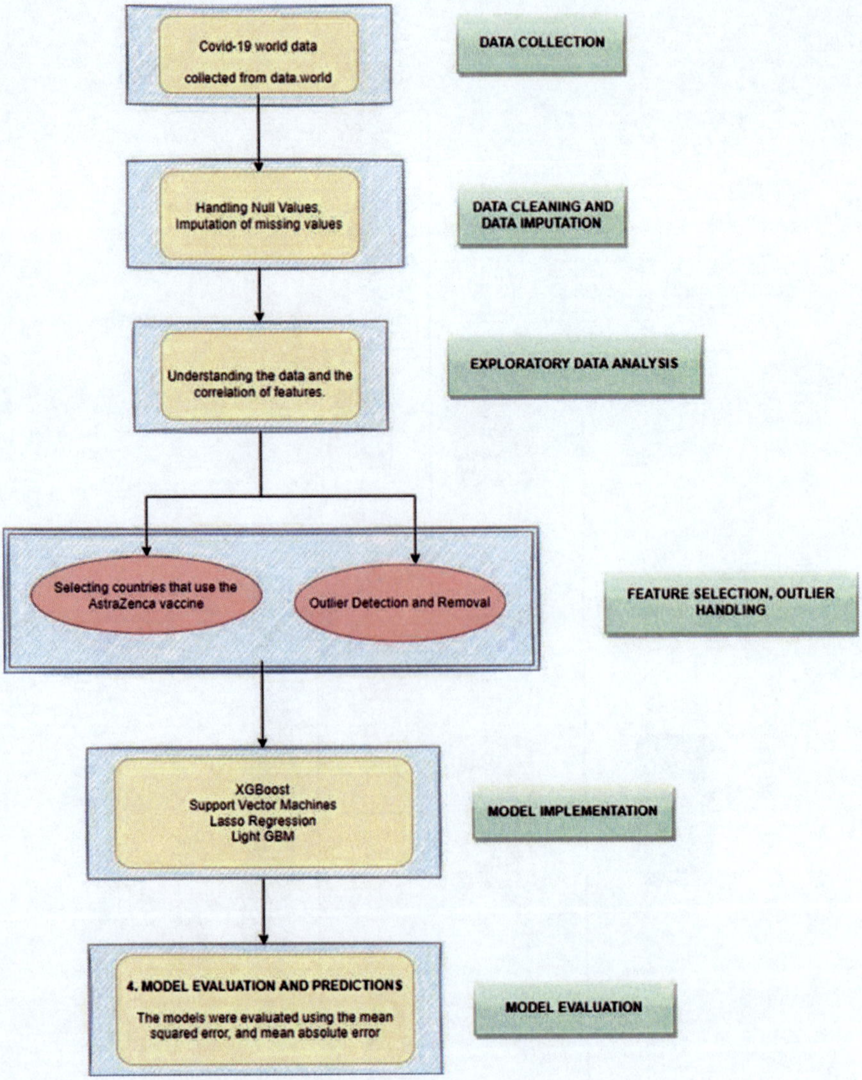

Fig. 3 System architecture for prediction of spread of COVID-19 based on socio-economic factors

in the dataset. These values can be imputed using various methods which include statistical methods such as mean, mode, median along with methods such as end of tail imputation and arbitrary value imputations. These methods are significantly used with data that consists of numerical variables. In case of categorical variables, methods such as frequent category imputation are performed. Since the data in picture was mostly numerical, the mean and mode methods were used to impute the data. Mean imputation is done by imputing the missing values by the mean of the observed value for each variable and mode imputation is done by imputing the missing values by the mode of each variable which necessarily mean the value of the data point that has occurred the most.

6 Exploratory Data Analysis

Correlation analysis is done to measure the relationship between two variables to understand their dependence and association with each other. It is done to understand the economic behaviour of the data and critically examine the dependency of each feature over other features. Being a statistical method, there are various ways to perform correlation analysis. In this project, Spearman correlation has been used to understand the dependency of variables. The values range from −1 to 1 demonstrating a negative and positive correlation, respectively. The value of 0 means that there is no dependency.

$$\rho = 1 - \frac{6\sum d_i^2}{n(n^2 - 1)} \tag{1}$$

In Eq. (1), ρ refers to the Spearman's rank correlation coefficient and d_i is the difference between the ranks of each data point in the feature column and n is the number of observations.

From the above heatmap in Fig. 4, significant positive correlation can be seen between new cases and new deaths. This proves to be correct since the data that was used to perform this correlation analysis was before vaccination and since there was no external immunity that was provided, then the number of deaths rose with the number of new cases. Also, it is seen that there is a significant negative correlation between hospital beds per thousand in a particular area and the number of deaths which suggests that if the availability of hospital beds increases the number of deaths decrease.

Some more correlations and dependencies are discussed in Figs. 5 and 6.

Line graphs and bar graphs were plotted using matplotlib and seaborn for an in-depth exploratory data analysis. The graphs give a much clearer picture about the correlation of the widespread of the disease with the quality of services provided by a country and the economic state of that country. Several socio-economic factors were considered, while plotting the graph and some of them showed a very strong correlation with the widespread. In Asia countries, like Pakistan and Indonesia which have a comparatively higher population and scarcity of hospital beds reported most new deaths whereas countries like Armenia and Kazakhstan on the other hand having much lower population and better facilities in hospitals reported the least deaths. Moreover, it was also found that countries which report a comparatively higher human development index reported much lesser number of total cases.

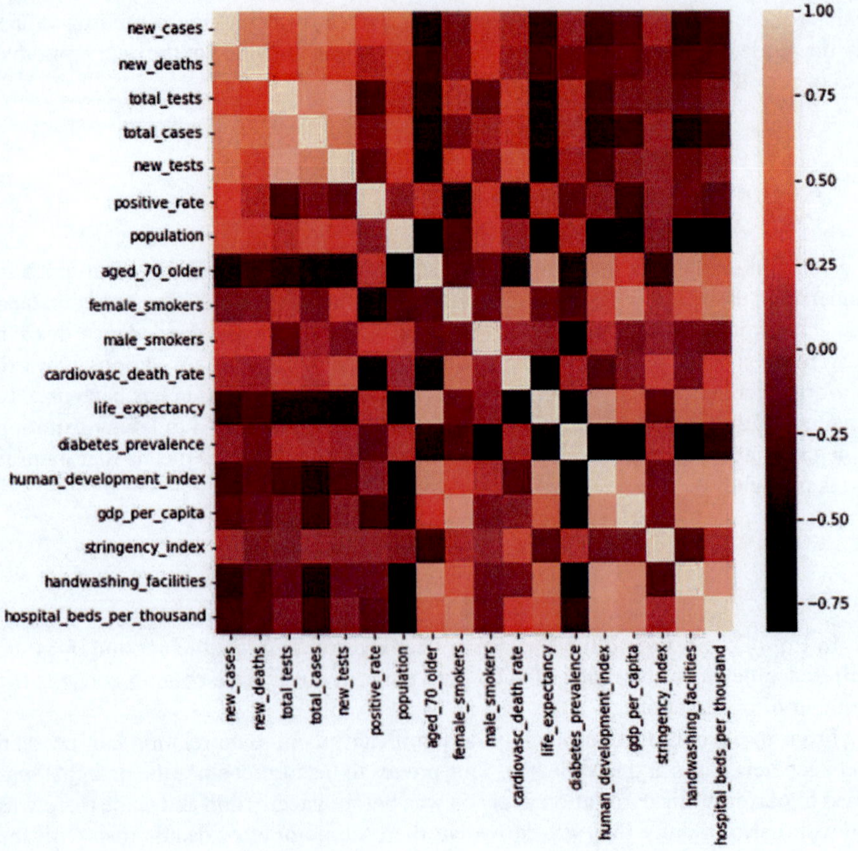

Fig. 4 Correlation heatmap of all the features

In South America, we noticed that Columbia which has a comparatively higher population but lacks in terms of handwashing facilities reported the greatest number of new deaths whereas countries like Ecuador and Paraguay which have a smaller population but have much better sanitization facilities reported comparatively much lesser new deaths. It was also noticed that countries that have higher GDP per capita conduct much more tests as compared to countries that report a comparatively lower GDP.

Figure 5 describes the relation between various factors that were considered for this study. Figure 5a helps us understand the correlation between human development index of a country and the total cases reported by the country. It is noticed that countries with a higher human development index usually sum up to a higher number of total, and Fig. 5a shows a negative correlation after a point between the positivity rate reported by the country and the quality of handwashing facilities available in

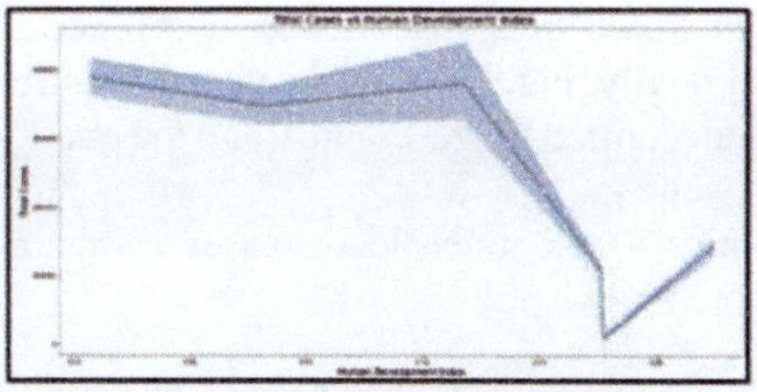

a. Total Cases vs Human Development Index

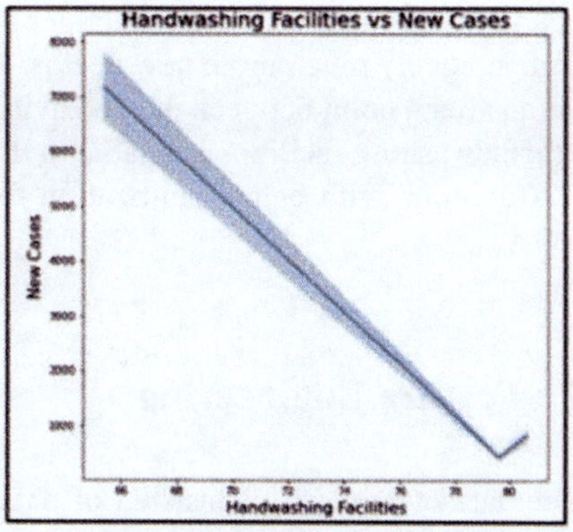

b. New Cases vs Handwashing Facilities

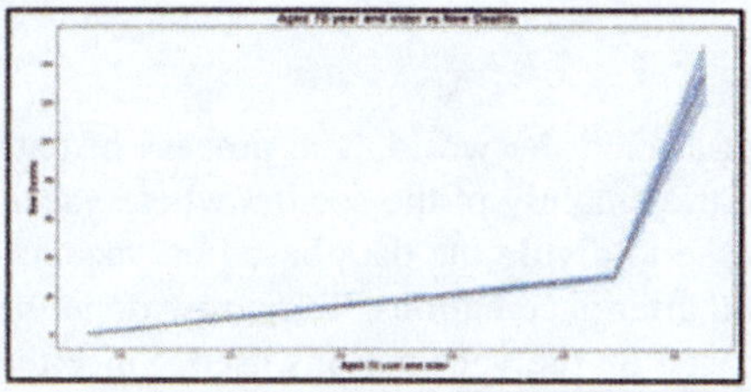

c. New Deaths vs Aged 70 year and older

Fig. 5 Line plots between different features/factors

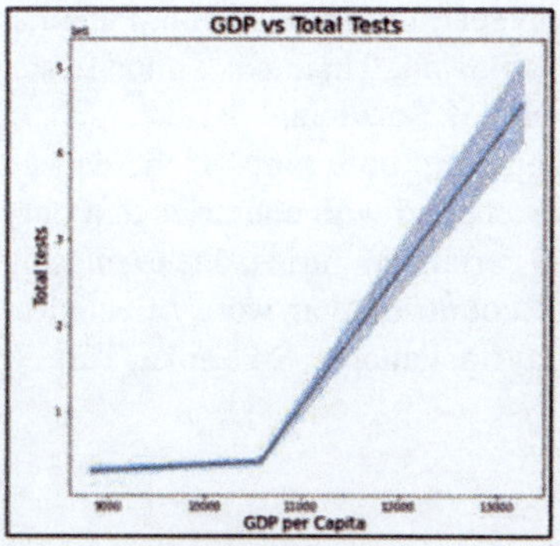

(a). GDP vs Total Tests

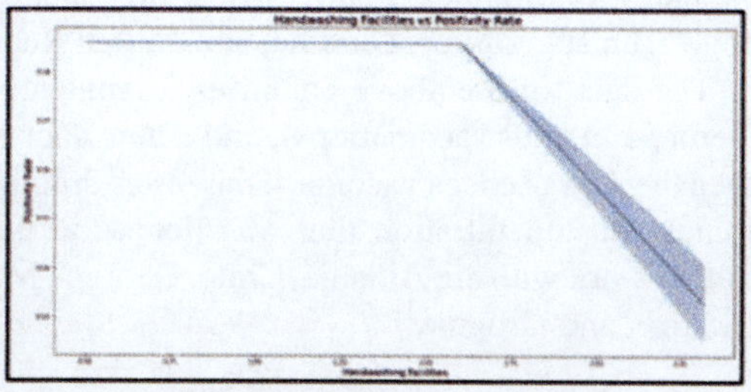

(b). Handwashing Facilities vs Positivity Rate

Fig. 6 Line plots between different features/factors

that country. Countries with better sanitization facilities report much lesser cases comparatively.

Similarly, Fig. 5b shows a negative correlation between handwashing facilities available in a country and new cases reported by that country. It is seen that countries with better handwashing facilities report much lesser cases as compared to countries which do not have the appropriate infrastructure for sanitization facilities.

Figure 6 describes the relation between various factors that were considered for this study. Figure 6a shows a positive correlation between the new deaths reported by a country and the number of people who are aged 70 year and older in that country. Countries which have a larger population with age 70 or older have reported comparatively much more new deaths. And finally, Fig. 6b, shows a negative correlation after a point between the positivity rate reported by the country and the quality of handwashing facilities available in that country.

Countries with better sanitization facilities report much lesser cases comparatively.

7 Feature Engineering

The dataset primarily consisted of data all around the world. The process of data cleaning led to the dropping of many countries mainly in the section where vaccination data was included. It only made sense to divide the data based on vaccinations, thus dividing the data into before and after vaccinations. To narrow done the data a bit more, countries were selected based on the vaccinations used. Since the most common vaccine at the point was AstraZeneca, it became the centre point of selecting the countries. The countries that have significantly used the AstraZeneca Vaccine are Albania, Armenia, Azerbaijan, Bangladesh, Brazil, Cambodia, Chile, China, Colombia, Dominican Republic, Ecuador, Egypt, El Salvador, Georgia, Hong Kong, Indonesia, Kazakhstan, Malaysia, Mexico, Nepal, Oman, Pakistan, Panama, Paraguay, Philippines, South Africa, Sri Lanka, Tajikistan, Thailand, Timor-Leste, Togo, Tunisia, Turkey, Ukraine, and United Republic of Tanzania.

The data for the above countries was intersected from both parts of the dataset (before and after vaccinations), and a new data was created with countries that only used the AstraZeneca vaccine. Thus, after dropping certain countries, due to missing values and the filtration that was done, the final countries that were selected to further work with are Albania, Chile, Georgia, Malaysia, Panama, Sri Lanka, Turkey, Ukraine, and Uruguay.

8 Outlier Detection and Removal

Considering new cases per day as the target variable, it was very substantial that it had a huge number of outliers. Considering the fact that many factors would have such visible outliers, they were treated using isolation forest algorithm. Isolation trees can be defined as a simple process of separating an instance from the rest of the instance [12]. To put it in other words, we can also say that anomalies and explicitly identified instead of having them recognized as normal data points and is like any other method, an ensemble method. Random split between the minimum and maximum value of the selected feature.

The following Fig. 7 shows the distribution of new cases that were recorded each day after the process of vaccination had begun. It is fairly evident that there existed some days where the cases were above the normal average. The cases ranged between

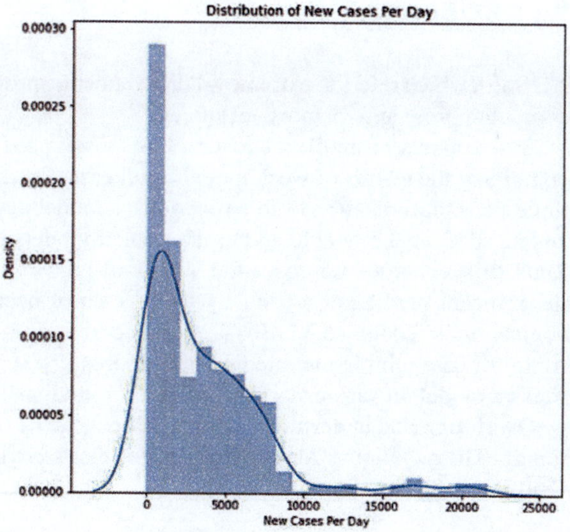

Fig. 7 Distribution of new cases per day

0 and 5000 on an average, but there clearly existed some days where the number of cases that was recorded each day crossed more than 20,000 and went up to nearly 25,000 with a very low density.

Isolation forest algorithm works with the principle of a decision tree that detects algorithms by isolating them by randomly selecting features and values.

9 Model Execution

This section talks about the models that have been tested on the available data to predict the new COVID cases after vaccinations had begun on countries that have extensively used the AstraZeneca vaccine. XGBoost, light GBM, support vector machines, and Lasso regression were used. The main reason behind selecting these algorithms was the huge size of the training data, and the memory usage of the algorithms like XGBoost and light GBM is comparatively lower since this experiment was done on personal systems. SVM is known for giving high prediction accuracy in the case of regression problems and is robust to outliers. And finally, Lasso regression can produce simpler models and the models which are more interpretable that incorporates only a reduced set of the predictors.

9.1 XGBoost

XGBoost which refers to extreme gradient boosting provides features such as efficient computing time and memory resources.

Based mainly on gradient boosting XGBoost is used to predict target variability by combining the results of weak models with ease. Gradient boosting mostly includes three steps: optimization of loss functions, a model that is weak to make predictions and an additional model to add to the weaker models to minimize the loss function. Thus, this technique improves the quality of predictions that have been done using insignificant prediction models by using a set of decision trees [6]. Many Kaggle competitions recognize XGBoost as an accurate, fast, and reliable predicting algorithm for data mining and prediction purposes [7]. It is a supervised algorithm that trains a model on various targets and further predicts a target variant.

Overfitting and underfitting with XGBoost can be handled using hyperparameter tuning. The techniques for hyperparameter that were used for this experiment were GridSearchCV and RandomSearchCV.

9.2 Support Vector Machines

When it comes to classification accuracy support vector machines (SVM), seem to have given the most recommendable results. These use multiple supervised learning algorithms for classification and regression [8]. The kernel trick technique is used to change data, and based on these changes, an optimal boundary is found and decides the possible outputs. Since SVM solves both classification and regression, it can capture multiple dependencies and relationships between data points without having to perform transformations individually.

9.3 Lasso Regression

Lasso regression and ridge regression are similar to each other. In ridge regression, the sum of the squared residuals is added to the constant (lambda) times the slope square is minimized. It may happen at times that the ridge regression line does not fit the training data as well as the line plotted with the least squares.

$$\beta = \left(X^T X\right)^{-1} X^T y \tag{2}$$

In Eq. (2), $\hat{\beta}$ is the ordinary least squares estimator, X is the matrix regressor variable, T is the matrix transpose, and y is the vector of the value of the response variable.

In such cases, we can say that the ridge regression line has a low bias and a very high variance. Now instead of squaring the slope like it is done while minimizing ridge regression, if we take the absolute value, we have Lasso regression.

9.4 Light GBM

It can be said that light GBM is a variant of XGBoost and is said to be more accurate and lighter. Light GBM is a fast, high performance based on the mechanism of gradient boosting which is the decision tree. Thus, it works like XGBoost and random forest. The tree is split according to the leaf whereas other algorithms do this tree wise or level wise. Splitting the tree leaf wise can lead to overfitting which can be minimized by defining the depth of the splitting. Choosing what should be the correct parameters for feeding the light GBM model can be selected using hyperparameter tuning.

10 Results and Discussions

Optimal values that fit the model were found using hyperparameter tuning for hyperparameters such as max_depth that signifies the minimum weights of all the observations required in a child, and colsample_by_tree which signifies the fraction of columns to be randomly used as samples for each tree, etc., by creating a dictionary with the key as the name of the hyperparameter and the value as a list of set of probable values of those hyperparameters, and then, they were passed in algorithms such as GridSearchCV and RandomSearchCV which provide as an output the best set of hyperparameters.

Thus, after providing the best set of hyperparameters, the training data was used to train the model to predict corresponding outputs based on the testing data. Accuracy of these models was checked using the mean squared error and scatter plots between real values of the target variables which was number of new cases each day and the predicted values of the same target variable.

Evaluation metrics such as mean squared error and mean absolute error were used. Mean squared error tells us about the difference between the actual and predicted value. Thus, it can be said that the mean squared will tell us about the variance and bias of the actual values. When we subtract the observed value from the predicted values, we get a residual that allows to understand the predictability or accuracy of the model.

$$\mathrm{MSE} = \frac{1}{n}\sum_{i=1}^{n}\left(Y_i - \widehat{Y_i}\right)^2 \tag{3}$$

Table 1 Comparison of evaluation metrics

Models	Mean squared errors	Mean absolute errors
Light GBM	1,300,260.30	330.94
Lasso regression	12,462,358.37	335.81
Support vector machines	70,101,038.72	2273.25
XGBoost	1,218,630.45	289.92

In Eq. (3), MSE refers to the mean squared error, n is the number of data points, and Y_i and $\hat{Y}_i$ are the observed and predicted values of the model.

The mean absolute error is the arithmetic mean of all the absolute errors where the absolute error refers to the difference between the actual and predicted values of the model. It is a convenient evaluation metric for data with continuous variables.

$$\text{MAE} = \frac{\sum_{i=1}^{n} |y_i - x_i|}{n} \tag{4}$$

In the above equation, MAE refers to the mean absolute error, n is the total number of data points, and y_i and x_i are the real and predicted values of the model.

Table 1 is a comparison of the mean squared errors and mean absolute errors that were provided by XGBoost, support vector machines, Lasso regression, and light GBM.

There cannot possibly be any acceptable upper or lower limit for mean squared error and mean absolute values that can tell us about the accuracy of the predictions. The range for both the evaluation metrics ranges for 0 to ∞. Accuracy over here will tell us about the exact match or difference between the actual and predicted values. Thus, whichever value approaches zero, it is a better mean squared or mean absolute error value.

In the above case, it is quite clear that the mean squared error and mean absolute error of the implementation of XGBoost are the most near to zero, thus making it visible that XGBoost outperformed the other three models.

Tables 2, 3, 4, and 5 show a comparison between five randomly selected real and predict values of given by the models. These values show that there is not much difference between values given by XGBoost, whereas other models such as light GBM, Lasso regression, and support vector machines show a much larger difference between them.

This above point can be made clear using the scatter plots that were plotted between real values of the target variables which was number of new cases each day and the predicted values of the same target variable as well.

Figure 8a–d shows the scatter plots of real and predict values of light GBM, Lasso regression, support vector machines, and XGBoost.

Table 2 Comparison between actual and predicted values: XGBoost

Actual value	Predicted value	Difference
434	330	104
777	450	327
3322	3142	180
4187	4311	−124
8216	8098	118

Table 3 Comparison between actual and predicted values: support vector machines

Actual value	Predicted value	Difference
434	1322	−888
777	1328	−551
3322	1387	1935
4187	4387	2800
8216	1398	6818

Table 4 Comparison between actual and predicted values: Lasso regression

Actual value	Predicted value	Difference
434	619	−185
777	598	209
3322	3036	286
4187	4393	−206
8216	7009	1207

Table 5 Comparison between actual and predicted values: light GBM

Actual value	Predicted value	Difference
434	365	69
777	439	338
3322	3070	252
4187	4429	−764
8216	8158	58

11 Conclusion and Future Work

From the above plots and mean squared error values, it can be deduced that XGBoost has outperformed the other three models quite significantly. Also, many factors such as availability of hospital beds, age, positivity index, handwashing facilities, and GDP per capita of a particular place play a significant role in the increase or decrease of COVID-19 cases on a daily basis. However, the results do not give any clear information about people who have contracted the disease after being fully or partially vaccinated. Accurate datasets for certain socio-economic factors like several smokers,

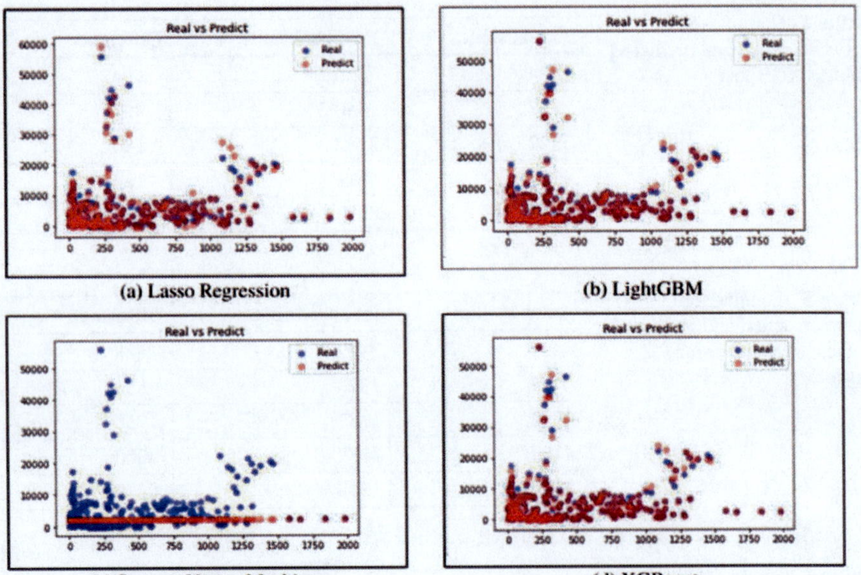

(a) Lasso Regression

(b) LightGBM

(c) Support Vector Machines

(d) XGBoost

Fig. 8 Real value versus predicted value plots of the models

diabetic patients, etc., were not available which could have helped in getting better results.

Further, the project focused only on countries which have extensively used the AstraZeneca vaccine and other vaccines.

With the availability of a more continuous data, the performance of these models can be taken into consideration, a proper prediction output can be deduced. Given the intensive distribution of vaccines, and occurrence of *n* number of variants, the severity of the virus seems to be going down. On taking these factors under the hood, we believe the patterns and behaviour of this virus can be understood in a more clear and specific manner.

References

1. Dowd et al (2020) Demographic science aids in understanding the spread and fatality rates of COVID-19. Proc Natl Acad Sci
2. Upadhyaya A et al Factors affecting COVID-19 mortality: an exploratory study. J Health Res
3. Bashir MF et al (2020) Correlation between climate indicators and COVID-19 pandemic in New York, USA. Sci Total Environ 728:138835. ISSN 0048-9697
4. Anderson RM et al (2020) How will country-based mitigation measures influence the course of the COVID-19 epidemic? Lancet 395(10228):931–934. ISSN 0140-6736
5. Black et al COVID-19: the case for health-care worker screening to prevent hospital transmission. Lancet 395(10234):1418–1420

6. Chen T, Guestrin C (2016) XGBoost. In: Proceedings of the 22nd ACM SIGKDD international conference on knowledge discovery and data mining—KDD'16
7. Ali J, Khan R, Ahmad N, Maqsood I (2012) Random forests and decision trees. Int J Comput Sci Issues
8. Vapnik V (1995) The nature of statistical learning theory. Springer, NY
9. Mihoub A et al (2020) Predicting COVID-19 spread level using socio-economic indicators and machine learning techniques. In: 2020 first international conference of smart systems and emerging technologies (SMARTTECH)
10. Coelho et al Assessing the spread of COVID-19 in Brazil: mobility, morbidity and social vulnerability. PLOS One 15(9):e0238214
11. Liu FT, Ting K, Zhou Z-H (2009) Isolation forest. 413–422. https://doi.org/10.1109/ICDM.2008.17
12. Bhadri Naarayanan P et al (2020) Comparing the performance of anomaly detection algorithms. Int J Eng Res Technol (IJERT) 9(7)
13. Chaudhry R et al (2020) A country level analysis measuring the impact of government actions, country preparedness and socioeconomic factors on COVID-19 mortality and related health outcomes. EClinicalMedicine 25:100464. ISSN 2589-5370
14. Hartley DM, Perencevich EN (2020) Public health interventions for COVID-19: emerging evidence and implications for an evolving public health crisis. JAMA
15. Hassan MM et al (2020) Assessment of epidemiological determinants of COVID-19 pandemic related to social and economic factors globally. J Risk Finan Manag
16. Yoosefi Lebni J, Abbas J, Moradi F et al (2021) How the COVID-19 pandemic effected economic, social, political, and cultural factors: a lesson from Iran. Int J Soc Psychiat
17. Wang J, Tang K et al (2020) Impact of temperature and relative humidity on the transmission of COVID-19: a modeling study in China and the United States, 9 March 2020
18. Farseev A, Chu-Farseeva Y-Y, Yang Q, Loo DB Understanding economic and health factors impacting the spread of COVID-19 disease. medRxiv 2020.04.10
19. Politis I, Georgiadis G, Nikolaidou A et al (2021) Mapping travel behavior changes during the COVID-19 lock-down: a socioeconomic analysis in Greece. Eur Transp Res Rev 13:21
20. Zohner YE, Morris JS (2021) COVID-TRACK: world and USA SARS-COV-2 testing and COVID-19 tracking. BioData Min. 2021 Jan 20.
21. Kotlar B, Gerson E, Petrillo S et al (2021) The impact of the COVID-19 pandemic on maternal and perinatal health: a scoping review. Reprod Health 18:10
22. McBride O, Murphy J, Shevlin M et al (2021) Monitoring the psychological, social, and economic impact of the COVID-19 pandemic in the population: context, design and conduct of the longitudinal COVID-19 psychological research consortium (C19PRC) study. Int J Methods Psychiat Res

India's COVID-2019 Epidemic Data Analysis Using Machine Learning Techniques: A Case Study of SIR Model

Ramjeet Singh Yadav

Abstract On January 30, 2020, the first patient of coronavirus was found in the Indian State of Kerala, which came from Wuhan city of China. Since then, till date, 3 phases of coronavirus (COVID-2019) disease have arrived in India. Currently, the third phase of coronavirus is going on. This phase in India has started due to the omicron variant of the COVID-2019 pandemic. The third phase has started in India from 1st January, 2021. Thus, an understanding widespread curve is very significant to forecast the growth of this COVID-2019 pandemic and optimize the best prevention strategies later. At present time, the number of coronaviruses in India is increasing very fast due to the coronavirus named omicron. The present study has been conducted to estimate the parameters of the COVID-2019 pandemic using the (SIR) model. The data of COVID-2019 from 27st December, 2021 to 20th January, 2022 has been used to do this pilot work. With the help of this proposed SIR model, the prediction of the peak of the COVID-2019 epidemic in India and the date of the end of the epidemic has also been found out. The results obtained from this study showed that the epidemic would reach its peak on 26th March, 2022, and the overall quantity of infected individuals at the peak would exceed 224,659,882. This study also suggests that the end of the COVID-2019 pandemic will be on 7th November, 2022. Also, at peak of epidemic, more than 421,500,197 people will be susceptible, and the reproductive number (R_0) is estimated at 3.3. Reproductive number (R_0) more than 3 means that one COVID-2019 infected person can infect more than 3 persons. The results obtained from this study can prove to be of great help to the Indian government, hospitals, doctors, and medical authorities for the prevention of the COVID-2019 epidemic and also the stages of disintegration of the coronavirus in future.

Keywords COVID-2019 pandemic · Regression analysis · Least square method · SIR model · Reproductive number

R. S. Yadav (✉)
Department of Business Management and Entrepreneurship, Dr. Rammanohar Lohia Avadh University, Ayodhya, UP 224001, India
e-mail: ramjeetsinghy@gmail.com

© The Author(s), under exclusive license to Springer Nature Singapore Pte Ltd. 2023
J. K. Mandal and D. De (eds.), *Frontiers of ICT in Healthcare*, Lecture Notes in Networks and Systems 519, https://doi.org/10.1007/978-981-19-5191-6_34

1 Introduction

COVID-2019 is a breathing viral illness that was initial conveyed in the Chinese town of Wuhan in 31st December 2019 and became a global pandemic [1]. The disease has affected more than 328 million people worldwide, causing over 5.54 million deaths [2]. The first patient of COVID-2019 was found on 30 January 2020 in the State of Kerala, and the disease is still spreading very fast in India with a total of 37,380,253 patients as of 10 January 2022. Initially, the virus was called SARSCoV, however, the WHO named it as COVID-2019 pandemic and stated it a worldwide epidemic on 11th March, 2020 [3, 4]. Currently, this virus is present in practically every corner of the planet, and due to its high infectivity, a great number of people have already succumbed to it [5]. SARSCoV-2 contagion represents one of these. Therefore, this disease is the biggest challenge for humanity.

Since then, till date, 3 phases of coronavirus (COVID-2019) disease have arrived in India. Currently, the third phase of coronavirus is going on. In the last two phases in India, it was observed that quantity of cases (patients) appeared to be decreasing steadily subsequently the highest of COVID-2019. This could be due to the policies that went into effect on 24th March, 2020 and beginning of May, 2021. These involvements included boundary restrictions, institute closures, social distancing, and the withdrawal of all communal crowds. However, the first phase of COVID-2019 saw a very rapid increase in the number of COVID-19 patients from mid-May to July, 2020. The delta variant in its second phase saw a high number of daily reported cases of COVID-19 patients from April, 2021 to July, 2021. In the second phase, the number of COVID-2019 patient deaths in India were also much higher than in the first phase. Enlarged figures have been reported due to a variety of features, plus a growth in daily examinations, nonetheless likewise a significant reduction of containment measures involving the elimination of containment measures and lighting. Despite all the measures taken by the Government of India for prevention of COVID-2019, this number is still increasing very fast. As such, it is of great importance for public authorities (Government of India and COVID Warriors) to predict the development of COVID-19 in order to provide information that can support them implement or read their preclusion procedures.

Several prediction approaches have been used to investigate and forecast the forthcoming trends of COVID-2019 (logistic growing method, susceptible–infectious–recover/removed (SIR) model, susceptible exposed infectious–recover)/removed (SEIR) model), statistical-based SIR model, and natural growth model [6–10]. In the present study, SIRs were used to predict the number of cases, rate of transmission, reproductive number (R_0), size and date of extinction in India for COVID-19 pandemic.

2 SIR Model

In the present study, the SIR model has been used for data analysis of the COVID-2019 pandemic. Kermack and McKendrick created the model in the 1920s, and it has a significant and long-lasting impact as an epidemiological model. Here, we divide the population of India into 3 groups: (1) Susceptible (S): Those who are susceptible. (2) Infected (I): Those who are contagious. (3) Remove/Recover (R): Those who die or recover. Anyone who can become infected is considered susceptible. Infected is a person who has the disease and can transmit it to others. Anyone who can no longer contract the disease, either because of immunity after having the disease and recovering or because of death, is considered to have been relapsed. Our presented model follows naturally from the above description. In the present study, let N be the total population of India, S is the population of persons who are susceptible, I am the population of persons who are infected, and R is the population of persons who have died or recovered from the disease. Since every person in the population must fall into one of these three categories, so we have the following fundamental equality:

$$N = S + I + R \tag{1}$$

In all situations, we study, in order to progress on our model, we must first make simplified assumptions, and we do our best to clarify those assumptions so that others can criticize or modify them. The population of india has remained stable during the intial phase of pandemic. In other words, we can say that no one has taken birth, no one has died, and no one has migrated. Another assumption of this model is that our population is homogeneously mixed. The flow diagram of SIR model is represented by Fig. 1.

Since the susceptible can only drop the series, we should expect that the graph for S will only decrease with time. Similarly, we should expect that the graph for R will only grow because people can only move in that box. To really start building a model based on a flow diagram, we need to label the arrows, that is, we need to determine how many people move from one compartment to another each day. This would involve the incorporation of two basic parameters based on two properties that have a significant impact on the severity of the pandemic:

1. How easily this disease is transmitted from an infected to a susceptible person?
2. How long does the infected person remain infected?

We quantify point 1 by introducing a parameter called the transition rate or infection rate, which we denote by the Greek letter beta, β. We define β as the average

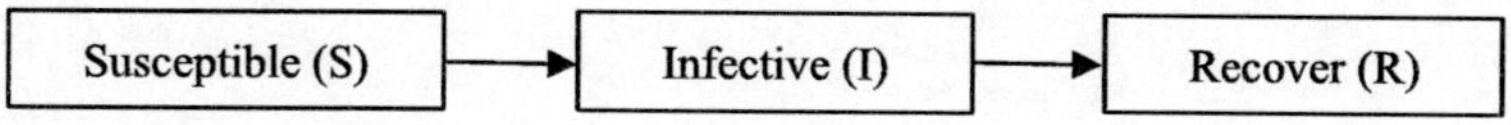

Fig. 1 Flow diagram structure for the (SIR) model

number of contacts per day that an infected person sufficiently transmits the disease. Thus, β is a quantitative measure of how easily the disease spreads. In practice, the parameter β proves to be extremely difficult to measure directly. Hence, in the present study, we have used the regression and least square method to estimate the value of infection rate (β). If we examine the definition, we see that β depends on social factors such as cleanliness, population density, and social customs or social distancing. We measure point 2 by introducing a parameter known as the recovery rate, and we denote it with the Greek letter γ. It is defined as the recovery rate. In the present study, both the parameters infection rate (β) and recovery rate (γ) have been calculated through direct observation COVID-2019 data of India in between 27th December, 2021 and 20th January, 2022. Three differential equations are used in the SIR model. These equations are given below:

$$\frac{dS}{dt} = -\frac{\beta}{N}SI \tag{2}$$

$$\frac{dI}{dt} = \frac{\beta}{N}SI - \gamma I \tag{3}$$

$$\frac{dR}{dt} = \gamma I \tag{4}$$

where $N = S + I + R$ denotes total population size independent of time (t), β denotes infection rate, and γ denotes recovery/removal rate.

3 Experimental Result

3.1 *Estimation of Infection Rate*

Almost the entire population is susceptible ($S \approx N$) in India at the start of the COVID-19 infection. After substituting $S = N$ in differential Eq. 3, we get a new equation which is given below:

$$\frac{dI}{dt} = \beta I - \gamma I = I(\beta - \gamma) \tag{5}$$

The solution of above differential Eq. 5 is given below:

$$I = I_0 e^{mt}, \text{ where } m = \beta - \gamma \tag{6}$$

Here, we have obtained the value of the constant m by using Eq. 6 and least square method from India's COVID-2019 datasets. The estimation of infection rate (β)-related parameter m and experimental results is shown in Table 1. Figure 2 describes input data with exponential growth log plot (estimation of m).

Taking log both sides of Eq. 6, we get

$$\ln I = \ln I_0 + \ln e^{mt} \Rightarrow \ln I = \ln I_0 + mt \tag{7}$$

After plotting the best fit by using Eq. 7, we have got the value of m (0.156670959) (India COVID-2019 Data from 27 December, 2021 to 20 January, 2022). The log plot and exponential model equation (Eq. 8) are given below:

Table 1 Estimation of infection rate (β)-related parameter m and experimental results

Date	Time (day)	Daily new case (I)	$Y = \ln(I)$	Predicted new case (Y)	Square error
27-Dec-21	1	6358	8.757469141	9.504529764	0.558099573
28-Dec-21	2	9195	9.126415137	9.661200722	0.285995622
29-Dec-21	3	13,154	9.484481174	9.817871681	0.11114923
30-Dec-21	4	16,764	9.726989009	9.97454264	0.0612828
31-Dec-21	5	22,775	10.03341872	10.1312136	0.009563838
1-Jan-22	6	27,553	10.2238667	10.28788456	0.004098286
2-Jan-22	7	33,750	10.4267357	10.44455552	0.000317546
3-Jan-22	8	37,379	10.52886433	10.60122647	0.00523628
4-Jan-22	9	58,097	10.96986931	10.75789743	0.044932075
5-Jan-22	10	90,928	11.41782326	10.91456839	0.253265466
6-Jan-22	11	117,094	11.67073231	11.07123935	0.359391809
7-Jan-22	12	141,986	11.86348374	11.22791031	0.403953587
8-Jan-22	13	159,632	11.98062645	11.38458127	0.355269854
9-Jan-22	14	179,723	12.09917206	11.54125223	0.311274536
10-Jan-22	15	168,063	12.03209419	11.69792318	0.11167026
11-Jan-22	16	194,720	12.17931791	11.85459414	0.105445523
12-Jan-22	17	168,063	12.03209419	12.0112651	0.000433851
13-Jan-22	18	264,202	12.48446924	12.16793606	0.100193254
14-Jan-22	19	268,833	12.50184565	12.32460702	0.031413532
15-Jan-22	20	268,833	12.50184565	12.48127798	0.000423029
16-Jan-22	21	271,202	12.51061921	12.63794894	0.016212859
17-Jan-22	22	258,089	12.46105977	12.7946199	0.11126236
18-Jan-22	23	238,018	12.38010158	12.95129085	0.326257186
19-Jan-22	24	282,970	12.55309616	13.10796181	0.307875888
20-Jan-22	25	317,532	12.66833388	13.26463277	0.355572368

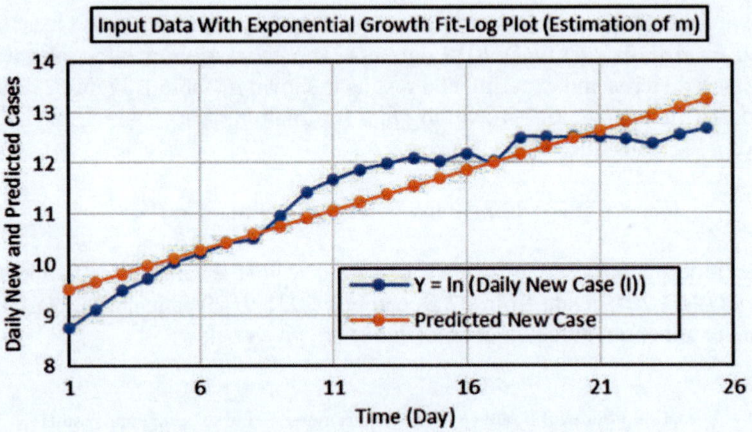

Fig. 2 Input data with exponential growth model: log plot (estimation of m)

$$
\begin{aligned}
Y &= 9.34785881 + 0.15667096t \\
I &= 11474.2e^{0.15667096t}
\end{aligned} \tag{8}
$$

R^2 is calculated to be 0.88 in this case. As a result, we infer that the R^2 of 88% indicates that the regression model fits 88% of the COVID-2019 data. In general, a greater R^2 suggests a better model fit.

3.2 *Estimation of Recovery Rate* (γ)

We have derived the value of recovery rate using differential Eq. 4 and estimate the value of recovery directly from India's COVID-2019 data. The procedures are given below: We know that from Eq. 4,

$$\frac{\mathrm{d}R}{\mathrm{d}t} = \gamma I \tag{9}$$

From the initial conditions $I = I_0$ and $R = 0$ at $t = 0$, the solution of above differential Eq. 9 is given below:

$$R(t) = \gamma I_0 t \tag{10}$$

If the COVID-19 pandemic takes T days to recover, then

$$R(T) = I_0, \quad \gamma = \frac{1}{T} \tag{11}$$

This is the recovery period of COVID-2019 pandemic (Eq. 11). The recovery rate of India can be estimate directly from the COVID-20019 dataset by using the following Eq. 12:

$$\gamma = \frac{R(t+1) - R(t)}{I} \tag{12}$$

Using the equation $\beta = m + \gamma$, we have been got the value of infection rate.

$$\gamma = 0.069061363,\ \beta = 0.225732321,\ R_0 = 3.268576125.$$

The calculation of doubling time of COVID-2019 epidemic of India is given by the following Eq. 13:

$$t_D = \frac{\ln 2}{(\beta - \gamma)} = 4.424223 \approx 4 \tag{13}$$

Thus, here, we can say that the doubling time COVID-2019 epidemic in India at the present time is four days. Currently, due to the Omicron variant in India, it is being seen that the number of infected with the COVID-2019 epidemic is doubling in 3–4 days. Table 2 shows the estimation of recovery rate estimates (γ) directly from India's COVID-2019 data. Figure 3 depicts the of recovery rate estimates (γ) directly from India's COVID-2019 data.

3.3 *Calculation of Infection for All Time*

At the beginning of transition of COVID-2019, infection (I) is minor while $S = N$ (total population size). Consequently, at time $t = 0$, there will be $I = 0$ and $S = N$. We can determine COVID-2019 infection for all time using following Eq. 14:

$$I = N - S + \frac{\gamma N}{\beta} * \ln\left(\frac{S}{N}\right) \tag{14}$$

This is the equation (Eq. 14) valid for all times. In general, the infection initially progresses rapidly and reaches a peak and gradually comes back to zero. Here, some questions will be arisen. These questions are as follows:

1. Can we find out maximum number of sick people ($I_{\max}$) at the peak of infection?
2. Can we find $S_\infty = \lim_{t\to\infty} S(t)$, i.e., the number of susceptible remains after the infection has passed?

Both the above questions can be answered with the help of Eqs. 3 and 14. Here, we assume that $S = N * s$, $I = N * i$, $R = N * r$, where *s*, *i*, and *r* represent fraction susceptible, fraction of infected, and fraction of recover, respectively. Substituting

Table 2 Estimation of recovery rate estimates (γ) directly from India's COVID-2019 data

Date	Time (day)	New case	Recover	γ
27-Dec-21	1	6358	7434	0.017301038
28-Dec-21	2	9195	7544	0.007721588
29-Dec-21	3	13,154	7615	0.006918048
30-Dec-21	4	16,764	7706	0.017000716
31-Dec-21	5	22,775	7991	0.486981339
1-Jan-22	6	27,553	19,082	−0.113127427
2-Jan-22	7	33,750	15,965	−0.148
3-Jan-22	8	37,379	10,970	0.426977715
4-Jan-22	9	58,097	26,930	−0.127355974
5-Jan-22	10	90,928	19,531	0.223594492
6-Jan-22	11	117,094	39,862	0.011247374
7-Jan-22	12	141,986	41,179	7.74724E-05
8-Jan-22	13	159,632	41,190	0.034554475
9-Jan-22	14	179,723	46,706	0.130923699
10-Jan-22	15	168,063	70,236	−0.055860005
11-Jan-22	16	194,720	60,848	0.048212818
12-Jan-22	17	168,063	70,236	0.2345787
13-Jan-22	18	264,202	109,660	0.050817178
14-Jan-22	19	268,833	123,086	0
15-Jan-22	20	268,833	123,086	0.057876079
16-Jan-22	21	271,202	138,645	0.049704648
17-Jan-22	22	258,089	152,125	0.021721189
18-Jan-22	23	238,018	157,731	0.129683469
19-Jan-22	24	282,970	188,598	0.126808496
20-Jan-22	25	317,532	224,481	0.08817694
Average (γ)				0.069061363

the values of *S*, *I,* and *R* in Eqs. 3 and 12, we have been got Eqs. 15 and 16:

$$\frac{\mathrm{d}i}{\mathrm{d}t} = i(\beta s - \gamma) \tag{15}$$

$$i = 1 - s + \frac{\gamma}{\beta} \ln s \tag{16}$$

The value of $\frac{di}{dt}$ will be zero at the peak of COVID-2019 pandemic, then Eq. 15 becomes Eq. 17.

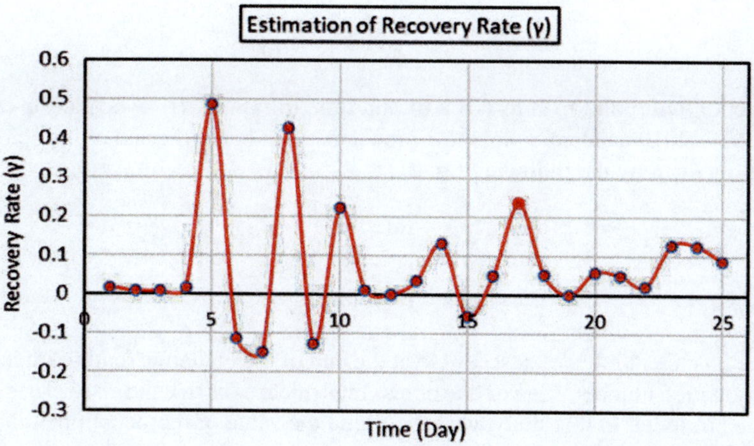

Fig. 3 Estimation of recovery rate estimates (γ) directly from India's COVID-2019 data

$$s = \frac{\gamma}{\beta} \tag{17}$$

Then, we find that

$$i_{\max} = 1 + \frac{\gamma}{\beta}\left(\ln \frac{\gamma}{\beta} - 1\right) \tag{18}$$

Putting the value of infection rate (β) and recovery rate (γ) in Eq. 18, we get

$$i_{\max} = 0.331710699 \approx 0.33$$

Therefore, at the peak of COVID-2019 in India, 33% of the total population will be infected. We will take $i \to 0$ and $t \to \infty$ to get the number of susceptible at the end of the COVID-2019 pandemic (Eq. 19).

$$i = 1 - s_{\infty} + \frac{\gamma}{\beta} \ln s_{\infty} = 0 \tag{19}$$

The value of s_{∞} can be obtained by numerically solving the above Eq. 19. Solving this equation by Newton Raphson method, we will get the value of s_{∞} ($s_{\infty} = 0.99$). Therefore, about 99% of the population remains susceptible at the end of the infection, and 1% of the population becomes infected at some point. The ratio of infection rate and recovery rate is called reproductive number (R_0), i.e., $R_0 = \frac{\beta}{\gamma}$. It epitomizes the number (average) of persons that infect person. On writing Eq. (18) in terms of the reproductive number (Eq. 20):

$$i_{\max} = 1 - \frac{1}{R_0}\left(1 - \ln\frac{1}{R_0}\right) \tag{20}$$

Infection will point to zero ($i \to 0$) and time to infinity ($t \to \infty$) at the end of the COVID-2019 pandemic. So, the reproductive number at the end of the epidemic will be obtained by the following Eq. 21:

$$R_0 = \frac{\ln(s_\infty)}{s_\infty - 1}$$
$$R_0 = 1.005033585 \tag{21}$$

where s_∞ is the number of susceptible at the end of the epidemic (end of infection). A reproduction number value of one or less than one means that the disease has come to an end in India. In this study, we have found the value of reproduction number to be 1.00503359.

3.4 *Simulation of SIR Model*

Here, we have used the Euler's method for solving SIR model's differential equations. This method is given below:

$$S(t_i + h) = S(t_i) - h\frac{\beta S(t_i)I(t_i)}{N} \tag{22}$$

$$I(t_i + h) = I(t_i) + h\frac{\beta S(t_i)I(t_i)}{N} - h\gamma I(t_i) \tag{23}$$

$$R(t_i + h) = R(t_i) + h\gamma I(t_i) \tag{24}$$

The above three Eqs. 22, 23, and 24 are Euler's method for solving the SIR model's differential equations. This experiment has been done by using Microsoft Excel. The simulated results with initial condition ($N = 1{,}380{,}000{,}000$, $S(0) = 1{,}379{,}993{,}642$, $\beta = 0.225732321$, $\gamma = 0.069061363$, $I(0) = 6358$, $R(0) = 7434$, $h = 1$) of projected SIR typical are revealed in Fig. 4. This result shows that after about 90 days from today, the widespread in India will be at its peak. Apart from this, in the last week of November 2022, this epidemic will end. Here, the estimated value of reproductive number is around one.

It is clear from Fig. 4 that after about 90 days (March 26, 2022), the COVID-2019 pandemic will be at its peak in India, and the disease will end in the last week of October 2022.

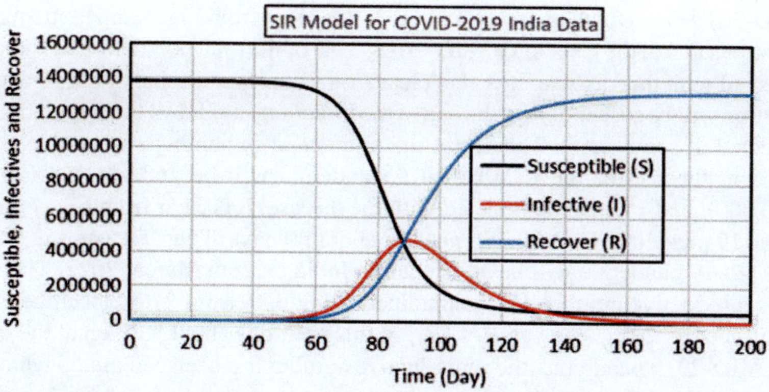

Fig. 4 Simulated result of SIR model with initial conditions condition ($N = 1{,}380{,}000{,}000$, $S(0) = 1{,}379{,}993{,}642$, $\beta = 0.225732321$, $\gamma = 0.069061363$, $I(0) = 6358$, $R(0) = 7434$, $h = 1$)

3.5 Calculation of Herd Immunity

To prevent the COVID-19 pandemic in India, the proportion of the vaccinated population should be atleast $1 - \frac{1}{R_0}$. From the threshold theorem, we know that if the vulnerability ratio drops below $\frac{1}{R_0}$, the COVID-19 pandemic will end. Because the vaccination program removes people from the susceptible compartment. We should vaccinate enough people in India to reduce the remaining susceptible ratio to less than $\frac{1}{R_0}$. This means that the immunization ratio should be greater than $\left(1 - \frac{1}{R_0}\right)$. In the present study, the calculated value of the reproductive number during the COVID-2019 pandemic is around 3. Therefore, the percentage of herd immunity (vaccination percentage) in India is given by the following calculation:

$$\text{Herd Immunity (\%)} = \left(1 - \frac{1}{R_0}\right) * 100 = \left(1 - \frac{1}{3}\right) * 100 = 66.67\%$$

Therefore, here, we can say that at the present time, 66.67% people has been vaccinated of the total population of India. This is the very big achievement Indian people as well as Indian Government to prevent the COVID-2019 pandemic.

4 Results and Discussion

In this study, we have used the (SIR) model to estimate the parameters related to the rising COVID-2019 epidemic curve in India and make individual estimates (such as pandemic prediction, peak and end of epidemic, and percentage of vaccination program). The value of infection rate (β) and the obtained constant (m) is shown in Fig. 2. We have estimated the value of recovery rate (γ) directly from India's

COVID-2019 data which is depicts in Fig. 3. It is clear from Fig. 4 and mathematical calculations that at the peak of COVID-2019, 33% of the total population of India will be infected with this disease. It is also clear from these studies that about 99% of the population will be susceptible at the end of the infection, and 1% of the population will be infected at some point. Therefore, the number of remaining susceptible people in India at the end of the COVID-2019 pandemic will be 260,481,478 (99% of 13,800,000), and 1% will be infected with the disease. It is clear from Fig. 4 that the COVID-19 pandemic in India will peak in about 90 days. Thus, we can say that the COVID-2019 pandemic will be at its peak in India on 26th March, 2022. The value of the reproductive number (R_0) is obtained using data from 27th December, 2021 to 20th January, 2022. The value of (R_0) in this period is about 3. Even at the end of the COVID-2019 pandemic, the reproductive number has been calculated which has a value of around 1.

We have taken India's COVID-2019 data from the Ministry of Health of India and Johns Hopkins University for experimental work and analysis purpose. The proposed SIR model has been shown that the COVID-2019 pandemic will reach its peak in India on 27th March, 2021. Apart from this, the epidemic will end after 90 days, i.e., on end of October, 2022. The estimated value of the reproductive number is 3, i.e., one person will infect at least three people. In conclusion, these parameters have been estimated using only RT-PCR confirmed case. If we manage to vaccinate at least 50% of India's population, we can stop the COVID-19 pandemic. I would like to point out to the Government of India and the people that the higher the value of the reproductive number, the more difficult it is to control COVID through the vaccination program.

5 Conclusion

In this study, we have studied the infection rate, recovery rate, epidemic peak, epidemic end, prediction, reproductive number, and vaccination program of this epidemic by using the India's COVID-2019 data from 27th December, 2021 to 20th January, 2022 and SIR model. This data has been taken from the Ministry of Health of India and Johns Hopkins University. The SIR model showed that the pandemic would peak in India 90 days after the onset of the COVID-19 pandemic. The presented model estimated that 1% of India's total population would be affected by the pandemic, and the remaining vulnerable would be around 99% after the end of the infection. The doubling time of this disease at the beginning of the COVID-2019 epidemic is about 3–4 days. Currently, due to the Omicron variant in India, it is being seen that the number of infected with the COVID-2019 epidemic is doubling in 3–4 days. Lastly, this type of study has the advantage that (in the case of India) strict government intervention and spreading awareness among people living in the city and village can significantly reduce the incidence of epidemics.

References

1. Lunis M (2020) Descriptive study of the current situation of COVID-19 in Algeria. Electron J General Med 17(6):253. 1–4
2. Johns Hopkins University of Medicine (JHUM). Accessed on 12 August 2020. Coronavirus Resource Center: https://coronavirus.jhu.edu/map.html.
3. De Leon UA-P, Pérez ÁGC, Avila-Vales E (2020) A SEIARD pandemic model for COVID-19 in Mexico: mathematical analysis and state-level forecasting. medRxiv [preprint]. https://doi.org/10.1101/2020.05.11.20098517
4. Khatua D, De A, Kar S, Samant E, Mandal SM (2020) A dynamic optimal control model for SARS-CoV-2 in India. Available at SSRN 3597498. https://doi.org/10.2139/ssrn.3597498
5. Bhattacharya A, Bhowmik D, Mukherjee J (2020) Prediction and interpretation of daily affected people during the 21-day lockdown due to the COVID-19 pandemic in India. medRxiv [preprint]. https://doi.org/10.1101/2200.04.22.20075572
6. Zou Y, Pan S, Zhao P, Han L, Wang X, Hemerik L, Knops J, van der Werf W (2020) Outbreak analysis with logistic growth model illustrating the COVID-19 suppression dynamics in China. Plus One 15(6):e0235247. https://doi.org/10.1371/journal.pone.0235247
7. Bagal DK, Rath A, Barua A, Patnaik D (2020) Estimating the parameters of the susceptible-infected-recovered model of COVID-19 cases in India during the lockdown period. Chaos Soliton Fractals. https://doi.org/10.1016/j.chaos.2020.110154
8. Alasaid A, Sadir H, Kamil R, Sari H (2020) Prediction of epidemic peak and infected cases for the COVID-19 disease in Malaysia, 2020. Int J Environ Res Public Health 17:4076. https://doi.org/10.3390/ijerph17114076
9. Huang NE, Qo F (2020) Data-driven time-dependent transmission rates for tracking an epidemic: a case study of 2019-nCoV. Sci Bull 65(6):425–427. https://doi.org/10.1016/j.scib.2020.02.005
10. Chu J (2020) A statistical analysis of the novel coronavirus (COVID-19) in Italy and Spain. PLOS One 1–25. https://doi.org/10.1371/journal.pone.0249037

Fine-Tuned Predictive Models for Forecasting Severity Level of COVID-19 Patient Using Epidemiological Data

Shweta A. Tikhe and Dipti P. Rana

Abstract HealthCare Data Analytics is the analysis technique using current and historical data related to the health domain to improve outreach, predict trends, and manage health-related matters. Severity level prediction will help battle the COVID-19 pandemic by providing early predictions for the treatment. Features are very significant for classification, so here this research is proposing to improve the model performance with the handcrafted features like severity level and weather category. Supervised machine learning models like random forest, decision tree, AdaBoost, K-Nearest Neighbors, and naïve Bayes analyzed the epidemiological dataset of COVID-19 to predict the severity level of COVID-19-positive patients. Various sampling techniques and feature selection techniques like feature score, feature importance, and correlation matrix are used to minimize the execution time and to improve and fine-tune the model. The result of the performance evaluation measure of the machine learning models showed that the random forest classifier has the best results of accuracy as 98.32% and a precision value as 97.52% followed by the decision tree classifier with SMOTE over-sampling technique when used the handcrafted features.

Keywords Data mining · Data analysis · COVID-19 · Feature engineering · Machine learning

1 Introduction

COVID-19 infection has outburst in more than hundreds of countries in a very short span. It is a contagious virus infection that started from Wuhan, China. Due to the exponential increase in cases day by day, the pandemic has been declared all

S. A. Tikhe (✉) · D. P. Rana
Sardar Vallabhbhai National Institute of Technology, Surat, Gujarat, India
e-mail: shweta.tikhe@gmail.com

D. P. Rana
e-mail: dpr@coed.svnit.ac.in

© The Author(s), under exclusive license to Springer Nature Singapore Pte Ltd. 2023
J. K. Mandal and D. De (eds.), *Frontiers of ICT in Healthcare*, Lecture Notes in Networks and Systems 519, https://doi.org/10.1007/978-981-19-5191-6_35

over the world, and human lives came into danger. As this pandemic was an unexpected outbreak for the whole world, medical systems were not enough to handle the situation. Hence, a number of researchers started to find solutions to control the spread. Many studies were focused on predicting positive–negative cases, the early-stage discovery of patients, finding needed recovery days for a patient, severity of COVID-19 patient, and many other studies. Data-driven businesses or different sectors/domains make choices based on data because of which they can be more efficient and confident in their actions or implementation for better results [1]. HealthCare is the maintenance and enhancement of one's health by prevention, finding, diagnosis, therapy, treatment, recovery, or healing of a disease, illness, injury, and other physical and mental disabilities in individuals [2]. Healthcare data analysis is able to show a big picture of an individual's health. And this helps in proper care and treatment according to the need. Supervised machine learning (ML) algorithms are achieving very good results over the last decades. It is showing a lot of promising performance results in the health domain. Due to quick resulting systems using ML algorithms, it is giving early detections and helps in early diagnosis and treatment for a patient. Using different data pre-processing, feature engineering, and data analysis techniques will help in understanding the effect and prediction of the COVID-19-related information by enhancing the model. Real-world data is usually inaccurate, imperfect, noisy, or unreliable. Data preprocessing helps in transforming raw data into meaningful, useful, and effective datasets. Feature engineering is the method of mining beneficial and useful features from raw data using domain information. The key purpose of data analysis is to find significant insights from the data to gain the knowledge from data to make significant decisions. This study will find informative COVID-19 data insights like COVID-19 related findings, patterns, understanding of the dataset and attributes, model, and visualization of the COVID-19 data. In this research, supervised ML techniques are analyzed and then improve prediction models using epidemiology labeled confirmed COVID -19 cases dataset with various severity levels. Various supervised learning algorithms like decision tree, AdaBoost, K-Nearest Neighbors, naïve Bayes, and random forest are used on the dataset having novel handcrafted features. This study will improve the performance of the predictive model by fine-tuning the models, help to enhance the medical systems, and decrease the execution time for early predictions by applying different techniques. The COVID-19 dataset available on GitHub is used for the experimental study. Results of this experiment work will provide a supervised ML model with better performance results, less execution time, and different visualization for the COVID-19 dataset.

1.1 Objective

The objective of the work is to predict the findings, patterns, understanding, modeling, and visualization to derive informative insights from the COVID-19 data. Supervised machine learning models were analyzed for predicting the severity level of COVID-19-positive patients by generating handcrafted features. The first handcrafted feature is severity which is generated with the help of symptom's feature, and another handcrafted feature is season which is generated based on country and date of confirmation features. This study will help in understanding the impact and predicting COVID-19 cases' severity level. The effect of the several COVID-19 data attributes will also be studied for better performance. A good supervised machine learning model with good results will help the medical expert in the current pandemic situation, and also fine-tuned model will provide intelligence to the machine.

2 Literature Survey

A large amount of research has already been done using various data analysis techniques and ML models for diagnosing and predicting infection of COVID-19 as well as for treatment and recovery of the patient.

Iwendi et al. [3] proposed a random forest classification model fine-tuned by boosting the AdaBoost algorithm. The study showed a positive relationship between patients' deaths and gender and indicated that the majority COVID-19 positive patients are aged between 20 and 70 years. Sakr et al. [4] proposed a comparison and performance evaluation of seven popular ML techniques on estimating all-cause mortality (ACM). Muhammad et al. [5] proposed work with learning algorithms containing both positive and negative corona patients. The performance of the models indicated that the decision tree model gained highest accuracy, naïve Bayes model gained highest specificity, and the support vector machine model gained highest sensitivity. Muhammad et al. [6] developed data mining models for prediction using epidemiological data of COVID-19 patients in South Korea. The results showed that with decision tree model is more effective than other models when compared with the accuracy. Onari et al. [7] proposed self-assessment decision support system (DSS) for differentiating the severity of the COVID-19 positive cases to improve the healthcare system. Choudhury et al. [8] proposed a Type-2 Fuzzy logic system which is designed to provide an initial analysis on how likely the symptoms of a patient having illness are caused by COVID-19 infection.

Hamzah et al. [9] proposed a CoronaTracker online platform which provides the latest news related to corona. Using predictive modeling, this research predicted the COVID-19 confirmed cases, losses, and recoveries. In the research by Khanday et al. [10], they applied ensemble and traditional ML approaches on clinical reports for classification of the patient into, namely, SARS, ARDS, COVID-19, and both (ARDS, COVID-19). Feature engineering was applied on the data. According to Sun et al. [11], chest computed tomography (CT) shows effective results in the diagnosis of corona virus. In the research of El-kenawy et al. [12], two optimization algorithms are proposed for COVID-19 classification and feature selection using CT images of positive and negative cases. Narin et al. [13] applied convolutional neural network-based models, namely, InceptionV3, ResNet50, and Inception-ResNetV2 on chest

X-ray radiographs with fivefold cross-validation. Ho [14] proposed a method to build tree-based classifiers whose capacity can be expanded to improve the accuracy for training and testing data.

To address informational crisis, Samuel et al. [15] identified sentiments with the help of tweets related to COVID-19 pandemic. This research study provided insights into coronavirus fear sentiment increase among people. Zhang et al. [16] proposed a new deep learning-based model for deep anomaly detection which is a faster and reliable model for screening of COVID-19. Alam et al. [17] suggested a feature ranking-based approach for classification of the medical data. Prediction results of the proposed method have performance better than the baseline method. Khanam et al. [10] focused on the data visualization and analysis. Based on the data, the increase in the COVID-19 positive patients is found to show exponential curve.

The related literature surveys that have been considered, studied, and reviewed so far show that data analysis, data mining, ML techniques, and various data science fields have important roles in detection, prediction, treatment, and diagnosis of the COVID-19, which can benefit limited healthcare systems to battle COVID-19 pandemic. To the best of our acquaintance and understanding, very limited work has been reported until now for the severity of the patient's condition together with the impact of the season based on the location by applying feature engineering using an epidemiologic dataset. Therefore, this study intends to work on these gaps.

3 Theoretical Background

3.1 *Data Preprocessing*

It is a data mining technique used to convert raw data into efficient and useful data.

- Data Cleaning: It is the approach of correcting and identifying the inaccurate or unusable data values in a dataset. There can be missing data or noisy data.
- Data Editing: It is the process which involves correction or adjustment of the data after reviewing the dataset.
- Data Transformation: It is the procedure of transforming and mapping raw data into appropriate and suitable format for data processing.
- Data Reduction: It is the process to reduce dataset and the analysis cost in order to increase efficiency and reduce hardship of the huge data analysis.

3.2 *Feature Engineering*

Feature engineering is the techniques or process of gathering features from the raw dataset which better represent the problem, resulting in improved model performance.

- Attribute and Feature: Feature is an attribute which is significant and meaningful in the context of a problem. All features are attributes but vice versa are not true.
- Feature Importance: The score of the feature is calculated by how the feature is correlated with the target variable.
- Feature Extraction: Feature extraction automatically reduces the dimensionality of big/long types of feature values into a smaller set that can be used to model machine learning model [18].
- Feature Selection: It is the method of choosing a subset of the features which are useful features for the problem.
- Feature Construction: It is the method to create new features from available raw data features for the model usability.
- Feature Learning: It is a collection of techniques that allow automatic finding of the representations required for feature classification or feature detection from raw data.

3.3 Encoding and Over-Sampling Techniques

OneHot encoder and Label encoder are used in this study for encoding categorical features and target feature.

Over-sampling [19] techniques are used for balancing the imbalanced dataset by increasing the samples of minority class for adjusting the class distribution. Various techniques, namely, Random, Synthetic Minority Over-sampling Technique (SMOTE), SMOTE for Nominal and Continuous (SMOTENC), SMOTE for Nominal (SMOTEN), bSMOTE1 and bSMOTE2 (Borderline SMOTE Type-1 and Borderline SMOTE Type-2), Support Vectors Machines SMOTE (SVM-SMOTE), Adaptive Synthetic Sampling (ADASYN), and KMeans-SMOTE are used for comparison.

3.4 Correlation Matrix (Heatmap) and Machine Learning Models

The cell with (i, j) position in the matrix defines the association between the ith and jth feature of the dataset. The features in the dataset are said to have a linear relationship, when the data points follow an approximately straight line trend. The correlation between features tells the linear association strength between them.

Random forest algorithm, decision tree algorithm, AdaBoost algorithm, K-nearest neighbors algorithm, and Gaussian naïve Bayes algorithm are used for experimentation.

4 Proposed Workflow and Methodology

Figure 1 shows the essential step-wise proposed framework to improve the supervised learning predictive model.

Using COVID-19 dataset and country geographic data, dataset is prepared. Data preprocessing techniques like cleaning, editing, transforming, and data reducing are applied for generating the meaningful dataset.

Handcrafted feature generation block defines the target features generation to prepare the dataset with handcrafted features to analyze the performance improvement of the classification models:

- Severity feature is created by considering the different scenarios and by using 'Symptoms', 'ChronicDiseaseQ', 'ChronicDiseases', 'DischargedQ', 'DeathQ', and 'DateOfDeath' features of dataset. Severity feature is added in the original dataset by considering the facts: If there is a death of a patient, then 'Severe'. If a patient is discharged, then 'Less Severe'. Together with this, if the patient has "ChronicDiseases", i.e., Non-null_Value or "ChronicDiseaseQ" is equal to True, then 'Severe'. If there is only one symptom in a patient, then 'Less Severe'. If COVID-19-related symptoms, and respiratory symptoms are there, then 'Severe'. If more than five symptoms in a patient, then 'Severe'. If values are unknown or no decidability for the severity factor, then 'Moderate Severe'.
- The geographical data like country-wise hemisphere [20] and month-wise seasonal data by each month [21] are mapped along with longitude, and latitude column by each country to generate the seasonality feature.

The next classifications block applies the several supervised machine learning algorithms on the prepared dataset with handcrafted features to classify the symptoms as of high (2), moderate (1), and low (0) severity levels.

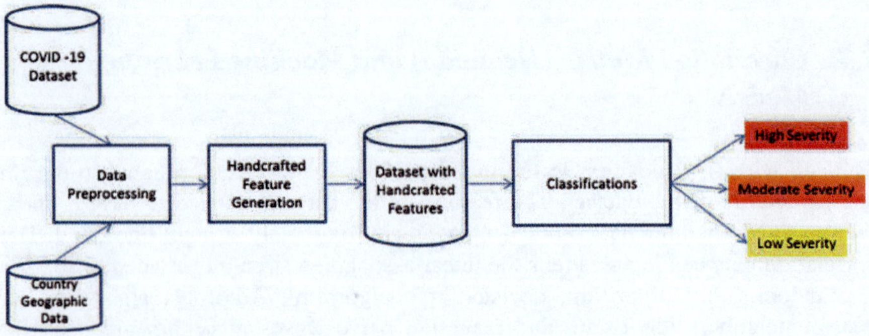

Fig. 1 Proposed workflow

5 Experimental Setup and Implementation

5.1 Data Collection

- COVID-19 Dataset: The dataset is collected from the GitHub repository [22] which consists of the gender, symptoms, age, etc. Rows: 6508, Columns: 12.
- Country and Hemisphere Data: The work in this study combines the information of COVID-19 patient with the hemisphere information [19] which tells the hemisphere its country resides in. Rows: 248, Columns: 2.
- Month-Wise Data of Hemisphere and Season: Season-wise information [21] in this dataset gives the information according to northern hemisphere and southern hemisphere. Rows: 12, Columns: 4.

These three datasets are utilized to generate the handcrafted features to create the final dataset essential for the study.

5.2 Data Preprocessing on Raw Data

- Data Cleaning: Symptoms feature-values like 'Quantity[—]' or 'Interval[[]]' are removed and 'fever' value is added in that cell if not present. Age feature–Age intervals are replaced with the mid value of the interval. Null values are filled with mean values for that particular feature. Gender feature-Blanks updated to 'Male' value as count for 'Male' value is more than the 'Female' value.
- Data Editing: ChronicDiseases feature value-If non-null then TRUE otherwise FALSE. DateOfOnsetSymptoms feature-Column value separated to three columns each for year, month, and date. DateOfConfirmation feature-Column value separated to three columns each for year, month, and date. All NaN values changed to 'na' because Python3 considers NaN value as null value and ignores it in the data processing.
- Data Transformation: ChronicDiseaseQ feature-If feature value is 'na' then it has been changed to FALSE. Gender feature: If cell value is 'Male' then changed to 0, and if cell value is 'Female' then changed to 1 using the Label Encoder.
- Data Reduction: Discharge, Symptom, Chronic disease, ID, and Date Of Confirmation_Year columns are removed. Country column is removed because longitude and latitude columns are added in the feature for better performance of the model.

5.3 Handcrafted Feature Generation

- Attribute and Feature: Important attributes are selected as a feature and other attributes, i.e., 'ID' is removed from the dataset.

- Feature Extraction: OneHot encoding is applied on symptom's feature.
- Feature Construction: As explained in the methodology, the handcrafted features are generated and prepared them for the classification model.

  Severity feature—This handcrafted feature is an ordinal feature. Therefore, values are transformed according to their order, i.e., 'Less Severe' → 0, 'Moderate Severe' → 1, and 'Severe' → 2.
  Country_Hemosphere feature-If cell value is 'NorthenHemisphere' then changed to 0, and if cell value is 'SouthernHemisphere' then changed to 1 using Label Encoder. And features like Country, and Season have more than 2 class values, therefore, OneHot Encoder can be applied.

- Feature Importance and Selection: Scores for each feature have been calculated with different methods. Subsets of features are selected which have highest scores in the learning model.

Also, performed different over-sampling methods applied to adjust the imbalanced dataset.

5.4 Dataset Analysis and Visualizations

See Figs. 2 and 3.

6 Prediction and Result Analysis

The raw dataset is preprocessed, and feature engineering is applied on the preprocessed data. The supervised ML models were applied on the prepared COVID-19 dataset. The dataset used in this work is imbalanced dataset; thus, applied different over-sampling techniques and found better results with SMOTE over-sampling technique, so utilized it for the further experiment (Figs. 4 and 5).

The experiments show that random forest algorithm with SMOTE over-sampling technique provides the best result with data preprocessing and feature engineering with accuracy as 98.32% and precision value as 97.52% followed by decision tree algorithm with accuracy as 97.90% and precision value as 96.74% (Fig. 6).

7 Conclusion

COVID-19 pandemic is a public medical emergency declared by the World Health Organization. Therefore, non-clinical techniques like machine learning, deep learning, etc. are being used by the researchers to help medical systems to early detect,

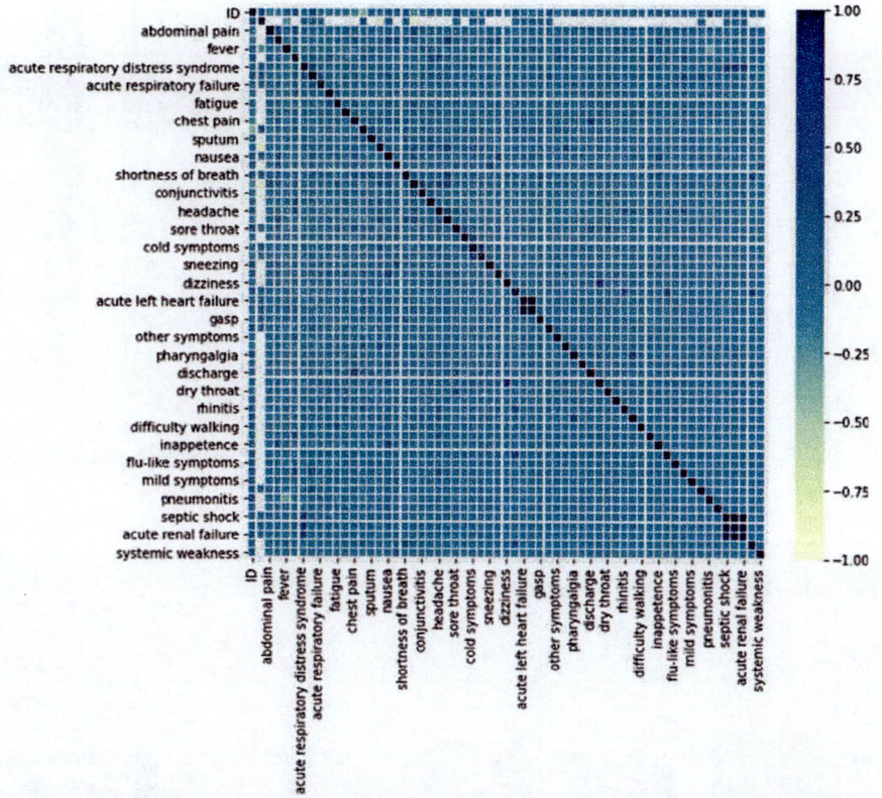

Fig. 2 Original dataset correlation matrix

predict severity, and treat patients to reduce burden on health domain. In this study, multiple classification algorithms are used on the COVID-19 dataset where dataset is prepared using various data preprocessing steps, and many feature engineering techniques like generating novel handcrafted and fine-grained features. Severity feature has been generated and labeled as target variable. Also, weather feature is generated to check if it is affecting the severity or not. Feature importance scores show that weather information affects the COVID-19 case. The experiments depict that the random forest algorithm provides better result with the handcrafted features.

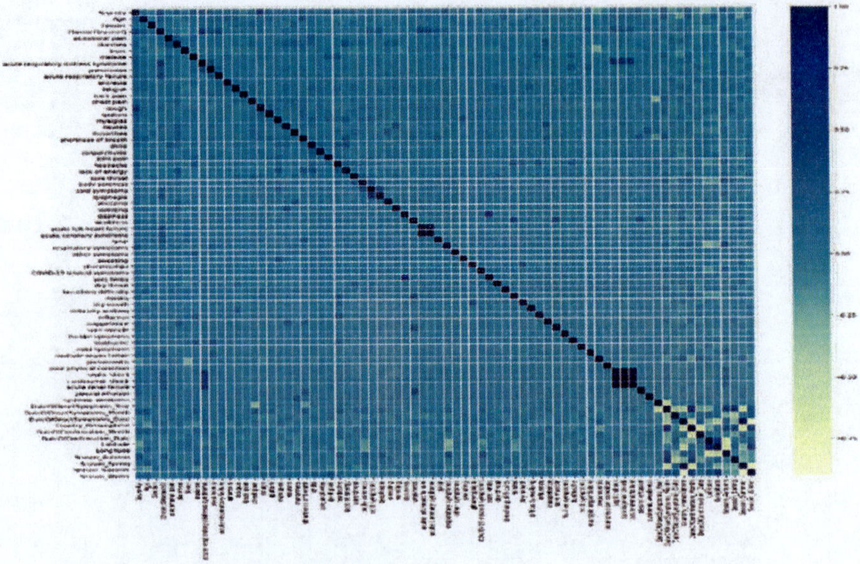

Fig. 3 Preprocessed dataset correlation matrix

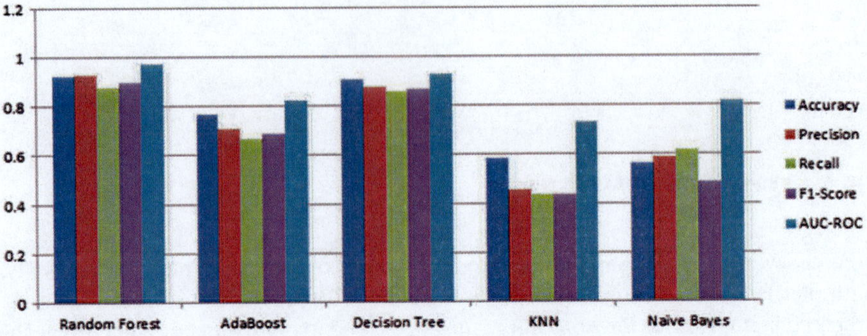

Fig. 4 Comparative study of performance evaluation before preprocessing the dataset

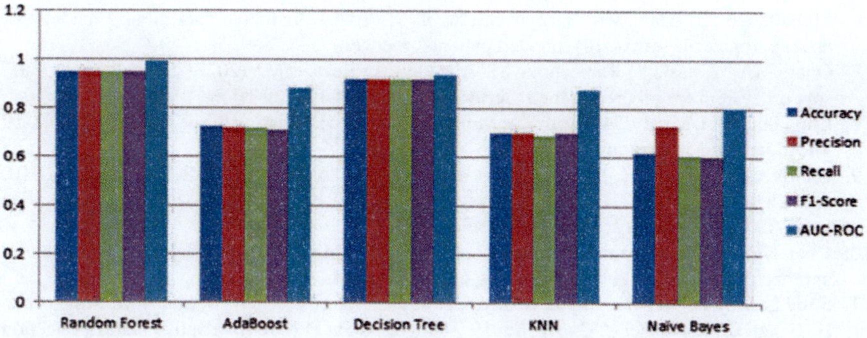

Fig. 5 Comparative study of performance evaluation after preprocessing the dataset

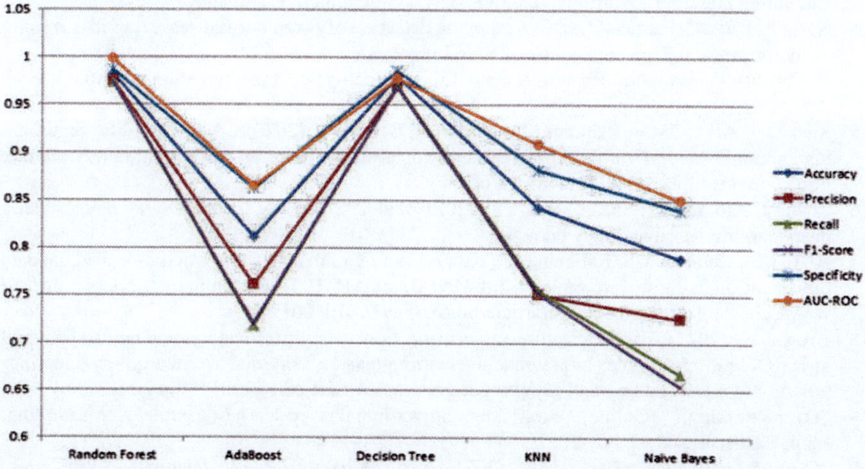

Fig. 6 Comparative performance analysis of supervised machine learning models

References

1. "Data analysis: what, how, and why to do data analysis for your organization," October 2019. [Online]. Available: https://www.import.io/post/business-data-analysis-what-how-why/
2. "Health care," [Online]. Available: https://en.wikipedia.org/wiki/Healthcare. Last accessed 12 July 2021
3. Iwendi C, Bashir AK, Peshkar A, Sujatha R, Chatterjee JM, Pasupuleti S, Mishra R, Pillai S, Jo O (2020) Covid-19 patient health prediction using boosted random forest algorithm. Front Public Health
4. Sakr S, Elshawi R, Ahmed AM, Qureshi WT, Brawner CA, Keteyian SJ, Blaha MJ, Al-Mallah MH (2017) Comparison of machine learning techniques to predict allcause mortality using fitness data: the henry ford exercise testing (fit) project
5. Muhammad LJ, Algehyne EA, Usman SS, Ahmad A, Chakraborty C, Mohammed IA (2020) Supervised machine learning models for prediction of covid-19 infection using epidemiology dataset

6. Muhammad LJ, Islam MM, Usman SS, Ayon SI (2020) Predictive data mining models for novel coronavirus (covid-19) infected patients' recovery
7. Onari MA, Yousefi S, Rabieepour M, Alizadeh A, Rezaee MJ (2021) A medical decision support system for predicting the severity level of covid-19
8. Choudhury SH, Mitaly TA, Aurin ZA, Mollah S, Rafi AA, Predicting the possibility of covid-19 infection using a fuzzy logic system
9. Hamzah FAB, Lau CH, Nazri H, Ligot DV, Lee G, Tan CL, Shaib MKBM, Zaidon UHB, Abdullah AB, Chung MH, Ong CH, Chew PY, Salunga RE (2020) Coronatracker: world-wide covid-19 outbreak data analysis and prediction
10. Khanday AMUD, Rabani ST, Khan QR, Rouf N, Din MMU (2020) Machine learning based approaches for detecting covid-19 using clinical text data
11. Suny L, Moy Z, Yany F, Xiay L, Shany F, Dingy Z, Songy B, Gaoy W, Shaoy W, Shi F, Yuan H, Jiang H, Wu D, Wei Y, Gao Y, Sui H, Zhang D, Shen D (2020) Adaptive feature selection guided deep forest for covid-19 classification with chest CT. IEEE J Biomed Health Inform 24(10):2798–2805
12. El-kenawy ESM, Ibrahim A, Mirjalili S, Eid MM, Hussein SE (2020) Novel feature selection and voting classifier algorithms for covid-19 classification in CT images
13. Narin A, Kaya C, Pamuk Z (2020) Automatic detection of coronavirus disease (covid-19) using x-ray images and deep convolutional neural networks
14. Ho TK (1995) Random decision forests. In: Proceedings of 3rd international conference on document analysis and recognition, vol 1, pp 278–282
15. Samuel J, Ali GGMN, Rahman MM, Esawi E, Samuel Y (2020) Covid-19 public sentiment insights and machine learning for tweets classification. Information 11(6). [Online]. Available: https://www.mdpi.com/2078-2489/11/6/314
16. Zhang J, Xie Y, Li Y, Shen C, Xia Y (2020) Covid-19 screening on chest x-ray images using deep learning based anomaly detection
17. Alam MZ, Rahman MS, Rahman MS (2019) A random forest based predictor for medical data classification using feature ranking. Inf Med Unlock 15:100180. [Online]. Available: https://www.sciencedirect.com/science/article/pii/S235291481930019X
18. Brownlee J (2021) Discover feature engineering, how to engineer features and how to get good at it. [Online]. Available: https://machinelearningmastery.com/discover-feature-engineering-how-to-engineer-features-and-how-to-get-good-at-it/. Last accessed 12 July 2021
19. "Over-sampling," [Online]. Available: https://imbalanced-learn.org/stable/over_sampling.html. Last accessed 12 July 2021
20. "Country and hemisphere data," 2021, List of countries by regional classification. [Online]. Available: https://meta.wikimedia.org/wiki/List_of_countries_by_regional_classification , Last accessed 12 July 2021
21. "Month wise data of hemisphere and season," 2021, last accessed 12 July 2021, Season. [Online]. Available: https://en.wikipedia.org/wiki/Season, Last accessed 12 July 2021
22. "Patient medical data for novel coronavirus covid-19," 2020, data retrieved from the Wolfram Data Repository, C19-Prediction-via-Symptoms-with- Fuzzy-Logic: Prospective Predictions Are the Future Joseph Paul Cohen and Paul Morrison and Lan Dao and Karsten Roth and Tim Q Duong and MarzyehGhassemi arXiv:2006.11988, https://github.com/Namerlight/C19-Prediction-via-Symptoms-with-Fuzzy-Logic/tree/master/data. [Online]. Available: https://github.com/Namerlight/C19-Prediction-via-Symptoms-with-Fuzzy-Logic/blob/master/data/WolframPatients.csv

An Ensemble Machine Learning Model to Detect COVID-19 Using Chest X-Ray

Somenath Chakraborty and Beddhu Murali

Abstract The COVID-19 which is caused by the severe acute respiratory syndrome coronavirus 2 or SARS-CoV-2, has taken a lot of human life and still continuing, and significantly disrupting the healthcare system. Due to challenges and controversies to testing for COVID-19, improved, alternative cost-effective, and machine learning methods are needed to detect the disease and related data analysis. For this purpose, machine learning (ML) approaches emerge as a strong forecasting method to detect a disease including COVID-19. Our proposed ensemble machine learning (EML) is a technique that leverages multiple deep learning models and then combines them to produce improved results. In this paper, we proposed an EML approach to detect COVID-19 using chest x-ray images. Radiographic images are readily available, which can be used as an effective tool compared to other expensive and time-consuming pathological tests, but not to replace pathological tests but rather give alternative extra confirmation and more detailed analysis to the medical fraternity. In conclusion, automatic computational machine learning models allow for rapid analysis of chest X-ray images and thus enable radiologists to filter potential candidates in a time-effective manner to detect COVID-19. Our proposed approach has very promising results with an average detection accuracy of 93.56% and a sensitivity of 91.24%, and an F1 score is 0.91.

Keywords COVID-19 · SARS-CoV-2 · Chest X-Ray · Ensemble machine learning model (EML)

1 Introduction

The Severe Acute Respiratory Syndrome Coronavirus 2 (SARS-CoV-2) causes the disease named COVID-19, which has created the greatest pandemic in recent times

S. Chakraborty (✉)
Department of Computer Science and Information Systems, Leonard C. Nelson College of Engineering and Sciences, West Virginia University Institute of Technology, Beckley, USA
e-mail: somenath.chakraborty@mail.wvu.edu

B. Murali
Computer Science and Engineering, University of North Texas, Denton, USA
© The Author(s), under exclusive license to Springer Nature Singapore Pte Ltd. 2023

J. K. Mandal and D. De (eds.), *Frontiers of ICT in Healthcare*, Lecture Notes in Networks and Systems 519, https://doi.org/10.1007/978-981-19-5191-6_36

and already traumatized the whole world. COVID-19 was reportedly started in Wuhan city of China in December 2019 [1, 2]. The World Health Organization (WHO) reported on their website that the total number of cases as of January 28, 2022 is 366,694,109 in the world. The total number of deaths in the world as of this date is 5,656,642, and the number is still increasing with a new growing fear of the Omicron coronavirus variant (B.1.1.529). COVID-19 is a disease which is initially affecting the respiratory organs, like the lungs [3]. As it is a highly transmittable viral infection, people are dying all over the world, and many severely suffering patients do not find hospital accommodation due to overloading with the existing COVID-19 patients. The critical care facility is also very limited in some countries. As the situation in the early 2020 was already started deteriorating and new cases are growing at an exponential level. The World Health Organization (WHO) declared it as a pandemic on March 11, 2020 [4]. The WHO distinguishes the variant of coronavirus into two categories: one is a variant of Interest, and another one is a variant of concern. According to the transmissibility and detrimental effects, the variant of concern coronavirus is more dangerous compared to the variant of interest. The detection of COVID-19 is one of the primal aspects to fight against this coronavirus. Initially, the detection was very critical and error-prone due to a lack of knowledge of the virus genome, but then the test named reverse transcription-polymerase chain reaction (RT-PCR) [5], which is still now a golden standard for detection of COVID-19 in spite of many challenges still remain in this COVID-19 detection research. The RT-PCR sensitivity rate is 60–70%, which is very low. In Fig. 1, the COVID-19 locality of interest region is shown in the X-ray images.

There are two accurate ways exist for the diagnosis of COVID-19: one is using a chest X-ray, and another is a chest CT scan [6, 7]. We propose to build the model from chest X-ray images using an artificial intelligence approach, which includes an ensemble machine learning (EML) model. Radiographic images such as X-ray images are inexpensive and less time-consuming to produce compared to other clinical approches. So, a chest X-ray is a very useful early detection tool to test whether a patient has COVID-19. Machine learning approaches allow for rapid analysis of chest X-ray images and thus enable radiologists to filter potential candidates in a

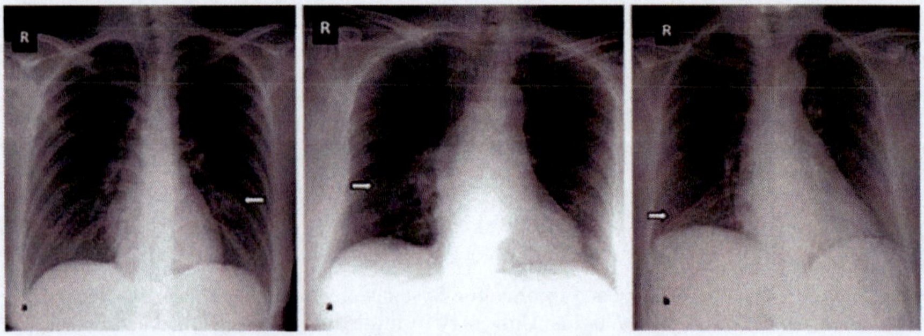

Fig. 1 COVID-19 pneumonia is characterized primarily by increased attenuation in the lung area

time-effective manner. Deep learning methods [8, 9] revolutionize the field of artificial intelligence and due to their application in medical diagnosis and prognosis system, millions of human life and labor have been saved.

2 Literature Review

The convolutional neural network (CNN) with effective deep layers is the fundamental building block of any deep learning framework. It is widely used for different types of computational problems as well as image classification problems [10–12]. There are many applications that were implemented in different research papers with the help of deep neural networks. Due to the advancement of different deep neural networks, like ResNet18, ResNet50 [13], AlexNet [14], DenseNet [15], VGG16 [16], etc., we can make a very sophisticated machine learning model which can detect COVID-19 from CXR, CT images, sometimes a combination of both. Previously, a handcrafted feature generation technique was used where the heuristic approach was used a lot. Prior to COVID-19, Rajpurkar et al. [17] describe a model named as CheXNet where they use a deep neural network to classify 14 kinds of Pneumonia disease. Their model uses more than 100,000 frontal view X-ray images with 14 diseases to develop their model. It is a very promising research work that can greatly influence the study of COVID-19 research using ML. Wang et al. [18] develop a machine learning model, they name it as COVID-Net using 13,975 CXR images. They had a total of 8066 patient cases who have no pneumonia, i.e., normal cases and 5538 patient cases who have non-COVID19 pneumonia. They have only 266 COVID-19 patient cases which makes their dataset have data imbalance issues. Minace et al. [19] develop their model using 5000 Chest X-rays. They use the transfer learning technique to use the pre-trained weights in their model. The main disadvantage of this kind of transfer learning weight is that the original deep learning network did not actually use a medical dataset, more especially the COVID-19 dataset, so the weights may lead to bias prediction to some extent. Khan et al. [20], named their model as CoroNet which consists of 310 normal images, 330 cases of Pneumonia Bacterial, 327 Pneumonia Viral, and only 284 COVID-19 sample images. Their research was done in early April 2020, and hence their model was built with such a lower number of sample cases.

3 Materials and Methodology

3.1 Collecting the Data-Source

First, we need to collect the CXR images from different sources [21–25]. Then we study the analysis process of CXR using a machine learning model. Then we need to collect the segmentation mask [26, 27] to get the segmented lung contour of the CXR images. We use U-Net, a Convolutional Networks for Image Segmentation Models framework [28], which is a semantic segmentation algorithm. This proposed model used a dataset of 6641 samples, of which 1684 had COVID-19, 1845 had pneumonia, and 3112 were healthy individuals.

The original chest X-ray images are resized to 224 × 224 to be compatible with the pre-trained model used in this research. All the images in the dataset used for training, validation, and testing are normalized using deep learning programming code. We used data augmentation to increase each data sample. The images were first proposed with some basic preprocessing technique, then they were horizontally flipped, magnified, and rotated for augmentation. After all these processes, we have the increased amount of data image samples in training, validation, and testing while maintaining the balancing property of the sample.

3.2 Methodology

We collect the data from different sources. Then data annotations and preprocessing have been done. After getting the segmented mask contour, then we build up an ensemble machine learning model (EML) which is a combination of many deep learning models and produces the optimum value for each stage of classification. We use different kinds of deep neural network architecture to improve the model which can filter out the error and generate the optimum results. The following Fig. 2 shows the functional flowchart, Fig. 3 is the abstract representation, and Fig. 4 is the architecture details of our proposed EML model.

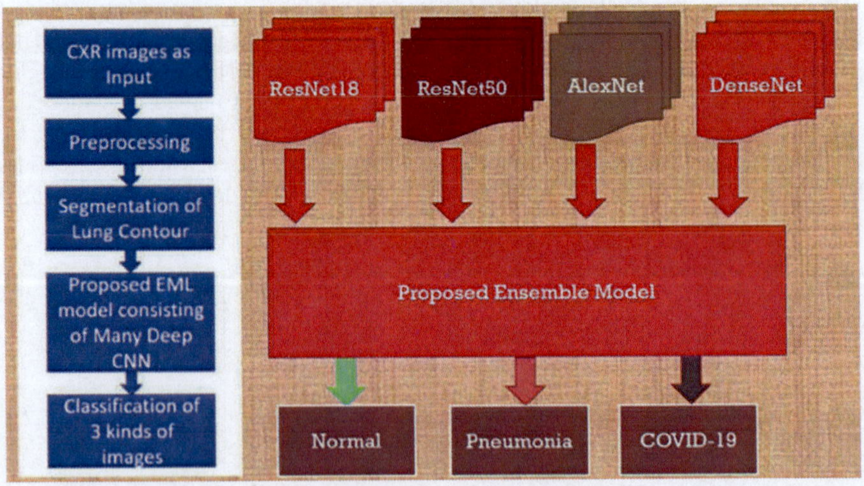

Fig. 2 Functional flowchart of the ensemble machine learning (EML) model

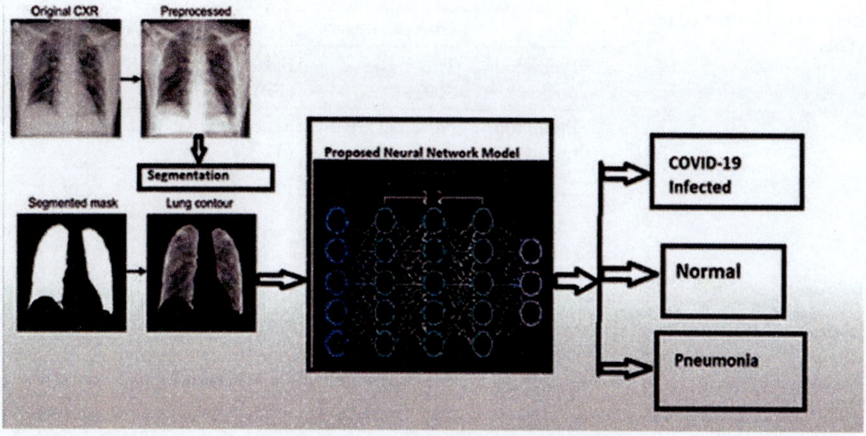

Fig. 3 The block diagram representation of the ensemble machine learning (EML) model

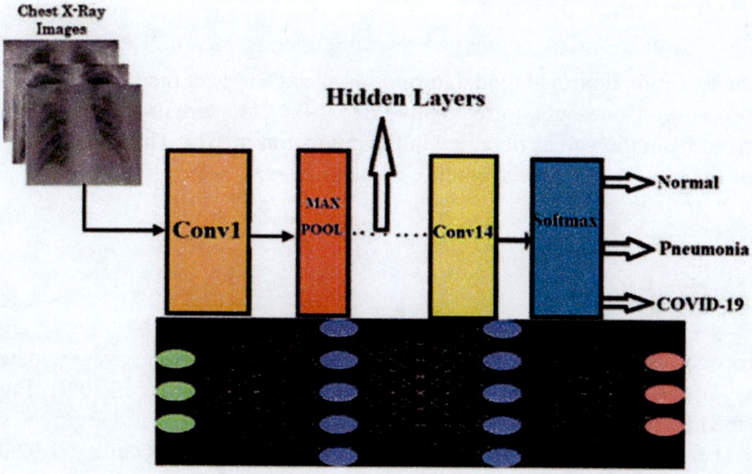

Fig. 4 Our proposed ensemble machine learning (EML) model architecture

Our EML model integrates many deep learning models and reduces the error with an optimum deep network that builds up with 46 layers. 14 convolution layers, 23 hidden layers, 4 Max-pooling layers, 2 average pooling layers, 2 dropout layers, and one SoftMax layer.

Table 1 Performance test details

	Disease present	Disease absent	Total
Predicted positive	True positive (TP)	False positive (FP)	TP + FP
Predicted negative	False negative (FN)	True negative (TN)	FN + TN
Total	TP + FN	FP + TN	TP + FP + FN + TN

Sensitivity or Recall = TP/(TP + FN)
Specificity = TN/(FP + TN)
Positive Predictive Value or Precision = TP/(TP + FP)
Accuracy = (TP + TN)/(TP + FP + FN + TN)
The weighted average of precision and recall, known as F1 Score = 2*(Recall * Precision)/(Recall + Precision)

4 Results

4.1 *Performance Metrics*

To evaluate a computational model, terminology such as accuracy, sensitivity, specificity, precision, F-measure, false positive rate (FPR), etc., are used. These measures are derived from the values obtained in the confusion matrix. This matrix is used to describe the classification performance of a model on a dataset (Table 1).

4.2 *Derived Results*

The proposed Ensemble Machine Learning (EML) model had an average detection accuracy of 93.56% and a sensitivity of 91.24%, and the F1 score is 0.91. Figure 5 shows the loss curve which is clearly evident the loss decreases, and Figure. 6 shows the test and train accuracy. The train accuracy is 97% and test accuracy is 92%.

Table 2 shows the comparative analysis with other existing models.

5 Conclusion

The research presented in this paper having concerning impact as we are still living in the pandemic scenario and new variants are coming day by day. If we could have automated detection techniques available everywhere then we may have some control over the COVID-19 spreading as this virus is asymptomatic in some cases and due to lacking testing, proliferating of the virus in communities is widespread. This EML model would help the medical practitioner to take decisions more confidently and

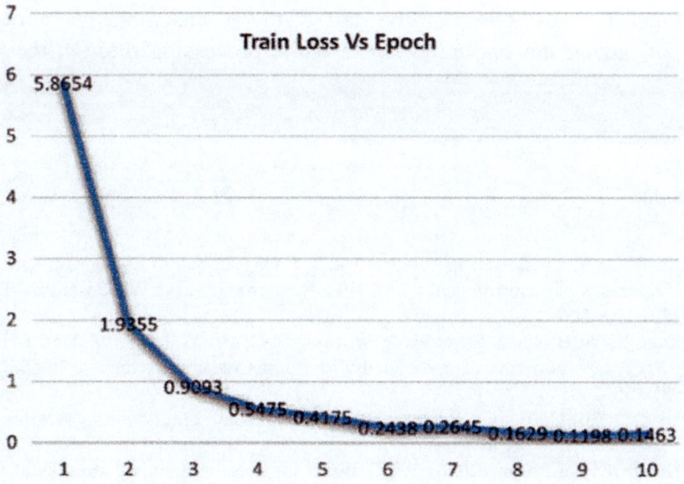

Fig. 5 Training loss versus Epoch

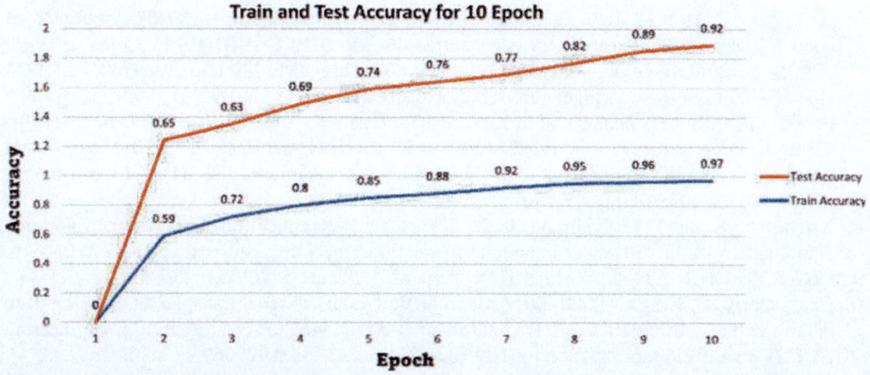

Fig. 6 Train and test accuracy

Table 2 Comparison Analysis with other existing models

Name	Accuracy	Sensitivity	Specificity	F1-Score
Proposed Method	93.56	91.24	0.95	0.91
Wang et al. [18]	92.04	90.41	0.94	0.87
Minaee et al. [19]	90.49	92.08	0.91	0.88
Khan et al. [20]	92.89	91.85	0.92	0.90
Das et al. [29]	92.41	91.29	0.92	0.89
Civit-Masot et al. [30]	93.12	90.89	0.94	0.88
Altan et al. [31]	91.85	92.42	0.89	0.85

speedy manner. It is also based on the state-of-the-art ensembles technique which is capable of having the optimum values while processing through the different networks.

References

1. Huang C, Wang Y, Li X, Ren L, Zhao J, Hu Y, Zhang L, Fan G, Xu J, Gu X et al (2020) Clinical features of patients infected with 2019 novel coronavirus in Wuhan, China. The Lancet 395(10223):497–506
2. Wu F, Zhao S, Yu B, Chen Y-M, Wang W, Song Z-G, Hu Y, Tao Z-W, Tian J-H, Pei Y-Y et al (2020) A new coronavirus associated with human respiratory disease in China. Nature 579(7798):265–269
3. McIntosh K (2020) Coronavirus disease 2019 (COVID-19): epidemiology, virology, clinical features, diagnosis, and prevention
4. World Health Organization (2020) WHO director-general's opening remarks at the media briefing on COVID-19
5. Wang W, Xu Y, Gao R, Lu R, Han K, Wu G, Tan W (2020) Detection of SARS-cov-2 in different types of clinical specimens. JAMA 323(18):1843–1844
6. Ai T, Yang Z, Hou H, Zhan C, Chen C, Lv W, Tao Q, Sun Z, Xia L (2020) Correlation of chest CT and RT-PCR testing for coronavirus disease 2019(COVID-19) in China: a report of 1014 cases. Radiology 296(2):E32-E40. https://doi.org/10.1148/radiol.2020200642.LNCS Homepage http://www.springer.com/lncs. Last accessed 21 Nov 2016
7. Fan L, Li D, Xue H, Zhang L, Liu Z, Zhang B, Zhang L, Yang W, Xie B, Duan X, Hu X, Cheng K, Peng L, Yu N, Song L, Chen H, Sui X, Zheng N, Liu S, Jin Z (2020) Progress and prospect on imaging diagnosis of COVID-19. Chin J Academic Radiol 3(1):4–13. https://doi.org/10.1007/s42058-020-00031-5
8. Krizhevsky A, Sutskever I, Hinton GE (2012) Imagenet classification with deep convolutional neural networks. In: Advances in neural information processing systems, pp 1097–1105
9. LeCun Y, Bengio Y, Hinton G (2015) Deep learning. Nature 521(7553):436–444
10. Chakraborty S, Zhang C (2020) Survival prediction model of renal transplantation using deep neural network. In: 2020 IEEE 1st international conference for convergence in engineering (ICCE), pp 180–183. https://doi.org/10.1109/ICCE50343.2020.9290695
11. Chakraborty S, Murali B (2022) A novel medical prognosis system for breast cancer. In: Mandal JK, Buyya R, De D (eds) Proceedings of international conference on advanced computing applications. Advances in intelligent systems and computing, vol 1406. Springer, Singapore. https://doi.org/10.1007/978-981-16-5207-3_34
12. Chakraborty S (2021) Category identification technique by a semantic feature generation algorithm. In: Deep learning for internet of things infrastructure. CRC Press, pp 129–144
13. He K, Zhang X, Ren S, Sun J (2016)Deep residual learning for image recognition. In: 2016 IEEE conference on computer vision and pattern recognition (CVPR), pp 770–778. https://doi.org/10.1109/CVPR.2016.90
14. Krizhevsky A, Sutskever I, Hinton GE (2017) ImageNet classification with deep convolutional neural networks. Commun. ACM 60(6):84–90. https://doi.org/10.1145/3065386
15. Huang G, Liu Z, Van Der Maaten L, Weinberger KQ (2017)Densely connected convolutional networks. In: 2017 IEEE conference on computer vision and pattern recognition (CVPR), pp 2261–2269. https://doi.org/10.1109/CVPR.2017.243
16. Zhang X, Zou J, He K, Sun J (2016) Accelerating very deep convolutional networks for classification and detection. IEEE Trans Pattern Anal Mach Intell 38(10):1943–1955. https://doi.org/10.1109/TPAMI.2015.2502579

17. Rajpurkar P, Irvin J, Zhu K, Yang B, Mehta H, Duan T, Ding D, Bagul A, Langlotz C, Shpanskaya K, Lungren MP, Ng AY (2017) CheXNet: radiologist-level pneumonia detection on chest Xrays with deep learning. arXiv:1711.05225. [Online]. Available: http://arxiv.org/abs/1711.05225
18. Wang L, Lin ZQ, Wong A (2020) COVID-Net: a tailored deep convolutional neural network design for detection of COVID-19 cases from chest X-ray images. Sci Rep 10:19549. https://doi.org/10.1038/s41598-020-76550-z
19. Minaee S, Kafish R, Sonka M, Yazdani S, Jamalipour Sou G (2020) Deep-COVID: predicting COVID-19 from chest X-ray images using deep transfer learning. Med Image Anal 65:101794
20. Khan AI, Shah JL, Bhat MM (2020) CoroNet: a deep neural network for detection and diagnosis of COVID-19 from chest X-ray images. Comput Meth Programs Biomed 196:105581
21. Shiraishi J et al (2000) Development of a digital image database for chest radiographs with and without a lung nodule. Amer J Roentgenol 174(1):71–74. https://doi.org/10.2214/ajr.174.1.1740071
22. Praveen (2020) Corona hack: chest X-Ray-Dataset. [Online]. Available: https://www.kaggle.com/praveengovi/coronahackchest-xraydataset. Accessed 21 Mar 2020
23. Paul Cohen J, Morrison P, Dao L (2020) COVID-19 image data collection, arXiv:2003.11597. [Online]. Available: http://arxiv.org/abs/2003.11597
24. Paul CJ (2020) Covid-19 image data collection. https://github.com/ieee8023/covid-chestxray-dataset
25. Paul M (2020) Kaggle chest X-ray images (pneumonia) dataset. https://www.kaggle.com/paultimothymooney/chest-xray-pneumonia
26. van Ginneken B, Stegmann MB, Loog M (2006) Segmentation of anatomical structures in chest radiographs using supervised methods: a comparative study on a public database. Med Image Anal 10(1):19–40
27. Jaeger S, Candemir S, Antani S, Wáng Y-XJ, Lu P-X, Thoma G (2014) Two public chest X-ray datasets for computer aided screening of pulmonary diseases. Quant Imag Med surgery 4(6):475
28. Ronneberger O, Fischer P, Brox T (2015) U-Net: convolutional networks for biomedical image segmentation. arXiv:1505.04597
29. Das NN, Kumar N, Kaur M, Kumar V, Singh D (2020) Automated deep transfer learning-based approach for detection of COVID-19 infection in chest X-rays. Ing Rech Biomed. https://doi.org/10.1016/j.irbm.2020.07.001.
30. Civit-Masot J, Luna-Perejón F, Morales MD, Civit A (2020) Deep learning system for COVID-19 diagnosis aid using X-ray pulmonary images. Appl Sci 10(13):4640
31. Altan A, Karasu S (2020) Recognition of COVID-19 disease from X-ray images by hybrid model consisting of 2D curvelet transform, chaotic salp swarm algorithm and deep learning technique. Chaos, Solitons Fractals 140:110071

Prediction of COVID-19 Cases Using the ARIMA Model and Machine Learning

Akash Pal, Garima Jain, Ishita Roy, and Sumit Sharma

Abstract In both the first and second waves of COVID-19, India suffered many casualties at the hands of the infectious virus in the ongoing pandemic. As the days passed, the number of daily cases steadily increased, with most cases reported from large cities and outbreaks in rural areas. In this proposed paper, we tried to explore the effects of the previous data on the number of daily new cases using the ARIMA Model in machine learning. To forecast COVID-19 spread, we analyzed the effectiveness of multiple machine learning approaches. The accuracy of models was compared using the root mean squared error (RMSE), mean absolute error (MAE), R2 coefficient of determination (R2), and represent fundamental percentage error (MAPE) parameters. The primary goal of this research is to figure out how these new COVID-19 instances will influence the rest of the globe and how many people will be affected by the pandemic. This paper works with the ARIMA Model to predict the accurate growth rate and COVID-19 cases, which can help the government and various organizations plan their systematic strategies. In this paper, we use the ARIMA Model to analyze the growth rate and different factors related to the COVID-19. The model deployed accurately predicts the confirmed cases with an accuracy of 98.97%.

Keywords COVID-19 · Pandemic · Machine learning · ARIMA model · Global pandemic

1 Introduction

In today's world, almost every work sector produces some data. Various industries can use this data to get proper knowledge related to it. The data analysis is done

A. Pal (✉) · G. Jain · I. Roy · S. Sharma
Department of Computer Science and Engineering, Noida Institute of Engineering and Technology, Gr. Noida 201310, India
e-mail: apal62214@gmail.com

G. Jain
e-mail: garimajain@niet.co.in

© The Author(s), under exclusive license to Springer Nature Singapore Pte Ltd. 2023
J. K. Mandal and D. De (eds.), *Frontiers of ICT in Healthcare*, Lecture Notes in Networks and Systems 519, https://doi.org/10.1007/978-981-19-5191-6_37

on multiple levels to obtain appropriate and desirable results. For example, a businessman is interested in finding out the likelihood of sales in the years to come. He can use this predicted data to adjust the production factors in his business to profit. It could also lead to the avoidance of unsold products and good production quality.

When statistical data is collected over time at regular intervals, this kind of data is called a "time-series". When we observe data at different points in time, the set of observations is called a "time-series". Time is not fixed here permanently; it can be a set of intervals which can be a year, months, days, hours, minutes, or even seconds [1]. Time is one of the essential factors in the time-series analysis as it is directly connected to a single variable.

1.1 The Utility of Time Series

- By observing the data, we can analyze the transformation that happened in the past.
- It helps us form plans for future work.
- It helps in evaluating the current events.

1.2 Covid-19

At the end of 2019, a sudden outburst of a new disease with symptoms similar to the common cold was noted in a particular part of China. The number of victims of this disease has increased rapidly in the leading country and its surroundings. In the following three months, the disease was well known to be the harbinger of death and was feared across the world [2, 3]. Even today, in 2021, we are witnessing the various variants of the COVID-19 taking their toll on multiple countries. Though vaccines and proper medications have been discovered for COVID-19, there is still no cure available to assure 100% safety of the patient. Recently, the Omicron variant has been feared more than the previous variants of COVID-19 as it is a mutation of the previous ones. Due to a lack of accurate information, it is irrelevant to say anything about the current variant of COVID-19.

1.3 Research Objective

In this research, we are trying to accurately predict the increase in the number of cases of COVID-19, i.e., daily confirmed cases, using machine learning techniques. We will be analyzing the data through the ARIMA Model. Through this predicted data, hundreds of lives can be saved.

1.4 Research Motivation

The motivation for this research was to develop efficient techniques to accurately predict the data, so that we can help the general public in terms of providing sufficient supplies in the COVID-19 era.

1.5 Research Contribution

The contribution in this paper are as follows:

- The paper contributes towards the implementation of the ARIMA Model to the dataset of COVID-19 cases.
- The paper effectively predicts the future values of the dataset with accuracy of 98.97%.

1.6 Road Map

The rest of the chapter is organized as follows. The first section introduces the time-series analysis and its usage, and COVID-19 pandemic to the paper. Section II gives the literature review and previous works that has been done in the prediction and analysis of the COVID-19 cases. The introduction to the ARIMA Model and its general characteristics with the algorithm is described in section III. The results of this study are explained in the section IV. Finally, section V concludes the paper.

2 Literature Review

2.1 Genetic Programming

The suggested prediction models are provided with precise formulae, and the importance of prediction variables is investigated. The developed models were analyzed and tested using statistical parameters and metrics. As per the findings, the suggested GEP-based models for time-series prediction of COVID-19 cases in India employ simple linkage functions and are highly reliable [4].

The ERP models used in the proposed paper are highly consistent in the prediction of both daily COVID-19 cases and the daily death cases in India, satisfying all the external conditions [5]. The solution in the proposed paper is highly dependable as the RSME and R-value of all cases are higher and are close to the factor of 1 [5]. The prediction variables that are used in the model only depend on one or two variables, thus making the model less reliable than the prediction models. The essential characteristic of GEP models is their ability to deal with fewer time-series data while still generating consistent results. In the early days of the pandemic, it was instrumental in analyzing and forecasting the course of cases. The problem develops when the volume of data increases. An optimization of GEP models is usually required. They are optimized using highly effective algorithms. This model can be used to forecast the spread of a pandemic in its early stages.

2.2 *ARIMA-WBF Models*

The main objective of using this model in the paper "Real-time forecasts and risk assessment of novel coronavirus (COVID-19) cases: A Data-driven analysis" [6] is to counter two main issues.

(a) Short-term real-time forecasting of new COVID-19 cases and deaths for various nations.
(b) To predict the disease's fatality rate using the demographic characteristics of the country's topography and the characteristics of COVID-19 diseases.

In the second edition, we use an optimal regression tree algorithm to identify variable root causes that significantly impact death rates in different countries. Various constraints are taken on the dataset used to analyze COVID-19 cases in problem (b) and projection of the future possibilities in the problem (a). These constraints or assumptions are:

1. The virus's mutation rate is the same across all countries.
2. When a person recovers from the virus, the recovered person will attain permanent immunity.
3. The effects of climate change are not taken into consideration. Since this model can be presented as a real-time forecasts system, thus the actual data can be updated regularly. This model can be used efficiently to adjust the lockdown period according to the actual time predictions.

2.3 *Two-Piece Scale Mixture Normal (TP-SMN)*

Two-piece scale mixture standard (TP-SMN) distribution model. The suggested time-series models surpassed standard Gaussian and symmetry models and were first adjusted to past COVID-19 datasets. [1] After that, the time series with the best match to each dataset is picked. Finally, the models chosen will be used to forecast the number of confirmed cases and the global death rate from COVID-19. The proposed algorithm model showed us that it could closely predict the potential forthcoming confirmed cases based on the various constraints and the historical data is present to be used.

2.4 *Dynamic Statistical Techniques*

In the proposed paper "Investigating the cases of novel coronavirus disease (COVID-19) in China using dynamic statistical techniques" uses the dynamic statistical techniques and use of the formation of the time-series model and data panel models to make and investigate the relationship between death cases and confirmed cases and recovered cases and the confirmed cases [7]. The study on the paper reveals that the effect of the confirmed COVID -19 cases on the accountable deaths due to the COVID -19 is heterogeneous. The relationships between the confirmed fatalities and the confirmed cases across mainland China and Wuhan are linear, while the same for the confirmed recovered cases and the confirmed cases are nonlinear. The models also show that the increase in the confirmed cases by 1% also results in the rise of confirmed deaths due to the COVID-19 by approximately 0.1–0.7%.

3 Methodology

ARIMA Model or Autoregressive Integrated Moving Average Model is a statistical model used to analyze univariate and multivariate time-series data to enhance the understanding of the datasets and predict the future outcomes of a problem. It is used to predict future values based on the previous values. 'An autoregressive (AR) model is a sort of random model used to describe predictable time-varying phenomena in nature, among other things. The future value in an AR(*p*) model is predicted to be a linear mixture of p prior observations, a constant, and a random error term. The AR(*p*) model may be stated mathematically as process:'

The moving average (MA) model is a technique for modeling univariate time series in time-series analysis, as shown by Eq (1). According to the moving-average model, the output variable is influenced by the current and numerous previous values of incorrect parameters. The MA(*q*) model may be expressed mathematically as process:

An AR (*p*) model is often delineated as:

$$Y_t = c + \varphi_1 Y_1 + \varphi_2 Y_2 \ldots + \varphi_p Y_p + Z_t, \tag{1}$$

where $Z_t \sim (0, 2)$,

Equation (2) shows that c associate unknown constant term, and φ_i, $i = 1 \ldots p$, are the parameters of the AR Model. A MA(*q*) Model is often described as:

$$Y_t = c + Z_t + \theta_1 Z_{t-1} + \ldots + \theta_q Z_{t-q}, \tag{2}$$

where $\{Z_t\}$ denotes a only random process with zero mean and variance σ2*z*.

3.1 Understanding ARIMA Model and Its Components

An autoregressive integrated moving average model is a statistical analysis that measures the strength of one dependent variable concerning other variables that change their values.

- Autoregression (AR) Model: A model in which a changing variable reverts to its previous values.
- Integrated (*I*) Model: An integrated model represents the differentiation of raw observations for the time series to become stationary.
- Moving Average (MA) Model: A moving average model integrates an observation's dependence on an estimation error from a moving average model applied to delayed readings.

3.2 Stationarity of Data in ARIMA Model

Seasonality is where data exhibits consistent and predictable patterns that reoccur for a calendar year and may damage the regression model. Many of the computations during the process cannot be made with great accuracy if a trend arises and stationarity is not visible.

The data in an autoregressive integrated moving average model are differenced to make it stationary. A stationarity model demonstrates that the data is consistent throughout time.

Equations (3), (4), and (5) show an ARIMA (*p*, *d*, *q*) model of the nonstationary random method $Y(t)$ is expressed as

$$\Phi(B)(1 - B)^\wedge dX^t = \theta(B)Z^t \tag{3}$$

with an AR operator

$$\Phi p(B) = 1 - \phi 1B - \ldots - \phi^{\mathrm{p}}\mathrm{Bp} \tag{4}$$

and a MA operator

$$\Theta q(B) = 1 - \theta 1B - \ldots - \theta^{\mathrm{q}}\mathrm{Bq} \tag{5}$$

where ϕ^p *is* *p*th AR coefficient, θ^q the *q*th MA coefficient, Z^t noise, X^t Rain attenuation. [8–10]. For stationary processes, Eq. (6) shows define autocorrelation between any two observations which can depend on the Time Lag *h* between them.

The autocorrelation for lag h is given by:

$$\rho_k = \mathrm{Corr}(y_t, y_{t-h}) = \frac{y_h}{y_0}, \tag{6}$$

3.3 ARIMA Model Parameters and Notations

Each component in the ARIMA Model function is a component of the observed data in the time series. In ARIMA Model [11], a standard notation would be p, d, and q to denote the numeric values that are substituted in place of argument to indicate the type of ARIMA Model used in the prediction.

The Notation is:

- The notation, p, denotes the number of lagged readings in the model; this is generally referred to as the lag order.
- The notation, d, denotes the count of the differenced raw readings, also known as the degree of difference.
- The notation, q, denotes the size of the moving average window; also referred to as the order of the moving average.

From Eq. (6), we define a (0) as a lag 0 covariance, i.e., the unconditional variance of the process. Confounding can explain as the distortion in the estimated measure of association where two variables can result from a mutual linear dependence on other variables.

3.4 Forecasting with ARIMA Model

ARIMA forecasting is accomplished by entering time-series data for the variable of interest. Statistical model and program will determine the proper number of delays or amount of differencing to the data and verify for stationarity. It will then produce the findings, which are frequently interpreted in the same way as a multiple linear regression model [10, 12, 13].

3.5 Dataset

In the ongoing pandemic, nation-wise data for confirmed cases for COVID-19 were obtained for India. The daily confirmed cases denote the total number of persons tested positive for COVID-19 in a single day. The dataset that is used in the section

Table 1 Dataset information

Variables in dataset	Variable type	Mean (in thousands)	Variance (in millions)	Min. value	Max. value
Daily confirmed	Numerical	7.79	132.44	0	50072
Total confirmed	Numerical	213.52	113404.08	1	1387088
Daily recovered	Numerical	4.98	62.59	0	37125
Total recovered	Numerical	123.24	44885.93	0	887124
Daily deceased	Numerical	0.18	0.07	0	2004
Total deceased	Numerical	5.88	75.79	0	32123

can be found at "https://www.kaggle.com/imdevskp/covid19-corona-virus-india-dataset?select=nation_level_daily.csv" for reproducibility of this work. The dataset contains variables such as Daily Confirmed Cases, Total Confirmed Cases, Total Recovered cases, Daily Confirmed Cases, Total Deceased Cases, and Daily Deceased Cases, which can be found in the mentioned dataset [14] (Table 1).

Algorithm

```
# IMPORT All the statistical libraries used for ARIMA Model and
Machine Learning
# IMPORT Visualization Libraries
# Read the data set "MAIN_DATASET.CSV" and CONVERT it in form of
DATAFRAME NAMED "DF"
# PRINT THE FIRST 5 ROWS OF DATAFRAME DF
# PRINT THE LAST 5 ROWS OF DATAFRAME DF
# CREATE A NEW DATAFRAME TO GET COLUMN "Daily Confirmed" for ANALYSIS
# PLOT THE GRAPH OF NEW DATAFRAME "NEW_DF" USING VISUALISATION
LIBRARIES
# USE ML LIBRARIES TO GET THE DIFFERENCED VALUE OF THE DATASET
"NEW_DF"
# DO THE ABOVE STEP AGAIN TO GET SECOND DIFFERENCED VALUE OF THE
DATASET
# PLOT THE BOTH THE "DIFF1" AND "DIFF2" TO CHECK FOR STATIONARITY OF
DATASET
# USE THE ARIMA FUNCTION OF THE ML LIBRARIES TO GET THE P, R, Q VALUES
OF THE ARIMA MODEL ANALYSIS DONE ON THE DATASET
# PREDICT THE VALUE OF THE FUTURE COVID-19 CONFIRMED CASES USING THE
ARIMA MODEL ANALYSIS
# PLOT THE GRAPH OF THE DATASET AND THE PREDICTED VALUE TO COMPARE
THEM TO CHECK ACCURACY OF THE PREDICTION.
In this paper, we use various matplotlib, scikit-learn, stats, ARIMA
libraries in the code part of the project to the apply the above algo-
rithm using the python programming language. We analyze the data,
get the required coefficients for the ARIMA Model. And try to predict
the future outcome using the same.
```

4 Result

From the above code and visualization, we can see that the forecast of the number of daily cases in the COVID-19 crisis is nearly correct with a minor error of $\pm$ 500 points, which is not significant given the large dataset on which the work is in processing. The graph and values of the predicted data show that the forecast is nearly accurate, with a prediction rate of 98.97%.

Figure 1 shows the initial dataset we were working on, it shows the first five and last five entries of the dataset.

Graphs are one of the best visualization tools to show the trends of a variable. We used Python matplotlib library to successfully plot the trends of COVID-19 cases in form of graph (Fig. 2).

```
          Date  Daily Confirmed  ...  Daily Deceased  Total Deceased
0   30 January                1  ...               0               0
1   31 January                0  ...               0               0
2  01 February                0  ...               0               0
3  02 February                1  ...               0               0
4  03 February                1  ...               0               0

[5 rows x 7 columns]
         Date  Daily Confirmed  ...  Daily Deceased  Total Deceased
173  21 July            39170  ...             671           28772
174  22 July            45601  ...            1130           29902
175  23 July            48443  ...             755           30657
176  24 July            48888  ...             763           31420
177  25 July            50072  ...             703           32123

[5 rows x 7 columns]
```

Fig. 1 Shows the start and end of the main dataset to begin with

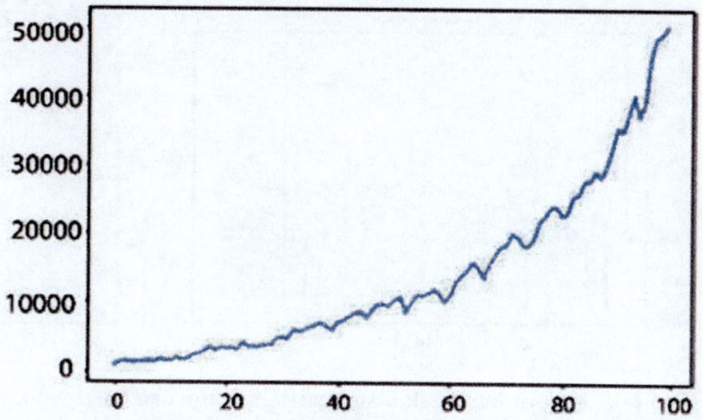

Fig. 2 This figure shows the dataset used in analyzing with its visualisation

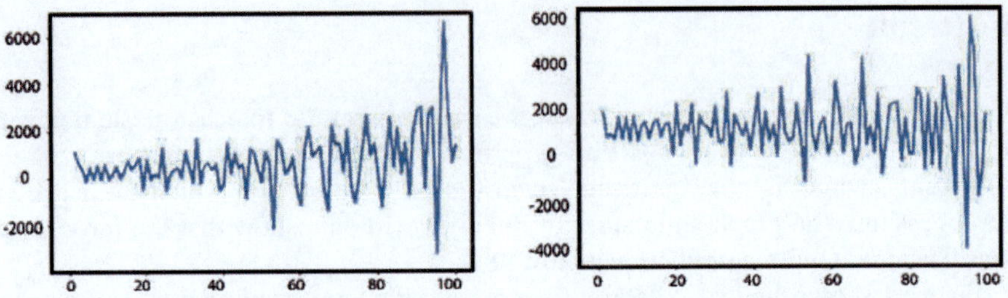

Fig. 3 This graph shows the difference between previous and current values for the ARIMA Model

The given dataset is checked for stationarity. The univariate time-series data of COVID-19 cases is checked for stationarity by differencing the current value from the previous values until the data is approximately stationary [15, 16]. The following figures show the differenced values of the univariate data for first time and second time, respectively (Fig. 3).

The following line graph shows the autocorrelated values of the dataset used in the prediction. This autocorrelated value is then used as a parameter in the ARIMA Model.

Autocorrelation refers to how much the value of dataset is correlated with its previous values. Partially Autocorrelated value is the statistical relationship between the readings of the dataset with the previous values of the dataset, where lagged observations are removed [17] This Autocorrelation plot shows the correlation between the various points of the dataset (Fig. 4).

The following table shows the result of the ARIMA Model obtained after applying the various functions. It returns values such as p-value, AIC value, BIC value, and HQIC values of the dataset. It is further used to predict the accurate results in ARIMA Model Analysis (Fig. 5).

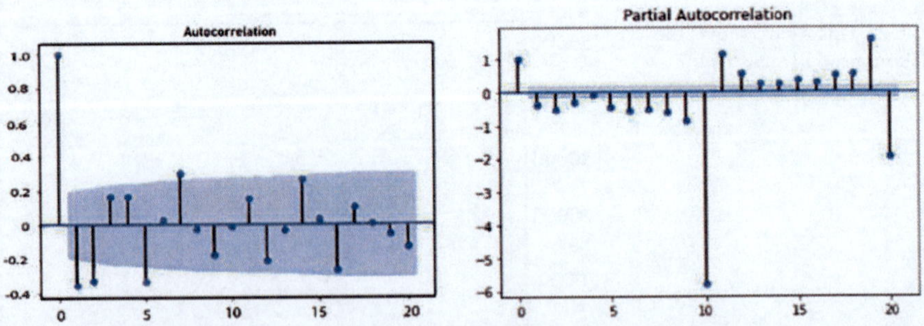

Fig. 4 Autocorrelated value and partially autocorrelated values of the dataset

ARIMA Model Results

Dep. Variable:	D2.Daily Confirmed	No. Observations:	98
Model:	ARIMA(5, 2, 1)	Log Likelihood	-815.659
Method:	css-mle	S.D. of innovations	972.009
Date:	Fri, 10 Dec 2021	AIC	1647.317
Time:	06:18:17	BIC	1667.997
Sample:	2	HQIC	1655.682

	coef	std err	z	P>|z|	[0.025	0.975]
const	18.2107	7.887	2.309	0.023	2.753	33.668
ar.L1.D2.Daily Confirmed	-0.3179	0.095	-3.345	0.001	-0.504	-0.132
ar.L2.D2.Daily Confirmed	-0.6111	0.094	-6.499	0.000	-0.795	-0.427
ar.L3.D2.Daily Confirmed	-0.4491	0.108	-4.164	0.000	-0.660	-0.238
ar.L4.D2.Daily Confirmed	-0.3725	0.100	-3.727	0.000	-0.568	-0.177
ar.L5.D2.Daily Confirmed	-0.5613	0.097	-5.813	0.000	-0.751	-0.372
ma.L1.D2.Daily Confirmed	-0.7492	0.067	-11.182	0.000	-0.880	-0.618

Roots

	Real	Imaginary	Modulus	Frequency
AR.1	0.6419	-0.8771j	1.0868	-0.1495
AR.2	0.6419	+0.8771j	1.0868	0.1495
AR.3	-0.3620	-1.0497j	1.1104	-0.3029
AR.4	-0.3620	+1.0497j	1.1104	0.3029
AR.5	-1.2233	-0.0000j	1.2233	-0.5000
MA.1	1.3348	+0.0000j	1.3348	0.0000

Fig. 5 ARIMA model result

The following Fig. 6 shows the proper value of the dataset of COVID-19 as compared with the predicted value generated by the ARIMA Model in the form of graph. It shows that the data are approximately similar with minor difference within the range of $\pm$ 500. The ARIMA Model generates the predicted data at an accuracy of approximately 98.97%.

5 Conclusion

The study's conclusion was that the daily growth of COVID-19 cases in the country could be predicted reliably. The forecast accuracy of 98.97% is considered satisfactory. This forecast can be used to take a variety of precautionary measures to prevent the virus from spreading. It can also be used to prepare hospital beds and to begin the production of various medications that can be used to combat the infection.

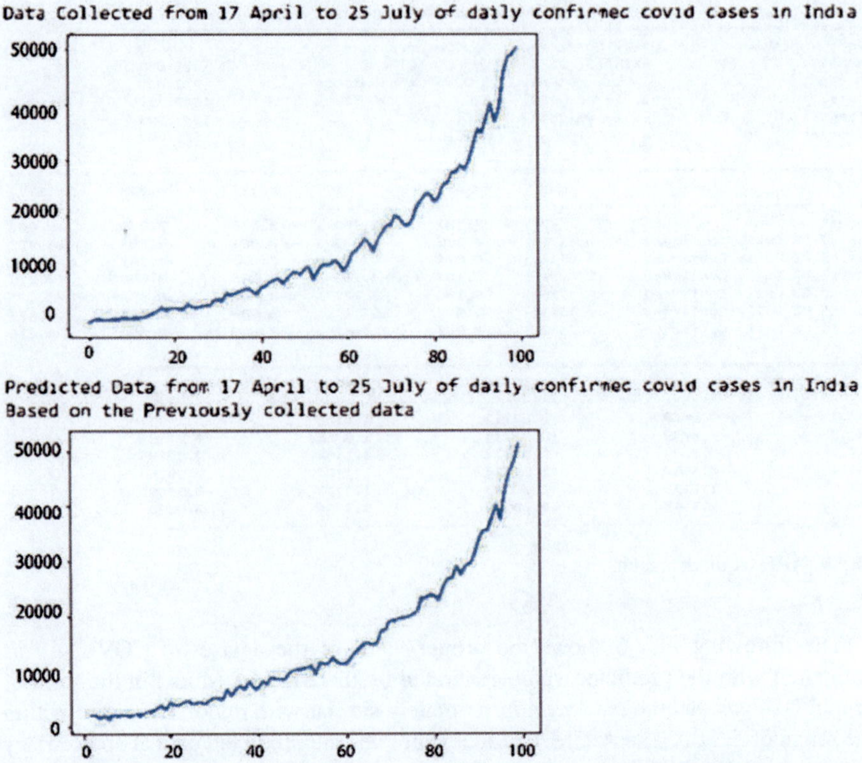

Fig. 6 Graphs of both the actual data and predicted data are approximately similar

References

1. Athiyarath S, Paul M, Krishnaswamy S (2020) A comparative study and analysis of time series forecasting techniques. SN Comput Sci 1:1–7
2. Tian J, et al (2020) Modeling analysis of COVID-19 based on morbidity data in Anhui, China. Math Biosci Eng 17(4):2842–2852
3. Zhuang Z, Zhao S, Lin Q, Cao P, Lou Y, Yang L, He D (2020) Preliminary estimation of the novel coronavirus disease (COVID-19) cases in Iran: a modelling analysis based on overseas cases and air travel data. Int J Infect Dis 94:29–31
4. Singh S, et al (2021) Time series analysis of COVID-19 data to study the effect of lockdown and unlock in India. J Institut Eng (India): Series B
5. Qi H, et al (2020) COVID-19 transmission in Mainland China is associated with temperature and humidity: a time-series analysis. Sci Total Environ 728:138778
6. Chakraborty T, Ghosh I (2020) Real-time forecasts and risk assessment of novel coronavirus (COVID-19) cases: A data-driven analysis. Chaos, Solitons Fractals 135:109850
7. Sarkodie SA, Owusu PA (2020) Investigating the cases of novel coronavirus disease (COVID-19) in China using dynamic statistical techniques. Heliyon 6(4):e03747
8. Jain G, Mallick B (2017) A study of time series models ARIMA and ETS. Available at SSRN 2898968
9. Jain G (2018) Time-Series analysis for wind speed forecasting. Malaya J Matematik 1:55–61

10. Garima J, Bhawna M (2016) A review on weather forecasting techniques. Int J Adv Res Comput Commun Eng 5(12):177–180
11. ArunKumar KE et al (2021) Forecasting the dynamics of cumulative COVID-19 cases (confirmed, recovered and deaths) for top-16 countries using statistical machine learning models: auto-regressive integrated moving average (ARIMA) and seasonal auto-regressive integrated moving average (SARIMA). Appl Soft Comput 103:107161
12. Chyon FA et al (2021) Time series analysis and predicting COVID-19 affected patients by ARIMA model using machine learning. J Virolog Meth 114433
13. Rahimi I, Chen F, Gandomi AH (2021) A review on COVID-19 forecasting models. Neural Comput Appl 1–11
14. The dataset used in the paper can be found publicly at https://www.kaggle.com/imdevskp/covid19-corona-virus-india-dataset?select=nation_level_daily.csv
15. Jain G, Prasad RR (2020) Machine learning prophet and XGBoost algorithm: analysis of traffic forecasting in telecom networks with time series data. In: 2020 8th international conference on reliability infocom technologies and optimization (trends and future directions) (ICRITO), pp 893–897
16. Ghafouri-Fard S, et al (2021) Application of machine learning in the prediction of COVID-19 daily new cases: a scoping review. Heliyon 7(10):e08143
17. Maleki M, et al. (2020) Modeling and forecasting the spread and death rate of coronavirus (COVID-19) in the world using time series models. Chaos, Solitons Fractals 140:110151
18. Benvenuto D, et al (2020) Application of the ARIMA model on the COVID-2019 epidemic dataset. Data Brief 29:105340
19. Kucharski AJ, et al (202) Early dynamics of transmission and control of COVID-19: a mathematical modelling study. Lancet Infect Diseases 20(5):553–558
20. Nishiura H, Linton NM, Akhmetzhanov AR (2020) Serial interval of novel coronavirus (COVID-19) infections. Int J Infect Dis 93:284–286
21. Kamarudin ANA, et al (2021) Prediction of COVID-19 Cases in Malaysia by using machine learning: a preliminary testing. In: 2021 international conference of women in data science at Taif University (WiDSTaif). IEEE

Travelling Guidance Using ACO and HBMO Techniques in COVID-19 Pandemics: A Novel Approach

Shashwat Saket, Shivam P. Mishra, Vandana Bhattacharjee, and Kamta Nath Mishra

Abstract The dynamic implementation of meta-heuristic and evolutionary algorithms has transformed computational intelligence's panoramic view. Considering the applicability of Nature-Inspired Algorithms in the view of the COVID-19 pandemic, the authors implemented the Honeybee Mating Optimization (HBMO), and Ant Colony Optimization (ACO) for efficiently travelling from different cities in vulnerability zone areas. The pheromone matrix and cost matrix were formulated using the HBMO algorithm and fed the aftermaths to map into the Ant Colony Optimization algorithm. The higher COVID-19 regions are denoted with less pheromone level, and the paths with a lower risk of getting infected comprise higher pheromone levels and vice versa. The authors featured the travel guide mapping of several cities of India and calculated the travelling probabilities for ensuring risk-free journeys. The four different threshold criteria maintained for the travelling probabilities are extremely safe conditions, moderately safe conditions, just safe conditions, and not safe conditions.

Keywords Ant colony optimization · Corona virus-19 · Pheromone matrix · Honeybee mating optimization · Meta-heuristic · Travelling paths

---

S. Saket · S. P. Mishra · V. Bhattacharjee · K. N. Mishra (✉)
Department of Computer Science and Engineering, Birla Institute of Technology, Jharkhand, India
e-mail: mishrakn@yahoo.com

S. Saket
e-mail: shashwat.saket46@gmail.com

S. P. Mishra
e-mail: shivambit65@gmail.com

V. Bhattacharjee
e-mail: vbhattacharya@bitmesra.ac.in

© The Author(s), under exclusive license to Springer Nature Singapore Pte Ltd. 2023
J. K. Mandal and D. De (eds.), *Frontiers of ICT in Healthcare*, Lecture Notes in Networks and Systems 519, https://doi.org/10.1007/978-981-19-5191-6_38

1 Introduction

The continuous use of nature-inspired computing algorithms has provided a paradigm for optimization in various engineering and technology fields. With the broad applicability, utility while service, and optimality while obtaining the global optima, the nature-inspired algorithms put a petrographic step towards the implementation of various meta-heuristics in the field of mathematical operational problems. The pandemic time has limited the travelling around several states blocking many routes. Thus, it is strenuous to travel from one city to other cities with dynamic constraints such as the spread of the virus, rate of change of infection, number of possible paths. The meta-heuristic algorithms based on swarm intelligence bolsters the computational intelligence such as Ant Colony Optimization, Honeybee Mating Optimization, Bee Algorithm, Simulated Annealing, Cuckoo Search, Particle Swarm altered the pre-existing dynamics of computation. These algorithms ensure an optimized paradigm for solving different problems based on mathematical engineering. This paper implements the meta-heuristic approaches for mapping the travelling probabilities in COVID-19 affected regions. The report considered several elements of real-world scenarios of COVID-19 with multimodal optimization using nature-inspired computing algorithms like HBMO and ACO.

Since most problems in the real-world scenario have multiple constraints and factors, thus the optimization goal is multimodal [1]. Several meta-heuristics and swarm intelligence algorithms are available to ease the applicability, such as Ant Algorithm, Bee Algorithm, Simulated Annealing, Cuckoo Search, Particle Swarm, and many more [2]. The bee-inspired algorithm enacts the behavioural features of the honeybee living in a colony. There are many variants of the famous bee algorithm, viz. Artificial Bee Colony Optimization, Honeybee Algorithm, Honeybee Mating Algorithm, Virtual Bee Algorithm, and others [3, 4]. The Honeybee Mating Optimization (HBMO) algorithm was developed by Bozorg-Haddad et al. [5] to analyse non-convex optimization problems. The Honeybee Mating Optimization (HBMO) algorithm is one of the significant swarm-based modus operandi in variegated optimization approaches. It ensures the mating behaviour observed in the case of honeybees. This algorithm can be used to model various clustering problems. Some of the impressive features of HBMO include its adaptability in abrupt alterations in the environmental factors; the ability to minimize the probability of risk factors, including notable tolerance endeavours; implementation of the algorithm in highly noisy data containing a colossal population; and its ease of performance without compromising the integral functions of the system [6, 7].

The simulated annealing developed by Andy et al. [8] can be understood as the grafting of physical annealing in computational references. It functions as a trajectory-based random search technique for obtaining the global optima. It stimulates the process of physical annealing, where the solids are firstly heated and then cooled to get the best fit solution for the arrangements of the crystals. It provides a prototype for procuring results from bound constraints as well as the unconstrained

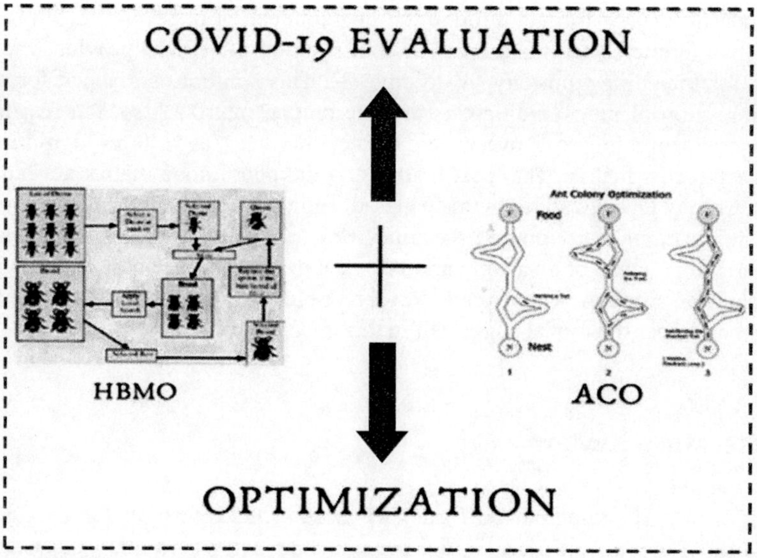

Fig. 1 Optimization using ant colony optimization (ACO) and honeybee mating optimization (HBMO) algorithms

problems of optimization. The new points are randomly engendered after the simulated annealing of each loop. The calibre of Simulated Annealing to avoid the hindrances caused by being trapped in local optima is mitigated an idiosyncratic amongst other algorithms. The algorithm propels the optimization with the decrease in the temperature, which acts as its controlling factor.

Figure 1 illustrates the COVID-19 evaluation using the simulation of Honeybee Mating Optimization and Ant Colony Optimization. The amalgamation of these algorithms under the factors such as simulated annealing provides the desired outcome.

Another meta-heuristic approach used in this paper is Ant Colony Optimization proposed by Dorigo et al. [9], which mimics the foraging behaviour observed in the colonies maintained by the ants. While travelling through an itinerary, the ants deposit a chemical on the path, namely pheromone, which turns out to be the indicator for other ants to follow the same direction. This approach fosters the ants to effectively reach towards the food or their colony destination providing the optimized solution using the variance in the concentration of pheromone deposits.

This paper maps the advantages of the Honeybee Mating Optimization algorithm and Ant Colony Optimization under the surveillance of Simulated Annealing and another ensemble. Its implications for finding the optimized solution for travelling in COVID-19 affected countries are several means of transportation but restricted because of hotspots of disease infections. The amalgamation of these algorithms put up creativity for solving the travelling problem arising due to varied rates of spread of COVID-19. The HBMO algorithm optimizes the possible paths available in the decision space formed through the interconnection of several locations in a country using intersected mapping. The trail solution of HBMO provides the best fit path for travelling from city 'A' to city 'B'. This solution is mapped for every interconnection of cities and acts as the pheromone matrix. Also, the feasibility, average transportation cost, one-to-one connection enact as features significant to generate the cost matrix. This cost matrix and the pheromone matrix are fed into the Ant Colony Optimization. In this paper, the humans represent the ants travelling from one destination to another; the itineraries followed up during the travel are considered the matrix of decision variables used to optimize the best path available in the decision space. A person would travel more feasible ways, thus releasing more pheromone as per the model suggested in this paper.

2 Literature Review

Bozorg et al. [5] presented the Honeybee Mating Optimization for solving the single reservoir problem. Further, the behaviour of honeybees mating concerning environmental features were simulated for developing the marriage-based algorithms observed in honeybees to optimize the performance using lucidly indicated mathematical functions with nonlinear benchmarks. The authors Dorigo et al. [9] presented the Ant Colony Optimization for solving the multi-reservoir and other problems. Selvi et al. [10] implemented the HBMO algorithm for mapping the effective clustering of nodes concerning the sensor networks. They minimized the energy consumption and further optimized the routing path whilst the heads of the cluster nodes signified the routing process. The primary factor making this algorithm a practical approach is the minimization of consumption of energy and maximization in the throughput of the communication-based routing. Mojarrad et al. [11] proposed a Multi-objective Modified Honeybee Mating Optimization to solve the Multi-objective Economic Emission Dispatch (MEED). They formulated a nonlinear constrained multi-objective optimization and implemented the evolutionary algorithms. They maintained a finite-sized repository of non-dominated solutions to generate the optimal set.

Jianlian et al. [12] amalgamated the ideation of neural networks to associate with the simulated annealing procedure to perform the network training with objective functions. They compared their model to other primitive neural networks following the gradient-based approaches to enter through the optima along with its feature of avoiding the risk of being stuck at the local optima. The authors ZeinEldin et al. [13] proposed simulated annealing to solve the constrained-based optimization problems. The aftermaths obtained in this paper provide the lucid indication that the improved simulated annealing (ISA) approach offers a better perspective for getting the optimal solution in many cases of constrained-based optimization problems outshining the results procured from other methods.

Jadon et al. [14] proposed an efficient method to optimize the modified ant colony optimization problems. They further ensured another step describing the adaptive mutation for advancing the algorithm to avoid the factors restricting the solution to get stuck in the local optima values. Moreover, they presented the experimental results for justifying the approach's performance when compared with the previous model. Chen et al. [15] proposed exploration control particle swarm optimization to solve the grid task scheduling. They integrated the ant colony optimization with the particle swarm optimization to obtain the grid samples' search efficiency. Xiang-yang Deng et al. [16] proposed an algorithm model named ACO +, which is an improved version of Ant Colony Optimization. They presented an effective modus operandi to update the pheromone matrix. They suggested that the algorithm has the calibre to calibrate further the functions of global exploration capability in association with the better convergence rate giving rise to a new approach with better robustness and performance under given metrics.

Collings et al. [17] proposed a novel decentralized peer-to-peer approach. At the same time, they propelled their experiment towards implementing Ant Colony Optimization on the set of variegate distributive memory clusters. They combined this algorithm with a fuzzy logic-based controller for determining the significance of various parameters in a distributive memory environment. Dewantoro et al. [18] proposed a coalescence of Ant Colony Optimization with Tabu Search for solving the travelling salesman problem. They formulated a method to find the best routes and further added to find out the better running time through this approach. They further compared the performance of hybrid Ant Colony Optimization (ACO-TS) with the pre-existing Ant Colony Optimization (ACO). They deduced that the hybrid method procured better performance on the metrics of finding the better running time. Guevara et al. [19] proposed implementing algorithms based upon the computational intelligence for reducing the spread of COVID-19 and mitigating the risk of reach in the local arena. They implemented the algorithm on the New York State dataset. They further implemented the clustering approach to obtain the hotspots based on COVID-19.

3 Proposed Mathematical Model

The evolutionary and meta-heuristic algorithms have fostered its way towards solving numerous mathematical problems which were earlier assumed as fallacy in computational beliefs. In this paper, the authors have proposed the model for travelling in COVID affected country. Firstly, they enlisted the symbols used in this paper in Table 1.

Firstly, the authors found the pheromone for travelling from each city other corresponding city. The decision variables used for the calculation of the pheromone matrix is given in the Table 2. Now, the authors considered K number of different paths that can be used to travel from city 'A' to city 'B'. Using the decision variables mentioned in Table 1, the authors formulated the initial population as given in Eq. 1.

Table 1 Nomenclature used for the mathematical model in this paper

Sl. No.	Symbols used	Description
1	Pop	Population used for mapping the decision variables
2	k	Number of possible paths for travelling from city A to city B
3	ς	The function used for finding the solution using simulated annealing
4	F	The fitness functions
5	X_b	Best path found till now
6	X_p	p th possible path found in the decision space
7	λ	The learning parameter
8	t	Number of iterations
9	ε	Trial solutions
10	Θ	Selection criterion
11	m	The number of days after which the paths are calculated again
12	$X_i^{'}$	Solution for new path generated after m days
13	y_i	Best solution in present iteration
14	$y_i^{'}$	Best solution in previous iteration
15	L	Lower bound
16	U	Upper bound
17	P_{A_i,B_j}	The pheromone added for travelling from city A_i to city B_j
18	C_{A_i,B_j}	The cost for travelling from city A_i to city B_j

$$\text{Pop} = \begin{bmatrix} x_1 \\ x_2 \\ \vdots \\ x_{k-1} \\ x_k \end{bmatrix} = \begin{bmatrix} x_{1,1} & x_{1,2} & x_{1,3} & x_{1,4} & x_{1,5} & x_{1,6} & x_{1,7} \\ x_{2,1} & x_{2,2} & x_{2,3} & x_{2,4} & x_{2,5} & x_{2,6} & x_{2,7} \\ \vdots & \vdots & \vdots & \vdots & \vdots & \vdots & \vdots \\ x_{k-1,1} & x_{k-1,2} & x_{k-1,3} & x_{k-1,4} & x_{k-1,5} & x_{k-1,6} & x_{k-1,7} \\ x_{k,1} & x_{k,2} & x_{k,3} & x_{k,4} & x_{k,5} & x_{k,6} & x_{k,7} \end{bmatrix} \quad (1)$$

Now, the authors targeted to obtain better condition for travelling from Kth using simulated annealing. They used the formula given in Eq. 2 for obtaining the best solution in terms of the paths available in the decision space.

$$\zeta\left(X_b, X_p\right) = e^{-\frac{|F(X_b)-F(X_p)|}{\lambda}} \quad (2)$$

The trial solution for the paths were obtained using the formulae given in Eq. 3 using the honeybee algorithm.

$$\varepsilon = \left\|F\left(X_b^{(t)}\right)\right| - \left|F\left(X_p^{(t-1)}\right)\right| \quad (3)$$

Table 2 The decision variables used for the calculation of the pheromone matrix

S. No.	Decision variables	Description
1	x_1	Spread of COVID in City 'A'
2	x_2	Spread of COVID in City 'B'
3	x_3	Rate of change of COVID in City 'A'
4	x_4	Rate of change of COVID in City 'B'
5	x_5	Number of possible paths
6	x_6	Highly infected regions in the path
7	x_7	Rate of infection during the travel

The selection criteria for the path can be parameterized by Θ. If the value of $\in \geq \Theta$, then the solution is selected and if the value of $\in < \Theta$, then the solution is not selected.

After '*m*' days, in accordance with the condition of the COVID, a new set of possible paths were obtained using one-point crossover, two-point crossover, and uniform crossover.

The path that was rejected must be reconsidered after improvement of the rates of COVID spread or further changes found in it. The generated new path can be found out using the Eq. 4.

$$x_i' = \{\phi(\delta)^2.G(y_i, \phi(\delta))\} + (1 - \phi(\delta)^2).\{\phi(\sigma)^2.G(x_i, \phi(\sigma)) + (1 - \phi(\sigma)^2).x_i\} \tag{4}$$

Here,

$$G(a, b) = \frac{1 + b}{2}\{\text{Rand}(a, x_i^U)\} + \frac{1 - b}{2}\{\text{Rand}(x_i^L, a)\} \tag{5}$$

$$\sigma = y_i - x_i \tag{6}$$

$$\delta = y_i - y_i' \tag{7}$$

The rejected path after the improvement of rates in the COVID scenario, were again put into the Eq. 2 and subsequently the best solution was found for each path in the decision space. Now, the best solution has been obtained for travelling from city A to city B with the paths available in the decision space. Let the solution for addition of pheromone whilst travelling from city A to city B be $P_{A,B}$.

The best possible path for travelling from all the cities to different cities can be mapped. The pheromone matrix can be drawn for travelling from every city.

Table 3 The variables used in this paper for the calculation of cost matrix from city 'A' to city 'B'

	Decision variable	Description
1	f_1	Average travelling expense
2	f_2	Time to travel from city A to city B
3	f_3	Connection in relativity
4	f_4	Means of transportation and preferences

$$\text{Phermone Matrix} = \begin{bmatrix} P_{A_1,B_1} & \cdots & P_{A_1,B_n} \\ \vdots & \ddots & \vdots \\ P_{A_n,B_1} & \cdots & P_{A_n,B_n} \end{bmatrix} \tag{8}$$

Now, the authors used decision variables given in Table 3 for the formation of the cost matrix.

Now using the equations given in Eqs. 2–7, the authors found the best solution for city A to city B as $C_{A,B}$. They further mapped the cost matrix for travelling from all the cities to different city as given in the Eq. 9.

$$\text{Cost Matrix} = \begin{bmatrix} C_{A_1,B_1} & \cdots & C_{A_1,B_n} \\ \vdots & \ddots & \vdots \\ C_{A_n,B_1} & \cdots & C_{A_n,B_n} \end{bmatrix} \tag{9}$$

The pheromone matrix and the cost matrix given in Eqs. 8 and 9, respectively, can be used to solve the shortest path possible for travelling from city A_i to city B_j using the Ant Colony Optimization algorithm.

4 Algorithmic Representations

The algorithm steps representation of proposed travelling guidance algorithm using Ant Colony Optimization (ACO) and HBMO techniques in COVID-19 pandemics is presented in Fig. 2.

Figure 2 denotes the algorithmic representation for COVID based travelling using Honeybee Mating Optimization and Ant Colony Optimization under the surveillance of simulated annealing. The dataset is gathered from the official Ministry of Health and Family Welfare, Government of India. The dataset is fed into the mathematical model formulated in this paper. The best paths are solved and subsequently considered for travelling under several circumstances, such as just safe, moderately safe, and highly safe conditions.

Algorithm COVID_Based_Travelling( )
{
Step 1: Enlist all the decision variables possible for the calculation of pheromone matrix and cost matrix.
Step 2: Generate the initial population as the path followed during the travel from city 'A' to city 'B' after considering the constraints of table 2 and table 3.
Step 3: Use simulated annealing for obtaining the better condition and parameter ϴ for checking if the solution crosses the threshold.
Step 4: Form the trial solution using the Honeybee Mating Optimization algorithm.
Step 5: Check for the improvement of condition of COVID after m- days and generate new path.
Step 6: Find the cost matrix and pheromone matrix using the optimization approach.
Step 7: Find the best possible path for travelling from city 'A_i' to city 'B_j' using the Ant Colony Optimization algorithm.
Step 8: End of the algorithm. }

Fig. 2 Algorithmic representation of the steps of proposed algorithm

5 Results and Discussions

The authors took six cities from India viz. Ranchi, Delhi, Mumbai, Bangalore, Chennai, Kolkata, and their corresponding data for the spread of COVID-19, COVID-19 change rate, number of possible paths, highly infectious regions between them, and rate of infection during the travel. Further, the authors calculated the trial solution using the Honeybee Mating Optimization for the possible paths for each city to the corresponding other towns. The authors generated the pheromone matrix as given in Eq. 8. Similarly, authors formulated the matrix for the cost of travelling as shown in Eq. 9 from all the cities to other cities, choosing different permutations of paths obtained in the Pheromone and cost matrix. The authors developed the travelling probability using ACO approach for travelling from city 'A' to corresponding city 'B' through a specified path via different cities available in the search space.

Table 4 and Fig. 3 represent the *safe travelling probability* when the person travels from city 'A' to city 'B' via any other city as available in the decision space of paths. The extremely safe paths are represented with green colour, the moderately safe conditions are denoted with yellow colour, the just safe conditions are denoted with orange colour, and the not safe conditions are represented with red colour in Table 4 and Fig. 3. It can lucidly be indicated from Table 4 and Fig. 3 that if a person needs to travel from Ranchi to Delhi, then the best route available to him is to travel directly to Delhi, which obtains a 90% chance of getting to the destination safely. The second-best path in the reference is via Kolkata, securing an 84% chance of getting to the destination without putting up the risk of getting the disease. The authors in this paper observed similar results for travelling from other cities. Table 4 and Fig. 3 foster the calculation for travelling via different routes, e.g. for calculating the probability for safe travel from city Ranchi to city Bangalore, via Delhi and Mumbai, the probabilities for each trip will be added and then normalized.

$$\text{Probability}(\text{Ranchi, Bangalore}) = \frac{0.54 + 0.71 + 0.92}{3} = 0.73 \tag{10}$$

Table 4 The general travelling probabilities from city 'A' to city 'B' via other cities

From	Via						To
	Ranchi	Delhi	Mumbai	Bangalore	Chennai	Kolkata	
Ranchi	–	0.90	0.79	0.62	0.48	0.84	Delhi
Ranchi	–	0.69	0.82	0.78	0.42	0.66	Mumbai
Ranchi	–	0.54	0.71	0.92	0.71	0.63	Bangalore
Ranchi	–	0.40	0.72	0.84	0.93	0.69	Chennai
Ranchi	–	0.62	0.53	0.44	0.28	0.98	Kolkata
Delhi	0.78	–	0.76	0.62	0.56	0.82	Mumbai
Delhi	0.63	–	0.74	0.84	0.46	0.67	Bangalore
Delhi	0.69	–	0.67	0.54	0.88	0.61	Chennai
Delhi	0.88	–	0.71	0.49	0.63	0.76	Kolkata
Mumbai	0.36	0.64	–	0.84	0.63	0.42	Bangalore
Mumbai	0.57	0.38	–	0.84	0.78	0.34	Chennai
Mumbai	0.78	0.83	–	0.46	0.42	0.69	Kolkata
Bangalore	0.16	0.08	0.74	–	0.86	0.56	Chennai
Bangalore	0.85	0.61	0.49	–	0.37	0.91	Kolkata
Chennai	0.87	0.38	0.64	0.75	–	0.96	Kolkata

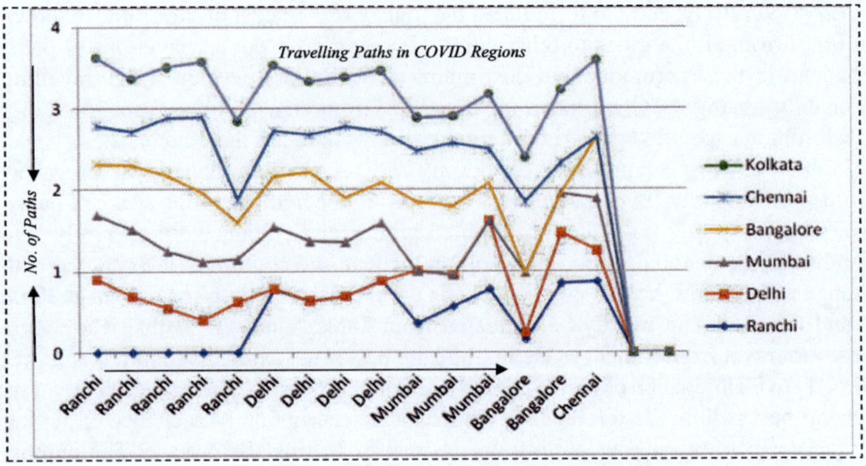

Fig. 3 The paths of general travelling probability from city 'A' to city 'B'

It can be deduced from Eq. 10 that the probability for safe travel from Ranchi to Bangalore via Delhi and Mumbai is obtained to be 73%. It gives the inference that if a person travels from Ranchi to Bangalore via Mumbai and Delhi, then he/she has a 73% chance of arriving at the destination without having any risk of being affected by the COVID-19 virus.

$$\text{Safety Threshold Value Matrix} = \begin{bmatrix} \text{Below 18} & 0.00 - 0.40 \\ 18 - 45 & 0.40 - 0.60 \\ 45 - 60 & 0.60 - 0.80 \\ \text{Above 60} & 0.80 - 1.00 \end{bmatrix} \quad (11)$$

The Eq. 11 represents the safety threshold for different travelling probabilities as per the given age factors provided in the domains of the age groups associated with Indian premises.

Figure 4 describes the mapping for travelling from Ranchi to Bangalore via Delhi and then Mumbai under the factors involved in COVID-19 affected regions. Using the Ant Colony Optimization, the travelling can be determined and further enhanced for travelling from different cities.

Table 5 and Fig. 5 define the paths that are *just safe* for travelling in a COVID-based regions. Just safe determines that the way is considered safe for fully fit people. The threshold value for the path being just safe is 0.40. Thus, the ways having 40% of safety are eligible for travelling with extreme precautions. The tracks below 40% of security are discarded in this table and henceforth considered unsafe paths for travelling.

Table 6 and Fig. 6 define the *moderately safe* paths for travelling under the effect of COVID affected regions. The courses having a threshold value of more than 0.60 are considered in this criterion. These paths are safe for the general public with moderately reasonable precautions. These paths allow travelling based on conditions for safety such as masks, COVID shields, sanitizers.

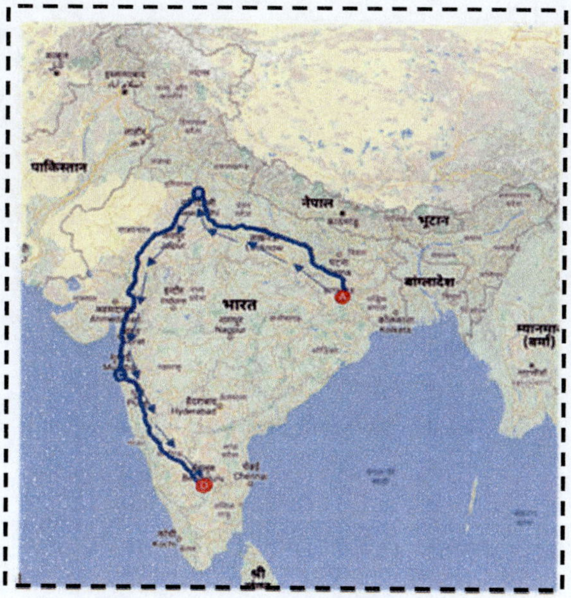

Fig. 4 Travelling representation from Ranchi to Bangalore via Delhi and Mumbai

Table 5 The probability for travelling with *just safe condition* from city 'A' to city 'B' via different cities

From	Via						To
	Ranchi	Delhi	Mumbai	Bangalore	Chennai	Kolkata	
Ranchi	–	0.90	0.79	0.62	0.48	0.84	Delhi
Ranchi	–	0.69	0.82	0.78	0.42	0.66	Mumbai
Ranchi	–	0.54	0.71	0.92	0.71	0.63	Bangalore
Ranchi	–	0.40	0.72	0.84	0.93	0.69	Chennai
Ranchi	–	0.62	0.53	0.44	–	0.98	Kolkata
Delhi	0.78	–	0.76	0.62	0.56	0.82	Mumbai
Delhi	0.63	–	0.74	0.84	0.46	0.67	Bangalore
Delhi	0.69	–	0.67	0.54	0.88	0.61	Chennai
Delhi	0.88	–	0.71	0.49	0.63	0.76	Kolkata
Mumbai	–	0.64	–	0.84	0.63	0.42	Bangalore
Mumbai	0.57	–	–	0.84	0.78	–	Chennai
Mumbai	0.78	0.83	–	0.46	0.42	0.69	Kolkata
Bangalore	–	–	0.74	–	0.86	0.56	Chennai
Bangalore	0.85	0.61	0.49	–	–	0.91	Kolkata
Chennai	0.87	–	0.64	0.75	–	0.96	Kolkata

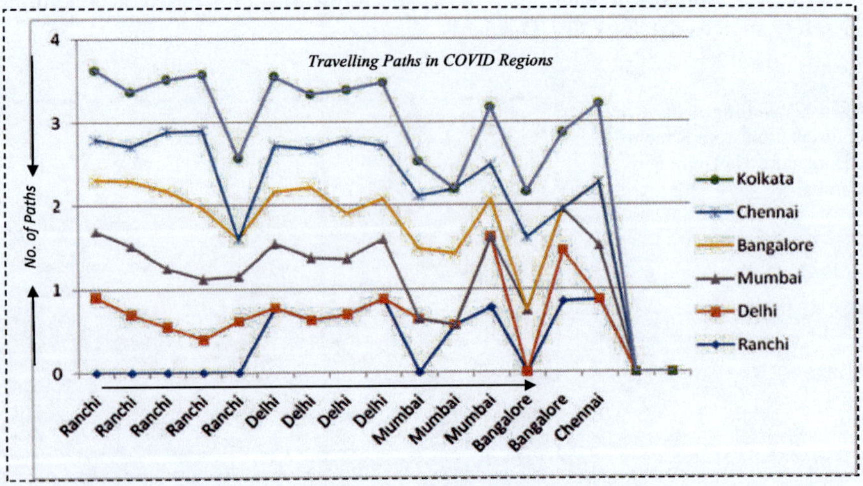

Fig. 5 Probability of travelling from every-city to every-other-city with *just safe condition*

Table 6 The probability for travelling with moderately safe conditions from city 'A' to city 'B' via different cities

From	Via						To
	Ranchi	Delhi	Mumbai	Bangalore	Chennai	Kolkata	
Ranchi	–	0.90	0.79	0.62	–	0.84	Delhi
Ranchi	–	0.69	0.82	0.78	–	0.66	Mumbai
Ranchi	–	–	0.71	0.92	0.71	0.63	Bangalore
Ranchi	–	–	0.72	0.84	0.93	0.69	Chennai
Ranchi	–	0.62	–	–	–	0.98	Kolkata
Delhi	0.78	–	0.76	0.62	–	0.82	Mumbai
Delhi	0.63	–	0.74	0.84	–	0.67	Bangalore
Delhi	0.69	–	0.67	–	0.88	0.61	Chennai
Delhi	0.88	–	0.71	–	0.63	0.76	Kolkata
Mumbai	–	0.64	–	0.84	0.63	–	Bangalore
Mumbai	–	–	–	0.84	0.78	–	Chennai
Mumbai	0.78	0.83	–	–	–	0.69	Kolkata
Bangalore	–	–	0.74	–	0.86	–	Chennai
Bangalore	0.85	0.61	–	–	–	0.91	Kolkata
Chennai	0.87	–	0.64	0.75	–	0.96	Kolkata

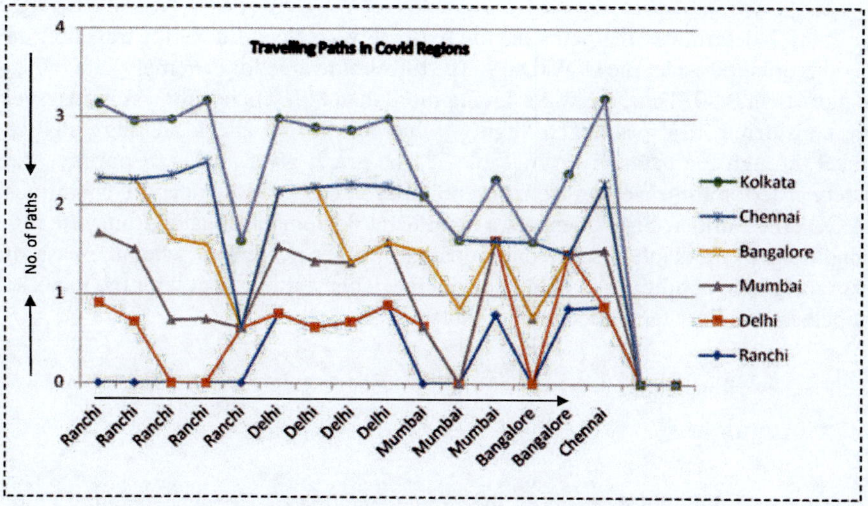

Fig. 6 Travelling in moderately safe condition from city 'A' to city 'B'

Table 7 Probability for travelling with *extremely safe conditions* from city 'A' to city 'B' via different cities

From	Via						To
	Ranchi	Delhi	Mumbai	Bangalore	Chennai	Kolkata	
Ranchi	–	0.90	–	–	–	0.84	Delhi
Ranchi	–	–	0.82	–	–	–	Mumbai
Ranchi	–	–	–	0.92	–	–	Bangalore
Ranchi	–	–	–	0.84	0.93	–	Chennai
Ranchi	–	–	–	–	–	0.98	Kolkata
Delhi	–	–	–	–	–	0.82	Mumbai
Delhi	–	–	–	0.84	–	–	Bangalore
Delhi	–	–	–	–	0.88	–	Chennai
Delhi	0.88	–	–	–	–	–	Kolkata
Mumbai	–	–	–	0.84	–	–	Bangalore
Mumbai	–	–	–	0.84	–	–	Chennai
Mumbai	–	0.83	–	–	–	–	Kolkata
Bangalore	–	–	–	–	0.86	–	Chennai
Bangalore	0.85	–	–	–	–	0.91	Kolkata
Chennai	0.87	–	–	–	–	0.96	Kolkata

Table 7 determines the paths having extremely safe conditions for travelling in regions affected under the COVID-19. The threshold value for extremely safe routes is more than 0.80. Thus, the ways having more than 80% chance for risk-free travel are considered. The passengers highly vulnerable to the attack are suggested to travel through the paths given in Table 7. The graph given in Fig. 7 portrays the safety criterion for travelling from several cities to other cities under the conditions of COVID. Further, Fig. 7 denotes a significant decrement in paths from *just safe* conditions to moderately safe conditions and further decrement when the case of extremely safe conditions is being considered. This signifies that with the increase of paths, the safety factor decreases (Table 8).

6 Conclusions

In this paper the authors fostered the implementation of Honeybee Mating Optimization for updating the cost matrix and pheromone matrix in the Ant Colony Optimization algorithm. Safety criterions were portrayed whilst a person travels from one city to another simulated around the regions and paths affected by the virus. Furthermore, the proposed approach prepares the chart based on safety, considering the person's age. It was observed that the experiment with the conditions of different travelling probabilities like *not safe* with threshold of 0.00–0.39, *just*

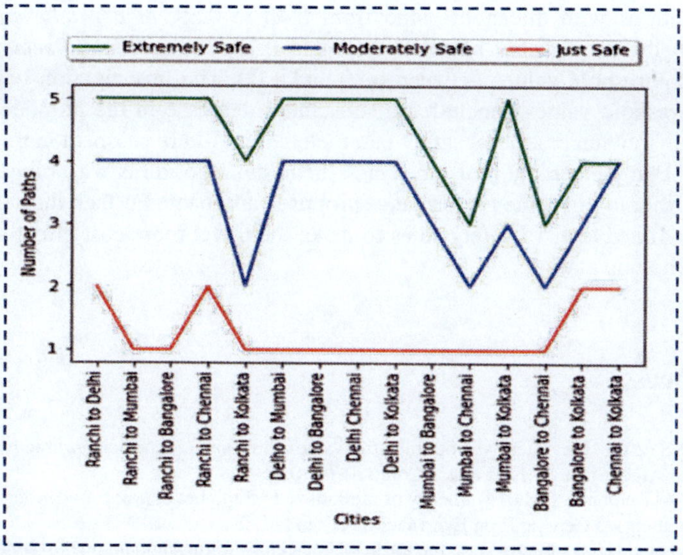

Fig. 7 Travelling paths available for *just safe*, *moderately safe*, *extremely safe* regions

Table 8 Performance comparison of various existing algorithms on metrics of various technologies

	Algorithm name	Classifier taken/technologies used	Results/observation
1	ECPSO [15]	ACO, PSO, scheduling	Implemented an algorithm to solve grid scheduling using ACO, PSO, scheduling
2	ACO + [16]	ACO, discrete combinatorial optimization, pheromone traits	Proposed a model for solving the travelling salesman problem with variants of ant colony optimization
3	Decentralized ACO [17]	Ant colony optimization, fuzzy logic, memory clusters	Proposed a decentralized approach to solve TSP using the amalgamation of ACO, fuzzy logic based on memory clusters
4	ACO-TS algorithm [18]	Ant colony optimization, tabu search	Generated a model for solving the travelling salesman problem using meta-heuristic approaches
5	Intelligent infectious disease algorithm [19]	Clustering, intelligent computing,	Performed the surveillance routing of COVID-19 using the intelligent computing model based on clustering
6	*Proposed approach*	*ACO, HBMO, SA*	*Solved the travelling problem based on effects of COVID-19 in several cities*

safe conditions with threshold value from 0.40 to 0.59, *moderately safe* conditions with threshold value between 0.60 and 0.79, and *extremely secure* conditions with threshold values between 0.80 and 1.00. The investigation based upon several threshold values concluded a substantial decrease in the number of paths when compared under several safety parameters. The future prospect in this work is through the implementation of other meta-heuristic algorithms with bigger dataset we can further improve the performance proposed approach. Further, the authors can propose a mixed level of safety so as to make the travel more cost effective for the real-life implementation.

References

1. Yang XS (2011) Meta-heuristic optimization: algorithm analysis and open problems. Int Symp On Exp Algo, Springer Lect Notes Comp Sc 6630:21–32
2. Auger A, Benjamin D (2014) Theory of randomized search heuristics: foundations and recent developments. J Genetic Prog Evo Mach 15(1):111–122
3. Akay B et al (2021) A survey on the artificial bee colony algorithm variants for binary, integer and mixed integer programming problems. Appl Soft Comp J 106:1–35
4. Karaboga, Dervis (2016) An idea based on honey bee swarm for numerical optimization. Technical report—TR16, Technical Report, Erciyes University, pp 1–10
5. Bozorg OH et al (2007) Honey-bee mating optimization (HBMO) algorithm for optimal reservoir operation. J Franklin Inst 344(5):452–462
6. Tovey C (2004) On honey bees and dynamic server allocation in internet hosting centers. Adapt Behav 12(3–4):223–240
7. Zhenwu W et al (2021) A comparative study of common nature-inspired algorithms for continuous function optimization. Entropy 23:1–40
8. Andy S et al (2009) The Kirkpatrick model: a useful tool for evaluating training outcomes. J Intell Dev Disabil 34(3):266–274
9. Dorigo M, Birattari M, Stutzle T (2006) Ant colony optimization. IEEE Comp Intell Mag 1(4):28–39
10. Selvi M et al (2016) HBO based clustering and energy optimized routing algorithm for WSN. In: 8th international conference on advance computer (ICoAC), pp 89–92
11. Mojarrad HD, et al. (2014) A novel multi-objective modified honey bee mating optimization algorithm for economic/emission dispatch. In: 19th Iranian conference on electronic engineering, pp 43–56
12. Jianlan G, Yuqiang C, Xuanzi H (2010) Implementation and improvement of simulated annealing algorithm in neural net. In: International conference on computer intelligence and section, pp 519–522
13. ZeinEldin RA (2012) An improved simulated annealing approach for solving the constrained optimization problems. In: 8th International conference on information and system (INFOS), pp BIO-27-BIO-31
14. Jadon RS, Datta U (2013) Modified ant colony optimization algorithm with uniform mutation using self-adaptive approach for travelling salesman problem. In: 4th international conference on computer, communication and net tech (ICCCNT), pp 1–4
15. Chen R, Shen Y, Wang C (2016) Ant colony optimization inspired swarm optimization for grid task scheduling. In: International symposium on computer, consumer and control (IS3C), pp 461–464
16. Xiang YD, et al (2012) A new ant colony optimization with global exploring capability and rapid convergence. In: Proceeding of 10th world congress on intel control and automation, pp 579–583

17. Collings J, Kim E (2014) A distributed and decentralized approach for ant colony optimization with fuzzy parameter adaptation in traveling salesman problem. In: IEEE symposium on swarm intelligent, pp 1–9
18. Dewantoro RW, Sihombing P, Sutarman (2019) The combination of ant colony optimization (ACO) and tabu search (TS) algorithm to solve the traveling salesman problem (TSP). In: 3rd international conference on election, telecomm and computer engineering (ELTICOM), pp 160–164
19. Guevara C, Peñas MS (2020) Surveillance routing of COVID-19 infection spread using an intelligent infectious diseases algorithm. IEEE Access 8:201925–201936

Restoration and Enhancement of COVID-19 Variants Using CT Images

R. Ranjani and R. Priya

Abstract Covid (COVID-19) is an irresistible illness brought about by the SARS-CoV-2 virus. Initially, it was first found in China and began to spread quickly all around the world causing numerous deaths and defeats in practically all fields. Computed tomography (CT) images are popularly being used in the field of computer vision to aid the medical experts to diagnose various diseases. This work aims to pre-process raw CT images which contain noises and disturbances which need to be filtered and enhanced for various medical applications. In this paper, we propose pre-processing steps (restoration and enhancing) of its variants utilizing CT scan images. Lung computerized tomography (CT) images can be viably utilized for early identification of COVID-19 patients. These CT images are handled utilizing computer aided diagnosis (CAD) procedures by the use of reasonable calculations. The first and fundamental stage for any sort of image is to restore and improve them. In this paper, the restoration algorithms used are a combination of two traditional algorithms (bilateral + anisotropic) thus naming it Improved Anisotropic Diffusion Bilateral Filter (2D IADBF). The efficiency of the proposed techniques is exhibited through comparison between traditional algorithms like 2D median filter, 2D log filter, and 2D frequency domain wavelet filter for restoration. The enhancement algorithm utilized is 2D edge preservation efficient histogram improvement (2D EPEHI) algorithm which is ensemble of Edge preservation and histogram processing which focuses on methods like contrast limited adaptive histogram equalization (CLAHE), 2D adaptive mean adjustment, and image coherence improvement, and the results are efficient.

Keywords COVID-19 · Variants · Enhancement · Restoration · CAD · CT image

---

R. Ranjani (✉) · R. Priya
Vels Institute of Science, Technology and Advanced Sciences (VISTAS), Chennai 600117, Tamilnadu, India
e-mail: ranji010794@gmail.com

R. Priya
e-mail: priya.scs@velsuniv.ac.in

© The Author(s), under exclusive license to Springer Nature Singapore Pte Ltd. 2023
J. K. Mandal and D. De (eds.), *Frontiers of ICT in Healthcare*, Lecture Notes in Networks and Systems 519, https://doi.org/10.1007/978-981-19-5191-6_39

1 Introduction

Computed tomography (CT) images are popularly being used in the field of computer vision to aid the medical experts to diagnose various diseases. The CT images of the lungs can be used for the diagnosis of multiple diseases including lung cancer and COVID-19 [1]. The Covid-19 viruses have taken multiple forms ever since they were first discovered. Viruses constantly change due to mutation. When a virus undergoes one or more mutations, it is called a variant. Coronavirus has caused several variants across the globe. Once a virus enters the physical body, its genetic material enters the cells and starts making copies of it which may infect the other cells. Whenever a blunder occurs during this copying process, it triggers a mutation [2].

Early discovery of COVID-19 aids in the ideal arrangement of clinical consideration to the patients. This recognition is possible with the assistance of lung CT images. There are two fundamental ways for the discovery of COVID-19 [3]. The principal classification is the lab-based methodology. This approach includes the examination of tests of human like bodily fluid, throat swabs, and blood. These samples are exposed to testing which includes nucleic acid testing, antigen testing, point testing, serology testing, etc. [4]. In these tests, the swab materials are tested over paper strips that have counterfeit antibodies. The normal awareness of this technique is around 60–71%. The subsequent classification is the use of clinical imaging methods like CT examine, X-ray, and so forth. The raw CT images acquired are applied to imaging methods and are exposed to different algorithms [5]. The algorithms used in this work give imaging information and give efficient results.

The primary methods of image processing are pre-processing, segmenting, and clustering. The pre-processing includes steps like noise removal and enhancement [6]. Restoration is the initial step utilized for the evacuation of noise that is consolidated into the image during the image acquisition step. The image is enhanced and utilized for working on the Brightness and differentiation elements of the image. Proper plan of filtering and improvement algorithms is required to work on the exactness of infection diagnosis [7].

Subsequently, in this research, two novel calculations are proposed for the image filtration and enhancement of the CT images to analyze COVID-19. COVID-19 variants are divided into three types. They are Variant of Interest, Variant of Concern, and Variant of High Consequence [8]. Table 1 illustrates the different kinds of variants with its origin, symptoms, and countries of spread.

Table 1 Origin and symptoms of COVID-19 variants

Variant	Originated from	Month and year	Countries affected	Symptoms
Alpha Variant	United Kingdom	September 2020	Minimum of 173 countries such as the United Kingdom, Bulgaria, Wales, Ireland, United States	Chills, loss of appetite, headache, and muscle aches
Beta Variant	South Africa	May 2020	122 countries including United States	50% more transmissible, severe infections
Gamma Variant	Brazil	November 2020	62 countries including Canada, Italy, United States	Body aches, sore throat, diarrhea, conjunctivitis, and headache, loss of taste or smell
Delta Variant	India	2020	96 countries including Singapore, France, Spain, UK, USA	Persistent cough, headache, fever, and sore throat. Headache, sore throat, runny nose, and fever seem to be more common
Omicron variant	South Africa	2021	Minimum 50 countries which include south Africa, USA, Canada, Ireland, Australia etc	Start with body ache, generalized weakness, fatigue, headache and fever, cough /cold where there is water from the nose, sneezing, etc.

2 Literature Survey

Ref. Paper and Year	Authors	Purpose	Author's proposed system
1. "Imaging manifestations and diagnostic value of chest CT of coronavirus disease 2019 (COVTD-19) in the Xiaogan area," *Clinical. Radiology. Volume 75, Issue5, May 2020*, vol. 75. no. 5, pp 341–347, 2020, Elsevier,https://doi.org/10.1016/j.crad.2020.03.004 [9]	K. Wang, S. Kang, R. Tian, X Zhang, and Y. Wang	To Diagnose of covid-19 using chest images	To test the relationship between severity level of infection and lymphocyte ratio To test the oxygen level of patients
2. "Diagnosis of the Coronavirus disease (COVID-19); rRT-PCR or CT?," *European Journal of Radiology*, vol. 126, no March, p 108961, 2020. Mar 25, National library of medicine . doi ,https://doi.org/10.1016/j.ejrad.2020.108961 [10]	C Long et al.	To compare the diagnostic values of CT scans and RCT-PTR Test	Detection of covid-19 based on CT Real-time reverse transcriptase-polymerase chain reaction(RCT-PTR Test)
3. "COVID-19 pneumonia. A review of typical CT findings and differential diagnosis," *Diagnostic and Interventional Imaging, Volume 101, Issue 5, May 2020, Pages 263–268, Elsevier.* doi: https://doi.org/10.1016/j.diii.2020.03.014 [11]	C. Hani et al.	To find a review on CT findings for covid-19 case	Analysis of various microbiological tests in identification of covid-19 like RCT-PTR Test and sequencing tests
4 "Diagnostic performance between CT and initial real-time RT-PCR for clinically suspected 2019 coronavirus disease (COVID-19) patients outside Wuhan, China," *Respiratory Medicine J Jul* 2020 vol. 168, no. April, p. 105980, 2020, *National library of medicine*, https://doi.org/10.1016/j.rmed.2020.105980 [12]	J. L. He et al.	To compare the diagnostic values of CT scans and RCT-PTR Test	The outcomes had no statistical difference between the 2 methods

(continued)

(continued)

Ref. Paper and Year	Authors	Purpose	Author's proposed system
5. "Lung X-Ray Segmentation using Deep-CNN on Contrast-Enhanced Binarized Images", MDPI, Mathematics, June 2020 [13]	Hsin-Jui Chen And Yan-Tsung Peng	Automatic Locating of Lung Regions in CXR Images is important on CAD	Applying other image enhancement and binirizahon methods for training coverage

The literature survey obviously shows that chest CT is exceptionally compelling in the acknowledgment of COVID-19. Further, it was seen that the awareness achieved utilizing chest CT is higher than that of continuous converse transcriptase-polymerase chain response. Along these lines, chest CT information is utilized for the location Covid-19 in this research.

3 Existing Method and Its Limitations

The proposed methods for image filtration utilize either anisotropic diffusion or bilateral filtering separately. In this work, the proposed algorithm works as a combination of both frequency and spatial domain filtering, and thus simultaneous conservation of gradient data alongside the speckle noise (a type of noise found in images) decrease is impossible [14]. Further, the existing enhancement methods that perform histogram leveling bring about the blurring of the image because of the deficiency of edge data.

4 Proposed Method and Advantages

See Fig. 1.

4.1 2D Improved Anisotropic Diffusion Bilateral Filter (2D IADBF)

Image restoration is done to filter out the speckle noise from the lung CT images. This is done based on the combination of anisotropic diffusion model and the bilateral filter and was implemented using 2D Improved Anisotropic Diffusion Bilateral Filter (2D IADBF). The restoration algorithm is a combination of spatial and frequency domain making it a spacio-frequency domain (i.e., Bilateral + Anisotropic). The anisotropic algorithm is a spatial domain algorithm which removes noise and preserves gradient

Fig. 1 Illustration of proposed method

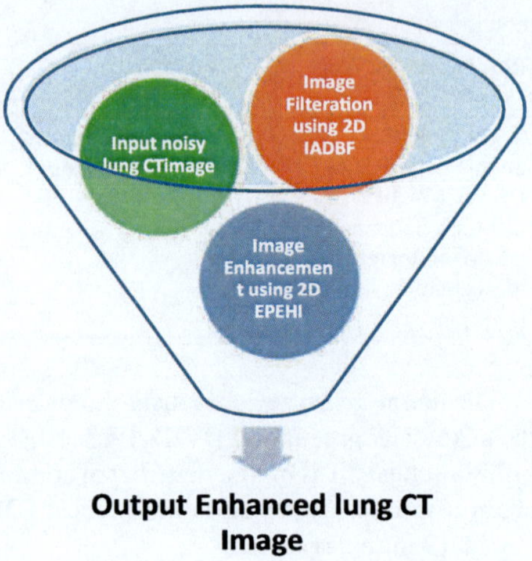

information. Similarly, the bilateral algorithm (frequency domain) is used in speckle noise detection is very high. To achieve the improved variation form of filtering is the 2D Improved Anisotropic Diffusion Bilateral Filtering algorithm is used. The algorithm is depicted below:

Algorithm 1: 2D Improved Anisotropic Diffusion Bilateral Filter (2D IADBF).

Input:

Input noisy CT lung image $I^{\mathrm{CT}} \in R^{p \times q}$.

Steps:

For the given input image define the anisotropic diffusion model using Eq. (1).

The diffusion coefficient is generated based on the gradient function using $DC^i(u, v) = gd(\Delta I)$.

The gradient function is modified using bilateral function as $gd(\Delta I) = \frac{1}{1+(|\Delta I|/\mathrm{BF})^2}$

The bilateral function is defined using the gradient function to enable accurate noise filtration using Eq. (4) [15].

Finally, the filtered image $F^{CT} \in R^{p \times q}$ is obtained using,

$$F_{t+1}^{\mathrm{CT}}(u, v) = F_t^{\mathrm{CT}}(u, v) + \frac{1}{4}[\mathrm{DC}^i(u, v) \cdot \sigma^2(u, v)]$$

Output:

Filtered image $F^{\mathrm{CT}} \in R^{p \times q}$.

4.2 2D Edge Preservation Efficient Histogram Improvement (2D EPEHI)

The next stage in the proposed system is the image improvement/enhancement which is oriented toward the general contrast and brightness of the image. The enhancement algorithm is utilized for a powerful edge protecting and an effective histogram giving a better outcome. The algorithm for enhancement is depicted below.

2: 2D Edge Preservation Efficient Histogram Improvement (2D EPEHI).

Input:

Filtered image $F^{\mathrm{CT}} \in R^{p \times q}$.

Steps:

- Divide the filtered image $F^{\mathrm{CT}} \in R^{p \times q}$ into sub-blocks of size $n \times n$.
- For each sub-block, compute the Tenengrad criterion using Eq. (6).
- Calculate the overall Tenengrad criterion for a particular block using $\mathrm{TCB} = \sum_{u \in w} \sum_{v \in w} [\mathrm{TC}(u, v)]^2$.
- Divide the image into 4 regions based on the Tenengrad criterion.
- Compute the weight function for each histogram using $wf(hm_i) = C(i)/\mathrm{MC}$.
- Compute the modified histogram using $\mathrm{MH} = \sum_{i=1,2,3} wf(hm_i) * hm_i$.
- Find the enhanced image $E^{\mathrm{CT}} \in R^{p \times q}$ using the modified histogram.

Output:

Enhanced image $E^{\mathrm{CT}} \in R^{p \times q}$.

5 Experimental Setup

All the experiments performed in this research were accomplished using MATLAB R2013b with Intel core i5 processor @4 GHz having8 GB RAM.

6 Results and Discussion

The proposed framework is implementation and results are discussed in this section.

7 Parameter Settings

The COVID-19 variant's lung CT images were obtained from the publicly available Imaging Archive dataset (https://www.mdpi.com/2076-3417/11/24/11902/html). The size of the sub-block $n \times n$ was chosen as 8×8.

8 Qualitative Analysis

The quantitative analysis of the proposed system was performed using four types of variant images, i.e., alpha, beta, gamma, and delta. These variant images are shown in Fig. 2. From the figure, it is evident that both the images have lesions around the periphery regions. However, the shape of the lesions varies in the images. The lesions are in patchy form in the COVID-19 images.

8.1 Qualitative Analysis on Covid-19 Images

Figure 3A shows the Alpha variant Covid CT lung input image filtered using 2D median filter (MF), 2D Adaptive Log Gabor filter (LOG), 2D Frequency domain wavelet filter (FDWF), and the proposed 2D IADBF filter. It is evident from Fig. 3 that the image is blurred in the case of 2D median filter. Similarly, the noise components are still prevalent in the 2D Adaptive Log Gabor filter. The contrast of the image filtered using 2D frequency domain wavelet filter is also poor. However, the proposed 2D IADBF filter produces best filtration results overcoming all the issues in the other filters.

Figure 4 shows the COVID-19 variant's CT lung filtered image enhanced using CLAHE, 2D AMA, Coherence adjustment and the proposed 2D EPEHI algorithm. The proposed 2D EPEHI algorithm achieves best enhancement results in which the

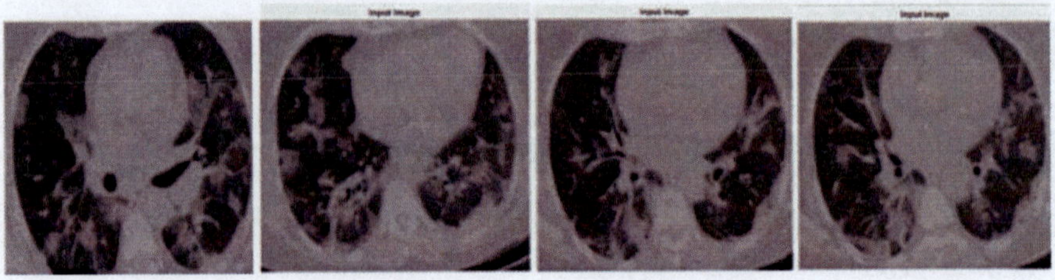

(a) (b) (c) (d)

Fig. 2 **a** Alpha variant, **b** beta variant, **c** gamma variant, **d** delta variant

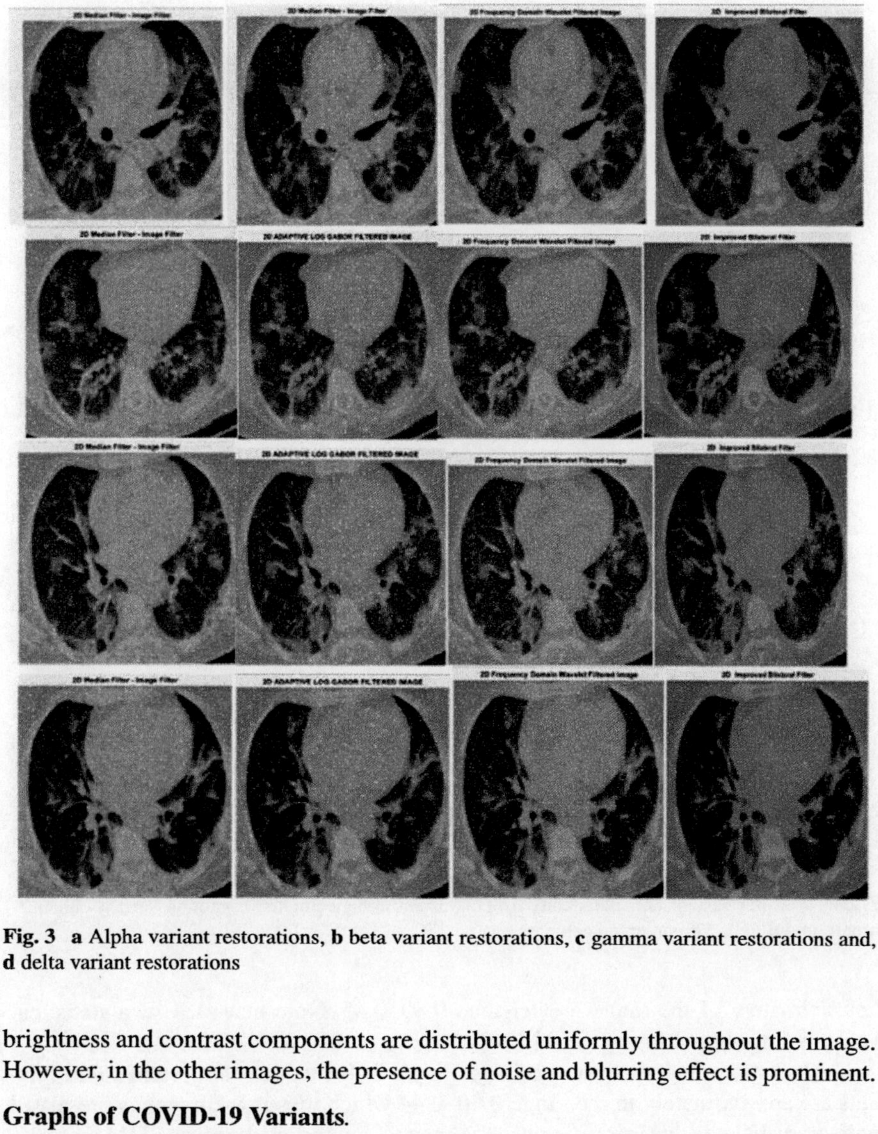

Fig. 3 **a** Alpha variant restorations, **b** beta variant restorations, **c** gamma variant restorations and, **d** delta variant restorations

brightness and contrast components are distributed uniformly throughout the image. However, in the other images, the presence of noise and blurring effect is prominent.

Graphs of COVID-19 Variants.

Figure 5 shows the comparison of processing time graph (*x*-axis—Diff algorithms; *y*-axis—processing time), RMSE graph (*x*-axis—Iterations: *y*-axis—Mean sqr values), and PSNR graph (*x*-axis—Algorithms; *y*-axis—PSNR in dB) for different filtering algorithms using COVID-19 variant's CT lung image (Table 2).

The above tabulation shows that the PSNR value of the proposed algorithm is in the range 35–38 i.e. image has been signalled and removed the noise (more the PSNR more the image is noise free). Similarly, the MSE values of the proposed algorithms of different variants show that there is almost no error in the image, i.e.,

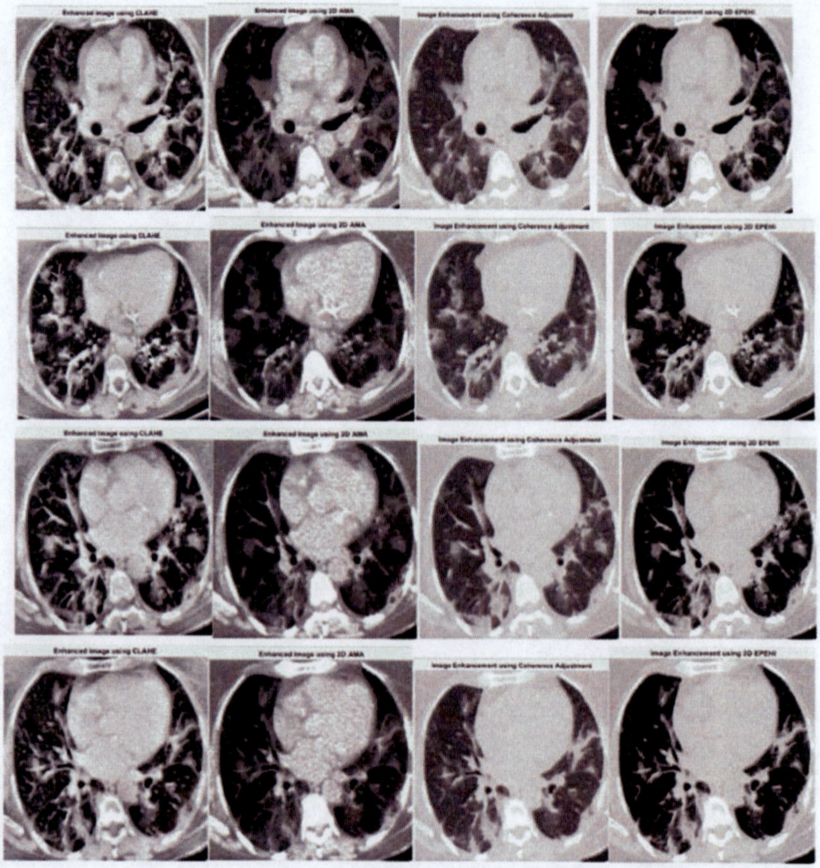

(a)
(b)
(c)
(d)

Fig. 4 **a** Alpha variant enhancements, **b** beta variant enhancements, **c** gamma variant enhancements, and **d** delta variant enhancements

approximately of the range greater than 0.80–0.85. Note that MSE is a statistical value and does not have any units [16].

Table 3 shows that the proposed algorithm's SSIM values of different covid variants are approximately in the range 0.40–0.44 which means the image is preserved with gradient and edge information in the specific range, i.e., the more SSIM more the image is preserved [17]. Similarly the AMBE values of the proposed algorithms of different variants show that image's average mean brightness error is approximately in the range 4.5–4.7. Note that both SSIM and AMBE are statistical values and does not have any units.

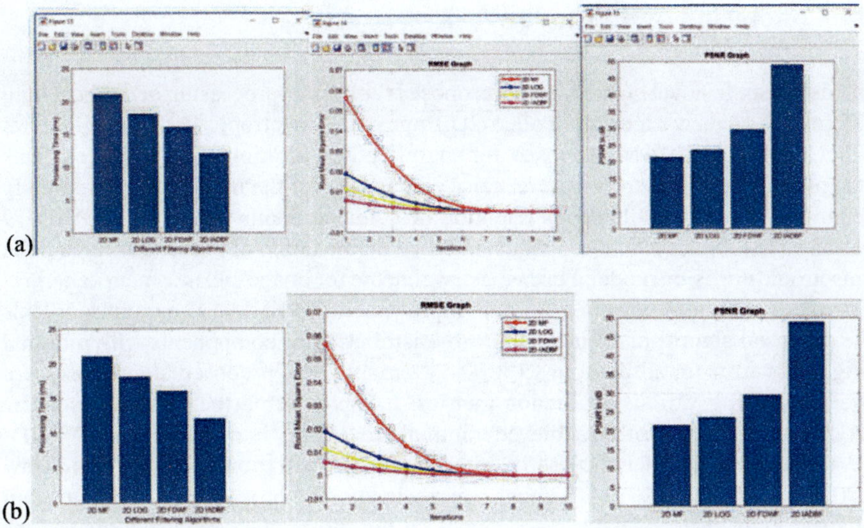

Fig. 5 **a** Alpha variant graphs, **b** beta variant graphs

Table 2 Comparison tabulation of Covid-19 variant's for restoration algorithms

Algorithm/Variant	Parameter (PSNR in dB)	2D AMA	2D LGF	2D FDWF	2D IADBF
Alpha variant	PSNR	20.35	27.93	19.98	38.75
	MSE	59.94	10.46	65.29	0.85
Beta variant	PSNR	19.84	27.82	19.52	37.84
	MSE	67.82	10.72	72.50	0.83
Gamma Variant	PSNR	19.95	27.88	19.60	38.00
	MSE	65.70	65.70	71.22	0.81
Delta variant	PSNR	19.85	27.89	70.91	38.01
	MSE	65.65	10.56	19.60	0.81

Table 3 Comparison Tabulation of COVID-19 variant's enhancement

Algorithm/Variant	Parameter	CLAHE	2D AMA	CIA	2D EPEHI
Alpha variant	SSIM	0.25	0.38	0.31	0.44
	AMBE	10.42	6.96	6.96	4.72
Beta variant	SSIM	0.19	0.41	0.38	0.43
	AMBE	9.48	5.93	7.23	4.70
Gamma variant	SSIM	0.38	0.42	0.35	0.48
	AMBE	7.52	5.46	6.8	0.71
Delta variant	SSIM	0.49	0.44	0.32	0.42
	AMBE	8.59	5.32	6.63	4.74

9 Conclusion and Future Work

In this research, novel algorithms are proposed for the pre-processing of medical lung CT images. A new algorithm called 2D Improved Anisotropic Diffusion Bilateral Filter (2D IADBF) was proposed for the effective filtration of CT images. This scheme was designed such that the noise components of the image were completely removed with the simultaneous retention of gradient details for all the COVID-19 variants [18]. This system was modeled based on the union of bilateral filter and the anisotropic diffusion model. Further, a new scheme for image enhancement called 2D Edge Preservation Efficient Histogram Improvement (EPEHI) is also proposed. Thus the proposed algorithm achieved uniform distribution of components with minimal brightness error for all the four COVID-19 variants. The proposed algorithms were evaluated using various evaluation metrics. It was inferred that the proposed 2D IADBF filtration algorithm achieved minimal processing time of 13 ms for COVID-19, respectively. Further, the RMSE of the 2D IADBF filtration algorithm was as low as 0.80 for the COVID-19 CT images, respectively. The proposed EPEHI algorithm attained high SSIM of 0.44, respectively. In the future, we can design algorithms for the segmentation and classification of these images for the effective diagnosis of COVID-19 Variants which can be used in medical applications.

References

1. Schofield R (2020) Image reconstruction: part 1—understanding filtered back projection, noise and image acquisition. J Cardiovasc Comput Tomography 14(3):219–225
2. Racine D (2020) Task-based characterization of a deep learning image reconstruction and comparison with filtered back-projection and a partial model-based iterative reconstruction in abdominal CT: a phantom study. Phys Med 76:28–37
3. Bhandary A (2020) Deep-learning framework to detect lung abnormality—a study with chest X-Ray and lung CT scan images. Pattern Recogn Lett 129:271–278. https://doi.org/10.1016/j.patrec.2019.11.013
4. Toğaçar M, Ergen B, Cömert Z (2020) Detection of lung cancer on chest CT images using minimum redundancy maximum relevance feature selection method with convolutional neural networks. Biocybern Biomed Eng 40(1):23–39
5. Mohamed Shakeel P, Desa MI, Burhanuddin MA (2020) Improved watershed histogram thresholding with probabilistic neural networks for lung cancer diagnosis for CBMIR systems. Multimedia Tools Appl 79(23–24):17115–17133
6. Zhang L et al (2020) Clinical characteristics of COVID-19-infected cancer patients: a retrospective case study in three hospitals within Wuhan, China. Ann Oncol: Official Eur J Oncol 31(7):894–901 (National Library of Medicine)
7. Li K et al (2020) CT image visual quantitative evaluation and clinical classification of coronavirus disease (COVID-19). Eur Radiol 30(8):4407–4416. https://doi.org/10.1007/s00330-020-06817-6
8. Mahase E (2021) Delta variant what is happening with transmission, hospital admissions, and restrictions? BMJ 373:n1513
9. Wang K, Kang S, Tian R, Zhang X, Wang Y (2020) Imaging manifestations and diagnostic value of chest CT of coronavirus disease 2019 (COVID-19) in the Xiaogan area. Clin Radiol

75(5):341–347. Long C et al (2020) Diagnosis of the Coronavirus disease (COVID-19): rRT-PCR or CT? Eur J Radiol 126:108961 (National Library of Medicine)
10. Hani C et al (2020) COVID-19 pneumonia: a review of typical CT findings and differential diagnosis. Diagnostic Interventional Imaging 101(5):263–268
11. He JL et al (2020) Diagnostic performance between CT and initial real-time RT-PCR for clinically suspected 2019 coronavirus disease (COVID-19) patients outside Wuhan, China. Respiratory Med 168:105980 (National Library of Medicine)
12. Chen H-J, Ruan S-J, Huang S-W, Peng Y-T (2020) Lung X-ray segmentation using deep convolutional neural networks on contrast-enhanced binarized images. Multidisciplinary Digital Publishing Institute, Mathematics
13. Chi J, Zhang Y, Yu X, Wang Y, Wu C (2019) Computed Tomography (CT) image quality enhancement via a uniform framework integrating noise estimation and super-resolution networks. Multidisciplinary Digital Publishing Institute, Sensors
14. Deng Y et al (2020) Usefulness of CT texture analysis in differentiating benign and malignant renal tumours. Clin Radiol 75(2):108–115
15. Ozsahin I, Sekeroglu B, Musa MS, Mustapha MT, Uzun Ozsahin D (2020) Review on diagnosis of COVID-19 from chest CT images using artificial intelligence. In: Computational and mathematical methods in medicine, vol 2020, 26 Sept 2020, Hindawi
16. Ranjani R, Priya R (2021) Efficient segmentation and classification of lung cancer diagnosis techniques using CT images: a review. Turkish J Comput Math Educ 12(10):2433–2440
17. Ranjani R, Priya R (2021) Filtering and enhancement of lung computerized tomography images for the diagnosis of Covid-19 and lung cancer. Des Eng 2021(07):13900–13918
18. Ranjani R, Priya R (2021) A comparison of image restoration techniques of lung CT Covid-19 images. Int J Mech Eng Kalahari J 6(3):15921593. ISSN: 0974-5823
19. Kumar A, Gupta PK, Srivastava A (2020) A review of modern technologies for tackling COVID-19 pandemic. In: Diabetes metabolic syndrome and clinical reservation, Revised Jul–Aug 2020, vol 14, no 4, pp 569–573. https://doi.org/10.1016/j.dsx.2020.05.008 (National Library of Medicine)
20. Chamola V, Hassija V, Gupta V, Guizani M (2020) A comprehensive review of the COVID-19 pandemic and the role of IoT, drones, AI, blockchain, and 5G in managing its impact. IEEE Access 8:90225–90265
21. Bose P, Roy S, Ghosh P (2021) A comparative NLP-based study on the current trends and future directions in COVID-19 research. IEEE Access 9:78341–78355

IoT in Healthcare

MediFi: An IoT-Based Health Monitoring Device

Saradwata Bandyopadhyay, Akash Kumar Singh, Sunil Kumar Sharma, Rajrupa Das, Arju Kumari, Angira Halder, and Sandip Mandal

Abstract This paper represents an IoT-based wireless portable healthcare device that examines the patient's heart rate, body temperature, SpO2, and tracks the number of steps of the patient. The sensors are clipped to a NodeMCU which reads the vitals of the patient and displays the output on the OLED display. This data is stored in the cloud storage for analysis and report generation. The mobile app empowers the medical representatives or family members to access obligatory information remotely. Thus, this device will reduce crowds in hospitals at rush hours. As a result, the doctors and the other healthcare representatives can give extra care to the patients.

Keywords IoT module · Health monitoring system · NodeMCU · SpO2 · WSN etc

1 Introduction

The advancement of technology has helped to bridge the distance between patient and doctor. The branch of IoT involved in medical field is called medical Internet of Things (mIoTs). Mankind has already been benefited from it and will be more benefitted in the near future. Internet of Things which is popularly known as IoT has the ability to connect technology with every aspect of our life, making our lives a lot easier.

Our health monitoring device "MediFi" was brought into vision during the advent of the deadly disease "Covid 19". The prevailing third wave of the pandemic along with other emerging diseases like mucor mycosis, yellow fungus, white fungus, etc. This device will be beneficial in several ways. Sensors are used to monitor the patient's health conditions and upload the patient's vitals to the cloud, making the vitals easily accessible via our application. The device provides continuous monitoring of patients without any human involvement, hence bridging the gap between patient, doctor, and patients' family.

S. Bandyopadhyay · A. K. Singh · S. K. Sharma · R. Das · A. Kumari · A. Halder · S. Mandal (✉)
University of Engineering and Management, Kolkata 700160, India
e-mail: sandip.mandal@uem.edu.in

© The Author(s), under exclusive license to Springer Nature Singapore Pte Ltd. 2023
J. K. Mandal and D. De (eds.), *Frontiers of ICT in Healthcare*, Lecture Notes in Networks and Systems 519, https://doi.org/10.1007/978-981-19-5191-6_40

2 Problem Statement

A lot of frontline health workers lost their lives worldwide daily because the techniques used in the past have failed miserably while treating communicable diseases. Patients with symptoms of influenza or with other pre-existing conditions like respiratory issues are facing a lot of trouble in getting their routine management as well as emergency healthcare due to COVID-19-related regulations. For enabling life toward getting near to normal, the first thing that must be made sustainable is the healthcare system. Hence, IoT devices equipped with sensors will make the patient monitoring much easier for the doctors.

Our healthcare system including both public and corporate getting challenged at every step, whether it is:

- Containment of disease
- Proper handling to emergencies due to non-COVID-19 chronic illness
- Protection of Health Care workers (HCWs)
- Sustainability

3 Literature Survey

Sathya et al. [1] manufactured a wearable device that can be embedded into the patient's body. Their health is continuously monitored, and the data that are collected, analyzed, aggregated, and mined to predict the possible diseases one might be affected with. The medical representative uses the processing algorithm for the personalization of the treatment, which actually makes the healthcare economical with improved outcomes.

Senthil Kumar et al. [2] proposed a system that can monitor the patient's body condition by reading the body parameters like temperature, humidity, pulse, and body movements uninterruptedly from anywhere in the world. Analysis of patients' health data is done against the normal situation to track physiological parameters and in emergency situations notifications will be sent to the doctors immediately.

Shiva Rama Krishan et al. [3] proposed system uses Arduino-Uno-connected body temperature and heart rate sensors to keep track of one's health. The LCD displays the results, and the readings are collected in a cloud server via Wi-Fi which tracks the real-time data. For any sudden changes in the patient's health, an alert is sent using IoT.

Rasseduzzaman et al. [4], made a system that collects a patient's pulse reading, body temperature and heartbeat and sends data into the IoT cloud platform by using Wi-Fi and are stored there. The medical representatives and authorized persons use the data to monitor the health of the patient.

Piyare et al. [5], proposed an Android-based mobile phone for monitoring home appliances. The home appliances are embedded with an Arduino-Uno board which could be controlled by a cellular device.

4 "MediFi"—The Wearable Device

IoT has transformed every aspect of our everyday lifestyle as it is a good match for healthcare solutions. Also, the popularity of wearable IoT devices is increasing day by day. Hospitals and other healthcare organizations are using wearable IoT devices to increase the comfort of the patients, reducing the chances of technical errors, decreased costs, better healthcare management, and safe environment both for healthcare workers and patients.

We have designed a Health Monitoring device—"MediFi" which monitors the patient 24 × 7 and uploads the data to the cloud, so that the hospital or family can easily access the data using the MediFi App. The device is motivated by the fitness devices that are trending in the market. Our device "MediFi" measures a patient's body temperature, heart rate, SpO2, and can also keep step counts. The patient's essentials uploaded to the cloud can be viewed from anywhere, anytime remotely. The doctors can easily recommend the accurate measures that can be taken at any point of time.

The app is designed keeping user experience at the top priority. The app actively monitors the patients and synchronizes the readings or vitals into the cloud server. The doctors and the patient's family can regularly monitor the patient's condition at their fingertips. Doctors can take appropriate steps based on the generated report and can create an e-prescription via the MediFi app.

5 System Architecture

The methodology adapted is to read the data using the sensors and then send it to the cloud servers. And the data can be viewed by the doctors and can be flagged as an alert if the readings are unusual.

Figure 1 shows the architecture of our proposed system for health monitoring of the patients remotely. Our MediFi wearable device can be firmly fitted on the wrist using the belt (Fig. 2)

The MediFi device mainly works in two parts. In the first part, the sensors take the vitals or the readings from the patient's body. The sensor MAX-30100 reads the heart rate and the SpO2 concentration, whereas the MPU-6050 records the steps of the patient. A LM-35 temperature sensor has been used to continuously record the body temperature of the patient. The patient's vital readings are then sent to the main processing device called NodeMCU. The NodeMCU takes those readings and does all the required calculations on the raw data that was just collected by the sensors. When the calculations are done, the NodeMCU displays the final readings on the OLED display mounted on the device. The NodeMCU also actively sends the patient's readings to the cloud through the internet. These patient's readings are regularly sent to the cloud server in real-time for future use.

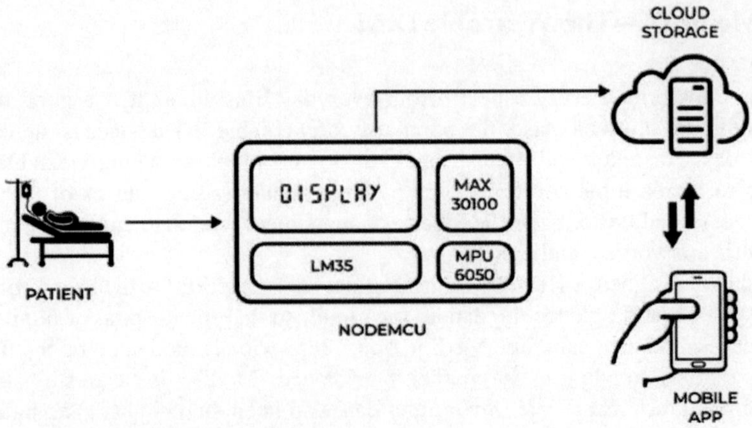

Fig. 1 Architecture of the proposed system

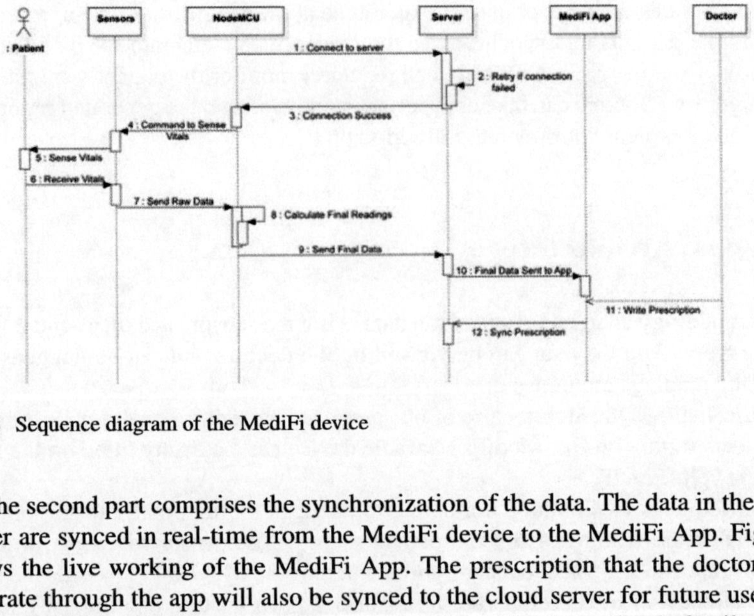

Fig. 2 Sequence diagram of the MediFi device

The second part comprises the synchronization of the data. The data in the cloud server are synced in real-time from the MediFi device to the MediFi App. Figure 3 shows the live working of the MediFi App. The prescription that the doctors will generate through the app will also be synced to the cloud server for future use.

The readings and the prescriptions can be viewed by the patient's family or the doctors from anywhere 24 × 7. This can be a great help for the family because they can instantly take measures as per the doctor's recommendation if the patient's condition is critical.

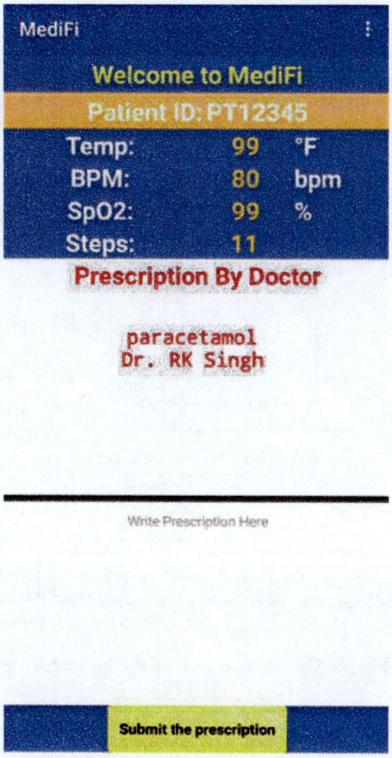

Fig. 3 The MediFi app displaying patients' data

6 Device Circuit and Working

Figure 4 shows how the sensors are connected on the NodeMCU development board.

Figure 5 shows the prototype of the device MediFi in working condition. This device works with the help of two concepts, IoT and Inter-Integrated Circuit Communication which is also known as I2C communication. I2C is a half-duplex communication protocol. This is a type of synchronous serial communication protocol.

The device has two wires for communicating between the device and sensors shown in (Fig. 6). SDA pin (Serial Data) is used to send requests and receive the raw data. SCL pin (Serial Clock) sends the clock pulse to the sensors. This communication has main two devices in general, the Master Device (NodeMCU) and Slave Device (I2C sensors). The device first tries to make communication with the server to transfer data, then the device tries to calibrate the sensors like accelerometer and gyroscope sensor. The device then starts sending the request to the sensors to fetch the data to the NodeMCU through I2C communication protocol. The sensors are triggered to send data at a particular time period. For the temperature, the sensor LM35 IC sends the raw data to the NodeMCU which through some mathematical calculations are converted into readable temperature readings. The calculated data is sent to the

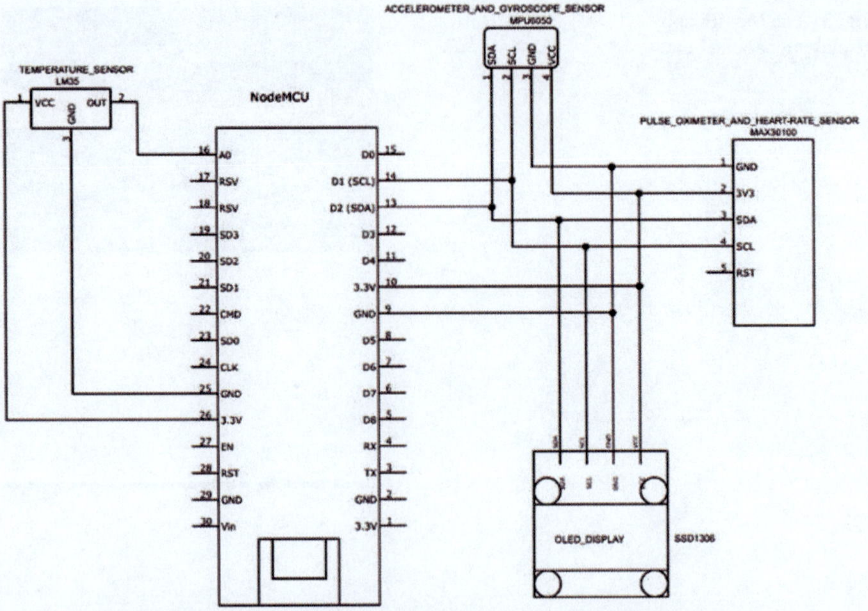

Fig. 4 Circuit diagram of the wearable device

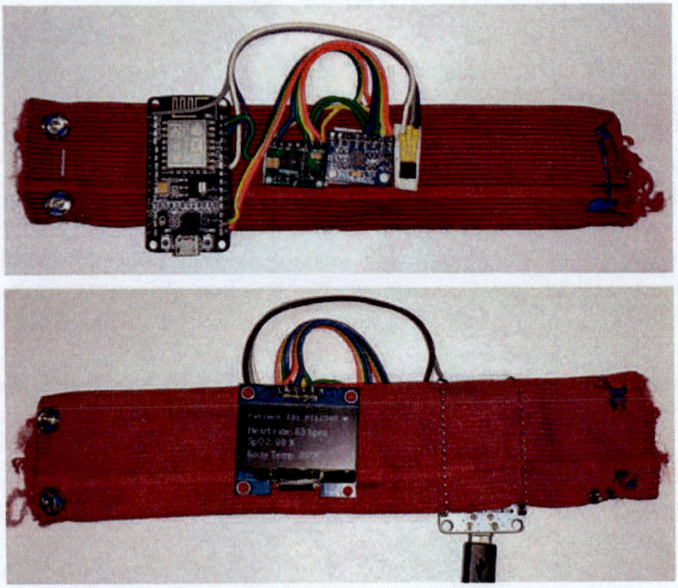

Fig. 5 MediFi device

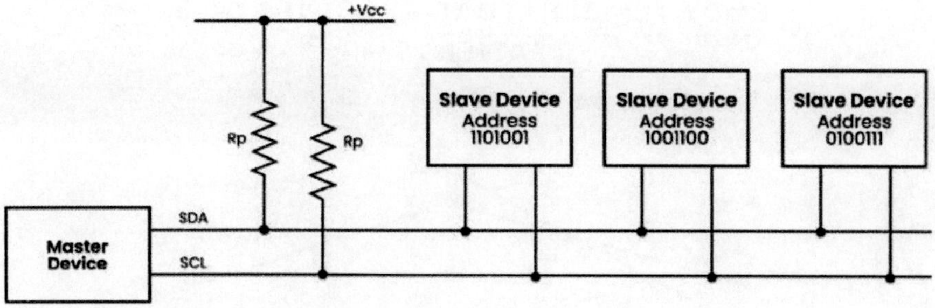

Fig. 6 I2C categorization of master and slave devices

server with the help of the IoT technology. Now through the server, the data can be fetched by our application for the user. In the MediFi app, the doctor can write the suggestions/prescription for the patient, patient's family, and for the hospital. The MediFi app data is also synchronized back to the server to save the information.

7 Simulation and Implementation Results

Since we already have a working prototype, we conducted a set of tests in order to present the readings of the device. We took data samples from three different people who were monitored over a course of three days constantly.

Table 1 shows the three different readings of body Temperature which are recorded over a period of three consecutive days from November 17, 2021 to November 19, 2021.

Figure 7 shows the graphical representation of the body temperature readings. The normal body temperature ranges from 97 °F (36.1 °C) and 99 °F (37.2 °C). Any value differing from the above-mentioned range should be considered abnormal by the doctors.

Table 2 shows the three different readings of SpO2 levels which are recorded over a period of three consecutive days from November 17, 2021 to November 19, 2021.

Figure 8 shows the graphical representation of the SpO2 readings. The SpO2 concentration of a healthy person should not be below 94%.

Table 1 Body temperature readings of the three patients

Sensor	Patient ID	Body temperature reading (°F)		
		Nov 17, 2021	Nov 18, 2021	Nov 19, 2021
LM-35	PT001	96.7	98.6	96.3
LM-35	PT002	97.5	95.2	95.1
LM-35	PT003	95.6	99.4	98.9

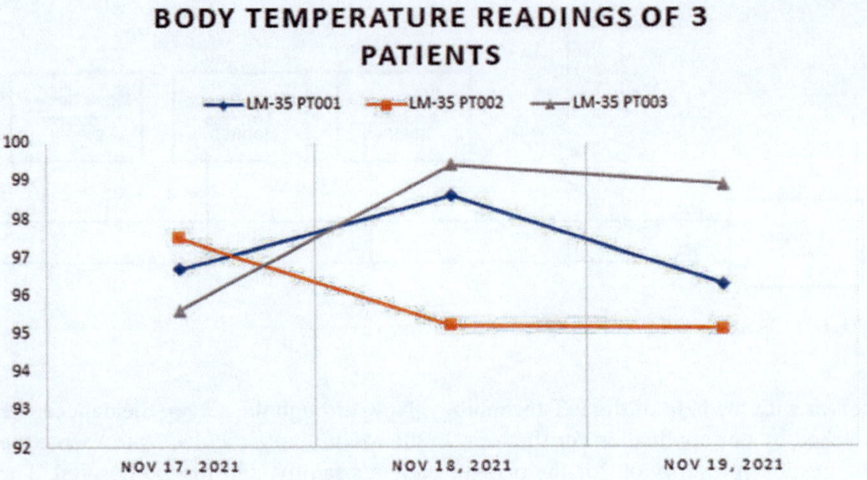

Fig. 7 Chart representing body temperature of 3 patients

Table 2 SpO2 readings of the three Patients

Sensors	Patient ID	SPO2 reading (%)		
		Nov 17, 2021	Nov 18, 2021	Nov 19, 2021
MAX30100	PT001	96	97	97
MAX30100	PT002	99	95	99
MAX30100	PT003	98	96	98

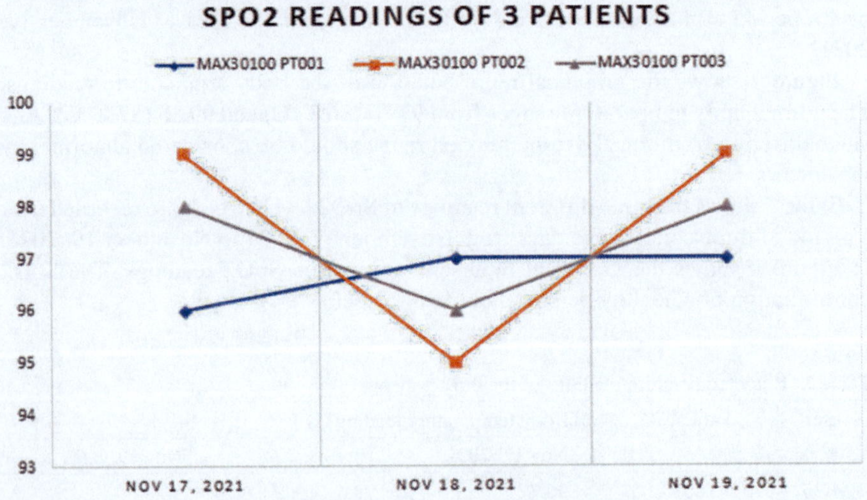

Fig. 8 Chart representing the SpO2 concentration of 3 patients

Table 3 Pulse readings of the three patients

Sensor	Patient ID	Pulse reading (bpm)		
		Nov 17, 2021	Nov 18, 2021	Nov 19, 2021
MAX30100	PT001	88	90	91
MAX30100	PT002	92	89	93
MAX30100	PT003	84	88	89

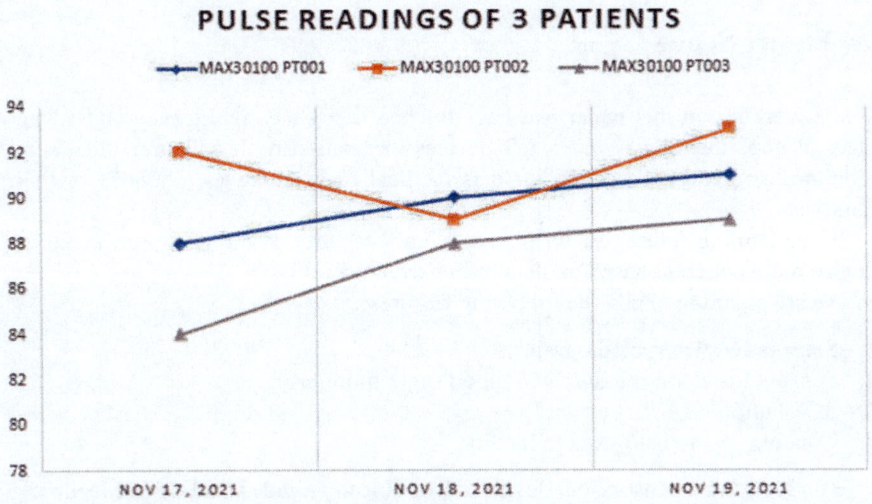

Fig. 9 Chart representing the pulse readings of 3 patients

Table 3 shows the three different readings pulse which are recorded over a period of three consecutive days from November 17, 2021 to November 19, 2021.

Figure 9 shows the graphical representation of the pulse readings of the three patients. The resting heart rate of any adult ranges from 60 to 100 bpm. The medical representatives can immediately take required actions if the readings come out to be abnormal or alarming

8 Benefits

Our device being an application of IoT has the following benefits:

- Real-time Remote Monitoring: Our IoT device can send smart alerts and can detect illness. Hence, it can save lives in case of a medical emergency.
- Prevention: Medical sensors examine health conditions and the environment around the patient and recommend preventive measures, thus will prevent the eventuality of the diseases and acute conditions.

- Medical Data Accessibility: Access of medical records allows patients and the concerned authorities to receive desired attention and help the authorities to take the required actions to prevent acute conditions.
- Reduction of healthcare costs: IoT reduces the overall expenditure of the medical bills and the visits, making it more affordable.
- Improved treatment management: IoT devices tracks the medical progress which results into an accurate treatment and management.

9 Future Scope

While working on this paper, we have tracked down the significance and advantages of implementing Wireless IoT devices for healthcare. It will strengthen basic monitoring for everyone, whether it is medical representatives, patient's or their families.

In the coming future, we wish to add more features to our device to make the device more coherent based on the current scenario.

We are planning to add the following features:

1. Sensors for electrocardiography.
2. Sensors for blood pressure and blood sugar monitoring.
3. SOS button.
4. Creating secure data storage facility.

By adding these sensors, our device will be able to provide a 360-degree feedback. The SOS emergency system that will send a signal to the healthcare representatives and to the patient's family if there is something wrong with the patient so that the patient gets immediate attention. We are very much aware of the fact that IoT devices perform notoriously when it comes to data privacy and security. So, we are working to make this device a lot more secure to provide the users with a secure and reliable environment.

10 Conclusion

Our research paper has proposed a medical IoT-based wearable device that can monitor patient's health. The proposed system can track the patient's vitals like the heart rate, SpO2, body temperature, and the steps with the help of various sensors mounted on the wearable device. The readings are actively uploaded to the cloud server so that it can be accessed anytime remotely via the MediFi App. This device can save a lot of time as the doctors can recommend treatment remotely. This proposed system will be a great resource to the medical world and will hugely support the healthcare field.

Acknowledgements We would like to express our gratitude to our beloved faculties for giving us the golden opportunity to showcase our talent and innovation via this project. Our respected professor, Dr. Sandip Mandal has been the light bearer throughout the entire process. He has guided us through thick and thin and encouraged us in taking up more responsibilities. Our esteemed institution, University of Engineering and Management, Kolkata has given us the recognition and support which helped us to reach our goal. Last but not the least, the effort of each and every member involved in this project has been the milestone towards making this paper a success.

References

1. Sathya M, Madhan S, Jayanthi K, Sagunthala (2018) Avadi: Internet of Things (IoT) based health monitoring system and challenges. Int J Eng Technol
2. Senthilkumar S, Brindra K, Charanya R, Kumar A (2019) Patients health monitoring system using IOT. Int J Public Health Res Dev
3. Shiva Rama Krishnan D, Gupta SC, Choudhary T (2018) An IoT based patient health monitoring system. In: International Conference on Advances in Computing and Communication Engineering (ICACCE)
4. Raseduzzaman Ruman Md, Jahan KR, Barua A, Jamil Roni Md, Rahaman W, Foyjur Rahaman Md (2020) IoT based emergency health monitoring system. In: 2020 International conference on industry 4.0 technology (I4Tech)
5. Piyare R (2013) Internet of Things: ubiquitous home control and monitoring system using android based smart phone. Int J Internet Things

Fog-Based Smart Road Safety Application Using IoT

Dougani Bentabet

Abstract Smart devices generate an unprecedented volume and variety of data. These volumes of data are most often intended to be processed and analyzed. Cloud computing paradigms are not really suited for the type and speed of data created by the Internet of Things in real-time (IoT). The fog computing model can be considered a technological innovation on the Internet. This new distributed computing system will have to be applied in multiple areas affecting the individuals lives to overcome the latency, bandwidth, and energy consumption limitations of IoT-Cloud models. Many applications can benefit from this infrastructure for processing data from sensors in a city or intelligent factory context. This work aims to model road safety and provide a timely response for road accident applications on fog-cloud infrastructures. We need to develop mechanisms for managing computing, storage, and network resources. The performance evaluation system and experiments have been conducted using Ifogsim simulator. The final findings demonstrate the efficiency of the model system in the hybrid fog cloud environment.

Keywords Internet of Things · Cloud computing · Fog computing · Smart road safety · Big Data

1 Introduction

Internet of Things is a global infrastructure that provides access to services by interconnecting objects (physical or virtual) [1]. Cloud computing provides the tools and services needed to access, store, and create IoT applications in various fields. However, cloud computing infrastructures are not adapted to the IoT needs due to their centralized architecture. The data centers' location far from users and connected objects does not allow them to respond with low latency. It makes its use incompatible in a certain number of cases for which this criterion is essential [2]. Some authors go so far as to say that the latency to reach a server located on a cloud computing site

D. Bentabet (✉)
Lab Smart Grids Renewable Energies, Tahri Mohammad University of Bechar, Béchar, Algeria
e-mail: douganibentabet@pg.univ-bechar.dz

© The Author(s), under exclusive license to Springer Nature Singapore Pte Ltd. 2023
J. K. Mandal and D. De (eds.), *Frontiers of ICT in Healthcare*, Lecture Notes in Networks and Systems 519, https://doi.org/10.1007/978-981-19-5191-6_41

is high and unpredictable [3]. Moreover, the increasing number of connected objects always increases the network load, especially on the links that converge, making the infrastructures difficult to scale [3]. Fog computing extends the cloud to get near to IoT devices. We can distribute the fog devices in any place with a network connection: in the factory, at the top of a power pole, along a railroad track, in vehicles, or on an industrial platform.

Fog nodes can be controllers, industrial switches, routers, or CISCO servers since they include computation, storage, and communications connectivity. Fog computing involves processing data closer to the origin. Common approaches were developed to the implementation of Fog in 2015 by OpenFog consortium [4]. The main area is the Internet of Things, which cannott be fully supported by only Cloud solutions. The development of the Internet of things has encountered the need to process and data should be filtered first sending it to the Cloud. As examples of applications of such features, applications that require low and predictable data latency over the network [5]. As examples of applications of such features, applications that require low and predictable data latency over the network [5, 6]. As well as applications that require real-time data processing.

With the rapid development of connected car concepts and autonomous vehicles and the increasing popularity of high-resolution surveillance in the streets, it is expected that the personal transportation field will usher in a revolution, including the reduction of traffic accidents, the reduction of road congestion, and ensure safety. In this study, a fog-cloud paradigm is produced to supply the safety in the roads by many services to the drivers and passengers and manage the data from various IoT objects in the streets. The attending purposes realize this: (a) a model of fog computing-based resource management, (b) The IoT objects are accessed through the Internet., collect and transmitting data to the fog devices, (c) The system process and analyzes the data to diagnose the status in the road, (d) Ifogsim-simulator [7] is used to simulate and estimate the performances. The rest of the paper is organized as follows. Section 2 reviews the related work of existing IoT applications, and Sect. 3 describes the proposed model and its variants. In Sect. 4, we report empirical results. We examine our approach in both IoT-cloud and IoT-fog-cloud systems. We conclude our paper in Sect. 5.

2 Related Work

Because wireless connections and intensive device deployment further complicate operations, achieving a seamless information flow between devices, infrastructure, cloud, and applications is one of the biggest IoT challenges [8, 9]. In the areas of public safety, emergency management, factory automation, self-driving vehicles, and the Health care, cloud computing can provide more computing power and storage for the connected devices. For example, the work in [10] makes a framework named SAaaS software as a service to deliver IoT devices in a cloud infrastructure. Advanced science and technology applied to accident detection, transportation, service control, and vehicle manufacture to increase the interaction between cars, roads, and users, leading to ensuring safety, improving efficiency, improving the environment, and saving human lives. In the study [10], the authors present an IoT-cloud solution to detect traffic flow parameters and notification of unexpected deceleration that can lead to an accident. The data is gathered by sensors installed in the vehicles and transmitted to a cloud server through 4G connections. In [11], the authors set out to avoid traffic accidents by creating a framework for detecting driver awareness. Entry data is captured by a camera positioned in advance of the driver to monitor head motions and eye nodding. The authors of [12] investigate the creation of a blind-spot detection system for smart vehicles. Three cameras installed outside a vehicle provide input for the proposed system. In [13], the authors develop a collaborative vehicle sensing approach by implementing collaborative vehicle perception. Where information can be exchanged among vehicles to prevent accidents, proposed systems designed in [14, 15] can be applied to road accident detection by detecting several objects from the image data. The detection of street elements in [16] can also support accident avoidance. Muhammad et al. [17] suggested a voice disease detection system using the IoT and cloud infrastructure. The patient's voice is detected by a sensor device and transmitted to the cloud for processing. He et al. [18] presented an IoT-based infrastructure known as FogCepCare, which integrates the sensors with the cloud level to measure patients' status. However, integrating cloud computing and the IoT requires novel reference models that consider both domains simultaneously. Fog computing is an architecture of horizontal resources that exists between IoT devices and traditional cloud or data centers. Figure 1 shows a global Fog computing architecture, in which the fog acts as middleware, extends the cloud, and provides resources to the various underlying IoT nodes. Compared to the traditional cloud, the fog is considered a micro data center with low capacity and resources than a cloud data center.

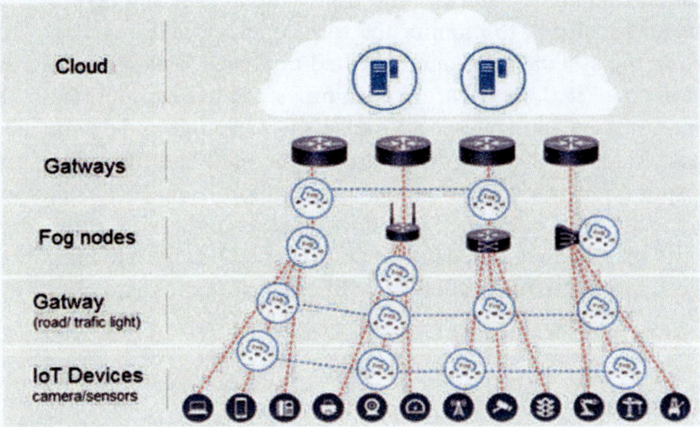

Fig. 1 Architecture-based fog computing

The fog also includes one or more gateways that contribute to a common communication and data exchange between the IoTs. The following challenges need to be addressed [19–21] to recognize IoT-based fog-assisted cloud computing's full capabilities. However, talking only about infrastructure is useless. The smart city concept makes no sense without the applications that are used in everyday life. In this article, we will mainly focus on applications that support activities related to road safety to show how technology can improve the lives of all if used in a planned way that is consistent with the growth prospects of large metropolises.

3 IoT Application Use Case

In this paper, we primarily consider a hierarchy with a single fog level, IoT devices at the edge of the network, a fog layer, and the cloud at the top of the scale (see Fig. 1). The use case of extended eCall services represents a major domain of the IoT [22]. Its objective is to increase road traffic services to road accidents on time and manage emergency services and ambulance services. The application can address several of the services mentioned above. These services can share data. For example, from the emergency, Warning messages can be sent to vehicle drivers to stop cars and or other nearby vehicles and passengers, notify them, provide medical assistance to the patient or injured passengers, as well as ambulance services (see Fig. 2).The system considered in this work consists of a generic scenario deployed in a fog-cloud type infrastructure. The devices consist of: cameras placed in the traffic lights for streaming video, measuring traffic flow, microphones, speakers, ambient sensors, and medical body-worn sensors used by drivers or passengers. IoT devices and sensors interact with fog nodes, which receive aggregated data through access points (i.e., Wi-Fi, 4G, LTE).

Data can be captured by sensors and transmitted to the fog layer for processing in real-time and analyzed to monitor the road, interact, and improve public safety. A fog node in the system can share collected traffic information to decrease traffic congestion in congested areas during peak times and to determine traffic accidents. Fog computing-based applications allow users to exchange and download data from their phones. Also, the monitoring system on the road and the ticketing system of public transportation can collect a lot of information from sensors and video data. A real-time analysis of edge data will then be realized based on fog computing to quickly notify users with detailed information to establish the regular flow and safety of passengers and pedestrians safety in public transportation and city.

4 Simulation and Results

In this section, we present the configuration with simulation and results. A summary of different used parameters is shown in Tables 1 and 2. All the parameters are

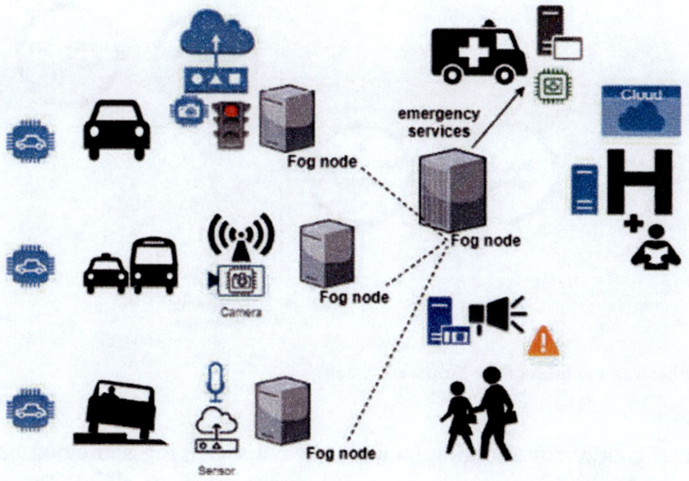

Fig. 2 Road safety use case

obtained from the references [23, 24]. Figure 3 represents the modeling of the application modules of the system.

IFogsim [7], simulates IoT devices, Fog nodes, cloud nodes, and network connections to test performance indicators. By using iFogsim, we can consider the model Sense-Process-Actuate. In this model, sensors publish data to the Internet of Things network, applications running on fog and cloud nodes subscribe to and process data from the sensors, and the final insights obtained are converted into actions that are forwarded to the actuator. The system consists of sensors, a gateway, and a cloud platform that functions to monitor the streets and provide real-time intervention and healthcare services in the workplace. In the experiment, we compared the IoT system after the introduction of fog computing with the traditional cloud computing IoT. The results of the simulation showed that the overall execution time of the IoT system with the introduction of fog computing was reduced by 31.1% (as seen in Fig. 4),

Table 1 Delay details in the system

Ressources	Delay (ms)
IoT device to fog device	2
Fog node to gateway	4
Gateway to cloud	100

Table 2 Configuration details in the system

Table head	CPU (MIPS)	RAM (GB)	Storage (GB)
IoT devices	1000	1	2
Fog device	2000	2	4
Cloud	4000	4	8

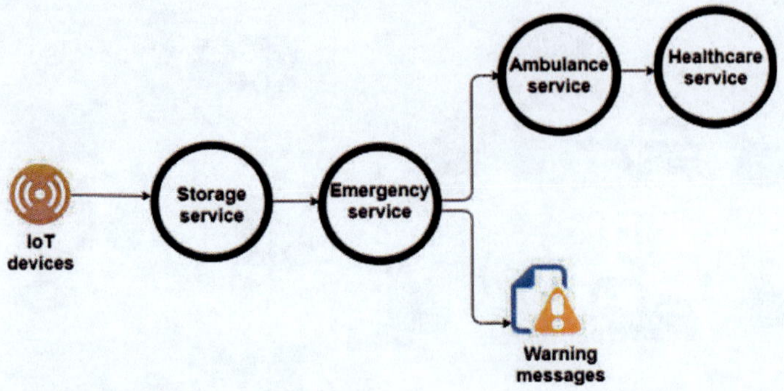

Fig. 3 Application modules of the proposed system

and the total energy consumption including IoT devices, fog and cloud nodes was reduced by 7.41–10.25% (as seen in Fig. 5) compared to the cloud. The estimated result of network usage for various IoT devices (as seen in Fig. 6) Fog reduces 85.9% average network usage time as compared to Cloud only.

Execution Time (MS)

See Fig. 4.

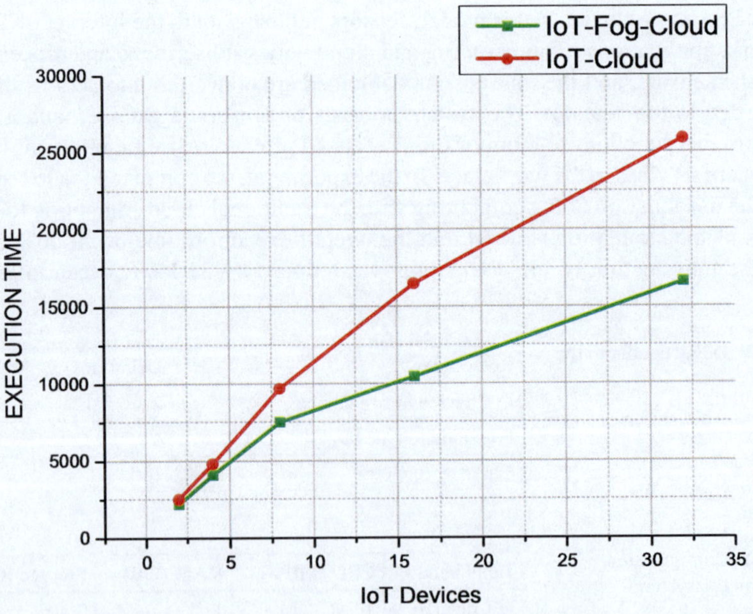

Fig. 4 Execution time

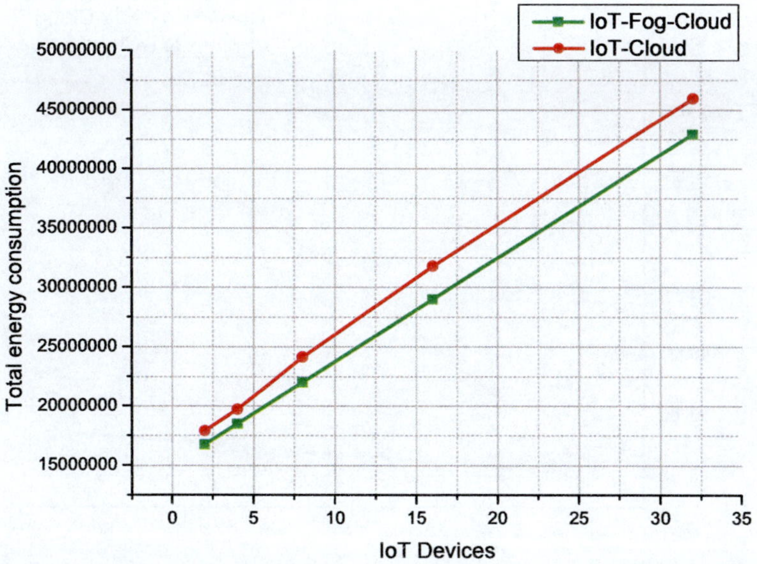

Fig. 5 Energy consumption

Energy (J)

See Fig. 5.

Network Usage (kb)

See Fig. 6.

5 Conclusion

In this paper, performance evaluation for smart road safety system was proposed. Fog computing was introduced into the traditional cloud-based IoT system, a local data processing algorithm was implemented at the sensor level, and simulated and validated under the iFogsim system. The results demonstrate that the introduction of fog computing. The overall amount of data transferred to the cloud platform is reduced by fog computing. By reducing data traffic, network scalability is improved. At the network node level, its greatest energy consumption is when sending and receiving data, so the reduction in data traffic also reduces the execution time, energy consumption of the network nodes, and usage network. In future research, we will further improve the data processing in the fog computing layer and try to apply scheduling problem of application modules on devices.

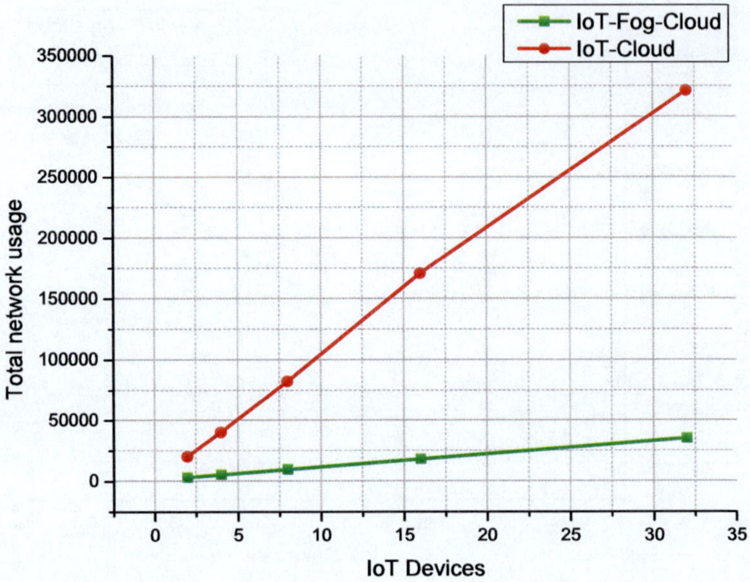

Fig. 6 Total network usage

References

1. Ray PP (2018) A survey on Internet of Things architectures. J King Saud Univ-Comput Inf Sci 30(3):291–319
2. Mukherjee M, Shu L, Wang D (2018) Survey of fog computing: fundamental, network applications, and research challenges. IEEE Commun Surv Tutorials 20(3):1826–1857
3. Rahbari D, Nickray M (2019) Low-latency and energy-efficient scheduling in fog-based IoT applications. Turk J Electr Eng Comput Sci 27(2):1406–1427
4. OpenFog Consortium (2017) OpenFog reference architecture for fog computing. Architecture Working Group, pp 1–162
5. Gill SS, Buyya R (2018) A taxonomy and future directions for sustainable cloud computing: 360 degree view. ACM Comput Surv (CSUR) 51(5):1–33
6. Huang C, Lu R, Choo KKR (2017) Vehicular fog computing: architecture, use case, and security and forensic challenges. IEEE Commun Mag 55(11):105–111
7. Mahmud R, Buyya R (2019) Modelling and simulation of fog and edge computing environments using iFogSim toolkit. In: Fog and edge computing: principles and paradigms, pp 1–35
8. Integration of Cloud Computing with Internet of Things: Challenges and Open Issues
9. Gill SS, Tuli S, Xu M, Singh I, Singh KV, Lindsay D, Pervaiz H et al (2019) Transformative effects of IoT, blockchain and artificial intelligence on cloud computing: evolution, vision, trends and open challenges. Internet of Things 8:100118
10. Celesti A, Galletta A, Carnevale L, Fazio M, Ĺay-Ekuakille A, Villari M (2017) An IoT cloud system for traffic monitoring and vehicular accidents prevention based on mobile sensor data processing. IEEE Sens J 18(12):4795–4802
11. Ghosh A, Chatterjee T, Samanta S, Aich J, Roy S (2017) Distracted driving: a novel approach towards accident prevention. Adv Comput Sci Technol 10:2693–2705
12. Kwon D, Park S, Baek S, Malaiya RK, Yoon G, Ryu JT (2018) A study on development of the blind spot detection system for the IoT-based smart connected car. In: Proceedings of the

2018 IEEE International Conference on Consumer Electronics (ICCE), Las Vegas, NV, USA, 12–14 Jan 2018, pp 1–4
13. Liu W, Kim SW, Marczuk K, Ang MH (2014) Vehicle motion intention reasoning using cooperative perception on urban road. In: Proceedings of the 2014 IEEE 17th international conference on Intelligent Transportation Systems (ITSC), Qingdao, China, 8–11 Oct 2014, pp 424–430
14. Ozbayoglu M, Kucukayan G, Dogdu E (2016) A real-time autonomous highway accident detection model based on big data processing and computational intelligence. In: Proceedings of the 2016 IEEE international conference on Big Data (Big Data), Washington, DC, USA, 5–8 Dec 2016, pp 1807–1813
15. Dogru N, Subasi A (2018) Traffic accident detection using random forest classifier. In: 2018 15th learning and technology conference (L&T), IEEE, pp 40–45
16. Munoz-Organero M, Ruiz-Blaquez R, Sánchez-Fernández L (2018) Automatic detection of traffic lights, street crossings and urban roundabouts combining outlier detection and deep learning classification techniques based on GPS traces while driving. Comput Environ Urban Syst 68:1–8
17. Muhammad G, Rahman SMM, Alelaiwi A, Alamri A (2017) Smart health solution integrating IoT and cloud: a case study of voice pathology monitoring. IEEE Commun Mag 55(1):69–73
18. He S, Cheng B, Wang H, Huang Y, Chen J (2017) Proactive personalized services through fog-cloud computing in large-scale IoT-based healthcare application. China Commun 14(11):1–16
19. Zeinab KAM, Elmustafa SAA (2017) Internet of things applications, challenges and related future technologies. World Sci News 2(67):126–148
20. Anawar MR, Wang S, Azam Zia M, Jadoon AK, Akram U, Raza S (2018) Fog computing: an overview of big IoT data analytics. In: Wireless communications and mobile computing
21. Andriopoulou F, Dagiuklas T, Orphanoudakis T (2017) Integrating IoT and fog computing for healthcare service delivery. In: Components and services for IoT platforms. Springer, Cham, pp 213–232
22. Höyhtyä M, Ojanperä T, Mäkelä J, Ruponen S, Järvensivu P (2017) Integrated 5G satellite-terrestrial systems: use cases for road safety and autonomous ships. In: Proceedings of the 23rd Ka and broadband communications conference, Trieste, Italy, pp 16–19
23. Gupta H, Vahid Dastjerdi A, Ghosh SK, Buyya R (2017) iFogSim: a toolkit for modeling and simulation of resource management techniques in the Internet of Things, edge and fog computing environments. Softw: Pract Experience 47(9):1275–1296
24. Taneja M, Davy A (2017) Resource aware placement of IoT application modules in fog-cloud computing paradigm. In: 2017 IFIP/IEEE symposium on integrated network and service management (IM), IEEE, pp. 1222–1228

Efficient Computing Resource Sharing for Mobile Edge-Cloud Computing Networks

Shashank Mishra, Aman Gupta, and K. Jairam Naik

Abstract To deliver better performance services to consumers, edge and cloud devices can be combined for mobile services. Edge servers can decrease computation delays by offering local computing services, whereas cloud servers can handle jobs that require a lot of processing power. When both edge and cloud servers are used together, it is possible to maximise computing resources while maintaining high Quality of Service (QoS). Edge-cloud computing business models rely on the ability to create effective collaboration between the edge and the cloud. This project develops a solid foundation for mobile edge-cloud computational networks that allows for effective resource exchange between the edge servers and the cloud server. Assign the administration of wholesale and buyback schemes to the edge servers and the determination of the wholesale price to the cloud server to maximise the utilisation of computing resources through the minimised computational delay. Then, using two techniques, proposed algorithms for optimising the computer resource sharing process. They are: (i) Zero profit exchange between the cloud server and the edge server. (ii) Profits transferring between the cloud server and the edge server.

Keywords Resource sharing · Mobile edge · Cloud computing networks · Computational delay · Energy consumption · Execution cost · Network usage

1 Introduction

Within mobile edge and cloud computing networks [1], edge devices work close to the mobile devices which in turn provide almost negligible delay to process the task for mobile devices hence the computation latency decreases and the cloud is responsible for processing huge tasks simultaneously. With the increase in computation requirements for the new coming applications and Internet of things (IoT), in recent years, e.g. Autonomous driving, natural language processing, interactive games, e-Health, Augmented Reality (AR) and Virtual Reality (VR), to provide Quality of

S. Mishra · A. Gupta · K. Jairam Naik (✉)
Department of CSE, National Institute of Technology Raipur, Raipur-492010, Chhattisgarh, India
e-mail: Jnaik.cse@nitrr.ac.in

© The Author(s), under exclusive license to Springer Nature Singapore Pte Ltd. 2023
J. K. Mandal and D. De (eds.), *Frontiers of ICT in Healthcare*, Lecture Notes in Networks and Systems 519, https://doi.org/10.1007/978-981-19-5191-6_42

Experience (QoE) for the user edge devices can be used so that latency to process a task decreases and use the cloud to fulfil the system requirement which are asked by this new recent year application by sharing resources between cloud and edge devices, both can be achieved at the same time. This can even help users to run multiple programmes at the same time which ask for huge computation resources without crashing of mobile devices with negligible latency.

The mobile edge server has a large net production and functioning cost due to its extensive use capabilities. Furthermore, the mobile edge server's profitability is poor since its processing needs are often time-varying and restricted, resulting in inefficient utilisation of computational power. The cloud server has a comparably cheap common production and operation value due to its centralised creation characteristics and high scale deployment. The rapidly expanding computational needs in the cloud, on the other hand, along with bringing an issue to the Quality of Service (QoS), but also significantly raises the operating price. In this scenario, the cloud server is constantly looking for low-cost computing resources, but the mobile edge server is looking for a higher profit and may give assured duty to the varying computational activity.

The following is a summary of the full project:

- Using the wholesale and buyback strategy, present an optimised technique for efficient computational resource sharing between the edge and cloud.
- The challenge is therefore defined as a problem of profit/gain maximisation, with the wholesale and buyback technique being used to efficiently manage computational assets between the edge and the cloud server.
- Then take two ways to resolving computing resource management issues: (i) maximising of general welfare through zero profit exchange between the edge and the cloud, and (ii) maximisation of profit for the mobile edge server and the cloud server through the efficient pricing and cloud computational asset management strategy.

2 Related Work

The relevant works are organised into two categories as given below:

2.1 System/Network Design

Liu et al. [3] has given a detailed analysis of mobile edge server structures, including architectural and technical enablers. Ceselli et al. [4] presented heuristic hyperlink-route formulations for designing mobile devices' access to networks in a small amount of time, and [5] devised a mobile edge server-based object detection structure using Wi-Fi for real-time monitoring apps. Considering into account the limited power supply, You et al. [6] offered a switch-based microwave power overall utility for mobile edge server to allow computing in low-complexity passive devices. To reduce the deployment cost of data centres, Liu and Shen [7] presented a heuristic technique below usage level limitations from the perspective of development cost. Yuan et al. [8] presents a dynamic edge-cloud placement infrastructure, integrating spot instance model of pricing and Machine Learning (ML) methods.

However, few studies take into account the combination of computational assets from the mobile edge server and the cloud server, which has the potential to dramatically improve system performance.

2.2 System Optimization

Wang et al. [9] proposed combining mobile edge server and wireless power transfer to improve device computing functionality and power supply while keeping the energy restriction in mind. Reference [10] proposed an energy-saving computation offloading control technique to reduce mobile device energy usage. Deng et al. [11] suggested a task allocation strategy that balanced energy intake and transmission delay; Zhang et al. [12] presented an energy-conscious offloading technique for concurrently optimising communication and computing usable resource allocation; and under latency restrictions, Sardellitti et al. [13] presented an offloading strategy to reduce overall consumer energy consumption. Reference [14] used a univariate search technique to construct a locally most suitable algorithm that reduced power consumption and execution delay.

There are also several other approaches for cloud service allocation, load management and scheduling were considered as the base sources for the QoS-based service management. Also, delay tolerant service management IoT and Fog in collaboration with the cloud service provisioning were clearly elaborated in [16–19]. These researches really guided this work for the service consolidation and efficient allocation of secure request processing with low delay.

However, how to improve the mobile edge server's and cloud's computing resource management while also increasing the use and profitability of computing resources is still a work in progress.

3 Proposed Methodology

3.1 System Model

In the following scenario: there are N1 edge servers and N2 cloud servers in a mobile edge and cloud computational network. Cloud is often scattered throughout the sector and provide computational power to faraway users through a network, whereas mobile edge servers are typically equipped with mobile base stations and

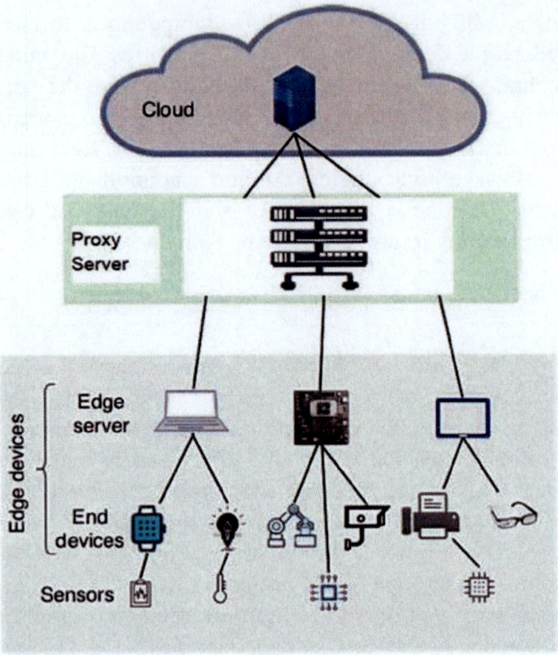

Fig. 1 The topology for edge and cloud computational networks

provide computational power to nearby mobile users. The number of computing tasks on the cloud is normally much larger than the number of computing jobs on each mobile edge servers, and their delay sensitivity is usually small. To offer Quality of Service, mobile edge servers must complete acquired computing responsibilities as quickly as possible, whereas the cloud desires to finish obtained computing duties as quickly as possible.

Figure 1 depicts the topology of edge and cloud computational networks.

3.1.1 Operation of Edge and Cloud Computational Networks

To control the computational assistance exchange procedures amongst the mobile edge servers and the cloud, an effective infrastructure is constructed for edge and cloud computational networks, as shown in Fig. 2. This machine has 2 distinct time frames: the time slot, and the time interval. A time interval can last hundreds of milliseconds, whereas a time slot might last many minutes. The mobile edge servers can sell a portion of their computational assets to the cloud server on wholesale during each time slot t. The edge servers can acquire a few computing assets lower back from the cloud at any time, as long as the cloud is pleased right now. As a result, the mobile edge servers wish to ensure the cloud's wholesaled computing assets and can change their buyback computational sources dependent on their computational needs. The cloud can use wholesaled computational assets from the edge server for

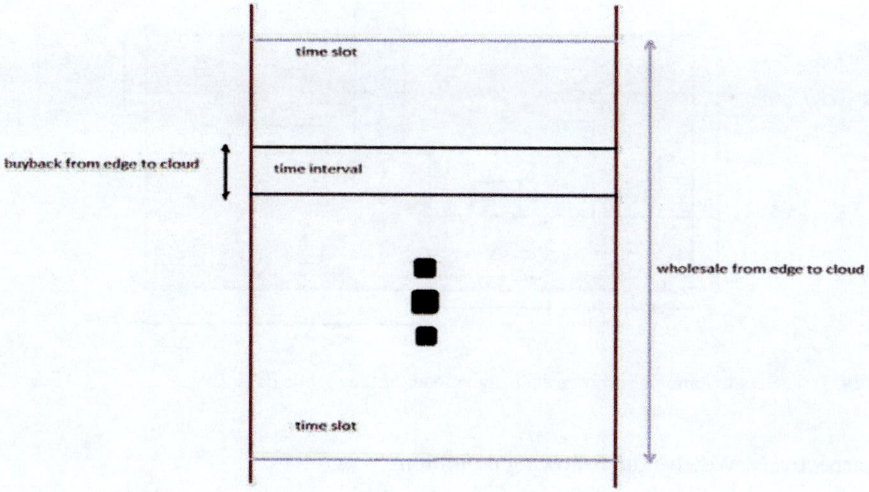

Fig. 2 The wholesale and buyback scheme of mobile edge servers

the duration of the time slot, but it must ensure repurchase computational assets for the edge servers at all times.

The letter t will be used to represent the t-th slot of time. Make 1slot of time into K time intervals, then during the duration of the slot, use k to represent the k-th interval of time slot. Due to the unique temporal differences of the wholesale and buyback schemes [2], the edge servers must recognise the wholesaled and buyback computing assets one by one. At the start of every slot of time, the cloud wishes to determine the wholesale and buyback value, as well as the cloud computing sources. For the sake of simplicity, let's suppose the repurchase price is fixed and the wholesale price is variable.

3.1.2 Model of Operation of Mobile Edge Servers

The computational assets of each mobile edge server may be classified into 2 groups. The 1st component resides with the mobile edge server and acts as a computational asset, managing the computational jobs allocated to it. The 2nd component is based on cloud and serves as a versatile computational server for cloud-based computing operations. Because computing activities are ad hoc, reserved computational assets might not be enough to execute all of them in a timely way, forcing the mobile edge server to promote some computational assets again to the cloud. As a result, the available computational assets of the mobile edge server are governed by the wholesale and buyback approach. Figure 3 depicts the computational resources available at each edge server.

At edge server e during t-th time slot, let $R_{e,t}$ signify total available computational assets, $R^{I}_{e,t}$ reserved computational assets, and $R^{C}_{e,t}$ wholesaled computational assets,

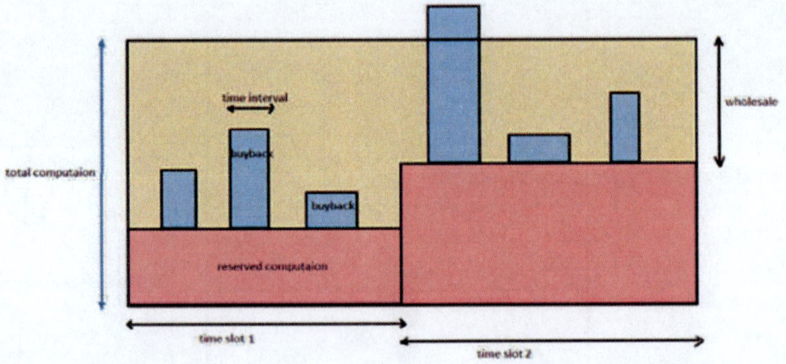

Fig. 3 The computational resource exchange model of the mobile edge server

respectively. We give the following definition:

$$R_{e,t} = R^{I}_{e,t} + R^{C}_{e,t} \tag{1}$$

Let $R_{e,k}$ and $R^{B}_{e,k}$ indicate the total available computational assets at edge server e throughout k-th time interval and the buyback computational assets at edge server e, correspondingly. As a result, we have the following:

$$R_{e,k} = R^{I}_{e,k} + R^{B}_{e,k} \tag{2}$$

Since the reserved computational assets are always accessible for the whole t-th slot of time, $R^{I}_{e,k} = R^{I}_{e,t}$.

3.2 *Algorithms Used*

3.2.1 Wholesale and Buyback Policy Without Profit Exchange

The profit transfers if all of the edge servers and the cloud belong to one organisation, e.g. $eI^{B}_{e,t} - I^{S}_{e,t}$, will not have an impact on the entity's total revenue. Consequently, the challenge of calculating useful aid manipulate can be framed in a number of ways. Integrating the wants and the restrictions in problems P_1 and P_2. It might be rephrased as

$$\boldsymbol{P1} : \min\ R^{C}_{e,t} R^{B}_{e,k} R_{c,t} t B(R_{c,t}) + I(X_{c,t}) \tag{3}$$

Task Scheduling

When the edge servers' calculation lags due to all of their computational responsibilities (including queuing delays) are within their tolerable postpone limits. Under the first-come, first-served (FCFS) coverage, all computational tasks may be completed. As a result, the common computation has been postponed for the time being, responsibilities at edge server e may be calculated using $\min\{X_{c,t}, X_{e,t}\}$. The long-term computing obligations in a non-shifting device are the same as the long-term computing responsibilities in a shifting device effective arrival charge on average $\lambda_{c,t}$ + $e\lambda_{e,t}$ increased as a result of the average time $X_{c,t}$ that a difficulty in computing consumes in the machine. Because there are no blocked jobs in the queue edge server mechanism, the general processing time $X_{c,t}$ the computational jobs that will be delivered to the cloud may be seen using.

$$X_{c,t} \approx X_{c,t}\left(\lambda_{c,t} + e\lambda_{e,t}\right) - e\lambda_{e,t} \min\left\{X_{c,t}, X_{e,t}\right\}\lambda_{c,t} \tag{4}$$

$X_{c,t}$ is a linear property of the common computation latency that may be dealt $X_{c,t}$.

$$\text{Let } O_k(k-1)\left(R_{c,t} + eR_{e,t}\right) \leq O_k \leq k\left(R_{c,t} + eR_{e,t}\right) \tag{5}$$

Computing resources are being repurchased $R^B_{e,k}$ may be set up to make sure that all computational jobs at the edge servers are finished ahead of schedule.

$$\begin{aligned} R^B_{e,k+De,t} &= L_{e,k}, \text{ if } k \geq X_{e,t}; \\ R^B_{e,k} &= L_{e,k}, \text{ otherwise.} \end{aligned} \tag{6}$$

when $L_{e,k} \leq R^C_{e,k}$.

We can rewrite the problem $P1$ by obtained $R^C_{e,t}$ and $R^B_{e,k}$.

$$P1' : \min R_{c,t}\, tB\left(R_{c,t}\right) + I\left(X_{c,t}\right) \tag{7}$$

$$\text{s.t.}0\ R_{c,t} R_{c,t}, \forall t, \tag{8}$$

$$X_{c,t} X_{c,t}, \forall t, \tag{9}$$

Algorithm 1: Task Scheduling

1. *Input provided:* ($\lambda_{e,t}$, Z_t, $X_{e,t}$) *for computing jobs,* ($R_{e,t}$, *T, K*) *for each mobile edge server, and* ($R_{c,t}$, $X_{c,t}$) *for the cloud server;*
2. *Output:* {$R_{c,t}$, $R^C_{e,t}\forall t$} *and* {$R_{B\,e}$,$k\forall k$};
3. *For every t-th time slot repeat the following:*
4. (a)$R^C_{e,t} = R_{e,t}$;

5. (b)*Find optimal* $R_{c,t}$ *by calculating P1′;*
6. (c)*For each k-th time interval repeat the following:*
7. (i) *Calculate* $R^{B}{}_{e,k}$ *by solving (Eq. 6);*
8. *end*
9. *End*

3.2.2 Wholesale and Buyback Policy with Profit Exchange

Figure 2 depicts the operating method for cell part-cloud computing networks. The cloud intends to charge the edge servers a wholesale price, the edge servers then decide on their wholesaled compute sources. To get to the bottom of these difficulties, we'll look at the relationship between the wholesaled computational assets from edge servers and the wholesale fee. Then, for the gold standard to be available computer sources, we create a critical scenario. Finally, we propose a top-rated pricing strategy and cloud computational asset management to maximise edge servers and cloud profitability simultaneously.

Optimal Pricing and Cloud Computational Asset Management

Because of the wholesale fee $f_{2,t}$, the cost of $_{e}(R^{C}_{e,t} - R^{B}_{e,t})$ is set in stone As a result, at any wholesale rate $f_{2,t}$,We can figure out which cloud computing suppliers are the most dependable. $R_{c,t}$ by resolving the ensuing snag:

$$\begin{aligned} &\boldsymbol{P2\_}1 : \min_{Rc,t} B\left(R_{c,t}\right) + I\left(X_{c,t}\right) \\ &\text{s.t. } 0 \le R_{c,t} \le R_{c,t}, \forall t, \\ &X_{c,t} \le X_{c,t}, \forall t. \end{aligned}$$

The goal is to keep the overall cost of local operations as low as possible as well as the cloud's Quality of Service (QoS) penalty, as well as the thresholds set for cloud computing sources $R_{c,t}$ and the lag in calculation $X_{c,t}$.

Algorithm 2: Optimal Pricing and Cloud Computational Asset Management.

1. *Input provided:* $(\lambda_{e,t}, Z_t, X_{e,t})$ *for computing jobs,* $(R_{e,t}, T, K)$ *for each mobile edge server, and* $(R_{c,t}, X_{c,t})$ *for the cloud server;*
2. *Output calculated:* $\{f^{*}{}_{2,t}, R^{*}_{c,t}, \forall t\}$;
3. *For each t-th time slot repeat the following:*
4. *(a). Put* $f_{2,t} = p_{c,t}(R_{c,t})$;
5. *(b). Find required* $R^{*}_{c,t}$ *by calculating P2_1;*
6. *(c). If* $R^{*}_{c,t} < R_{c,t}$*, Set* $f_{2,t} = 0$ *and* $f_{2,t} = f_{2,t}$*, then*
7. *(i). Set* $f_{2,t} = f_{2,t} + f_{2,t}{}^{2}$;
8. *(ii). Find optimal* $R^{*}_{c,t}$ *by calculating P2_1;*
9. *(iii). If* $p_{e,t}(f_{2,t}) < p_{c,t}(R^{*}_{c,t})$ *then*
10. *Put* $f_{2,t} = f_{2,t}$ *and go step 7;*

11. *end*
12. *if* $p_{e,t}(f_{2,t}) > p_{c,t}(R^*_{c,t})$ *then*
13. *Set* $f_{2,t} = f_{2,t}$ *and go step 7;*
14. *end*
15. *if* $p_{e,t}(f_{2,t}) = p_{c,t}(R^*_{c,t})$ *then*
16. $f^*_{2,t} = f_{2,t}$,
17. *Break;*
18. *end*
19. *End*
20. *If* $R^*_{c,t} = R_{c,t}$, *Set* $f_{2,t} = f_{2,t}$, *then*
21. *1) Put* $f_{2,t} = (1 +)a_{2,t}$ *and again set the* $I_{c,t}$*;*
22. *while* $I_{c,t}|f_{2,t} < I_{c,t}|f_{2,t}$ *repeat:*
23. *Put* $f_{2,t} = f_{2,t}$ *and again set* $I_{c,t}|f_{2,t}$ *by step 21;*
24. *end*
25. *2) Put* $f_{2,t} = f_{2,t}$ *when* $I_{c,t}|f_{2,t} \geq I_{c,t}|f_{2,t}$*;*
26. *3) Set* $f_{2,t} = (f_{2,t} + f_{2,t})/2$ *and again set the cost* $I_{c,t}$*;*
27. *if* $I_{c,t}|f_{2,t} > I_{c,t}|f_{2,t}$ *then*
28. *Set* $f_{2,t} = f_{2,t}$ *and go step 28;*
29. *end*
30. *if* $I_{c,t}|f_{2,t} < I_{c,t}|f_{2,t}$ *then*
31. *Set* $f_{2,t} = f_{2,t}$ *and go step 28;*
32. *end*
33. *if* $I_{c,t}|f_{2,t} = I_{c,t}|f_{2,t}$ *then*
34. $f^*_{2,t} = f_{2,t}$,
35. *Break;*
36. *end*
37. *end*
38. *Find the optimal* $R^{C*}_{e,t}$ *and* $R^{B*}_{e,k}$ *by EWBS given in* [2].
39. *End*
40. *Where* ε *is a negligible step*

4 Simulation and Performance Evaluation

4.1 Experimental Setup

We study the planned infrastructure in this part and give numerical results and analysis. For simulation of an edge-cloud computing network, we used a fog simulator named iFogSim 2.0. We first designed an edge-cloud infrastructure in a tree-like hierarchical structure. At the top level is the cloud server, one level below is the proxy server. Below the proxy server, multiple edge servers are attached. Each edge

Table 1 Parameters of edge-cloud framework

	Mips	RAM	upBw	downBw	ratePerMips	Busy power	Idle power
Cloud server	600,000	440,000	100	10,000	0.01	16*103	16*83.25
Proxy server	400,000	12,000	10,000	10,000	0.01	16	8
Edge server	35,000	1200	10,000	10,000	0.01	16	8
Devices	200	100	10,000	10,000	0	2	1

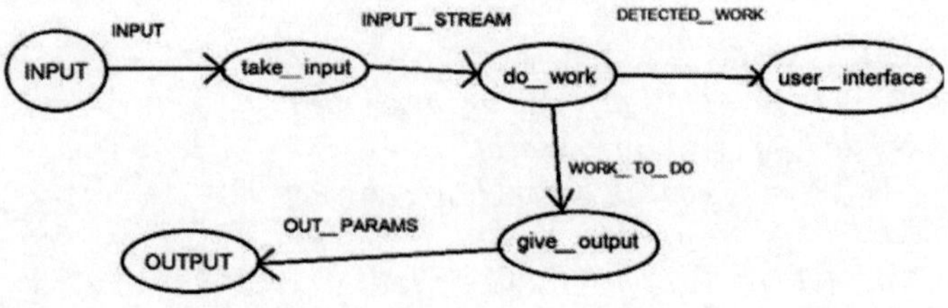

Fig. 4 Application model of the edge-cloud framework

server has multiple end devices (sensors) attached to it. The following is the evaluation setting: There are 40 edge Servers, each with 35,000 Million Instructions per Second (MIPS) of computing power, and each edge includes 20 end devices with 200 MIPS of processing power. The cloud server has 600,000 MIPS of processing power, whereas the proxy server has 400,000 Million Instructions per Second (MIPS) of processing power. Cloud computing resources are charged at a rate of 0.01 per MIPS. We assume that computational workloads arrive at edge servers at a rate of [5, 10] per second. Edge servers and cloud service pricing are considered to be the same. Table 1 lists out the various parameters of the framework.

We designed a model for the processing of various computational tasks in the network. The model consists of sensors named INPUT and actuators named OUTPUT along with four different App Modules namely, take_input, do_work, user_interface and give_output. All these modules are connected to each other through App Edges namely, INPUT, INPUT_STREAM, DETECTED_WORK, WORK_TO_DO and OUT_PARAMS. Figure 4 showing the above-mentioned model is given below.

4.2 *Performance Evaluation*

(A) *Simulation Results and Performance Analysis*

We altered the task arrival rates $\lambda_{e,t}$ at mobile edge servers and observed the values of parameters like Execution time, Energy consumed at cloud server, Execution cost at cloud server, Energy consumed at each edge server, Energy consumed at each end device and Network usage. The table of our measurements is given in Table 2.

Table 2 Measurement table

Task arrival rates $\lambda_{e,t}$	Execution time (in milliseconds)	Energy consumed at cloud (in watts)	Execution cost at cloud (in $)	Energy consumed at each edge (in watts)	Energy consumed at each end device (in watts)	Network Usage (in Mbps)
5	372	2,666,740	52,015	17,210	4000	11,782
6	362	2,666,419	45,928	17,019	3713	9936
7	340	2,666,195	41,668	16,883	3480	8854
8	310	2,665,783	33,850	16,780	3305	7146
9	284	2,665,224	23,238	16,700	3189	5196
10	268	2,665,364	23,993	16,639	3070	5232

With increase in task arrival rate at the edge node, edge node requires more computation resource hence it will reduce its buyback cost and wholesale resources to the cloud reduces. Hence the wholesale resources from edge server decrease cloud have to increase its wholesale cost. Hence less execution occurs at cloud/energy consume will be less/servers have to decrease its execution time to provide better Quality of Service (QoS) hence network uses also decreases.

We compare the proposed method with the 2 other algorithms as described below:

1. Resource Allocation Algorithm [15]:-In this algorithm minimum resources are allocated initially by keeping in account of users uses history that's why when there is a more requirement in between this method don't give us a better result.
2. Resource Management Algorithm [2]:-In this algorithm minimum resources is allocated to an edge server similar of algorithm 1 in addition to that Buyback and wholesale of resources occur to maximise profit at only edge server, because it is not considering the profit maximisation of cloud this is not as efficient as algorithm 3.
3. Proposed Algorithm:-In this algorithm both Algorithm 1 and Algorithm 2 have used in addition to the profit maximisation at the cloud server due to which it gives the most efficient result as compared to the previous two algorithms.

Table 3 for the measurements of the 3 algorithms is given below.

The performance comparisons for above measurement data are given below. Figure 5 shows execution time of the three algorithms. Figure 6 shows the energy consumed at cloud server, Fig. 7 displays the trends of execution cost at cloud server for the 3 algorithms. Figure 8 displays energy consumed at each edge server and Fig. 9 shows network usage for the 3 algorithms. Figure 10 shows the trend of energy consumed at each end device.

Table 3 Comparison of algorithms

Algorithms	Execution time (ms)	Energy consumed at cloud (watts)	Execution cost at cloud (in $)	Energy consumed at each edge (watts)	Energy consumed at each end device (in watts)	Network usage (Mbps)
Resource Alloc. Algo [15]	75,013	2,956,203.402	5,548,165.857	21,997.30286	4000	1,619,504
Resource Mngmt. Algo [2]	58,514	2,956,031.438	5,544,900.714	21,005.39429	3712.9	1,510,740
Proposed Algo	49,264	2,955,631.81	5,537,312.857	20,301.85143	3479.5	1,431,668

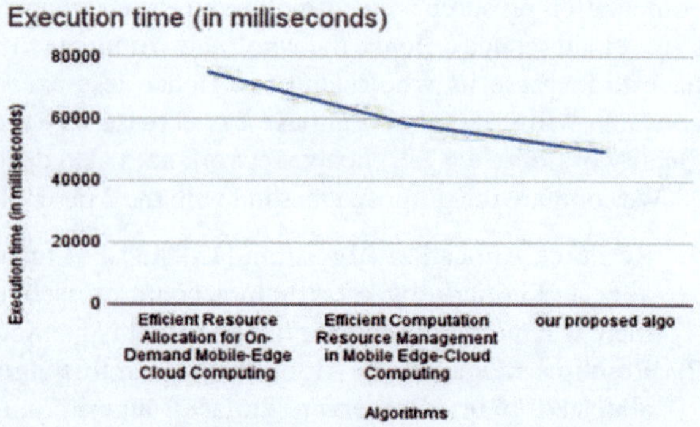

Fig. 5 Execution time in (milliseconds) for three algorithms

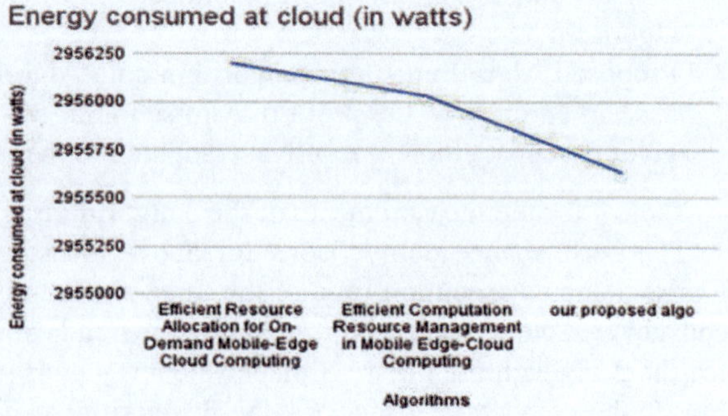

Fig. 6 Energy consumed at cloud server in (watts) for three algorithms

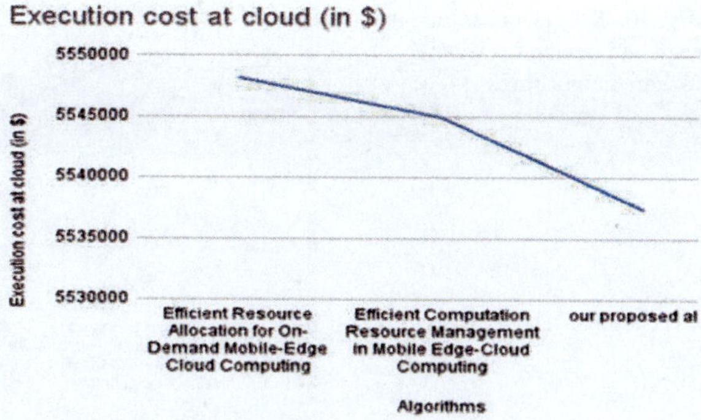

Fig. 7 Execution cost at cloud server in ($) for three algorithms

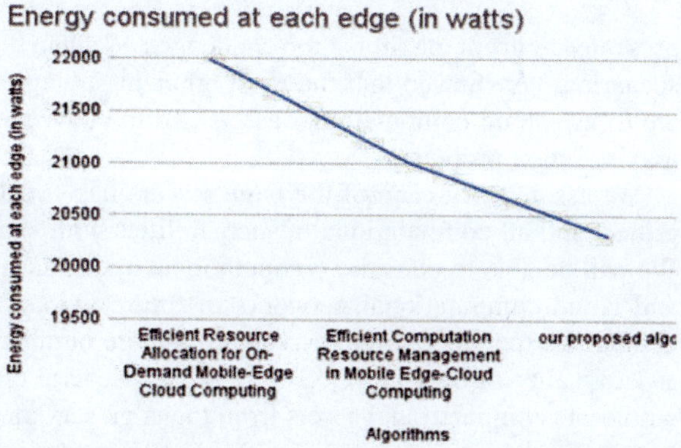

Fig. 8 Energy consumed at each edge server in (watts) for three algorithms

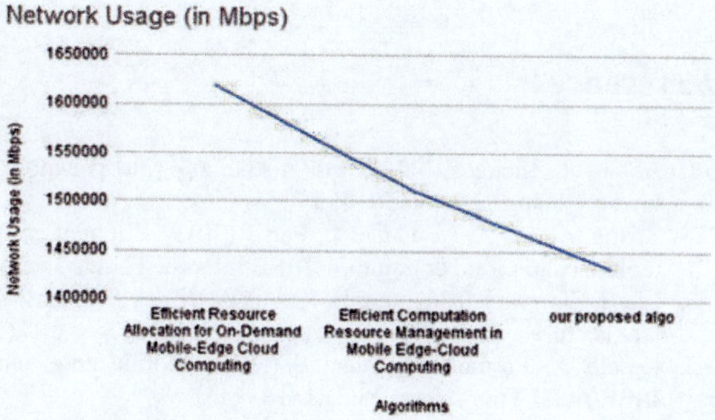

Fig. 9 Network usage in (Mbps) for three algorithms

5 Conclusion and Future Scope

For the edge server, we provided an effective architecture and in order to enhance income in this project, the cloud was used to distribute and share computer resources. The edge server's and cloud's computing resource management concerns were

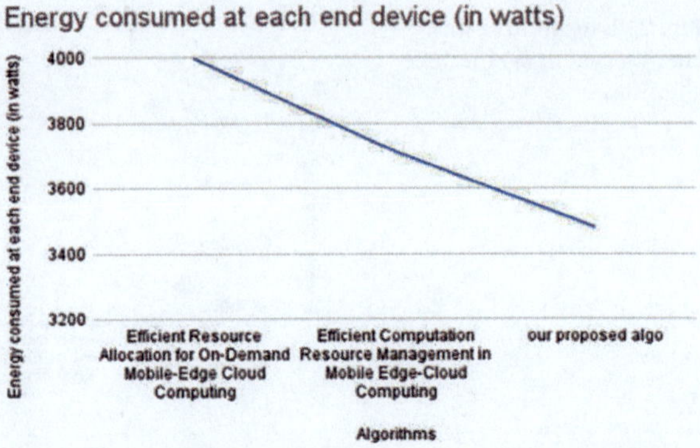

Fig. 10 Energy consumed at each end device in (watts) for three algorithms

presented as profit maximisation challenges. We then fix those concerns based on two scenarios. We showed that the most efficient strategies to maximise social welfare are to use cloud computational assets and the concave nature of the social welfare maximisation problem.

We assume that each of the edge servers has equal computational assets in this project and all computational responsibilities with similar Quality of Service need. We will be able to consider computational asset sharing in large-scale mobile edge and cloud computational networks in future works, if a number of edge servers belong to exceptional enterprises with a large number of computational assets and strict Quality of Service (QoS) criteria and several cloud servers will compete for wholesale computational assets from the edge servers at the same time. To increase revenues, the cloud server might impose various fees on different organisations.

References

1. Abbas N, Zhang Y, Taherkordi A, Skeie T (2018) Mobile edge computing: a survey. IEEE Internet Things J 5(1):450–465
2. Zhang Y, Lan X, Li Y, Cai L, Pan J (2019) Efficient computation resource management in mobile edge-cloud computing. IEEE Internet Things J 6(2):3455–3466
3. Liu H, Eldarrat F, Alqahtani H, Reznik A, de Foy X, Zhang Y (2018) Mobile edge cloud system: architectures, challenges, and approaches. IEEE Syst J 12(3):2495–2508
4. Ceselli A, Premoli M, Secci S (2017) Mobile edge cloud network design optimization. IEEE/ACM Trans Netw 25(3):1818–1831
5. Ren J, Guo Y, Zhang D, Liu Q, Zhang Y (2018) Distributed and efficient object detection in edge computing: challenges and solutions. IEEE Netw 32(6):137–143
6. You C, Huang K, Chae H (2016) Energy efficient mobile cloud computing powered by wireless energy transfer. IEEE J Sel Areas Commun 34(5):1757–1771
7. Liu G, Shen H (2017) Minimum-cost cloud storage service across multiple cloud providers. IEEE/ACM Trans Netw 25(4):2498–2513
8. Yuan X, Sun M, Fang Q, Du C (2019) DLECP: a dynamic learning-based edge cloud placement framework for mobile cloud computing. In: IEEE conference on computer communications workshops (INFOCOM WKSHPS), pp 1035–1036

9. Wang F, Xu J, Wang X, Cui S (2018) Joint offloading and computing optimization in wireless powered mobile-edge computing systems. IEEE Trans Wireless Commun 17(3):1784–1797
10. Guo F, Zhang H, Ji H, Li X, Leung VCM (2018) An efficient computation offloading management scheme in the densely deployed small cell networks with mobile edge computing. IEEE/ACM Trans Netw 26(6):2651–2664
11. Deng R, Lu R, Lai C, Luan TH, Liang H (2016) Optimal workload allocation in fog-cloud computing toward balanced delay and power consumption. IEEE Internet Things J 3(6):1171–1181
12. Zhang J et al (2018) Energy-latency tradeoff for energy-aware offloading in mobile edge computing networks. IEEE Internet Things J 5(4):2633–2645
13. Sardellitti S, Scutari G, Barbarossa S (2015) Joint optimization of radio and computational resources for multi cell mobile-edge computing. IEEE Trans Sign Inf Process Netw 1(2):89–103
14. Wang Y, Sheng M, Wang X, Wang L, Li J (2016) Mobile-edge computing: partial computation offloading using dynamic voltage scaling. IEEE Trans Commun 64(10):4268–4282
15. Chen X, Li W, Lu S, Zhou Z, Fu X (2018) Efficient resource allocation for on-demand mobile-edge cloud computing. IEEE Trans Veh Technol 67(9):8769–8780
16. Naik KJ, Naik DH (2020) Minimizing deadline misses and total run-time with load balancing for a connected car systems in fog computing. Scalable Comput: Pract Experience 21(1):73–84
17. Naik KJ, Vidya BV (2018) A group tasks scheduling algorithm for cloud computing network based on QoS. Int J Eng Technol 7(4):6
18. Naik KJ (2020) A co-scheduling system for fog-node recommendation and load management in cloud-fog environment (CoS_FRLM). In: 2020 International conference on data analytics for business and industry, 26–27 Oct 2020, University of Bahrain
19. Naik KJ (2020) A dynamic ACO-based elastic load balancer for cloud computing (D-ACOELB). In: Data engineering and communication technology. Advances in Intelligent Systems and Computing, vol 1079. Springer

Intuitionistic Fuzzy Stream Cipher for Privacy Preservation of Biometric Data in IoMT

Arun Sarkar, Rajdeep Chakraborty, and Malabika Das

Abstract The biometric data is inevitably used in Medical Things (IoMT) like fingerprints, retina scans, X-ray images, MRIs, and many more. In the medical system, it is generally collected by IoT devices like a scanner or by special machines like MRI scanners which are then transferred to a medical database using the Internet or local networking. Thus, security is must during the transmission of this data. An intuitionistic fuzzy system or set is defined with an unspecific boundary, it may have a random output for a specific input or it can be defined by the probability rather than yes/one or no/zero. Intuitionistic fuzzy system is a set theory in which the assessment of the member elements with two functions: for calculating the membership and also for calculating non-membership. In this paper, we proposed an intuitionistic fuzzy-based stream cipher for Privacy Preservation of Biometric Data in IoMT. Here, the linearity of LFSR is made nonlinear by the use of intuitionistic fuzzy system. We use two 64-bit LFSRs, which are initialized first by 128-bit session key / secret key, now, in each clock cycle, both produce 1-bit output, which is fed to the IF system, and finally, we apply the membership or non-membership function to get 1-bit output which is xored with 1-bit plaintext to produce 1-bit ciphertext. We also established that the stream of bits generated, say, 128-bit, is pseudorandom.

Keywords Intuitionistic fuzzy logic · Intuitionistic fuzzy set · Fuzzy stream cipher · Privacy preserving · Biometric data · IoMT

1 Introduction

There is a rapid development is on artificial intelligence, big data, mobile communication, and other technologies. Unfortunately, because of changing nature and

---

A. Sarkar · M. Das
Department of Mathematics, Heramba Chandra College, Kolkata 700029, India

R. Chakraborty (✉)
Department of CSE, Chandigarh University, Chandigarh, India
e-mail: rajdeep_chak@yahoo.co.in

© The Author(s), under exclusive license to Springer Nature Singapore Pte Ltd. 2023

J. K. Mandal and D. De (eds.), *Frontiers of ICT in Healthcare*, Lecture Notes in Networks and Systems 519, https://doi.org/10.1007/978-981-19-5191-6_43

nonability to make full use of correct information of any controlled object, conventional backstepping control will not be the better control performance than other control methods. A fuzzy system approximates a function through the covering of its all graphs with fuzzy that patches and averaging these patches that must overlap. The fuzzy system is basically a set of if–then–else rules that maps input to output. So, each of the fuzzy rules defines a fuzzy patch from these input–output state spaces of this function. So, the fuzzy set-based mathematical calculation is being used widely in many scientific fields and scopes such as physics, planning of transportation [1], optimization [2], business, finance, management [3], current flow, and control theory [4]. It is seen that more parameters or variables are real numbers found in understudy models.

Therefore, these parameters or variables usually take some uncertain values in practice. One of the approaches is to quantify with cope and the uncertainty there is using fuzzy numbers without and instead of real numbers. This paper discusses the fuzzy stream cipher design [10] and applications [12] on the Internet of Medical of Things (IoMT) and the extended fuzzy sets and logic, known as intuitionistic fuzzy set (IFS) and logics (IFLs) [5].

Figure 1 depicts an intuitionistic fuzzy system [4] as a whole here, and the input is classical bits say set of. The fuzzification is the process to convert the classical bits to an intuitionistic fuzzy system [6] and this system takes the classical bit input and the intuitionistic fuzzy rules, here described in detail in Sect. 2.1, and gives the combination to the inference engine. The inference engine is the one which converts the classical bits to the intuitionistic fuzzy values based on the inference rules. Now, the real world must need the classical bits as an output, so it is carried out by the defuzzification system and based on the inference rules.

Figure 2 depicts the basic diagram which is a stream cipher that encrypts bit by bit or byte by byte. The main component is the keystream generator which gives pseudorandom bits, and if it is so, it is called a one-time pad [13].

The main advantages of stream ciphers are as follows:

- It takes low computing power.
- It takes low memory.

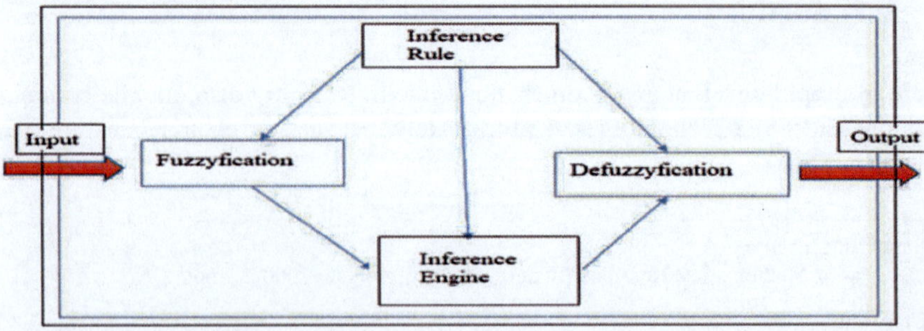

Fig. 1 The intuitionistic fuzzy system

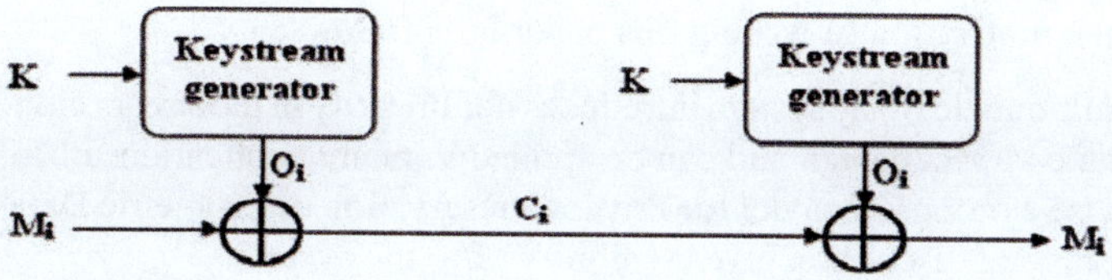

Fig. 2 The stream cipher

- Stream ciphers work well for large or small chunks of data.
- Stream cipher is equally secure than block cipher [11], and if it turns out to be a one-time pad, then it is most secured.

Section 2 gives a short literature review and motivation for writing this paper. Section 3 discusses the intuitionistic fuzzy system, Sect. 4 discusses the LFSR we have taken, Sect. 5 discusses the proposed intuitionistic fuzzy cipher, and Sect. 6 gives the result and discussion. Finally, Sect. 7 draws the conclusion, and the references are added at last.

2 The Literature Review and Motivation

The literature review is mainly based on the objectives of fuzzy systems, and the construction of stream cipher and fuzzy stream cipher. So, this section gives these three reviews in the subsequent three paragraphs.

Shounak Roychoudhury and Sujeet Shenoi [7] describe the fuzzy rule-based encoding techniques where a Knowledge Discovery (KDD) is designed where databases are enhanced by introducing common fuzzy rules. These fuzzy rules drive the database inference engine and bring with latest knowledge that are facts and with rules. This paper gives three techniques for generating rule-based KDD by combining other precise/fuzzy rules. Author also proposes database security through inference analysis and control.

In the second paper, Anikin and Alnajjar [8] describe a fuzzy stream cipher system, which is our main motivation for this paper. In this paper, the authors use NFSR (Non-Linear Feedback Shift Register) and fuzzy system to generate keystream. But the author claimed that the system is deterministic in nature and that it is used as same parameters as the fuzzy-based pseudorandom generator that gives the same random bits sequence.

The third paper, Sweedle Machado et al. gives an application of fuzzy stream cipher in their paper titled [9], and this paper secured ATM pins and also passwords that use fingerprint fuzzy-based secure vault system. The author(s) gave specific applications of biometric authentication systems using fuzzy-based encoding.

In the fourth paper, Sweedle Machado et al. describes one of the important application of fuzzy-based cryptography. Authors proposed the model of securing ATM pins and password through fuzzy-based vault system.

Thus, the motivation of writing this paper is as follows: -

- The intuitionistic fuzzy system introduces nonlinearity in the stream cipher design.
- This is a compact design and can be applied in many applications of IoMT.
- We devise a proposed model for Privacy Preservation of Biometric Data in IoMT.
- The result and discussion give credibility of/to the system.
- We also tested for randomness, and it is coming to be a pseudorandom design.
- We also calculated the memory requirements and minimum processing power.

3 Intuitionistic Fuzzy Set (IFS)

Atanassov [5] developed the notion of IFS for better capturing uncertainty by combining the concepts of non-membership and membership degrees [2].

Definition 1 Atanassov [5] Let X be fixed. An IFS $\mathcal{I}$ on X can be described by

$$\mathcal{I} = \{(x, \mu_{\mathcal{I}}(x), \nu_{\mathcal{I}}(x)) | x \in X\} \tag{1}$$

where the functions $\mu_{\mathcal{I}}$ and $\nu_{\mathcal{I}}$ are the membership degrees and non-membership degrees, respectively, of each $x \in X$ in $\mathcal{I}$ satisfying the condition that

$$0 \leq \mu_{\mathcal{I}}(x) \leq 1, \ 0 \leq \nu_{\mathcal{I}}(x) \leq 1 \ \ 0 \leq \mu_{\mathcal{I}}(x) + \nu_{\mathcal{I}}(x) \leq 1. \tag{2}$$

For convenience, Xu and Yager [6] called $\mathcal{I} = (\mu_{\mathcal{I}}(x), \nu_{\mathcal{I}}(x))$ as an intuitionistic fuzzy number (IFN); in short, an IFN may also be represented by $\mathcal{I} = (\mu_{\mathcal{I}}, \nu_{\mathcal{I}})$. For any IFN $\mathcal{I} = (\mu_{\mathcal{I}}, \nu_{\mathcal{I}})$, the score function $S(\mathcal{I})$ of $\mathcal{I}$ and accuracy function $A(\mathcal{I})$ of $\mathcal{I}$ are presented [6] as

$$S(\mathcal{I}) = \mu_{\mathcal{I}} - \nu_{\mathcal{I}}, \text{ where } S(\mathcal{I}) \in [-1, 1], \tag{3}$$

and $A(\mathcal{I}) = \mu_{\mathcal{I}} + \nu_{\mathcal{I}}$.

The space of considerations showing the membership space and non-membership space of an IFS is presented in Fig. 3.

In our intuitionistic fuzzy system, we used three variables as low, average, and high, and their interaction, inference rule, is shown in Fig. 4 to give the values 0 and 1 for the variables set $\{a, b, c, d, e, f, h\}$.

First, we obtain the result for g_0 and then calculate $|g_1 - g_2|$ and the membership value and non-membership value are calculated based on Golomb's conditions based on the membership function and non-membership functions. Then, the intuitionistic fuzzy inference engine based on this Fuzzy inference rule stated above must decide which LFSR's bit must be selected as the output bit of this fuzzy system. Figure 4 illustrates the membership function and non-membership functions of intuitionistic fuzzy variables g_0, $|g_1 - g_2|$.

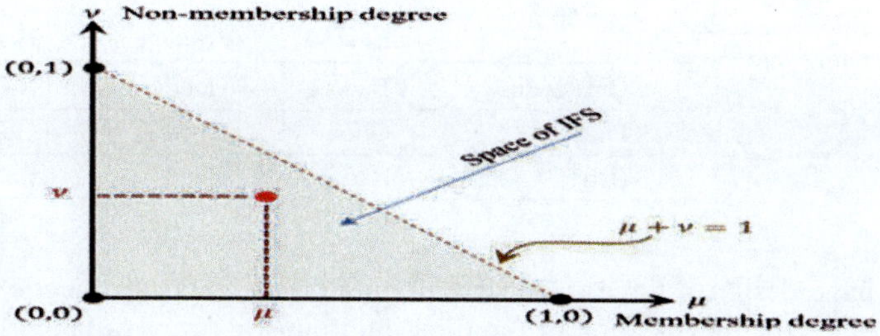

Fig. 3 Space of considerations of membership and non-membership of IFS

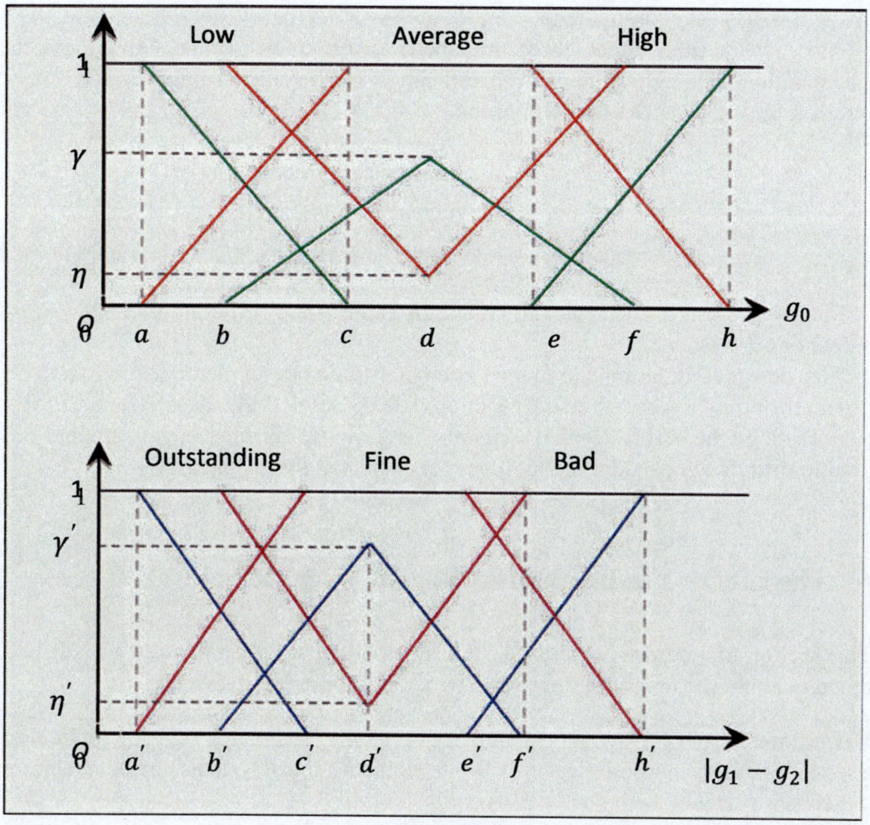

Fig. 4 Intuitionistic fuzzy variables with membership and non-membership functions

Table 1 Intuitionistic fuzzy states of the output variable

	Low	Average	High
Outstanding	Bad	Good	Bad
Fine	Good	Good	Good
Bad	Bad	Good	Bad

So we have designed three membership and non-membership functions (Low, Average, High) for fuzzification of the First intuitionistic fuzzy variable, g_0 (that is, the number of ones that exist in the buffer of size 8-bits) [3]:

(i) $g\_0 \in \{0,1,2\}$ is assigned to {Low}; (ii) $g\_0 \in \{3,4\}$ is assigned to {Average}; (iii) $g\_0 \in \{6,7,8\}$ is assigned to {High}.

Also, we design other three membership and non-membership functions (Outstanding, Fine, Bad) here the fuzzification of the second intuitionistic fuzzy variable, |g_1-g_2| as the following sets:

$$|g\_1 - g\_2| \in \{0\} \text{ is considered as } \{\text{Outstanding}\};$$
$$|g\_1 - g\_2| \in \{1, 2\} \text{ is considered as } \{\text{Fine}\};$$
$$|g\_1 - g\_2| \in \{3\} \text{ is considered as } \{\text{Bad}\}.$$

Finally, we use if–then rules as shown in Table 1 to get the intuitionistic fuzzy output of our system.

This designed intuitionistic fuzzy system has three output membership functions and three output non-membership functions (Best, Good, Bad). Thus, which LFSR's output will be the best is decided by using this. It is also selected as the output of the intuitionistic fuzzy pseudorandom binary sequence at the moment.

4 The Linear Feedback Shift Register (LFSR)

This section first defines what is LFSR mathematical and then the well-established theorem about the length of the stream generated for its tap selection.

Definitions 2 An LFSR with the length L over a finite automaton state Fq, producing a sequence of semi-infinite $Fq, s = (s_t)t \geq 0$, elements, that is to satisfy a linear relation which is recurrence with degree L over Fq

$$s_{t+L} = \sum_{i=1}^{L} c_i s_{t+L-i}, \quad \forall t \geq 0. \tag{4}$$

The L coefficients with c_1, c_2, to c_L are considered elements of Fq. They are also known as feedback coefficients of that LFSR.

Theorem 1 *Sequence that is generated as* $(s_t)t \geq 0$, *having an LFSR length and polynomial as L and P, respectively, iff,* $\exists$ *polynomial* $Q \in Fq[X]$ *and* $deg(Q) < L$, *is another polynomial,* $(s_t)t \geq 0$ *satisfies, and* $(s_t)t$ *is the generating function.*

$$\sum_{t \geq 0} s_t X^t = \frac{Q(X)}{P(X)}. \tag{5}$$

So, the polynomial Q must be determined by coefficients of all P and that initial state of this LFSR:

$$Q(X) = -\sum_{j=0}^{L-1} X^j \left(\sum_{k=0}^{k} s_k c_{j-k} \right) \quad \text{where } P(X) = -\sum_{i=0}^{L} c_i X^i.$$

So, it is a polynomial of degree < L iff. The second right-hand term becomes zero or vanishes.

$$\sum_{k=j-L}^{j} s_k c_{j-k} = 0 \tag{6}$$

So we can infer that coefficients in this polynomial should be 1's or 0's and also known as feedback polynomial.

Here, we use the LFSR of Eqs. (7) and (8)

$$X^{61} + X^{31} + X^{11} + X^7 + 1 \tag{7}$$

$$X^{53} + X^{23} + X^{17} + X^5 + 1 \tag{8}$$

This particular equation is chosen for the following reasons.

- It is already established that LFSR will give maximum-length output if the selected tap's number is even, so only 2 or 4 taps will be sufficient for extremely large sequences. Here, we use four taps.
- The selected set of taps should be relatively prime, and there will be no common divisor.
- So, it is one length more than maximum tap of sequences for a given LFSR length.
- Therefore, if one maximum-length tap sequence is found, then the other automatically follows.

Figure 5 depicts the generic LFSR where the function is defined by Eqs. (7) and (8), 0 <= n <= 63, Sn = {0,1}64 and Cn = {0,1}64 is the value after one rotation of S n.

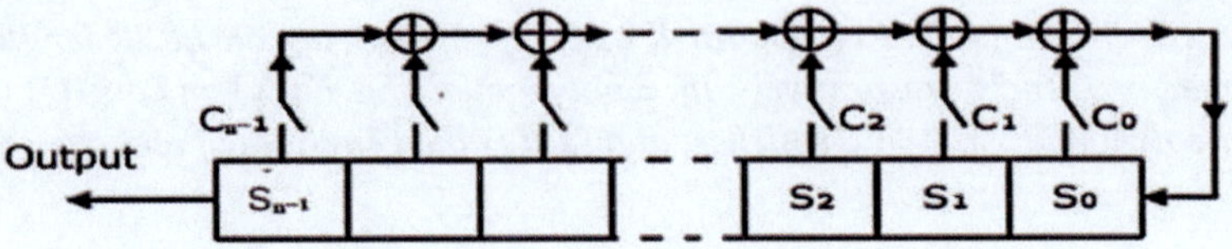

Fig. 5 The generic LFSR

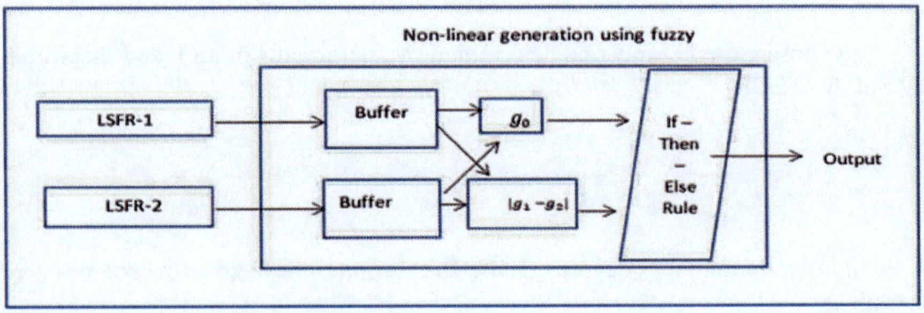

Fig. 6 The proposed stream cipher model

5 Proposed Intuitionistic Fuzzy Stream Cipher and IoMT Secure Model

The proposed system is basically a stream cipher that adds nonlinearity by intuitionistic fuzzy system. The proposed model is depicted below in Fig. 6.

The proposed stream cipher depicted the use of two LFSR as defined by Eqs. 7 and 8 and explained in Sect. 4 with Eqs. 4, 5, and 6. The intuitionistic fuzzy system is defined by the rules and descriptions given in Sect. 3 and Eqs. 1, 2, and 3. Therefore, the output is the pseudorandom bits generated in each clock cycle.

Figure 7 depicts the IoMT security modeling for privacy preserving. The biometric data is generated through the medical equipment or collector such as a thumbprint, then the data is encrypted with the proposed stream cipher and fed to the available network of the medical unit, and this data is decrypted in the receiver end. The receiver end may be a data repository like a database, or this data can be used in IoMT edge computing to infer some knowledge like cancer detection.

6 Result and Discussion

We performed the frequency mono-bit test, which is the most basic method of testing randomness. This test checks whether the pseudorandom number generator values are uniformly distributed or not. This test focuses on the ratio of zeros and ones present in the entire sequence S against the expectation that the sequences were truly

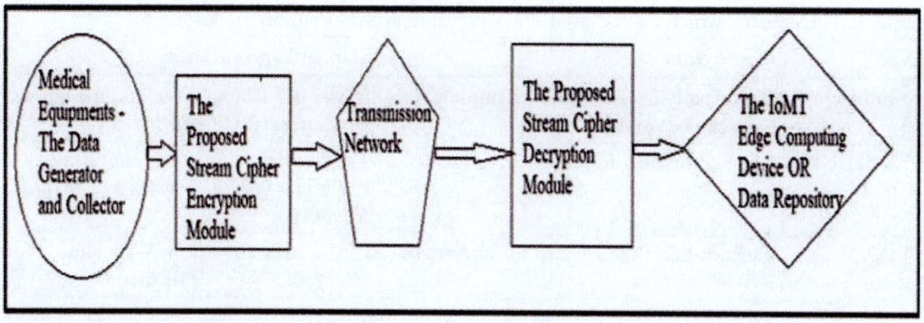

Fig. 7 Privacy preservation of biometric data in IoMT

random. It is expected that numbers of zeros and ones to be virtually the same. Let n_0 and n_1 be the number of zeros or ones in S. The test statistics can be defined as follows:

$$X_1 = \frac{(n_0 - n_1)^2}{2} \tag{9}$$

here X_1 represents a Chi-square test with one degree of freedom. Equation (9) shows that the higher value of X_1 generates a higher discrepancy between the observed and expected frequencies of zeros and ones. Table 2 depicts the frequency test results of ten samples. These ten samples are the bit sequence generated in each interval of 128-bits with a clock cycle of $128 \times 10 = 1280$ total clock cycles [1]. The result shows that the maximum sample passes this test.

Table 3 gives the most popular IoT devices which can be used for this proposed cipher implantation and Privacy Preservation of Biometric Data modeling in IoMT. So, it can be easily seen that the memory requirement and power consumption are quite low as compared to the conventional non-IoT system.

The poker test is another statistical randomness test. This test is mainly based on the frequency of certain digits that are repeated in a series of numbers. Table 4 gives the poker test and the passing and failed samples. Here, we got the more passing samples than failed samples.

Table 2 Monobit frequency test of output of the proposed cipher

Frequency test (with significance level alpha value = 0.05), Max. allowable value 3.84, F = failed (>3.84), P = passed (< = 3.84)

Sample no	1	2	3	4	5	6	7	8	9	10
Pass (P) or Fail (F)	P	F	P	F	P	P	P	F	P	P

Table 3 The devices which can be used for encryption and decryption module

Type	Description	Standard specification
Antminer	It is usually used for bitcoin mining and here can be used for cipher	It uses 1.5 KW in 24 h, and the basic version has 2 GB of Memory
Raspberry Pi	Most common single-board computer	The basic version consumes 30.66 KWh in a year, and it has 512 MB of Memory
FPGA	Custom-build FPGA unit for ciphers in IoT	FPGA uses 10–100 mW in Hour and has typically 6 MB of memory

Table 4 Poker test of the proposed system

Sample no	1	2	3	4	5	6	7	8	9	10
Pass (P) or Fail (F)	F	F	P	F	P	P	P	P	P	P

7 Conclusion

This paper starts by introducing the intuitionistic fuzzy system and stream cipher. Next, we give the details of the intuitionistic fuzzy system and the approach we used in this proposed system, and before that, we give three important literature surveys with motivation. Then, we discussed LFSR with definition and proof. After that, we proposed the intuitionistic fuzzy-based stream cipher and proposed model for Privacy Preservation of Biometric Data in IoMT. Then, we proved in the result section that the keystream generated by this stream cipher is pseudorandom and the platform where both models are given.

References

1. Sarkar A, Sahoo G, Sahoo UC (2012) Application of fuzzy logic in transport planning. Int J Soft Comput 3(2):1–21. A1
2. Youness EA, Mekawy IM (2012) A study on fuzzy complex linear programming problems. Int J Contemp Math Sci 7(19):897–908. A2
3. Bojadziev G, Bojadziev M (2007) Advances in fuzzy systems applications and theory. In: Fuzzy logic for business, finance and management, vol 23. 2nd edn, A3
4. Driankov D, Hellendoorn H, Reinfrank M (1996) An introduction to fuzzy control. Springer, Berlin Heidelberg, p A4
5. Atanassov KT (1986) Intuitionistic fuzzy sets. Fuzzy Sets and Syst 20:87–96 A5
6. Xu Z, Yager RR (2006) Some geometric aggregation operators based on intuitionistic fuzzy sets. Int J General Syst 35(4):417–433.A6
7. Roychowdhury S, Shenoi S (1997) Fuzzy rule encoding techniques. Research supported by MPO Contracts MDA904-94-C-6117 and MDA904-96-1-0114 and OCAST Grant AR2-002, 0-7803-3796-4/97/$10.0001997JEE.-
8. Anikin IV, Alnajjar K (2015) Fuzzy stream cipher system. In: 2015 International Siberian conference on control and communications (SIBCON), IEEE. 978-1-4799-7103-9/15/$31.00 ©2015

9. Machado S et al (2018) Securing ATM pins and passwords using fingerprint based fuzzy vault system. IEEE. 978-1-5386-5257-2/18/$31.00 ©2018
10. Sadkhan SB (2020) Complexity determination of stream cipher sequence based on discrete-time signal transformation. In: 2020 1st ınformation technology to enhance e-learning and other application IT-ELA, 2020, pp 144–147. https://doi.org/10.1109/IT-ELA50150.2020.9253070
11. Alnajjar K, Anikin I (2020) Secure gamma generation for stream cipher based on fuzzy logic. In: 2020 International conference on ınformation technology and nanotechnology (ITNT), 2020, pp 1—7.https://doi.org/10.1109/ITNT49337.2020.9253298
12. Wang X, Wang X, Zhao J et al (2011) Chaotic encryption algorithm based on alternant of stream cipher and block cipher. Nonlinear Dyn 63:587–597. https://doi.org/10.1007/s11071-010-9821-4
13. Shifa A, Naveed Asghar M, Ahmed A et al. (2020) Fuzzy-logic threat classification for multi-level selective encryption over real-time video streams. J Ambient Intell Human Comput 11:5369–5397. https://doi.org/10.1007/s12652-020-01895-2

Sleep Monitoring with Wearable Sensor Data in an eCoach Recommendation System: A Conceptual Study with Machine Learning Approach

Ayan Chatterjee, Andreas Prinz, Nibedita Pahari, Jishnu Das, and Michael Alexander Riegler

Abstract The collective effects of sleep loss and sleep disorders are correlated with many adverse health consequences, including increased risk of high blood pressure, obesity, diabetes, depressive state, and cardiovascular symptoms. Research in eHealth can provide methods to enrich personal health care with information and communication technologies (ICTs). An eCoach system may allow people to manage a healthy lifestyle with extended health state monitoring (e.g., sleep) and tailored recommendation generation. Using supervised machine learning (ML) techniques, this study investigated the possibility of classifying sleep stages at night for adults on hourly and daily basis. The daily total sleep minutes and hourly total sleep minutes for defined sleeping period served as input for the classification models. We first used publicly available Fitbit dataset to build the initial classification models. Second, using the transfer learning approach, we re-used the top five best-performing models on a real dataset as collected from the MOX2-5 wearable medical-grade activity device. We found that support vector classifier (SVC) with "linear" kernel outdated other classifiers with a mean accuracy score of 99.92% for hourly sleep classification and a K-nearest neighbor (KNN) outpaced other classifiers with a mean accuracy score of 99.47% for daily sleep classification, for the public Fitbit datasets. Moreover, to determine the practical efficacy of the classifier models, we conceptualized to use the classifier models in an eCoach prototype system to attain tailored sleep goals (e.g., a weekly goal of 49–63 h of sleeping).

A. Chatterjee (✉) · A. Prinz
Department of Information Technology, Center for eHealth, University of Agder, Kristiansand, Norway
e-mail: ayan.chatterjee@uia.no

N. Pahari
Department of Software Engineering, Knowit AS, Oslo, Norway

J. Das
Department of Library and Information Science, University of Calcutta, Calcutta, India

M. A. Riegler
Department of Holistic Systems, Simula Research Laboratory, Oslo, Norway

© The Author(s), under exclusive license to Springer Nature Singapore Pte Ltd. 2023
J. K. Mandal and D. De (eds.), *Frontiers of ICT in Healthcare*, Lecture Notes in Networks and Systems 519, https://doi.org/10.1007/978-981-19-5191-6_44

Keywords Sleep time · Sleep stage · Activity sensor · Machine learning · eCoach · Recommendation generation

1 Introduction

Sleep is a particular category of physical activity. Adults require 7–9 h of proper sleeping daily, while athletes may benefit as much as 10 h to maintain a healthy lifestyle [1, 2]. Sleep deprivation can increase the causes of memory issues, trouble with thinking and concentration, accidents, mood changes, weakened immunity, risk of diabetes, elevated blood pressure, weight gain, low sex drive, risk of heart disease, and body imbalance [1]. Unhealthy lifestyle practices, poor sleeping hygiene, sleep disorders, work pressure, and medical conditions may result in sleep deprivation [3]. In contrast, chronic oversleeping may cause cognitive loss, daytime sleepiness, lethargy, headaches, depressive mind, and trouble in falling or staying sleeping [4]. Research [4] in 2010 showed that staying up late for 20 to 25 h can affect individual concentration and performance, just as blood alcohol concentration (BAC) is 0.10%. In most places, people are considered legally drunk when their BAC is 0.08%. A study [4] in 2014 of 24,671 adults found evidence that more than 10 h of sleep a night or prolonged sleep is related to depression and obesity. Long-term sleep is also associated with high blood pressure and type 2 diabetes [4]. Therefore, sleep deprivation and excessive sleep may lead to the gradual development of chronic symptoms. Chronic diseases are the most common cause of death worldwide [5–7]. It is the leading unconditional probability of dying between ages 30 and 70 years [7]. Around 60−85% of the world's people live a sedentary lifestyle [5–7]. Regular physical activity has a significant impact on good sleep [4]. Still, more than 80% of the adolescent population in the world lack physical activity regularly [7].

Studies related to sleep monitoring can be classified into monitoring with wearable devices or non-wearable devices [8]. Polysomnogram (PSG) has been the gold standard to assess sleep psychology [9]. Health and the clinical market have enhanced real-world sleep mode indicator [9]. Longitudinal home monitoring avoids certain limitations of laboratory PSG, such as atypical sleeping environments and single-night snapshots. Sleep is a dynamic process that changes every day, so measuring sleep over multiple nights for medical, research, and health reasons is essential [9]. Home monitoring equipment may provide a more realistic platform to capture sleep data for many nights. Longitudinal data may prove invaluable for discovering internal patterns of sleep variability or linking sleep to the timing of various other activities. The personal health goal of sleep monitoring to optimize health also needs to be achieved through longitudinal monitoring and self-tracking. In multiple environments outside the field of sleep medicine, portable monitoring can accomplish this goal. Sleep can be monitored based on brain activity signals (e.g., EEG, EMG, and EOG), automatic alerts based on movements (e.g., actigraphy and body position), bed-sleep monitoring, heart-rate-variability (HRV), body temperature, galvanic skin response (GSR), sleep images, PSG, and touch-free remote tracking (e.g., LIDAR and

Wi-Fi) [9–11]. Relevant sleep monitoring devices are iBrain, Zeo, Heally Recording System, M1, Fitbit, MOX2-5, Lark, Sleep Cycle Alarm, Sleep Tracker, Up, Wake-Mate, Air Cushion, Early Sense Mattress, Emfit Bed Sensor, Home Health Station, Linen Sensor, Sleep Minder, Bio Harness, Health Vest, Magic vest, Radiofrequency monitor, and Wrist Care [9]. Baron et al. [8] developed a "Sleep Bunny" mobile app based on wearable technology for sleep behavioral intervention; however, the app suffers from personalization, effective reminder design, and notification generation. Stucky et al. [12] used Fitbit Charge 2 wearable device to estimate sleep using polysomnographic measures; however, it suffered from quantifying individual sleep episodes.

The idea of activity coaching may improve individual sleep health with daily and hourly sleep monitoring and tailored recommendation generation. In context, an electronic coach (eCoach) [13, 14] system may generate personalized activity recommendations based on the insight from sensory observation to reach personalized activity (e.g., sleep) goals. From the literature search, the eCoach concept in eHealth is in the nascent stage, and there is very little research conducted on actual sensor data using machine learning technology. In this study, we have conceptualized a novel, personalized, and data-driven eCoaching concept that can collect activity data from participants with wearable activity sensors, process those data with different ML models to classify sleep stages, and generate personalized recommendations on individual progress to attain personalized sleep goals (e.g., daily, weekly, or monthly based on preferences). The research questions for this study are—

(RQ-1) How to classify daily and hourly sleep time into different sleep stages?

(RQ-2) How to fit the classification models in an eCoach system for recommendation generation to attain personalized sleep goal?

To demonstrate the pertinency of the study, we described how to apply the classification model to achieve personalized weekly sleep goals. The remainder of the paper is structured as follows. In Sect. 2, we present the adopted methods. In Sect. 3, we discuss the experimental results, and the paper is concluded in Sect. 4.

2 Method

We used established statistical methods and ML models to analyze public and private sleep datasets for adults. Moreover, we assessed the performance of different ML classifiers against standard metrics to classify both hourly and daily sleep stages. The overall process includes data collection, data pre-processing, feature selection, data visualization, ML model training, testing, cross-validation, evaluation, and model re-use for personalized recommendation generation. In this study, we focused only on night sleep datasets for adults. Sleep data for the aged, children, athletes, bodybuilders, and pregnant women are beyond the scope of this study.

2.1 Data Collection

We used anonymous public Fitbit dataset for adult participants available in "Zenodo" [15] for initial ML model training and testing. The dataset has various features related to the activity; however, we selected the feature "sleep minutes" to maintain the focus of this study. We used the public dataset to discover the best performing classifiers with the defined feature in a multiclass classification problem.

Then, we applied the model to the actual dataset as collected with MOX2-5 wearable activity device [16] based on the transfer learning and incremental approach to proving the concept of personalized activity recommendation generation in an eCoach system to attain the personal sleep goal. Therefore, we collected anonymous nightly sleep data from two adults in Norway for one month using the MOX2-5 sensor following the ethical guidelines. The attributes of MOX2-5 sensor data are—timestamp, activity intensity (IMA), sedentary seconds, weight-bearing seconds, standing seconds, low physical activity (LPA) seconds, medium physical activity (MPA) seconds, vigorous physical activity (VPA) seconds, and steps per minute. IMA gives the impression if the activity is LPA or MPA or VPA. To associate the pre-trained model with the public dataset, we considered the "sedentary" feature from MOX2-5 for real-time classification. In MOX2-5 sensor, sedentary time refers to the non-activity duration, including leisure time and sleep time. Therefore, we considered ten hours of sleep data from two participants between 23:01:00 of day-(n-1) to 09:00:00 of day-n and calculated hourly and total daily sleep time. The relation between sedentary time and activity (LPA/MPA/VPA) time can be written as

$$\sum(\text{sedentary, active, weight} - \text{bearing, standing}) = 60\ \text{second}s\,(\text{sec.}).$$

During sleep time, sedentary minutes goes high ($\approx$58–60 s.) with IMA $\approx$ 0–20, step count ≈ 0, and activity time $= 0$. The IMA value can be correlated to the energy expenditure expressed in metabolic (MET) values. This makes it possible to classify:

$$\begin{aligned}
&\text{Low physical activity (LPA)}: \ \text{between 1.5 and 3 METS}\\
&\text{Moderate physical activity(MPA)}: \ \text{between 3 and 6 METS}\\
&\text{Vigorous physical activity(VPA)}: \ \text{6.0 or more METS}
\end{aligned}$$

For an upper leg sensor placement, the corresponding IMA thresholds are

$$\begin{aligned}
&4.5 < \text{LPA} \leq 11.9\ \text{cycles per seconds (cps)}\\
&11.9 < \text{MPA} \leq 26.8\ \text{cps}\\
&\text{VPA} > 26.8\ \text{cps}
\end{aligned}$$

2.2 Data Processing and Preparation

The collected activity data are continuous. All the data are numerical in format. For the classification, we converted the data from continuous to discrete by removing the timestamp feature. We also removed participants' data which are less than one month, noisy, incomplete, or missing. We decided data for 33 participants as they performed activities more than a month, resulting in 413 records for daily sleep stage classification and 2762 records for hourly sleep stage classification. Normality test with methods, such as Shapiro–Wilk, D'Agostino's K^2, and Anderson–Darling test [16] on each feature of the datasets revealed that data samples did not look like "Gaussian". The normality test was performed following the hypothesis testing method with P-value $>\alpha = 0.05$ (i.e., sample looks like Gaussian) [16].

For the feature selection, we performed methods, such as univariate (e.g., SelectKBest), recursive feature elimination, unsupervised principal component analysis or PCA, feature importance (e.g., ExtraTreesClassifier), modeling ML pipeline with PCA and SelectKBest, and the correlation analysis. The correlation analysis with the "spearman" method revealed the strength of the linear relationship between features [17–20]. We removed features if they showed a powerful dependency score ($r >=$ 0.6). In final, we selected the "sleep time" feature only. Afterward, we created a new feature class, "sleep stage" (on which classification would occur), based on the "sleep time" feature [4]. The "sleep stage" represents three classes—sleep deprivation (0), appropriate sleep (1), and excessive sleep (2) for daily sleep stage classification problem, and two classes—bad sleep (0) and good sleep (1) for hourly sleep stage classification problem. The rule for "sleep stage" feature class creation is defined in Table 1, based on the nature of MOX2-5 data. The feature, such as age, gender, weight, weight-bearing, and standing, is not in the scope of this study.

We used Python 3.8.5 supported language libraries, such as pandas (v. 1.1.3), NumPy (v. 1.21.2), SciPy (v. 1.5.2), Matplotlib (v. 3.3.2), Seaborn (v. 0.11.0), Plotly (v. 5.2.1), scikit-learn or sklearn (v. 0.23.2), and Graph Viz. (v. 2.49.1) to process data and build the machine learning models. We set up the intended Python environment in Windows 10 Enterprise system using Anaconda distribution and used the Spyder 5.x IDE for the development, debugging, and data visualization.

Table 1 Defined rules for "sleep stage" feature creation for this study

Classification type	Active class	Rule
Hourly sleep	Bad sleep	58 < sedentary minutes AND steps > 2
	Good sleep	58 <= sedentary minutes <= 60 AND 0 <= steps <= 2
Daily sleep	Sleep deprivation	Sleep time <7 h. / day
	Appropriate sleep	7 <= Sleep time <= 8 h. / day
	Excessive sleep	Sleep time > 7 h. / day

2.3 Model Training and Testing

In this study, all the selected machine learning models for classification are described in Table 2 with corresponding optimization methods. To better use data, initially, we shuffled the dataset, then split the dataset into training and testing with a random state integer value. To boost the performance of the machine learning model, we used k-fold cross-validation where $k >= 1$. Moreover, we adopted grid search parameter optimization technique for ML model tuning as appropriate selection of learning rate (alpha (α) and gamma (γ)) in gradient descent, and proper selection of components, such as PCA components, criterion, and max_depth is important for tree-based models. Ensembles [19] can give a boost to ML results in combination with several supervised models based on the approaches, such as parallel ensemble (bagging), sequential ensemble (boosting), and voting. Gradient descent follows a convex optimization technique.

We executed each ML classification model for five times and calculated their mean performance score for comparison. The general pseudocode is stated below:

Input: An instance of ML classifier model, mlcSleep
Input: A value-set to train from, value
Input: Necessary parameters for data splitting, param
Input: A value for cross validation, kfold
Input: A value-set for optimization technique, optValue
Input: Number of times model execution, count
Output: Predictions, classified_class, best_params, mean(best_score)
Begin

Table 2 Machine learning classifier models with optimization methods

Models	Optimization method
SVM (kernel = linear or rbf)	Gradient descent
Logistic regression	Gradient descent
Naïve Bayes (NB)	Gradient descent
Decision tree (DT)	Information Gain, Gini
K-nearest neighbor (KNN)	'auto', 'ball_tree', 'kd_tree', 'brute'
Random forest (RF)	Ensemble—bagging
Linear discrimination analysis (LDA)	Gradient descent
Bagging classifier	Ensemble—bagging
AdaBoost classifier (ADA)	Ensemble—boosting
Extra trees classifier (ET)	Ensemble—bagging
Gradient boosting classifier (GB)	Ensemble—boosting
Voting classifier	Ensemble—voting

```
    value ←shuffle_rows (value)
    X, y← split (value, param)
    arr← list ()
    While n < count do
        model←calculate (mlcSleep, optValue, kfold, 'accuracy')
        model.fit (X, y)
        arr.append(model.classified_class),
        arr.append(model.best_params)
        arr.append(model.best_score)
        n←n + 1
    end
    return top_five(arr)
end
```

2.4 Model Evaluation Metrics

In this study, performance of a ML-based classification models has been evaluated with discrimination measures. Discrimination metrics are—precision, recall, specificity, accuracy score, F1 score, classification report, and confusion matrix. A confusion matrix is a two-dimensional table ("actual" vs "predicted"), and both dimensions have "True Positives (TP)", "False Positives (FP)", "True Negatives (TN)", and "False Negatives (FN)" [17–20]. The equations for calculating metrices are [17–20]:

$$\begin{aligned}
&\text{Accuracy} = (\text{TP} + \text{TN})/(\text{TP} + \text{FP} + \text{FN} + \text{TN}),\\
&\text{Precision}(P) = \text{TP}/(\text{TP} + \text{FN}),\\
&\text{Recall}(R)\text{ or Sensitivity}(S) = \text{TP}/(\text{TP} + \text{FN}),\\
&\text{Specificity} = (1 - \text{Sensitivity}) = \text{TN}/\text{TN} + \text{FP},\\
&F1\text{ score} = (2 * P * R)/(P + R).
\end{aligned}$$

Also, we used cross-validation score to determine overfitting and underfitting and learning curve to visualize the convergence status of training score with the cross-validation score. We tested if the standardization technique on the entire dataset before learning can improve the performance of the models by reducing data leakage.

2.5 Transfer Learning for Recommendation Generation

The eCoach prototype system aims to collect individual activity data from wearable activity sensors at a daily level (day-n) and classify the sleep data into the identified three classes using machine learning models. In the procedure, participants can set personal preferences (e.g., daily goal, weekly goal, monthly goal, recommendation time, and the mode of recommendation) in the eCoach mobile app for tailored recommendation generation and its delivery. In this study, we have focused on daily sleep goal of 7–9 h. to achieve a weekly goal of 49–63 h. of sleeping. We considered a good hourly sleep as $\approx$ 58–60 min of sedentary time with IMA $\approx$ 0–20, step count $\approx$ 0, and activity time = 0. This study will help participants to identify their hourly sleep as well as daily sleep variation to achieve personalized sleep goals.

Different classification models are available; however, we cannot determine "a priori" which classifier will perform the best. It requires enormous data for training, validation, and testing. We collected real-activity data for two adults using the MOX2-5 activity sensor over thirty days. However, that volume of data is not sufficient to determine the accuracy of the best classifier. Therefore, we adopted the concept of transfer learning and incremental training approach. Initially, we trained all the potential classifiers (see Table 2) with public Fitbit data using K-fold = 10 and random_state = 7. Afterward, we selected the top five best performing classifiers and saved them as pickle files. Then, we used those pre-trained models for individual hourly and daily sleep stage classification. In this study, we classified the MOX2-5 sensor data with collected over 30-days from two participants. The sleep stage classification method entails two steps—a. training of pre-trained models with individual sleep data and model storing for individual participants, and b. sleep classification for day-n with individual models and re-train the models with the individual classification result of that day for the following day (day-n + 1) classification. Models trained with personalized sleep data are disjoint with the trained models for other participants. We selected the classification results from the individual classifiers with the highest mean accuracy. The process can be applied to other participant datasets.

3 Experimental Results and Discussion

This section describes—first, the analyses on public Fitbit datasets with ML classifier models, second, the selection of top five models with their best parameters to train MOX2-5 activity data for personalized sleep classification, and third, the representation of personalized sleep goal achievement in an eCoach prototype mobile app. We prepared public Fitbit data for hourly and daily sleep classifications with 21 different variants of classifiers and corresponding average accuracy scores for five passes described in Table 3. The SVM (kernel = "linear") outpaced other classifiers in the hourly sleep classification, and ExtraTreesClassifier outperformed different classifiers in daily sleep classification. The learning curves for both the highest-ranked classifiers in each category are depicted in Figs. 1 and 2. The result shows neither overfit nor underfit. The top five models in the respective category are bold in Table 3 and used for transfer learning as described in Sect. 2.

The best optimization parameters (as obtained with grid search method) for those top five models under each category are described in Tables 4 and 5. Furthermore,

Table 3 Performance of the machine learning classifier models for different classification approaches

ML classifier models with high level specification	Mean accuracy of hourly sleep classification	Mean accuracy of daily classification
SVC (kernel = 'linear')	**99.92**	**99.32**
SVC (kernel = 'rbf')	99.8	98.64
LogisticRegression ()	99.8	98.5
GaussianNB ()	95.6	95.1
BernoulliNB ()	85.3	53.0
ComplementNB ()	14.7	44.06
DecisionTreeClassifier (criterion = "gini")	99.8	99.18
DecisionTreeClassifier (criterion = "entropy")	99.8	99.18
RandomForestClassifier (n_estimators = 25)	99.8	99.18
RandomForestClassifier (n_estimators = 50)	99.8	99.18
RandomForestClassifier (n_estimators = 100)	**99.9**	99.18
KNeighborsClassifier (n_neighbors = 2)	99.8	**99.47**
KNeighborsClassifier (n_neighbors = 4)	99.8	99.47
LinearDiscriminantAnalysis ()	95.0	90.27
BaggingClassifier (base_estimator = DecisionTreeClassifier ())	99.8	99.18
AdaBoostClassifier (n_estimators = num_trees, random_state = seed)	**99.9**	**99.18**
ExtraTreesClassifier (n_estimators = 25, max_features = max_features)	**99.9**	99.28
ExtraTreesClassifier (n_estimators = 50, max_features = max_features)	99.9	**99.32**
ExtraTreesClassifier (n_estimators = 100, max_features = max_features)	99.9	99.22
GradientBoostingClassifier	**99.9**	99.17
VotingClassifier (estimators)	99.8	**99.42**

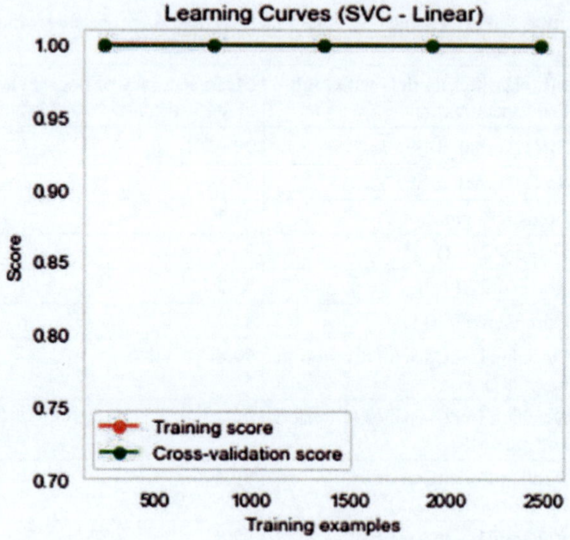

Fig. 1 Learning curve for SVC in hourly sleep classifications

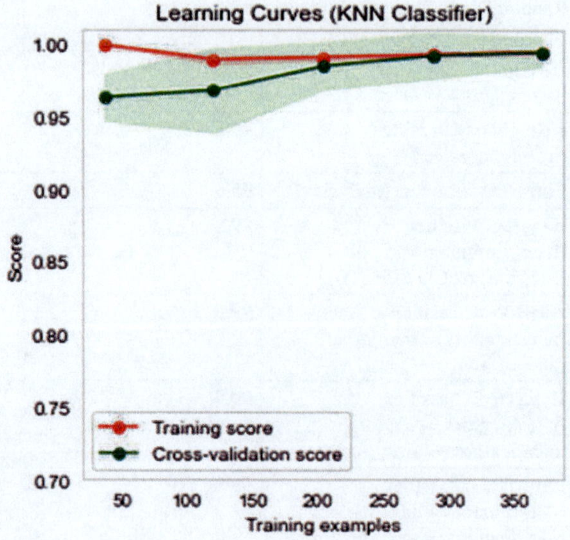

Fig. 2 Learning curve for KNN in daily sleep classifications

during training data preparation, we investigated if the pipeline execution concept can improve the performance of the ML classifiers or not! Thus, we created data preparation pipeline models for the best performing classifier. We tried to standardize the whole datasets in each data preparation pipeline and then classify the sleep data. However, the data preparation pipeline improved the performance of the models after addressing typical non-Gaussian nature of datasets. The results of SVC with linear kernel and KNN in pipeline execution are in Table 6.

To prove the practical usefulness of the classifier models, we conceptualized to use them in an eCoach prototype system to achieve personalized activity goals of active sleeping (7–9 h. of sleeping/day) for an entire week. We collected activity data from two adult participants over thirty days with the MOX2-5 activity sensor and measured sleep time from features, such as IMA, sedentary time, LPA, and steps.

Table 4 Optimized parameters for top five models in hourly classification

ML classifier models	Parameter list	Best parameter
ExtraTreesClassifier	Criterion = ['gini', 'entropy'] max_depth = [2, 4, 6, 8, 10, 12]	Max_depth = 8, criterion = 'gini'
SVC (kernel = 'linear')	Alphas (α) = [0.001, 0.01, 0.1, 1, 10] Gammas (γ) = [0.001, 0.01, 0.1, 1]	$\alpha = 0.01$, $\gamma = 0.001$
AdaBoostClassifier	Criterion = ['gini', 'entropy'] Max_depth = [2, 4, 6, 8, 10, 12]	Max_depth = 6, criterion = 'gini', $\alpha = 0.001$
RandomForestClassifier	Criterion = ['gini', 'entropy'] Max_depth = [2, 4, 6, 8, 10, 12]	Max_depth = 2, criterion = 'gini'
GradientBoostingClassifier	Criterion = ['gini', 'entropy'] Max_depth = [2, 4, 6, 8, 10, 12]	Max_depth = 4, criterion = 'gini', $\alpha = 0.01$

Table 5 Optimized parameters for top five models in daily classification

ML classifiers	Parameter list	Best parameter
SVC (kernel = 'linear')	Alphas = [0.001, 0.01, 0.1, 1, 10] Gammas = [0.001, 0.01, 0.1, 1]	$\alpha = 0.01$, $\gamma = 0.001$
ExtraTreesClassifier	Criterion = ['gini', 'entropy'] Max_depth = [2, 4, 6, 8, 10, 12]	Max_depth = 8, criterion = 'entropy'
KNN	Metrics: ['minkowski', 'euclidean', 'manhattan'] weights: ['uniform', 'distance'] n_neighbors: [2, 3, 4, 5, 6]	metrics = 'minkowski', weights = 'uniform', n_neighbors = 2
AdaBoostClassifier	Criterion = ['gini', 'entropy'] Max_depth = [2, 4, 6, 8, 10, 12]	Max_depth = 4, criterion = 'entropy', $\alpha = 0.001$
RandomForestClassifier	Criterion = ['gini', 'entropy'] Max_depth = [2, 4, 6, 8, 10, 12]	Max_depth = 2, criterion = 'gini'

Table 6 Result of pipelined ML model execution

Classifier type	Model	Accuracy score
Hourly data	SVC (kernel = 'linear')	99.93
Daily data	KNN	99.51

Table 7 Hourly sleep stage classification over a day (MOX2-5 dataset)

Participant	Set of hours (hrs.)	Classifier model with mean accuracy on day-29	Set of sleep stages
P-1 (Age:34, and normal weight)	{hr-1, hr-2, hr-3, hr-4, hr-5, hr-6, hr-7, hr-8, hr-9, hr-10}	SVC (kernel = 'linear') Mean accuracy = 99.966%	{0, 0, 1, 1, 1, 1, 1, 1, 0, 1}
Text recommendation		*"You had a good sleep of 7 h, which is optimal and initial 2 h the sleep was not perfect"*	
P-2 (Age:40, obese)	{hr-1, hr-2, hr-3, hr-4, hr-5, hr-6, hr-7, hr-8, hr-9, hr-10}	GradientBoostingClassifier Mean accuracy = 99.96%	{1, 1, 1, 1, 1, 1, 1, 1, 1, 0}
Text recommendation		*"You had a great sleep of 9 h, which is sufficient and every hour the sleep was proper"*	

Initially, we assumed that their goal was to maintain active sleeping for an entire week (i.e., the last seven days of the 30 days). Therefore, we used the top five classifiers mentioned in Table 3 to train, validate, and test MAX2-5 datasets for two participants and develop personalized ML models using an incremental approach. We divided 30 days into two parts—a. 23 days data for training and b. remaining seven days data for testing. Based on the training performance up to date-($n-1$), we classified individual sleep data for the day-(n) with the best classifier. Next, we trained each participant's five classifiers based on their sleep stage classification result on the day-(n). It helped for sleep stage classification on the day-($n + 1$). We repeated the same incremental process until the 7-days goal periods got over. The whole result has been captured for the nth day (e.g., $n = 30$) in Table 7 and the last seven days in Table 8.

A motivation with an eCoach may improve self-behavior by keeping up an active pace of sleeping over the day or weeks or months. The daily sleep stage will give a reflection on daily sleep status, and the hourly sleep stage classification will explain in which hour the sleep was good or bad. In real coaching, to attain a weekly sleep goal, the eCoach module will generate personalized recommendations based on the sleep outcome on each day and followed by a predictive analysis to achieve the weekly or monthly goal. In our future study, we will address it with more participants ($N > 15$).

4 Conclusion

This study has shown a direction to use ML technology to design and develop an intelligent eCoach system to generate automatic, meaningful, evidence-based, and tailored sleep recommendations to attain personal sleep goals. Improvement of physical activity in sequence with wearable activity sensors and digital activity trackers,

Table 8 Daily sleep stage classification over a WEEK (MOX2-5 dataset)

Participant	Set of days	Classifier model	Accuracy day-(n-1)	Sleep stage on day-n
P-1 (Age:34, normal weight)	Day-1	KNN	99.51	2
	Day-2	KNN	99.52	1
	Day-3	KNN	99.52	2
	Day-4	KNN	99.52	2
	Day-5	Random forest	99.52	2
	Day-6	KNN	99.53	2
	Day-7	KNN	99.53	1
Text recommendation		*"You have slept more than adequate sleeping hours for a week. Try to reduce your sedentary bouts for next week"*		
P-2 (Age:40, obese)	Day-1	Extra trees	99.52	1
	Day-2	KNN	99.51	1
	Day-3	KNN	99.52	1
	Day-4	KNN	99.52	2
	Day-5	KNN	99.52	2
	Day-6	KNN	99.53	2
	Day-7	KNN	99.53	2
Text recommendation		*"You have slept more than adequate sleeping hours for a week. Try to reduce your sedentary bouts for next week"*		

eCoach features can be encouraging. The concept, such as transfer learning, exists; its re-use with incremental training and testing approach in a sleep eCoaching concept is novel. Moreover, this is the first study conducted on MOX2-5 datasets on sleep monitoring and the conceptualization of tailored recommendation generation. This study has presented a detailed analysis of different ML classifiers on sleep data at a granular level. In the future study, we will focus on classifying leisure time and sleep time from sedentary time based on temporal feature analysis.

References

1. Carden KA (2020) Sleep is essential: a new strategic plan for the American academy of sleep medicine. J Clin Sleep Med 16(1):1–2
2. Vitale KC, Owens R, Hopkins SR, Malhotra A (2019) Sleep hygiene for optimizing recovery in athletes: review and recommendations. Int J Sports Med 40(08):535–543
3. Naitoh P, Kelly TL, Englund C (1990) Health effects of sleep deprivation
4. How Much Sleep Do I Need? Webpage. https://www.cdc.gov/sleep/about_sleep/how_much_sleep.html
5. The GBD 2015 Obesity Collaborators (2017) Health effects of overweight and obesity in 195 countries over 25 years. New England J Med 12 June 2017. https://doi.org/10.1056/NEJMoa1614362

6. GBD 2017 Diet Collaborators (2017) Health effects of dietary risks in 195 countries, 1990–2017: a systematic analysis for the global burden of disease study 2017. The Lancet. 2 Apr 2019. https://doi.org/10.1016/S0140-6736(19)30041-8
7. Physical activity. Webpage: https://www.who.int/news-room/fact-sheets/detail/physical-activity
8. Robbins R et al (2020) Four-year trends in sleep duration and quality: a longitudinal study using data from a commercially available sleep tracker. J Med Internet Res 22(2):e14735
9. Kelly JM et al (2012) Recent developments in home sleep-monitoring devices. International Scholarly Research Notices
10. Liu X et al (2014) Wi-sleep: contactless sleep monitoring via wifi signals. In: IEEE real-time systems symposium, pp 346–366
11. Hong H et al (2019) Microwave sensing and sleep: noncontact sleep-monitoring technology with microwave biomedical radar. IEEE Microwave Mag 20(8):18–29
12. Baron KG et al (2018) Technology-assisted behavioral intervention to extend sleep duration: development and design of the sleep bunny mobile app. J Med Internet Res 5(1):e3
13. Chatterjee A et al (2021) Human coaching methodologies for automatic electronic coaching (eCoaching) as behavioral interventions with information and communication technology: systematic review. J Med Internet Res 23(3):e23533
14. Rutjes H et al (2016) Understanding effective coaching on healthy lifestyle by combining theory-and data-driven approaches. PPT@ PERSUASIVE, pp 26–29
15. Crowd-sourced Fitbit datasets 03.12.2016-05.12.2016. Webpage https://doi.org/10.5281/zenodo.53894
16. MOX2 Bluetooth LE activity monitor. Webpage. https://www.accelerometry.eu/products/wearable-sensors/mox2/
17. Chatterjee A et al (2020) Identification of risk factors associated with obesity and overweight—a machine learning overview. Sensors 20(9):2734
18. Sklearn Page. Available online: https://scikit-learn.org/stable/supervised_learning.html
19. Chatterjee A et al (2021) Comparing performance of ensemble-based machine learning algorithms to identify potential obesity risk factors from public health datasets. In: Emerging technologies in data mining and information security, Springer, pp 253–269
20. Brandt S et al (1970) Statistical and computational methods in data analysis. North-Holland Publishing Company

LSEA-IOMT: On the Implementation of Lightweight Symmetric Encryption Algorithm for Internet of Medical Things (IoMT)

Sohail Saif, Priya Das, and Suparna Biswas

Abstract The Internet of Medical Things (IoMT) has made a monumental improvement in patient monitoring, early detection of diseases and treatment methods. This not only enriched the quality of living but also the healthcare cost and errors are minimized. This promising technology has greatly helped the patient and frontline healthcare workers. However, security and privacy breaches are one of the major concerns in IoMT due to wide variety of devices and communication network. The lack of security can affect a patient life since IoMT devices transmit patient data to a cloud-based medical server over insecure channel. Hence, maintaining the privacy and confidentiality becomes an utmost issue worth of further exploration and resolution. Cryptography is one of the primitive technologies which can ensure the confidentiality of a data; however, the complex solutions are not a good choice for resource-constrained IoMT device. Accordingly, we have designed a novel lightweight symmetric encryption algorithm (LSEA) for low-powered IoMT devices. Proposed algorithm uses 8-bit block ciphering technique using two 8-bit secret keys. Physiological parameter such as pulse rate of human body has been considered as one the secret keys while designing the algorithm. Security analysis shows that the algorithm is resilient to known plain text attack and known cipher text attack. LSEA has been tested in Arduino with varying payload. Experimental result depicts that it requires only 1.25 ms time for 16 byte and 7.4 ms for 512 byte data. Proposed algorithm has been compared to AES in a similar experimental environment.

Keywords IoMT · LSEA · Encryption · Decryption · Pulse rate

S. Saif (✉)
Department of Computer Applications, Maulana Abul Kalam Azad University of Technology, Kolkata, West Bengal, India
e-mail: sohailsaif7@gmail.com

P. Das
Department of Computer Science, Chakdaha College, Chakdaha, West Bengal, India

S. Biswas
Department of Computer Science & Engineering, Maulana Abul Kalam Azad University of Technology, Kolkata, West Bengal, India

© The Author(s), under exclusive license to Springer Nature Singapore Pte Ltd. 2023

J. K. Mandal and D. De (eds.), *Frontiers of ICT in Healthcare*, Lecture Notes in Networks and Systems 519, https://doi.org/10.1007/978-981-19-5191-6_45

1 Introduction

The Internet of Medical Things (IoMT) has become well-liked technology which facilitates remote monitoring of a patient health condition. Tiny sensors attached to patient body can collect several physiological information and send to a healthcare facility using internet connectivity. The physiological data is also known as electronic health record (EHR) which helps a doctor to diagnosis the patient remotely [1, 2]. With the integration of tiny sensors, smart devices, artificial intelligence using internet, the possibilities are endless [3]. This can upgrade the current focus of curative care to well-being and wellness. The burden of healthcare cost also can be reduced. IoMT is gaining momentum since it can provide real-time information on symptoms by continuous monitoring of patient's health conditions [4].

An architecture is shown in Fig. 1 which depicts the use of various biosensors used to collect health vitals such as blood pressure, ECG, heart rate. These sensor devices forward the collected data to a medical cloud database using a local processing unit (LPU) and internet. A cloud medical database stores the patient information which also delivered the data to the concerned user. A doctor can access these data and diagnosis the patient health condition. In a real-time scenario, patients' information should be available all the time in the server so that in case of any critical condition, medical team can take action as soon as possible. The patient data consists of the identity of a patient as well the health condition, and these information are private in nature and should not be disclosed.

Healthcare industry is facing security breaches at an alarming rate which includes cyberattacks on the IoMT devices. Patient data transmitted using internet is highly vulnerable to cybercriminals if proper data security is not ensured. One of the ways to prevent the cyberattacks against disclosure of sensitive information is to encrypt the data while transmitting and storing in cloud medical database [5]. Only trusted

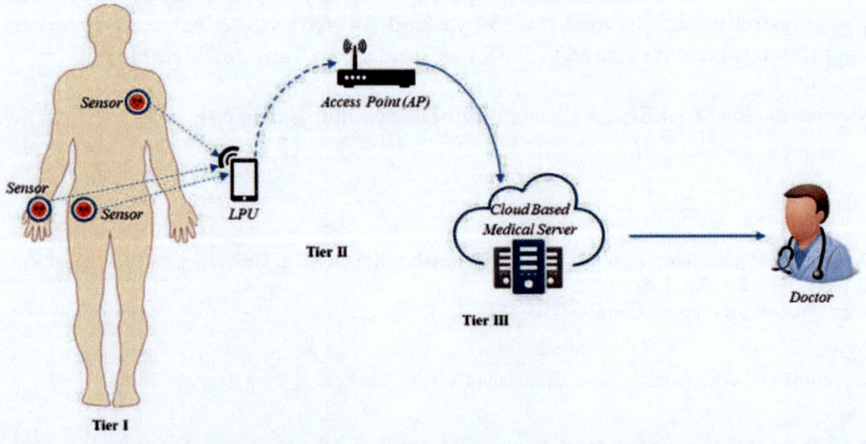

Fig. 1 Architecture of IoMT-based health monitoring system

parties having the decryption key can access the information. But, use of encryption algorithms in a resource-constraint IoMT device such as LPU is a biggest challenge. LPUs are mostly a small battery operated device having less computational ability. Typical encryption algorithms such as AES, RSA, ECC are complex in nature which need more computational resource [6]. In this paper, we have proposed a lightweight symmetric encryption algorithm (LSEA) which is specially designed for IoMT framework which uses physiological information of human body as a secret key. Rest of the paper is organized as following. Section 2 reports the recent related works on lightweight encryption algorithms. Proposed algorithm has been described in Sect. 3, while Sect. 4 presents the security analysis. Section 5 describes the performance analysis of the proposed algorithm. Finally, the research work is concluded in Sect. 6.

2 Related Works

Jabeen et al. [7] proposed a genetic-based encryption algorithm for wireless body area network which uses 8-bit key and 8-bit plain text for encryption. Author has used simple operation like 1's complement, XOR, S-Box and genetic operators such as cross-over and mutation in the algorithm. Key generation is performed in three steps: a random integer generation then conversion to binary afterward 1's complement and circular 2-bit right shift. The algorithm is implemented using MATLAB, and security analysis shows that it is free from man-in-the-middle attack and known plain text attack. Alshamsi et al. [8] used lightweight encryption algorithm (LEA) in their proposed architecture for secure transmission of patient data. Authors have added an encryption layer to the three-tier architecture of wireless body area network. Sensor captured data is sent to the mobile device of patient which has very limited memory. The architecture proved that LEA is most appropriate for restricted memory space with lesser power consumptions. LEA used simple operation such as XOR, rotation and addition. LEA used 128-bit block with three variable key sizes of 128, 192 and 256 bits. This algorithm is secure against well-known attack such as linear, differential, integral attacks. Prakasam et al. [9] developed enhanced energy efficient lightweight cryptography method (E3LCM) which works on 8-bit manipulation principal. Authors have applied this method on speech signal. The main focus of this algorithm is low power consumption and high speed. They have used linear feedback shift register to marginally alter the S-Box. This method consumed 202 mW power and 0.9 Kbytes on Sparten3E XC3S500E FPGA device. E3LCM is verified using histogram and correlation parameter. After validation, authors found that E3LCM consumes 18.18% less memory and 10.39% less power compared to method. Hong et al. [10] proposed a hardware-oriented block cipher named HIGHT (high security and lightweight). It is a lightweight cipher with 64-bit block and 128-bit key length. It has simple operation like addition, XOR, left bit rotation. Key generation process of HIGHT is consisting of two algorithms: whitening key generation and sub-key generation. HIGHT is an ultra-light and high security ciphering technique designed for RFID tags. One clock cycle is required for one round encryption. Experimental shows that HIGHT is faster than AES in 8-bit software implementation. Lim and Korkishko [11] developed a 64-bit block cipher called mCrypton with 64, 98, 128 bit key sizes. It is designed for low-cost sensor device and RFID tags which has compact implementation in software and hardware. mCrypton requires one clock cycle for each round. It requires 3500–4100 gates for both encryption and decryption while it requires 2400–3000 gates for encryption process only. An 8-byte block is represented in 4 × 4 nibble array in mCrypton. Encryption and decryption both consist of 12 repetitions of same round. Ensuring low-cost mCrypton is also a secure cipher that protects data from well-known attacks. Wu and Zhang [12] proposed a lightweighted block cipher called LBlock. It has 64-bit block and 80-bit key length. LBlock uses simple operation like substitution and permutation. Round function uses a SP-network, a 4 × 4 S-Box is used in confusion layer and a small 4-bit permutation function is used in diffusion layer. LBlock has both hardware and software implementations. An 8-bit microcontroller requires 3955 clock cycle for encryption. For hardware implementation, it requires 1320 GE on 0.18 μm and throughput is 200 Kbps at 100 kHz. This algorithm provides enough security against linear cryptanalysis and differential cryptanalysis. Aboushosha et al. [13] developed SLIM, an ultra-lightweighted cipher. It is a 64-bit symmetric block cipher where Feistel structure is used. It uses 80-bit key for encryption and decryption with 32 rounds. SLIM uses a S-Box with size 4 × 4 that works as a nonlinear component and works on 16-bit data. It has very simple implementation and appropriate for RFID tags and internet of health thing. SLIM can defend linear and differential cryptanalysis attacks. Usman et al. [14] proposed secure IoT (SIT), a symmetric key cipher with 64-bit plain text and key. SIT was designed with low computational cost and substantial security. Rounds of this algorithm are restricted in only five to improve efficiency. Mathematical operation is performed on 4-bit data of each round. It uses Feistel network of substitution–diffusion function to create maximum confusion and diffusion in data. Authors have applied this algorithm on image encryption. Suzaki et al. [15] proposed a versatile block cipher called TWINE. It is a 64-bit lightweighted block cipher with two key variants of 80 bit and 128 bit. TWINE has very small hardware implementation which is appropriate for embedded software. Algorithm was implemented both in software (8-bit microcontroller) and hardware (FPGA and ASIC). Experimental results show that 1500 GE is required for both encryption and decryption processes. 23-round TWINE-80 is appropriate for differential attack, and 24-round TWINE-128 defends from the most powerful attack. It is a fast cipher which is implemented within 0.8–1.5 Kbytes ROM. Beierle et al. [16] proposed a tweakable block cipher called SKINNY. It is flexible due to its variable block, key, tweak, size. SKINNY is very effective for threshold application and side channel protection. It has two versions: SKINNY-64 and SKINNY-128. SKINNY-64 uses 64-bit block and 64/128/192 bit key sizes with 32/36/40 rounds. SKINNY-128 uses 128-bit block and key variants of 128/256/384 bit with 40/48/56 rounds. It achieves very good efficiency in microcontroller and software implementations.

3 Proposed Algorithm

Here, we have proposed a low-cost symmetric encryption algorithm to protect the IoT-based healthcare data. Proposed algorithm is based on block ciphering technique where 8-bit block of plain text and two 8-bit secret keys are required to encrypt the data. Secret keys need to be shared with the receiver for the decryption of cipher text. Secret key 1 is a random integer between 1 and 10, and Secret key 2 is one of the vital parameters of patient body; here, we have considered pulse rate of the patient. In first step, each character of plain text is converted to its respective ASCII value. The second step of the encryption process is to check if the value is even or odd. If the value is even, then key1 (k1) is substituted from the value, and if the value is odd, then key1 (k1) is added to the ASCII value. Then, the new value is converted to 8-bit binary number. The third step of this encryption process is to perform permutation using P-Box. Table 1 shows the permutation table which is used to shuffle the bits of the binary number. Permutation table is an array of size 8 with an index from '0' to '7'. All of the binary bits are shuffled according to the array index. For example, binary data at index 0 is replaced by binary data at index 7. Shuffling process is performed reversed for decryption. XOR operation between second key (k2) and output of third step is performed in the fourth step. The fifth step is to perform substitution using S-Box. Table 2 presents substitution value for each 4-bit binary number. An 8-bit binary number (output of fourth step) is divided into two parts. First and second bits of each part are considered as row of S-Box. Third and fourth bits of each part are denoted the column of S-Box. After substitution, one hex number is generated for each 4-bit binary number. All of the five steps of encryption are performed in reversed direction for decryption to get the original plain text. Logic of the second step of encryption is opposite for decryption process. An 8-bit binary value obtained from permutation step is converted to decimal value; then, if the value is even, then key1 (k1) is added with this value, and if the value is odd, then key1 (k1) is substituted from this value. Finally, the ASCII value is converted to the plain text. Proposed algorithm is shown below.

Table 1 Permutation box (P-Box)

0	1	2	3	4	5	6	7
7	5	0	1	2	4	3	6

Table 2 Substitution box (S-Box)

S-Box	00	01	10	11
00	1	A	9	6
01	0	B	2	7
10	8	4	3	E
11	C	5	D	F

Proposed Encryption Algorithm

```
Input: plain_text, k1, k2
Output: cipher_text
k1 = random integer between 1 and 10
k2 = pulse rate
for i = 1 to length of plain_text
   Convert plain_text(i) to plaintext_dec
   if (plaintext_dec = even)
      plaintext_dec = plaintext_dec−k1
   else
      plaintext_dec = plaintext_dec + k1
   end if
   Convert plaintext_dec to 8-bit binary number (plaintext_bin)
   Perform permutation using P-Box on plaintext_bin
   plaintext_bin = plaintext_bin ⊕ k2
   perform substitution using S-Box on plaintext_bin
   cipher_text (i) = S-Box output
end for
Return cipher_text
```

Proposed Decryption Algorithm

```
Input: cipher_text, k1, k2
Output: plain_text
k1 = random integer between 1 and 10
k2 = pulse rate
for i = 1 to length of plain_text
   perform substitution using S-Box on cipher_text(i), return ciphertext_bin
   ciphertext_bin = ciphertext_bin ⊕ k2
   Perform permutation using P-Box on ciphertext_bin
   Convert ciphertext_bin to Ciphertext_dec
    if (Ciphertext_dec = even)
       Ciphertext_dec = Ciphertext_dec + k1
    else
       Ciphertext_dec = Ciphertext_dec−k1
    end if
   plain_text (i)= Ciphertext_dec
end for
Return plain_text
```

4 Security Analysis

While designing the algorithm, two well-known attacks such as known plain text attack and known cipher text attack have been considered as attack model. This section describes how the proposed algorithm can avoid both if this attacks.

4.1 *Known Plain Text Attack*

This is one of the popular attacks targeted to cryptographic algorithms. In this attack, an intruder is having a part of plain text and cipher text and tries to find out relationship between them to get complete plain text. The attacker applies several kinds of permutation and substitution process to find out the encryption algorithm that is used for encryption.

$$P(C(S, R)) = A(S, R) \tag{1}$$

Here, P is plain text that is encrypted and sent to sender S. Attacker A tries to find out the complete information from cipher text C. Our proposed algorithm is free from plain text attack since original plain text is never sent over the network. So, the attacker will not get the plain text and unable to decrypt the cipher text.

$$P(E_n(C(S, R))) = A(C) + R(E_n) \tag{2}$$

P is the original text that is sent after encrypted by our proposed encrypted algorithm E_n. So, the attacker can only get the cipher text C which is impossible to decrypt without the knowledge of decryption algorithm and secret keys. As C is only accessible by receiver R, so it can be decrypted by R using E_n.

4.2 *Known Cipher Text Attack*

In this attack, the attacker has only access the encrypted message (cipher text), but attacker has no idea about any part of plain text or secret key. Our proposed algorithm is free from this attack because proposed algorithm has two secret keys. It is impossible for attacker to find both keys and decrypt the cipher text to get original plain text. Proposed algorithm is also used permutation and substitution boxes for more diffusion.

$$P(S, R) + E_n + K_1 + K_2 = A(C) + R(E_n, C) \tag{3}$$

Sender S encrypts plain text P using encryption algorithm E_n and secret keys (K_1 and K_2) and send it to receiver R. Attacker A only has cipher text C but do not have knowledge about the encryption and decryption process. Hence proposed algorithm is safe against Know Cipher Text Attack.

5 Performance Analysis

Proposed algorithm has been implemented using C++ and tested in Arduino Uno microcontroller board. For our experiments, we have used a pulse sensor to collect pulse rate from human body. Pulse rate has been encrypted and decrypted using our proposed algorithm. For comparison, the same algorithm has been implemented in MATLAB and tested in a Laptop. Table 3 shows the software and hardware specifications of the experimental setup. Figure 2 shows the hardware prototype for pulse rate collection in encrypted format using our proposed algorithm.

For performance comparison, well-known symmetric algorithm AES has been considered. A 128-bit variant of AES has been also tested in Arduino and laptop. During experiments, data size of plain text has been varied and the execution time

Table 3 Hardware and software configurations of the experimental setup

Parameters	Arduino Uno	Desktop
CPU	ATmega328	Intel Core i3 2310
Clock speed	16 MHz	2.10 GHz
Storage	32 KB	500 GB
Ram	2 KB	4 GB
Software	Arduino IDE	MATLAB

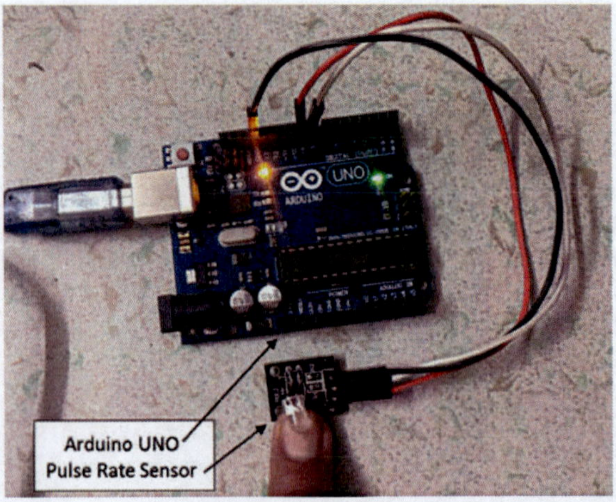

Fig. 2 Hardware test bed for pulse rate collection in encrypted format

Fig. 3 Execution time required in Arduino UNO

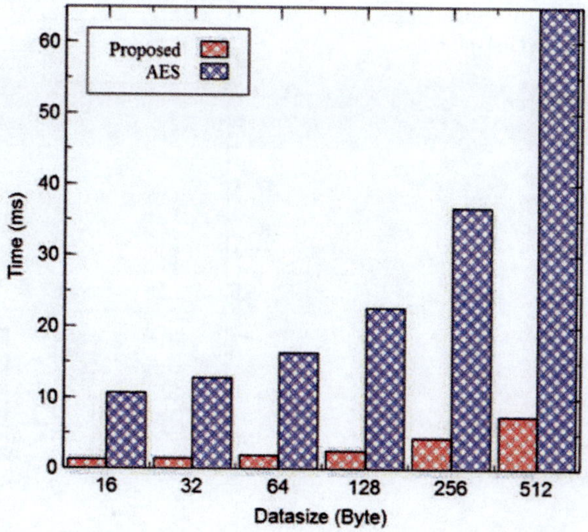

has recorded. Execution time depicts the time required to encrypt and decrypt the entire data. Figures 3 and 4 show the execution time required in Arduino UNO and laptop, respectively. It can be observed from Fig. 3 that it requires 1.25 ms time to complete the encryption and decryption processes for 16-byte data, while it requires 7.4 ms for 512 byte of data which is less than the time required for AES. Similarly, it requires 0.14 ms for 16 byte and 0.88 ms for 512 byte when executed in a laptop equipped with more hardware resources. Hence, the experimental results prove that our proposed lightweight symmetric encryption algorithm (LSEA) can execute in resource constrain device ensuring the security of the data.

6 Conclusion

With the rapid advancement of IoMT-based health monitoring systems, security of patient data has become a prime concern. Sensitive patient data must be protected from being disclosed to cyber criminals. Therefore, ensuring the confidentiality of the data is significant priority for IoMT framework. End-to-end security can be implemented in a low-powered IoMT device using lightweight block cipher encryption technique. This paper presents a novel lightweight symmetric encryption algorithm which requires block size of 8 bit and two secret keys of 8 bit. Pulse rate of human body has been considered as one of the secret key elements. Proposed LSEA has been tested over Arduino Uno device and laptop. Execution time has been recorded for different payloads. Experimental results show that the algorithms require less time than standard AES both in Arduino and laptop.

Fig. 4 Execution time required in laptop

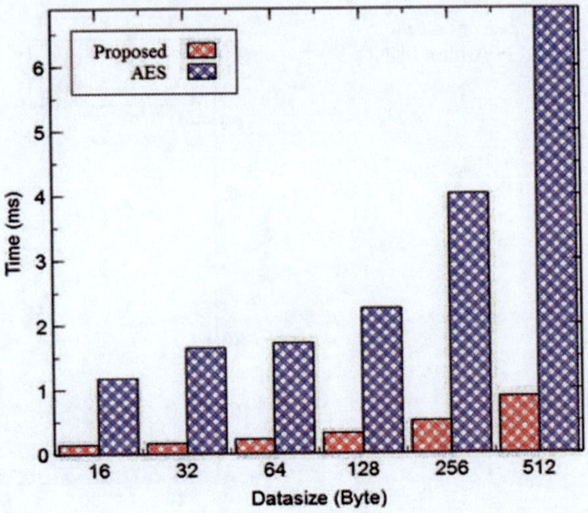

References

1. Girardi F, De Gennaro G, Colizzi L, Convertini N (2020) Improving the healthcare effectiveness: the possible role of EHR, IoMT and Blockchain. Electronics 9(6):884
2. Rubí JNS, Gondim PRL (2019) IoMT platform for pervasive healthcare data aggregation, processing, and sharing based on OneM2M and OpenEHR. Sensors 19(19):4283
3. Saif S, Jana M, Biswas S (2021) Recent trends in IoT–based smart healthcare applying ML and DL. In: Emerging technologies in data mining and information security, pp 785–797
4. Saif S, Saha R, Biswas S (2021) On development of MySignals based prototype for application in health vitals monitoring. Wirel Pers Commun, pp 1–18
5. Saif S, Biswas S (2019) Secure data transmission beyond tier 1 of medical body sensor network. In: Proceedings of international ethical hacking conference 2018. Springer, Singapore, pp 405–417
6. Saif S, Biswas S (2020) On the implementation and performance evaluation of security algorithms for healthcare. In: Proceedings of the 2nd international conference on communication, devices and computing. Springer, Singapore, pp 629–640
7. Jabeen T et al (2020) A lightweight genetic based algorithm for data security in wireless body area networks. IEEE Access 8:183460–183469
8. Alshamsi AZ, Barka ES, Serhani MA (2016) Lightweight encryption algorithm in wireless body area network for e-health monitoring. In: 2016 12th International conference on innovations in information technology (IIT). IEEE
9. Prakasam P et al (2021) An enhanced energy efficient lightweight cryptography method for various IoT devices. ICT Express
10. Hong D et al (2006) HIGHT: a new block cipher suitable for low-resource device. In: International workshop on cryptographic hardware and embedded systems. Springer, Berlin, Heidelberg
11. Lim CH, Korkishko T (2005) mCrypton–a lightweight block cipher for security of low-cost RFID tags and sensors. In: International workshop on information security applications. Springer, Berlin, Heidelberg
12. Wu W, Zhang L (2011) LBlock: a lightweight block cipher. In: International conference on applied cryptography and network security. Springer, Berlin, Heidelberg
13. Aboushosha, B et al (2020) SLIM: a lightweight block cipher for internet of health things. IEEE Access 8: 203747–203757

14. Usman M et al (2017) SIT: a lightweight encryption algorithm for secure internet of things. arXiv preprint arXiv:1704.08688
15. Suzaki T et al (2011) Twine: a lightweight, versatile block cipher. In: ECRYPT workshop on lightweight cryptography. vol 2011
16. Beierle C et al (2016) The SKINNY family of block ciphers and its low-latency variant MANTIS. In: Annual international cryptology conference. Springer, Berlin, Heidelberg

Image Processing in Healthcare

Cardiovascular Disease Prediction in Retinal Fundus Images Using ERNN Technique

M. Shahina Parveen and Savitha Hiremath

Abstract In recent years, heart disease increases the humanity rate transversely the world. So, it is required to extend a model to envisage the heart disease incident as early as feasible with an elevated rate of accuracy. In this study, cardiovascular disease is predicted by a novel method with the retinal image data. In this system, the retinal fundus image data are used to indicate heart disease occurrence. The cardiovascular disease gets detected from the changes in the microvasculature, which is imaged from the retina. The prediction of disease is by considering features like age, gender, smoking status, systolic blood pressure, diastolic blood pressure, and HbA1c that can be extracted using Improved GLCM approach. Then the pointed features can be selected using the ICA algorithm. Risk factors for heart disease occurrence are detected from the microvasculature of ERNN-classified retinal fundus image using MATLAB. The input image is taken from the UCI machine learning repository based on Cleveland datasets. The main objective of the proposed system is to predict the occurrence of heart disease from retinal fundus image with a higher rate of accuracy.

Keywords Heart disease · Improved GLCM · ICA · ERNN · MATLAB

1 Introduction

Nowadays, the distinct reason for demise among the human is cardiovascular disease (CVD) that has become the crucial impacts, and the probable survivability rate becomes less. Consequently, the cardiovascular disease (CVD) detection is extremely significant and sufficient to reduce the humanity rate. Numerous procedures are offered to perceive the incidence of CVD. So far, they are expensive to identify the CVD and also take much more time. The relationship between heart and eye is high. The blood vessels collection at the eye's backside also acknowledged as the retinal

M. Shahina Parveen (✉)
Computer Science Technology Department, Dayananda Sagar University, Bengaluru, India
e-mail: shahina-cst@dsu.edu.in

S. Hiremath
Department of Computer Science Engineering, Dayananda Sagar University, Bengaluru, India

© The Author(s), under exclusive license to Springer Nature Singapore Pte Ltd. 2023
J. K. Mandal and D. De (eds.), *Frontiers of ICT in Healthcare*, Lecture Notes in Networks and Systems 519, https://doi.org/10.1007/978-981-19-5191-6_46

vasculature, which is strongly attached to the health of the heart, which means the issues in the eye visualize directly. The related heart issues with the heart and the blood vessels in the human body [1]. The important feature in the eye is retina that can use in straight microcirculation. Retina gives a gap for prediction changes in microvasculature relating to the CVD improvement. So, the retinal fundus images are the vital factor to provide and predict the CVD with high prediction rate [2].

The prediction of risk methods can be CVD component prevention and control efforts because it can assist in recognizing the people at high danger factor of CVD, and it should assistance the majority from defensive interventions. Much more risk prediction methods expanded, usually estimating personality threat over ten years ago by use of measured stages of predictable risk factors for CVD. While to implement observance, and usual Physical Activity (PA) plans the preferred performance, consideration should be listening carefully to evaluate quantifiable results. Thus, CVD should be a solution variable of concern for the surgeons and patients correlated to the health [3]. Retinal fundus images play a considerable role in the recognition and CVD separation. Cardiovascular disease (CVD) can be anticipated by the occurrence of hemorrhage, micro aneurysms, exudates, and gyration arteries in the retinal fundus. The intense pixels in retinal fundus images, which damages its generalization to testing cases of retinal fundus imagery [4]. Retinal fundus imaging is a simple, non-invasive, and elevated resolution method, which produces the eye's 2D representation. In retinal imaging methods that recommend the amends or abnormalities predict in human retinal vasculature that has a sturdy relationship with diverse systemic conditions like hypertension, diabetes and CVD. Hence, the usual optical inspection is important for the retinal vascular abnormalities prediction to recognize human at high risk of these diseases for an initial stage and in-time medications.

Fundus imaging remains a vital imaging tool as it permits non-invasive examination of disease development over inbounds of time. The practical implications of CVD predictions associated with the risk factors by retinal fundus images that never point out the reorganization of patients at CVD risks and moment-to-experience investigation. To regard as the retinal fundus imaging for evaluating the patient's CVD risks based on mediocre conditions. The retinal fundus images, which might calculate cardiovascular disease (CVD) and differentiate the patients in CVD over the conservative risk aspects like FRS, diabetes, hypertension, dyslipidemia, and strengthening habits [5]. Significantly, such transforms herald the development of end-organ harms and adaptable appearances. Besides, microvascular dysfunction in marginal beds reflects a dysfunction in intuitive beds, which offering validation for imaging available microvessels. The ocular media transparency permits the straight visualization of the microvasculature, which may be exaggerated by systemic diseases [6]. In the interior plane of an eye, the retina gets placed that is the top acting layer. The optic nerve is worn to join the human's brain and the eye. The adaptation of light rays dropped in the eye into electrical signals, which is the majority of major step, and relocate these pulses to the brain by way of optic nerves in the eye. The retinal image is the lucid and available area of an optic disk (OD). The segmentation in the retinal fundus image is executed by the optic disk effectively that plays a prominent role in the automatic development of the CVD diagnosis system [7]. Nowadays, the heart-related problems arise to establish the several health-related issues also detriments the fatality to the human being.

The classification of the diseased region is the crucial task to utilize several distinct methods. The medical image processing had some demerits according to the techniques. As to overcome all the issues related to the CVD prediction, the improved method is necessary to initiate the CVD prediction based on the region-based accuracy prediction. Here, the improved accuracy based GLCM for feature extraction, ICA-based feature selection, and RNN-based classification to classify the accurate prediction of CVD-affected regions through the effective retinal fundus images. The proposed approach helps to identify the CVD with optimal accuracy based on its distinct features.

The remaining paper gets organized in the given formation as Sect. 2 provides the related works with other author experimental works. Section 3 represents the proposed methodology to enhance the resultant analysis. Section 4 offers the performance analysis of the proposed research work with its obtained results. Finally, Sect. 5 shows the conclusion about as concludes the research work.

2 Related Work

This section provides the related works about the several cardiovascular diseases (CVD) with retinal fundus images-based prediction given below: Ahiante et al. [8] proposed the retinal microvasculature and the macro vascular deterioration-based leptin in strong, black in young, and individuals in White. To established serum leptin, central retinal artery calculation, vein counterparts, and arterio-venous ratio. To evaluate the retinal vessel reactions to light glimmer aggravation. Zhang et al. [9] stated the electronic medical records-based CVD prediction through an Enhanced Character-level Deep Convolutional Neural Networks (EnDCNN) method. Depends on text region embedding and its vector unit enables through the down-sampling method to organize the training dataset. The free dimension-matching in training offers the capability to routinely clinical texts process for accurate prediction.

Patro et al. [10] provided the supervised learning-based CVD prediction with the consideration of health care and social care system. The heart disease problem-solves through IoT through the availability of the medical resource system. For the classification stage, K-nearest neighbors, Naive Bayes, support vector machine, Lasso, and ridge regression algorithms are used to enable the prediction of heart diseases with practical manner. Boscari et al. [11] proposed the premature cardiovascular disease that causes the type 1 diabetes (T1D) to reduce the survival rate of the human. The logistic regression method helps to estimate the steno T1D engine for cardiovascular disease (CVD) and also offers comprehensive information to the approximate risk. Rekha et al. [12] proposed to identify the heart disease occurrence with a high fatality rate of accuracy. The cardiovascular disease estimated from the fundus image data by utilizing the several features, which causes the risk factors for human. The numerous features help for detection and segmentation of microvasculature-enabled retinal fundus images.

Parameswari and Ranjani [13] stated that the atherosclerosis prediction through the efficient Machine Learning (ML) techniques. The early detection of atherosclerosis depends on the classification of arteries and veins through the morphological appearances. The proposed mixed algorithm helps to attain the accurate disease prediction and also enables the illumination correction of the blood vessels. The feature extraction and classification is the prime model. Here, the Enhanced Bayesian Arithmetic Classifier (EBAC) is used to classify the blood vessels that are also an effective approach. Wong et al. [14] provided the CVD prediction using deep learning (DL) method in clinical diagnosis. The DL method-based black box requiring knowledge provides the necessary information. The performance analysis of proper cardiovascular disease detection. CVD-based retinal fundus image classification, segmentation, and detection are improved here.

Lim et al. [15] offered the fundus imaging technique based on diabetic retinopathy predicted here. Manual screening is done by the diverse of Artificial Intelligence (AI) in specific of deep learning (DL) method. The diabetic retinopathy system establishment solved the issues on clinical deployment among the specific fundus imaging modalities.

Litjens et al. [16] stated the CVD analysis using DL approach from Cardiac Magnetic Resonance, CT (Computed Tomography), and single-photon emission-based Computed Tomography, to intravascular Optical Coherence Tomography (OCT) and echocardiography. The multiple ML approaches with the Convolutional Neural Networks (CNN) that provides a significant impact on clinical practice. Schmidt-Erfurth et al. [17] proposed the artificial neural network (ANN) method-based deep learning (DL) algorithm. AI image-based diagnostic system that has recently been approved by the FDA as a first of its kind in medicine. Benjamins et al. [18] allowed to progress patient mind and decrease healthcare costs. AI has the probable to improve traditional statistical analyzes significantly and to permit the 'hidden' information discovery in too complex datasets. AI can be an important value in the diagnosis and cardiovascular disease treatment that are unaware of the fundamentals at the back of artificial intelligence (AI) and predictable applications. Appaji et al. [19] stated the retinal microvasculature with the high vascular morbidity occurrence in SCZ and BD have analyzed. The retinal vascular caliber and have noticed and also increased retinal venular caliber in schizophrenia (SCZ). Retinal vascular tortuosity could provide a superior structural measure than caliber as it is static and less susceptible to pulse period variations.

3 Proposed Work

The prediction of heart disease based cardiovascular disease (CVD) provides an accurate forecast. The flow diagram of the proposed method is shown in Fig. 1. The

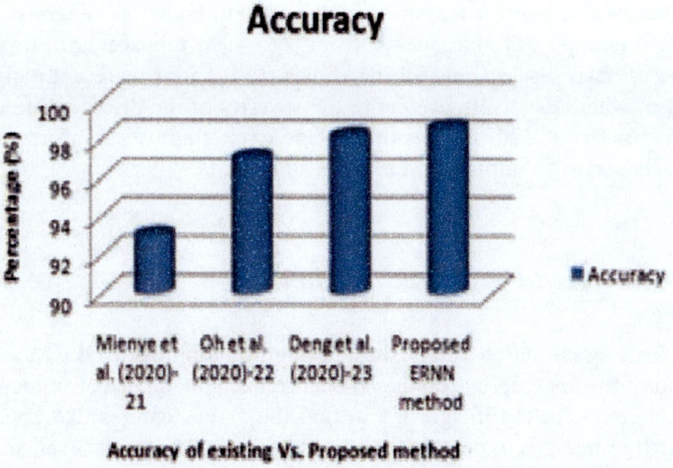

Fig. 1 Accuracy comparison of existing versus proposed method

heart disease prediction using retinal fundus images consists of following procedures such as:

- Preprocessing using adaptive median filter (AMF)
- Feature extraction using Improved GLCM
- Feature selection using ICA
- Classification using ERNN

Here, the proposed methodology performs better accuracy based Microvascular changes lead the medical appearance, and so its recognition should have predictive value. Indeed, ophthalmoscopic changes in retinal microvasculature structure have been identified as independent predictors for hypertension, diabetes, coronary disease, renal disease, and stroke.

3.1 Dataset Availability

To collect the heart disease data from the UCI machine learning repository. There are four datasets (i.e., Cleveland, Hungary, Switzerland, and the VA Long Beach). The Cleveland database was selected for this research because it is a commonly used database by machine learning researchers with records that are mostly complete. The dataset contains 303 records. Although the Cleveland dataset has 76 attributes, the dataset provided in the repository only includes information for a subset of 14 attributes. The data source of the Cleveland dataset is the Cleveland Clinic Foundation. 13 attributes feature in heart disease prediction, and one attribute serves as the output or the predicted attribute for the presence of heart disease in a patient. The

Cleveland dataset contains a feature named ‘num’ to show the diagnosis of heart disease in patients on different scales, from 0 to 4. In this scenario, 0 represents the absence of heart disease, and all the values from 1 to 4 represent patients with heart disease, where the scaling refers to the severity of the disease. The dataset is taken from Amin et al. [20] for identifying and extracting useful information from the clinical dataset with minimal user inputs and efforts.

3.2 GLCM Based Feature Extraction

Here, the feature extraction establishes through an improved GLCM technique. GLCM texture feature employs on the co-occurrence phenomena of immediate gray level and its counts in the image. It can find the given features like color, shape, size, and texture features to decrease the sources to portray the data set, so the classification process using fewer data can do. The GLCM texture feature is evaluated through a square matrix depends on the Region Of Interest (ROI) measurement of the total grayscale levels (N) in the X-ray images. GLCM well-identified method for 2nd-order statistical texture features extraction via numerical distributions of intensity values and the grouping at different locations comparative to every other in an image. Based on the total intensity points in an image, information is separated into first, second, and superior order. Higher orders statistics are hypothetically probable but not executed due to computation difficulty. The heart disease features include information concerning the structural collection of exteriors and their neighboring relationships. A total of heart disease features are evaluated and consist of given influenced factors that are: energy, entropy, contrast, correlation, homogeneity, and several factors. The corresponding definitions are formulated, as shown below: Let’s presume the Co-occurrence Matrix with ‘N’ measurement and a, b are its coefficients and manages of the factors. Energy is also referred to as ‘Consistency’ or ‘Angular second moment’. It provides the addition of square aspects in GLCM matrix. It is through the homogeneous areas to non-homogeneous areas. It is high when the frequency of repeated image pixel is high.

3.3 ICA Based Feature Selection

The extracted deceased images get to establish the selection stage. Here, independent component analysis (ICA) helps to select the optimal features. The ICA-based feature selection is supplementary helpful with individuals data that pursues non-Gaussian distributions of information. The aim is to discover a linear demonstration of non-Gaussian information so that the components are numerically independent, or as independent as potential.

3.4 Enriched Recurrent Neural Network (ERNN) Based Classification

Here, the classification performs through the concern of enriched recurrent neural network (ERNN). ERNN offers a better classification of the diseased area. RNN is a supervised machine learning (ML) method that is the collection of artificial neurons by way of one recurrent loop, also referred to as the feedback loop. The feedback loops pass on to the recurrent sequences that run eventually in a consecutive approach. The RNN training completed in a direct method that needs training datasets. A conventional recurrent neural network (RNN) steadily presumes that all the inputs and outputs are self-sufficient with every other. However, the sequential data output is linked to the preceding calculations. The neural network-based RNN consist with inside the loops, so facilitating data to persist for the sub-sequential outcomes. With any long data sequences, RNNs can memorize the information theoretically. The aim ERNN is used to decrease the dissimilarity between the yield and the targets. RNN has the ability to processing the consecutive inputs by adjusting a recurrent hidden position, whose commencement depends on the preceding step. From this manner, the network shows dynamic temporal performance. Moreover, the recurrent layer allows the information feeding of the preceding steps and joins the ensuing output with the input of the present time steps, which employs a central part in the processing. The algorithm permits the resultant output improvement and other intellectual with every new update. In different areas, the RNN is applicable. RNN is composed of three layers, which are the input layer, recurrent hidden layer, and output layer.

3.5 Pseudocode for ERNN Classification

- Step 1: To fix the input part, output part, booster to describe the network.
- Step 2: To normalize the input dataset into values from zero to one through Input.
- Step 3:Choose the training label size and consequently categorize the datasets.
- Step 4: intended for n *times and batch size do*
- *Step*5: *To train the network.*
- Step 6: End for
- Step 7: Run calculation via the trained network
- Step 8: Loss role calculation

4 Performance Analysis

The performance analysis establishes through the simulation of MATLAB software to enhance classification accuracy. Here, the classification accuracy offers the UCI

Table 1 Comparison table of existing methods versus proposed method

Mienye et al. [21]	93	91	93
Oh et al. [22]	97	92.5	98.1
Deng et al. [23]	98.13	98.19	98.09
Proposed ERNN method	98.56	98.60	98.4

machine learning repository based on Cleveland datasets. The Cleveland dataset has information concerning heart disease analysis. The collected data from the Cleveland Clinic Foundation and it is available at the UCI machine learning repository. The performance metrics such as classification accuracy, sensitivity, specificity values help to attain the heart disease prediction whether the given region diseased or not. The proposed method gets compared to the existing heart disease prediction methods are Mienye et al. [21], Oh et al. [22], Deng et al. [23] to evolve the several factors. The comparison table of existing methods Vs. proposed method illustrates in Table 1.

Figures 1, 2, and 3 represent the performance metrics such as accuracy, sensitivity, specificity values and compared to the existing heart disease prediction methods to the proposed method. Here, the several performance metrics values get drawn according to its respective performance. The enriched recurrent neural network (ERNN) classification attained the optimal classification accuracy results. The achieved classification accuracy is 98.56%, the sensitivity value is 98.60%, and the specificity value is 98.4% with efficient achievement.

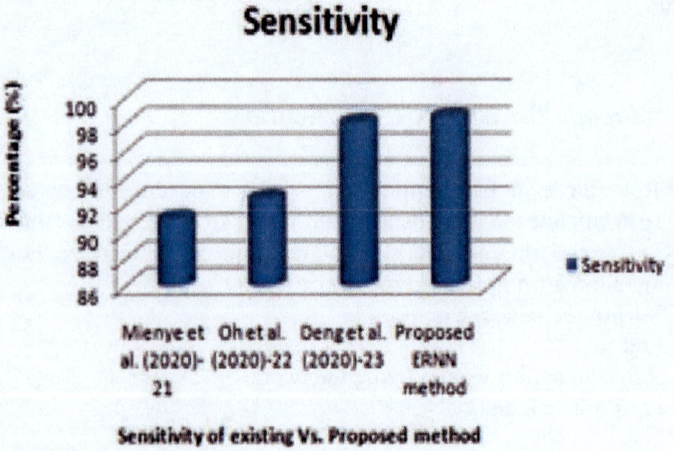

Fig. 2 Sensitivity comparison of existing versus proposed method

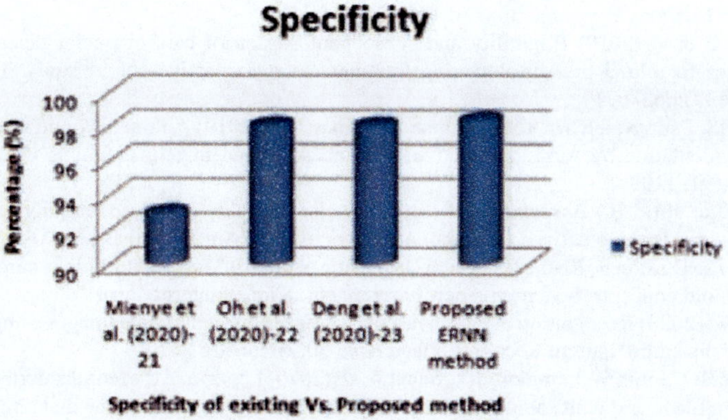

Fig. 3 Specificity comparison of existing versus proposed method

5 Conclusions

Heart disease has significantly become higher when contrast with the precedent decades and has driven out to be the leading cause of fatality. To identify quick and accurate identification, heart disease prediction extremely difficult for health-care experts. Consequently, it is necessary to execute computer proficiency in this investigation to assist healthcare experts in identifying in the early stages with improved prediction accuracy. Here, a prediction of heart diseases using retinal image datasets. By concerning from the UCI machine learning repository based on cleveland heart disease datasets helps to attain the best classification accuracy of cardiovascular disease (CVD). The prediction of CVD consists of given stages that are: Adaptive median filter (AMF) for preprocessing, gray level co-occurrence matrix (GLCM) for feature extraction, indiscriminant component analysis (ICA) for feature selection, and enriched recurrent neural network (ERNN) for classification of given input datasets. The aim to achieve this paper as, the better diagnosis of heart disease with accurate prediction according to its features. The proposed work attained 98.56% of classification accuracy, 98.60% of sensitivity, and 98.4% of specificity. The achieved results compared to the existing CVD prediction methods and the proposed development proves the accurate manner of detection based on the features, i.e., diseased regions.

References

1. Kaptoge S et al (2019) World Health Organization cardiovascular disease risk charts: revised models to estimate risk in 21 global regions. Lancet Glob Health 7(10):e1332–e1345
2. Hervella AS, Rouco J, Novo J, Penedo MG, Ortega M (2020) Deep multi-instance heatmap regression for the detection of retinal vessel crossings and bifurcations in eye fundus images.

Comput Methods Programs Biomed 186:105201
3. Herrett E et al (2019) Eligibility and subsequent burden of cardiovascular disease of four strategies for blood pressure-lowering treatment: a retrospective cohort study. The Lancet 394(10199):663–671
4. Naqvi SS, Fatima N, Khan TM, Rehman ZU, Khan MA (2019) Automatic optic disk detection and segmentation by variational active contour estimation in retinal fundus images. SIViP 13(6):1191–1198
5. Chang J et al (2020) Association of cardiovascular mortality and deep learning-funduscopic atherosclerosis score derived from retinal fundus images. Am J Ophthalmol
6. Farrah TE, Dhillon B, Keane PA, Webb DJ, Dhaun N (2020) The eye, the kidney cardiovascular disease: old concepts, better tools new horizons. In: Kidney international
7. Rajan SP (2020) Recognition of cardiovascular diseases through retinal images using optic cup to optic disc ratio. Pattern Recognit Image Anal 30(2):256–263
8. Ahiante BO, Smith W, Lammertyn L, Schutte AE (2020) Leptin and the retinal microvasculature in young black and white adults: the African-predict study. In: Heart, lung and circulation
9. Zhang Z, Qiu Y, Yang X, Zhang M (2020) Enhanced character-level deep convolutional neural networks for cardiovascular disease prediction. BMC Med Inform Decis Mak 20(3):1–10
10. Patro SP, Padhy N, Chiranjevi D (2020) Ambient assisted living predictive model for cardiovascular disease prediction using supervised learning. In: Evolutionary intelligence, pp 1–29
11. Boscari F et al (2020) Performance of the Steno type 1 risk engine for cardiovascular disease prediction in Italian patients with type 1 diabetes. In: Nutrition, metabolism and cardiovascular diseases
12. Rekha R, Brintha V, Anushree P (2019) Heart disease prediction using retinal fundus image. International conference on artificial intelligence, smart grid and smart city applications. Springer, Heidelberg, pp 765–772
13. Parameswari C, Ranjani SS (2020) Prediction of atherosclerosis pathology in retinal fundal images with machine learning approaches. J Ambient Intell Humanized Comput 1–11
14. Wong KK, Fortino G, Abbott D (2020) Deep learning-based cardiovascular image diagnosis: a promising challenge. Futur Gener Comput Syst 110:802–811
15. Lim G, Bellemo V, Xie Y, Lee XQ, Yip MY, Ting DS (2020) Different fundus imaging modalities and technical factors in AI screening for diabetic retinopathy: a review. Eye and Vision 7:1–13
16. Litjens G et al (2019) State-of-the-art deep learning in cardiovascular image analysis. JACC: Cardiovasc Imaging 12(8):1549–1565
17. Schmidt-Erfurth U, Riedl S, Michl M, Bogunovic´ H (2020) Artificial Intelligence in retinal vascular imaging. In: Retinal vascular disease. Springer, Heidelberg, pp 133–145
18. Benjamins J, Hendriks T, Knuuti J, Juarez-Orozco L, van der Harst P (2019) A primer in artificial intelligence in cardiovascular medicine. Netherlands Heart J 1–9
19. Appaji A et al (2019) Retinal vascular tortuosity in schizophrenia and bipolar disorder. Schizophr Res 212:26–32
20. Amin MS, Chiam YK, Varathan KD (2019) Identification of significant features and data mining techniques in predicting heart disease. Telematics Inform 36:82–93
21. Mienye ID, Sun Y, Wang Z (2020) An improved ensemble learning approach for the prediction of heart disease risk. Inf Med Unlocked 20:100402
22. Oh SL et al (2020) Classification of heart sound signals using a novel deep WaveNet model. In: Computer methods and programs in biomedicine, p 105604
23. Deng Y et al (2020) ST-Net: synthetic ECG tracings for diagnosing various cardiovascular diseases. Biomed Signal Process Control 61:101997

Medical Image Security Using RIW for Grayscale and Color Images

Aishi Pramanik, Aniket Banerjee, Dhrupadi Das, Debashis De, and Sudip Ghosh

Abstract In recent years, the application of reversible image watermarking (RIW) in the field of medical science has significantly increased. In order to ensure medical image security, reversible or lossless watermarking technique is very useful, as it enables the user to embed secret data (or payload), imperceptible to the naked eye, into the host or cover image while the host information is kept intact. As the term "reversible" suggests, it is possible to extract the embedded payload from the image with the watermark to retrieve host image. This becomes crucial for several applications including medical ones. This paper presents a new efficient reversible watermarking scheme that utilizes prediction-error expansion algorithm with the use of location map that has been implemented and tested on grayscale standard as well as special medical images. Further, a novel prediction-error expansion-based reversible watermarking technique with location map has been proposed for RGB color images. Experimental results have been shown on standard and special medical test images. Relevant plots are shown for grayscale as well as RGB color images to assess how well the algorithm performs which demonstrate promising results.

Keywords Reversible image watermarking (RIW) · Prediction-error expansion (PEE) · Location map · Medical image security · PSNR · SSIM · Color image

1 Introduction

Digital watermarking is the method of embedding important data (watermark) into digital image, video, audio to ensure copyright protection, content authentication, broadcast monitoring, etc. In present times, diagnosis using medical images has

A. Pramanik · A. Banerjee · D. Das · S. Ghosh (✉)
IIEST Shibpur, Howrah, West Bengal, India
e-mail: sudip_etc@yahoo.co.in

D. De
Maulana Abul Kalam Azad University of Technology (MAKAUT), Kolkata, West Bengal, India

© The Author(s), under exclusive license to Springer Nature Singapore Pte Ltd. 2023
J. K. Mandal and D. De (eds.), *Frontiers of ICT in Healthcare*, Lecture Notes in Networks and Systems 519, https://doi.org/10.1007/978-981-19-5191-6_47

Fig. 1 Context of a pixel

$m1$	$m2$
$m3$	p

become ubiquitous [1]. By embedding the watermark, distortion is inevitably introduced even if that is imperceptible to human eyes. However, in some specific applications, especially in medical data, even slight modifications in pixel values may be unacceptable [2]. Here comes the importance of reversible data embedding. Medical images such as MRI, CT, PET, X-rays are used in E-healthcare applications [3]. The main purpose of reversible embedding is to ensure a distortion-less or lossless data embedding where the watermark-embedding is performed in such a way that enables the decoder to perfectly restore the content of the original or the cover image along with watermark extraction. Without the use of metadata, this method provides with self-authentication.

The following parameters help in evaluating the performance of a reversible watermarking algorithm, (i) limit of payload capacity that represents the highest number of information bits possible to be embedded, (ii) visual standard that determines how much distortion has occurred after embedding and (iii) the complexity of the reversible data-embedding algorithm.

Section 1 is the brief introduction followed by the literature review of related works in Sect. 2. After that, in Sect. 3, the proposed work is elaborated. Section 4 gives a brief summary about the proposed algorithm for color images. Section 5 describes the experimental results and the analysis of the implementation details.

2 Literature Review of Related Work

Different approaches have been proposed to better the performances based on these parameters, as seen in existing literature. In order to ensure reversibility, additive spread-spectrum techniques based on modulo arithmetic have been deployed in the literature. The extensions of these watermarking techniques are known as type-I algorithm in the existing literature [4–7]. Another popular approach is expansion embedding, which is a reversible data-embedding algorithm with high embedding capacity. This method uses embedding of a bit into a feature element having a small magnitude created by the de-correlating operator. The bits are embedded by expanding these feature elements to create vacancies typically at the least significant bit position where the secret bits are embedded.

Tian proposed the first expansion embedding algorithm in his difference expansion (DE) algorithm [8]. As the name of this method suggests, the difference values of the adjacent pixels of a cover image typically known as high pass components are expanded. In a single pass, considerably larger amounts of data, 2 bpp and close to 0.5, can be embedded using this technique, which outperforms the earlier work in terms of distortion and payload sizes [9]. Tian's algorithm has been further extended by Alattar [10] who proposed DE method for integer transforms.

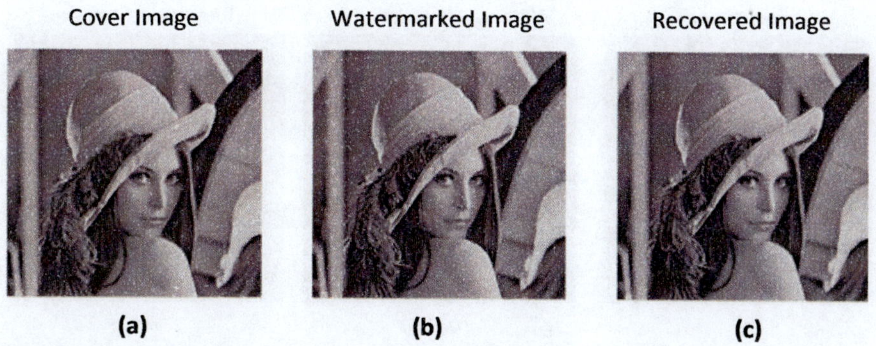

Fig. 2 (a) Grayscale Lena Test Images for Cover, (b) Watermarked and (c) Recovered Image

Thodi and Rodríguez presented a new reversible data-embedding scheme known as prediction-error (PE) expansion [9]. The main advantage of PE over DE is that the magnitude of the feature elements generated by a predictor in PE is smaller than the ones generated by a difference operator in DE [9]. Another advantage of this approach is the use of correlation present in the surrounding of a pixel, unlike difference operators that use the correlation only in the direction of pairing [9]. Hence, Thodi and Rodríguez prediction-error expansion exploits the correlation better than Tian's DE scheme. The better ability of a predictor to de-correlate in case of prediction-error algorithm gives rise to efficient data-embedding capacity, almost twice the maximum embedding capacity than that of the difference expansion algorithm [9]. The feature set also contains significantly large number of feature elements in PE algorithm.

In this paper, Thodi and Rodríguez prediction-error-based algorithm for grayscale image has been implemented. Since most of the medical image watermarking schemes available are for grayscale images, comparatively fewer watermarking algorithms exist in the literature for RGB color medical images [11]. In this paper, a novel prediction-error-based watermarking technique for RGB color images has been proposed and implemented, which is not available in the literature, according to the best of our knowledge.

3 Proposed Methodology

In this reversible watermarking algorithm, a predictor uses a particular algorithm that computes the predicted pixel value $\tilde{p}$ from the neighborhood of a pixel p. Taking the difference of the pixel intensity and the predicted pixel intensity results into the pixel difference d given by the following expression, $d = p - \tilde{p}$.

Now, an information bit b is embedded in the expanded prediction error d as given in the following expression, $d_w = 2d + b$.

Hence, the modified watermarked pixel value is $p_w = \tilde{p} + d_w$.

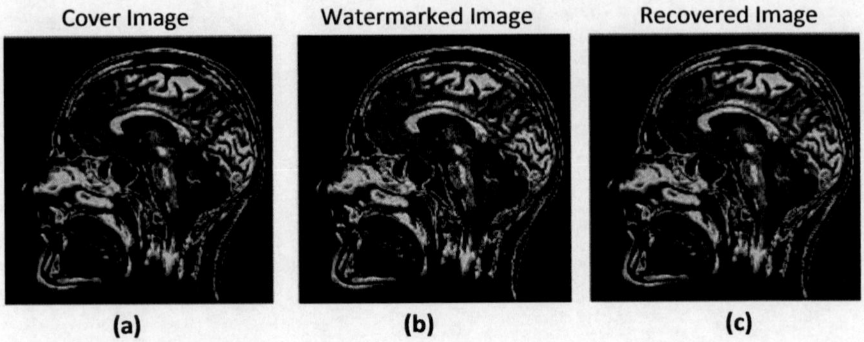

Fig. 3 (a) Medical Test Images for Cover, (b) Watermarked and (c) Recovered Image

3.1 Encoding Algorithm

With the help of this algorithm, predicted pixel value for each pixel is computed from its neighboring pixels defined as context. The complexity of this algorithm is low, and it operates on the pixels at the top-left $m1$, top $m2$ and left $m3$ of the present pixel p, shown in Fig. 1.

$$\tilde{p} = \begin{cases} \max(m2, m3), & \text{if } m1 \leq \min(m2, m3) \\ \min(m2, m3), & \text{if } m1 \geq \max(m1, m3) \\ m2 + m3 - m1, & \text{otherwise} \end{cases}$$

The predicted intensity of the first pixel is considered to be zero because it does not have a context. The context of all the pixels presents in the first row, and the first column has only one pixel. Their predicted intensities are considered to be the same as the pixel intensities of the context. In order to ensure that all the predicted error values are changeable, all the predicted values are set to the even integers.

$$\tilde{p} = 2\tilde{p}/2$$

3.2 Location Map

The predicted pixel intensity at every location is ensured to be an even integer that guarantees all prediction-error intensities are changeable. The prediction-error matrix is a matrix having the same length and width as that of the original image.

The region of invertibility $R_p()$ condition for PE algorithm for an n-bit image representation can be derived as follows:

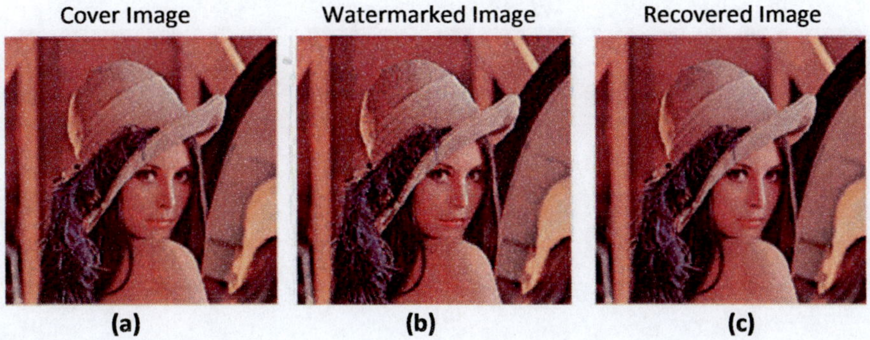

Fig. 4 (a) Colour Lena Test Images for Cover, (b) Watermarked and (c) Recovered Image

$$R_p(\tilde{p}) = \left[-\tilde{p}, 2^n - 1 - \tilde{p}\right]$$

$$|2d + b| \in R_p$$

$$|2d + b| \leq (2^n - 1 - \tilde{p}) \tag{1}$$

The prediction errors which satisfy the condition (1) are expandable prediction errors. Since all the prediction-error values in this matrix are changeable, therefore the matrix is segregated into two sets of prediction-error values.

1. $EN1$—All expandable prediction errors whose value is less than the threshold.
2. $EN2\_CN$—The set $EN2\_CN\_SET$ contains all expandable prediction errors whose value is greater than the threshold but they are treated as changeable prediction errors and set $EN2\_CN\_SET$ also contains all changeable prediction errors, which do not satisfy the condition mentioned in (1).

A 1-bit bitmap (or location map) is created with the expandable prediction-error values. The value 1 is assigned when the prediction-error value lies in the set EN1, and 0 is assigned when the prediction-error value lies in the set $EN2\_CN$. The location map bitstream is compressed losslessly using arithmetic encoding. All the original LSBs of the predicted error values are collected from the $EN2\_CN$ set and compressed using arithmetic encoding.

Total embedding capacity = bit length of $EN1\_SET$ + bit length of $EN2\_CN\_SET$.

Total payload = bit length of compressed local map vector + bit length of encoded LSBs.

The length of the watermark has to be adjusted to satisfy the following condition:

The bit length of the watermark = total embedding capacity − total payload − header length.

Now, all the bitstreams are concatenated to obtain the final embedding stream B as follows-

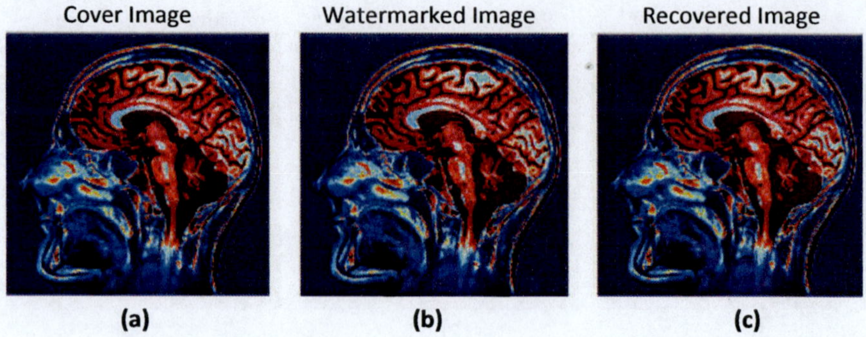

Fig. 5 (a) Colour Medical Test Images for Cover, (b) Watermarked and (c) Recovered Image

$B =$ [Header encoded local map vector encoded LSBs watermark padding].

3.3 Decoding Algorithm

The prediction algorithm used results in the predicted pixel value for any location being an even number. This implies that, in the binary format, the LSB of each predicted value is zero. Hence, in order to extract the embedded bitstream, we can just sequentially collect the LSB of each pixel.

The restoration process for the cover image should be as follows.

Step 1: We begin with restoring the location (1, 1) of the image. For this pixel, we had the predicted value as zero. Therefore, the value of this pixel in the watermarked image is $2d + b$ or $2d/2 + b$, where the error value d is the original pixel intensity. Also, keeping in mind whether the pixel was expandable or changeable, we can say

$$r_{(1,1)} = \frac{p_{w(1,1)}}{2} \quad \text{if expandable}$$

$$r_{(1,1)} = 2\frac{p_{w(1,1)}}{2} + \text{LSB} \quad \text{otherwise}$$

Step 2: In this step, we shall restore the values for the pixels on the top row and the column on the extreme left. For these pixels, we had just one context. For the top-most row, the context was the pixel to the immediate left. We have already restored the original context for the location (1, 2), i.e., the pixel (1, 1). And once we restore it, we have the required context for location (1, 3). This process can be repeated sequentially to have the pixels of the top-most row restored. And the same process is to be followed for the pixels on the left-most column. The computation can be stated as follows:

For the top-most row

$$r_{(1,j)} = \frac{p_{w(1,j)} - b + r_{(1,j-1)}}{2} \quad \text{if expandable}$$

$$r_{(1,j)} = 2\frac{p_{w(1,j)}}{2} + \text{LSB} \quad \text{otherwise}$$

For the top-most column

$$r_{(i,1)} = \frac{p_{w(1,j)} - b + r_{(i-1,1)}}{2} \quad \text{if expandable}$$

$$r_{(1,j)} = 2\frac{p_{w(i,1)}}{2} + \text{LSB} \quad \text{otherwise}$$

Step 3: Once the above two steps are successfully completed, we can just sequentially proceed from the location (2, 2) onwards. We shall observe that we have already restored the three pixels which constitute the context for this pixel. So, we can find the predicted value in the same way we had done before and subtract it from the pixel value in the watermarked image to get the expanded/changed error value. Then, we can restore the pixel intensity as follows:

$$r_{i,j} = \frac{p_{w(i,j)} - \tilde{p}}{2} + \tilde{p} \quad \text{if expandable}$$

$$r_{(i,j)} = 2\frac{p_{w(i,j)}}{2} + \text{LSB} \quad \text{otherwise}$$

Henceforth, we can move on the location (2, 3) and note that we can apply the above procedure to get back the original pixel intensity since we already have the required context. As we proceed to the right, we can keep restoring the pixel intensities of all the locations and then move on to the next row until we have completed restoring the entire picture.

$\boldsymbol{r}_{(x,y)}$ represents the restored image where x, y are the positions.

LSB refers to the least significant bit for the concerned pixel as obtained from the extracted bit stream.

b refers to the information bit obtained from the extracted bitstream that was embedded at the concerned location.

4 Proposed Methodology for RGB Color Images

In today's medical applications, color in medical images such as MRI, ultrasound and many more has drawn a lot of attention. Each color is used to convey some specific meaning in medical applications. In our proposed work for watermarking in RGB

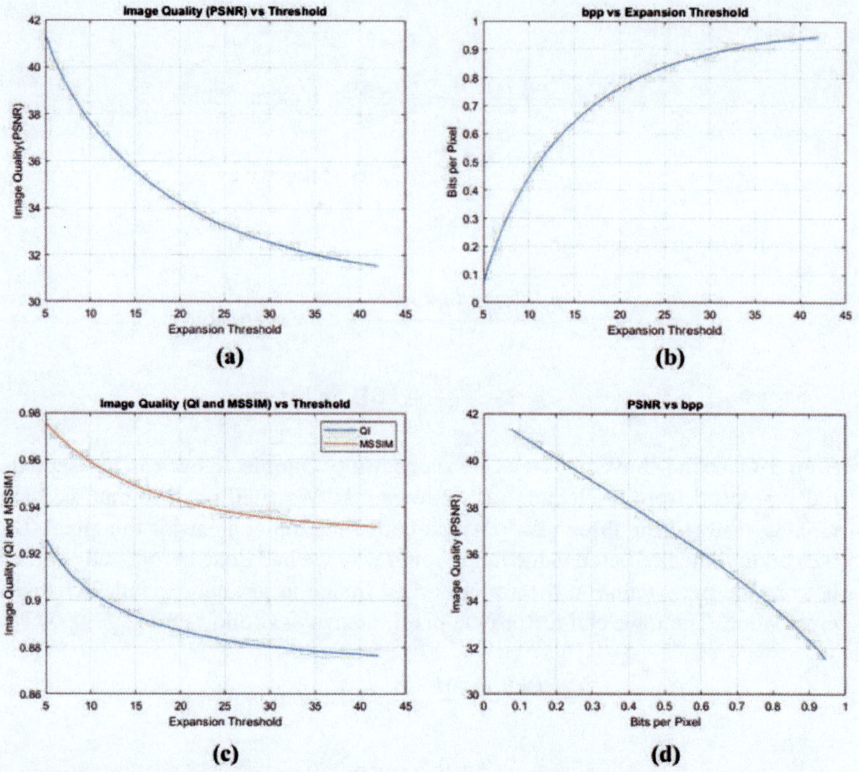

Fig. 6 Plots of grayscale Lena image using our algorithm implementation (512 × 512)

color images, each of the three channels was considered separately and treated like a grayscale image. Then, the PEE algorithm with location map mentioned previously was applied on each of the channels separately and concatenated together.

5 Implementation Details

In this paper, PEE algorithm using location map was implemented on both grayscale and RGB images. The experiments were conducted in MATLAB after embedding a randomly generated bitstreams and then decoding them.

5.1 Test Images

The algorithm was evaluated on standard Lena images (512 × 512) (Figs. 2a and 4a) and special MRI test images (512 × 512) (Figs. 3a and 5a) for both grayscale and RGB.

6 Result Analysis

In this section, PSNR versus expansion threshold (6(a) and 8(a), bits per pixel (bpp) versus expansion threshold (6(b) and 8(b)), image quality index (QI) and mean structural similarity index (MSSIM) versus expansion threshold (6(c) and 8(c)), image quality (PSNR) versus bits per pixel (6(d) and 8(d)) were plotted by varying the operating threshold. PSNR versus bits per pixel has also been plotted. All the plots were plotted using MATLAB for Lena (512 × 512) grayscale as well as RGB images. Comparison of the performances of the proposed algorithm, PEE-based algorithms using median edge detector (MED) predictor and gradient adjusted predictor (GAP) and the PEE-based algorithms proposed by Maity et al. [12] on Lena image gives a better result for the proposed work as shown in Table 1.

Thodi and Rodríguez algorithm [9] is based on prediction error using location map. At payload size of 0.2 bpp, Thodi and Rodriguez algorithm gives 39.07 dB PSNR whereas our implementation results in around 41 dB PSNR value for the grayscale image of Lena. Our algorithm implementation outperforms Thodi and Rodríguez implementation at lower bpp for grayscale Lena image.

From the plots (Figs. 6 and 8), it can be inferred that with increase in the expansion threshold, bits per pixel value increases and image quality gets distorted. It can be justified from the fact that with the increment of expansion threshold, number of expandable prediction error increases. Therefore, the distortion in the watermarked

Table 1 Comparative results of PSNR at different bits per pixel

	PSNR		
Bpp	Proposed work	GAP [12]	MED [12]
0.1	41.07	38.41	33.54
0.2	40.09	34.8	33.01
0.3	39.1	34.75	32.75
0.4	38.1	34.63	32.61
0.5	37.11	34.55	32.5
0.6	36.05	34.53	32.43
0.7	34.94	34.5	32.4
0.8	33.73	34.2	32.27
0.9	32.32	33.9	31.47

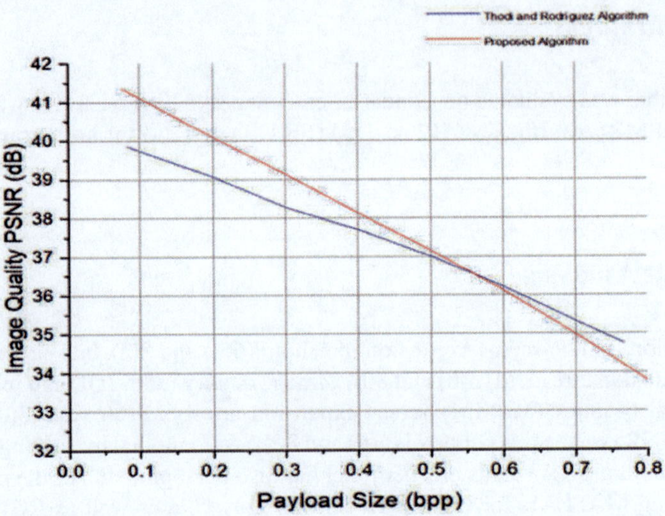

Fig. 7 Performance plot comparison of Thodi and Rodríguez algorithm [9] with our algorithm implementation for Lena grayscale image

image also increases. Again, with the increase of bits per pixel, the image quality (PSNR, QI, SSIM) reduces (Fig. 7).

7 Conclusion

In this paper, a new and efficient RIW technique that utilizes Thodi and Rodríguez prediction-error expansion with location map, has been implemented in MATLAB on grayscale standard test image. Special medical images (MRI scan of brain) have also been tested in this paper. Based on this prediction-error algorithm with location map, a novel reversible watermarking scheme for RGB color images has also been proposed and implemented in MATLAB. Relevant graphs have been plotted by varying the expansion threshold and bits per pixel to evaluate the performance, which shows promising results.

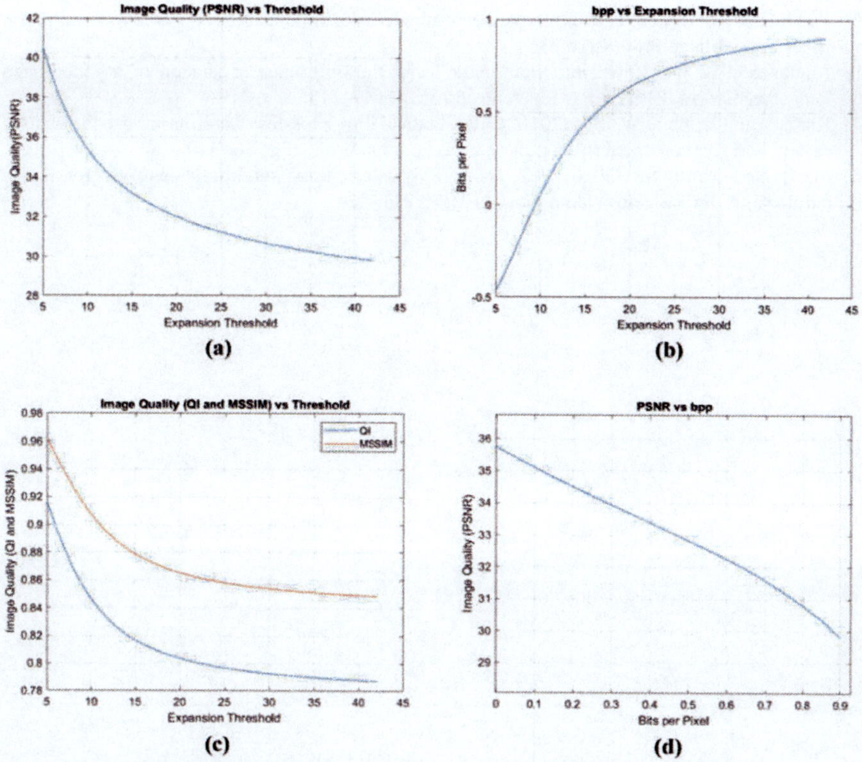

Fig. 8 Plots of RGB color Lena image using our proposed algorithm (512 × 512)

References

1. Kamal ST, Hosny K, Elgindy TM, Darwish M, Fouda MM (2021) A new image encryption algorithm for gray and color medical images. IEEE Access 99:1–1
2. Kelkar V, Tuckley K (2018) Reversible watermarking for medical images with added security using chaos theory. In: Proceedings of the international conference on communication and electronics systems (ICCES)
3. Sivananthamaitrey, Rajesh Kumar PP (2021) Teaching-learning based optimization of dual watermarking of color images
4. Bender W, Gruhl D, Morimoto N, Lu A (1996) Techniques for data hiding. IBM Syst J 35(3):313–336
5. Barton WJM (1997) Method and apparatus for embedding authentication information within digital data. U.S. Patent 5 646 997, 1997
6. Honsinger CW, Jones P, Rabbani M, Stoffel JC (2001) Lossless recovery of an original image containing embedded data. U.S. Patent 6 278 791
7. Macq B (2000) Lossless multi resolution transform for image authenticating watermarking. In: Presented at the European signal processing conference, Tampere, Finland
8. Tian J (2003) Reversible data embedding using a difference expansion. IEEE Trans Circ Syst Video Tech 13(8)

9. Thodi DM, Rodríguez JJ (2007) Expansion embedding techniques for reversible watermarking. IEEE Trans Image Process 16(3)
10. Alattar AM (2004) Reversible watermark using the difference expansion of a generalized integer transform. IEEE Trans Image Proc 13(8):1147–1156
11. Xia Z, Wang X, Zhou W, Li R (2018) Color medical image lossless watermarking using chaotic system and accurate quaternion polar harmonic transforms. Sig Proc 157
12. Maity HK, Maity SP (2016) PEE based RW using fuzzy conditional entropy for image partitioning. Int J Electron Commun (AEÜ)70:211–224

Feather-Light Vessel Segregation Model

Shirsendu Dhar, Sumit Mukherjee, Ranjit Ghoshal, and Bibhas Chandra Dhara

Abstract Ophthalmic disorders like glaucoma, diabetic retinopathy, hypertension can be easily identified by examining the vascular structure of the retina. This makes vessel segregation of fundus images very important for the detection and diagnosis of similar diseases. There are challenges, especially given a large amount of noise and the diverse structures of thin vessels. This article has created an innovative approach to the extraction of vascular structures for the detection and diagnosis of a wide variety of eye diseases. First, we use a variety of image processing techniques to help you extract the features you need. The next step is to build the model using the Extreme Gradient Boosting algorithm using the data extracted from different techniques earlier. All of these models are tested on other image sets and an accuracy rating is calculated. A larger model is prepared based on the accuracy rating. From that the less significant features are removed without compromising the performance. The model results are analyzed using standard scoring parameters and prove to be one of the best in the class.

Keywords Ophthalmic disorders · Retina · Vascular extraction · Extreme Gradient Boosting · Feature extraction

S. Dhar
Fractal Analytics, Bengaluru 560103, India

S. Mukherjee (✉)
Tata Consultancy Services, Kolkata 700156, India
e-mail: sum.mukherjee@gmail.com

R. Ghoshal
St. Thomas' College of Engineering and Technology, Kolkata 700023, India

B. Chandra Dhara
Jadavpur University, Kolkata 700098, India

© The Author(s), under exclusive license to Springer Nature Singapore Pte Ltd. 2023
J. K. Mandal and D. De (eds.), *Frontiers of ICT in Healthcare*, Lecture Notes in Networks and Systems 519, https://doi.org/10.1007/978-981-19-5191-6_48

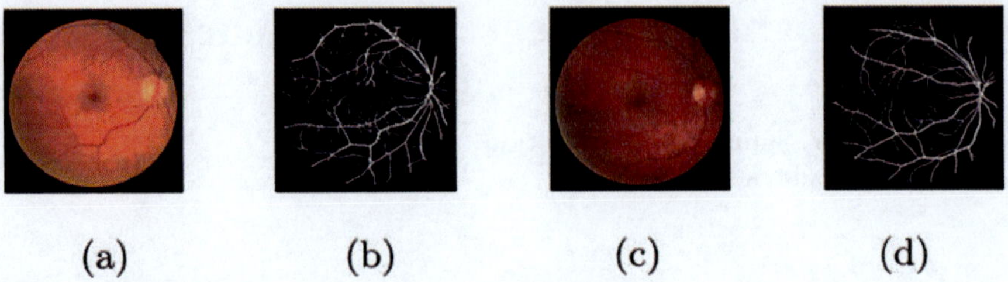

Fig. 1 **a**, **c** RGB retinal images, **b**, **d** associated ground truths

1 Introduction

An ophthalmoscopic examination (Fig. 1) uses an advanced ophthalmoscope to allow a doctor to examine the fundus and other components to analyze various eye problems. Structural orientation of retinal vessels is an important diagnostic indicator for many eye problems. Therefore, it is highly recommended to separate out blood vessels from images of the retinal fundus to obtain insight about eye-related diseases.

The presence of different components in small blood vessels with many structures complicates the technique of retinal blood vessel extraction. The purpose of this article is to solve these complex problems. Morphological techniques are used in traditional approaches to clear out noise from images, which destroy the granular characteristics of blood vessels and often alter the vascular structure. Therefore, morphological techniques can cause additional errors and are not recommended when making important decisions. Here, an attempt to build a lightweight model to extract blood vessels without affecting the granular structure so that important decisions could be made based on output without taking too much processing power.

Several techniques have been proposed, including matching filters [1], to enhance the contrast and separability of blood vessels from the background and facilitate continuous blood vessel recognition. Marin et al. [2] proposed deep learning to classify functions based on grayscale and moment invariants. Ricci et al. [3] to train support vector machines (SVMs). The proposition was to use two orthogonal line operators as feature vectors, the pixels were classified into vascular and non-vascular pixels using SVM. In a recent study by Frucci et al. [4], several directional map-based approaches were used. Oliveira et al. [5] employed a fully convolutional neural network (CNN) that can generate the astounding results.To convey semantic information between output layers, Guo et al. [6] proposed a deeply trained multi-scale and multilevel CNN with short links for vessel segregation, and short links were used. This article also showed a new formulation of a patch-based complete CNN that results in more accurate segmentation of retinal vessels. By using the skip CNN architecture, which has lost local entropy sampling and class balancing, full patch-based CNN training has been improved and the entire process has been accelerated. Liskowski et al. [7] used a deep neural network pre-processed with global contrast normalization, null phase whitening, and trained with a huge sample of examples enhanced with geometric correction and gamma correction with a recently monitored segmentation technique. In the proposed method, 41 different filters (32 Gabor filter variations, Canny Edge, Roberts Edge, Sobel Edge, Scharr Edge, Prewill Edge, Sigma 3 and 7 Gaussian, Sigma 3 and 7 Median and Variance filter was used on all the image. Then, along with the 41 filtered images above, the original and the ground truth image are expanded into one dimension matrix, from which a data-frame is formed. Here, the N models, each of their corresponding N image datase, are trained in their respective data-frames and applied to the remaining $N - 1$ images to calculate the corresponding accuracy of each model. Based on the results of these accuracies, the top $3N/4$ images were selected, the model was rated the best, and the final model was built using the XGBoost algorithm in the combined data-frame of these images. The following is a breakdown of the structure of this article. Image extraction by 41 methods is shown in Sect. 2. How XGBoost works is explained in Sect. 3. Section 4 describes the process of selecting and merging the top $3N/4$ (In this case 15) images and how to reduce the functionality to improve test time without impacting performance. Section 5 examines the performance of the proposed method. Section 6 concludes the article.

2 Feature Extraction

The proposed vessel extraction approach may be broken down into a few basic steps. To extract vessels from a retinal fundus image, first transform the image from RGB to green channels, which provides the best contrast for blood vessels (Fig. 2). The idea behind this method is that the original image will go through a series of filters and processing steps that will result in a final output that is close to the ground truth image. Weights will be assigned to the filters or processing that will allow this advised strategy to achieve the intended goal. Filers have been used in the proposed work listed below.

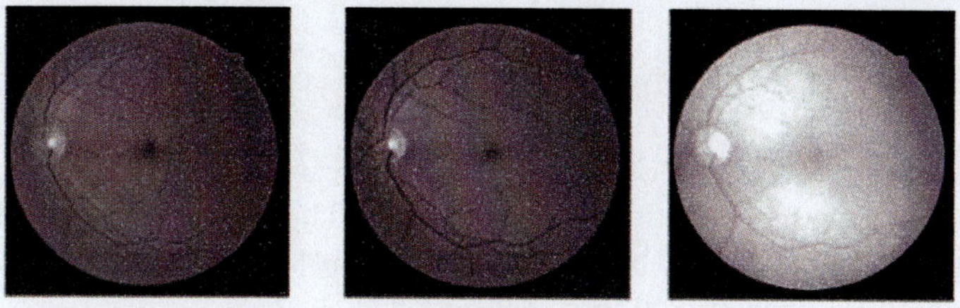

(a) (b) (c)

Fig. 2 **a–c** are the red, green and blue channels of the RGB image

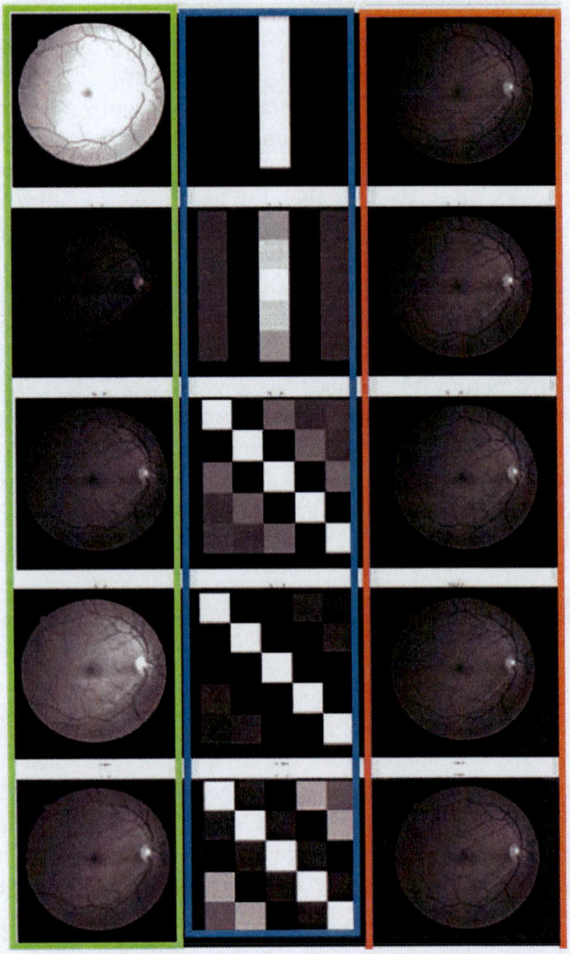

Fig. 3 Green channel of the Retinal Fundus images are in Lime marked box, Gabor kernels are presented in Turquoise marked box, corresponding images after using gabour kernels are in Orange marked box

2.1 32 Gabor Filters

Gabor Filters, in the context of image processing can be used in texture analysis, edge detection, feature extraction which can be used by machine learning algorithm for training purposes. The Gabor Filters are band pass filters, i.e., they will allow certain band of frequencies and reject others (Fig. 3).

1	0
0	-1

(a)

0	1
-1	0

(b)

Fig. 4 **a, b** are the 2 Robert Mask to detect the 2 diagonals

-1	0	1
-2	0	2
-1	0	1

(a)

1	2	1
0	0	0
-1	-2	-1

(b)

-1	0	1
-1	0	1
-1	0	1

(c)

1	1	1
0	0	0
-1	-1	-1

(d)

Fig. 5 **a, b** are the vertical and horizontal Sobel masks, **c, d** are the vertical and horizontal Prewitt masks

2.2 *The Different Edge Detectors*

Edge Detectors are simply used to locate areas in an image where there is an abrupt change in intensity or color. A high value indicates a steep change and low indicates shallow. The following figure represents PoI or Pixel of Interest, that would give idea about neighborhood, collection of pixels in matrix form.

Roberts Masks are used to detect the diagonals, which an improvement to the ordinary masks which detects only the horizontal and vertical masks. The masks representation are in Fig. 4. Being an even mask and having less neighborhood and small size (2×2), it carries a slight disadvantage.

To counter these disadvantages, Sobel and Prewitt masks comes (Fig. 5). The Sobel mask has two kernels (3×3 matrix), corresponding to horizontal and vertical direction. These two kernels are convoluted with the original image through which the edge points are calculated. This approach works through calculation of the gradient of the image intensity at every pixel within the image.

The Prewitt mask is similar to the Sobel but with minor difference. The Prewitt operator shall give the values which are symmetric around the center, unlike Sobel operator which gives more weight to the point which is closer to (x, y). The fig represents Prewitt x and y operator values.

Scharr Filter is a filtering method used to identify and highlight edges and features using the 1st derivative. Typically this is used to identify the gradients along the x-axis ($dx = 1$, $dy = 0$) and y-axis ($dx = 0$, $dy = 1$) independently. This is quite similar to the Sobel filter. Figure 6 shows edge filter effects.

Canny Edge, another edge detection technique, suppresses the noise while detecting the edges flawlessly, which is limited to gray scale images only. In this process,

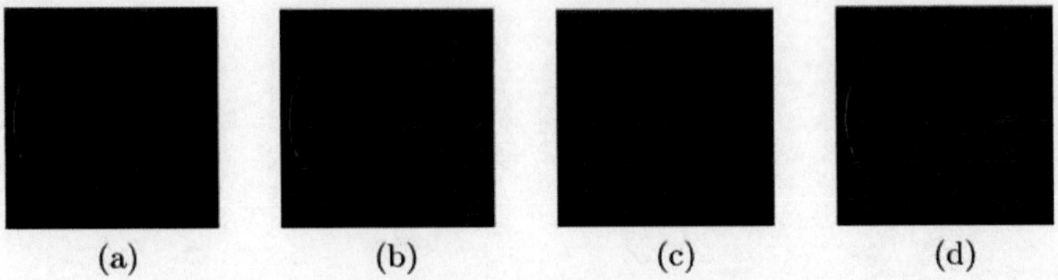

Fig. 6 **a–d** are the edge detected images by Prewitt, Sobel, Roberts and Scharr Masks, respectively

Fig. 7 **a** is the Retinal Fundus RGB image and **b** is the corresponding canny edge image

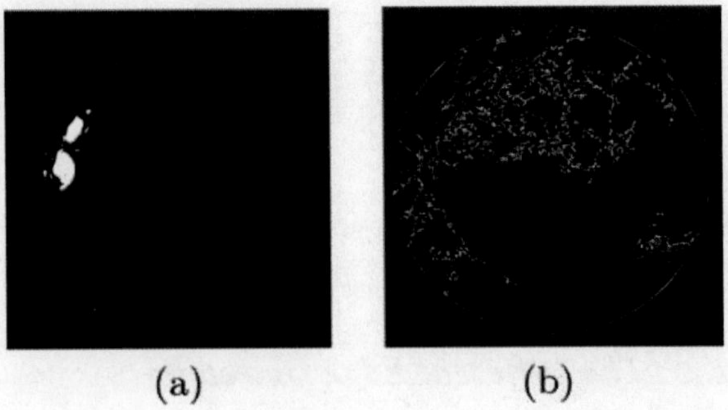

the image is processed by Gaussian Blur, which removes the noise, making it smooth and enabling further process to be flawless. The second step is Intensity Gradient Calculation. The Canny Edge transformation in Fig. 7.

2.3 *Blurring Methods*

Blur Filters, soften a selection of pixels or an image and are useful for retouching. They smooth the transition by averaging the color values. Gaussian Blur or smoothing is the result of blurring an image by a Gaussian function. The visual effect of this technique is a smooth blur resembling that of viewing through a translucent screen. The median filter is a noise reduction technique, used as a pre-treatment step to boost the outcomes of future approaches. It removes different noises from images and smooth them out. Neighborhood averaging can suppress isolated out-of-range noise, but the side effect is that it also blurs sudden changes such as line features, sharp edges and other details. It is an effective method that can, to some extent, distinguish out-of-range isolated noise from legitimate image features such as edge lines.

3 XGBoost

"Extreme Gradient Boosting" is a supervised-based algorithm, where the use of training data (with multiple features) x_i is used to predict a target variable y_i. It is built on decision trees concept. Decision tree ensembles models consists of a set of classification and regression trees (CART), where each leaf or node represents a test. The existing data is classified into different leaves and assign them the score on the corespondent leaf. In CART, which is a bit different decision trees, the leaves contain the real score associated with it, which gives us a richer interpretation that goes beyond classification.

Usually, a single tree is not found to be that effective in practice. So, instead of that, an ensemble model is used which sums the prediction of multiple trees together.

Both Random Forest and XGBoost shares Tree ensembles as their common feature.They differ in the manner in which they are trained. Boosting builds models from individual decision trees or "weak learners" in an iterative way. But unlike Random Forest, individual models are not completely built on random subsets of data or features. Instead, in boosting, more weight is put on individual models in a sequential way, in another words, learns from past mistakes. The name Gradient comes from Gradient Boosting, the same algorithm deep learning uses to find the minima in the loss function. Due to its high performance, in addition to less training time and size, its used as an alternative to deep learning algorithms. To optimize the normal boosting, it uses tricks like computation of 2nd order gradients to figure out the direction of gradients. It also uses L1 and L2 regularization to prevent over-fitting. Parallel computing makes this super fast.

4 Algorithm: Way of Working

As there are only 20 images in the DRIVE dataset, which is considerably low to train any model, so dataset is needed to be handled carefully. So at first 41 different filters or extraction techniques are defined. Each image is then processed through and then flattened out. Then for every image, a model was trained based on the cross-sectional data of that image. After creating 20 such models, each model was tested on the total set of images (20).

On the basis of the mean accuracy, the top $3N/4$ images (75 of the total set) was taking for the training set and rest 5 was for testing. With this approach the effects of outliers have been muted as much as possible. Upon building the model, further modifications were made to filter out the less significant features.

One of the many features of XGBoost it has over deep learning is its not a black box, and thus we can see how much each features importance is in the final model. This helps us to select a threshold (in this case 95%), and the features that contribute to that total will be kept, rest all are discarded. This helps boosting the training time

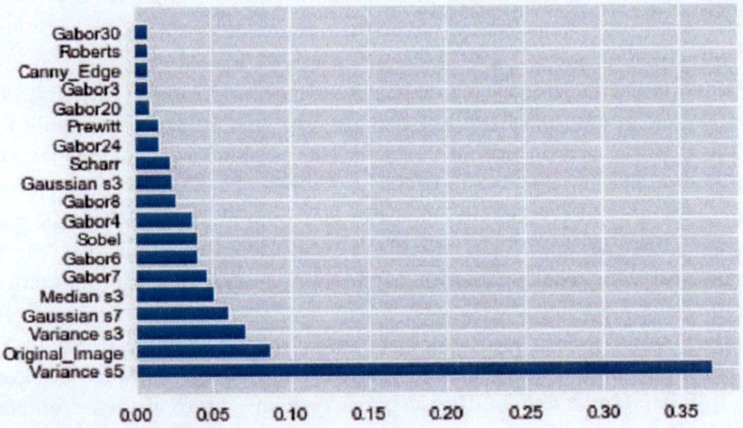

Fig. 8 Model feature importance of the top 19 features

further, also making the model size small in exchange of little accuracy. In Fig. 8 top 19 features that makes more than 95% of the model are shown.

The algorithmic steps are detailed out below:

1. Images are processed through 41 different filters as described in Sect. 2.
2. Then, output of the 41 filters, the original image and the ground truth image are unwrapped into a single dimension data-frame.
3. Now, N models, each of the those N images are trained on their respective data-frames.
4. Each model is fed with the rest of the $(N - 1)$ images and the corresponding accuracy is considered as score. On the basis of scores, the top $3N/4$ images, whose models scored the highest are selected, and the final model is built on by using the XGBoost classification on the combined data-frames of these images.
5. On the basis of feature importance, the top features having cumulative importance of 95% are kept, and the rest are discarded.

5 Analysis and Evaluation of Results

This experiment is conducted on globally available DRIVE dataset[1] of retinal fundus images. It includes 20 train and test images, as well as the ground truth result. The images were captured as part of a Dutch diabetic retinopathy screening program. This 40-image set is broken into two sets, each with 20 images: test and training.

[1] DRIVE dataset is available at http://www.isi.uu.nl/Research/Databases/DRIVE/download.php.

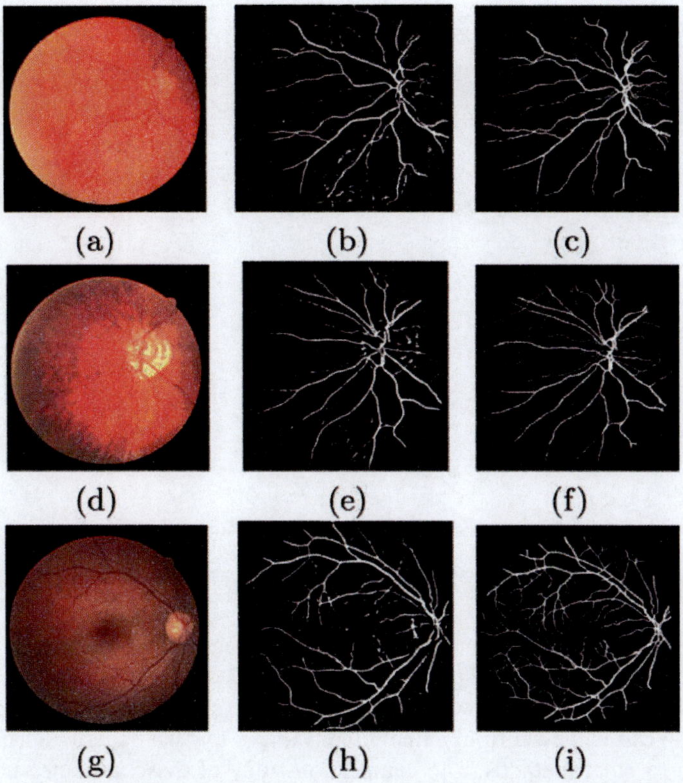

Fig. 9 **a**, **d**, **g** are the RGB images from DRIVE. **b**, **e**, **h** are the proposed model output. **c**, **f**, **i** are the respective Ground truth images

Output of the proposed method on some of the test images are shown in Fig. 9 with their corresponding RGB and ground truth images. To test the performance of the proposed method, following parameters have been considered: sensitivity, specificity and accuracy. The pixel classes are defined as follows:

Y: The pixel is $white$ on ground truth as well as on the model output
$\hat{Y}$: The pixel is $black$ on ground truth as well as on the model output
N: The pixel is $black$ on ground truth and $white$ on the model output
$\hat{N}$: The pixel is $white$ on ground truth and $black$ on the model output.

Based on the pixel distribution among classes $Y, \hat{Y}, N, \hat{N}$ the attributes sensitivity, specificity and accuracy are determined as:

$$\text{Sensitivity} = \frac{Y}{Y + \hat{N}}$$

Table 1 Vessel separation result comparison

References	Sensitivity	Specificity	Accuracy
Martin et al. [2]	0.7067	0.9801	0.9452
Miri et al. [8]	0.7155	0.9765	0.9435
Singh et al. [9]	0.7138	0.9801	0.9460
Fu et al. [10]	0.7603	N.A	0.9523
Oliveira et al. [5]	0.7810	0.9800	0.9543
Guo et al. (FS-DSN) [6]	0.7756	0.9802	0.9542
Guo et al. (S-DSN) [6]	**0.7893**	0.9789	0.9547
Proposed method	0.6464	**0.9886**	**0.9574**

$$\text{Specificity} = \frac{\hat{Y}}{\hat{Y} + N}$$

$$\text{Accuracy} = \frac{Y + \hat{N}}{Y + \hat{Y} + N + \hat{N}}$$

These proposed attributes are formulated to measure the similarity between ground truth map and a vessel probability map. The results of the experiments were compared with those of other works. On comparing, it shows that we have developed a method to extract vessel from retinal fundus image that has superior accuracy and specificity to other methods. The comparison study of these attributes have been presented in Table 1.

6 Future Prospects and Conclusion

The scheme proposed in this article uses a collection of 19 image filter and Extreme Gradient Boosting to segregate retinal vessels. This method is effective in removing most of the noise with high precision. But doing that it loses a bit of its ability to predict the vessels in some parts. The advantage of this method is that it builds the model by choosing the best images using a mixed data set of filters in a relatively very small dataset (20). This model provides 95% accuracy, which is quite good considering the dataset size, is very fast and lightweight (381 kB). In terms of its efficiency, strength and ease of use, the proposed method is a good candidate for introduction into pre-screening programs for the clinical prognosis of ophthalmic diseases.

References

1. Cinsdikici M, Aydin D (2009) Detection of blood vessels in ophthalmoscope images using MF/ant (matched filter/ant colony) algorithm. Comput Methods Prog Biomed 96:85–95
2. Marin D, Aquino A, Gegndez-Arias ME, Bravo JM (2011) A new unsupervised method for blood vessel segmentation in retinal images by using gray-level and moment invariants-based features. IEEE Trans Med Imaging 30(1):146–158
3. Ricci E, Perfetti R (2007) Retinal blood vessel segmentation using line operators and support vector classification. IEEE Trans Med Imaging 26(10):1357–1365
4. Frucci M, Riccio D, Sanniti di Baja G, Serino L (2016) SEVERE, segmenting vessels in retina images. Pattern Recogn Lett 82:162–169
5. Oliveira A, Pereira S, Silva CA (2017) Augmenting data when training a CNN for retinal vessel segmentation: How to warp? In: IEEE 5th Portuguese meeting on bioengineering (ENBENG), Coimbra, pp 1–4. https://doi.org/10.1109/ENBENG.2017.7889443
6. Guo S, Gao Y, Wang K, Li T (2018) Deeply supervised neural network with short connections for retinal vessel segmentation. arXiv:1803.03963v1 [cs.CV], 11 Mar 2018
7. Liskowski P, Krawiec K (2016) Segmenting retinal blood vessels with deep neural networks. IEEE Trans Med Imaging 35(11):2369–2380. https://doi.org/10.1109/TMI.2016.2546227
8. Miri MS, Mahloojifar A (2011) Retinal image analysis using curvelet transform and multi-structure elements morphology by reconstruction. IEEE Trans Biomed Eng 58(5):1183–1192
9. Singh D, Dharmveer, Singh B (2014) A new morphology based approach for blood vessel segmentation in retinal images. In: 2014 annual IEEE India conference (INDICON), Dec 2014, pp 1-6
10. Fu H, Xu Y, Lin S, Wong DWK, Liu J (2016) Deepvessel: retinal vessel segmentation via deep learning and conditional random field. In: International conference on medical image computing and computer-assisted intervention, pp 132–139

Hyperspectral Image Segmentation Using Balanced Entropic Thresholding

Radha Krishna Bar, Somnath Mukhopadhyay, and Debasish Chakraborty

Abstract Hyperspectral Image contains hundreds of continuous bands. This large number of bands leads to "Curse of dimensionality" problem. Segmentation of such hyperspectral image is a difficult task due to strongly co-related bands and ambiguous multiple regions of interest. In last few years a number of algorithms were proposed to segment Hyperspectral Image (HSI). In this paper we first reduce the bands in HSI using cuckoo search approach. Then the reduced banded HSI is segmented using the same approach. For the reduction of bands Band Co-relation (BS) is used as objective function. Tsallis Entropy (TE) and Rényi Entropy (RE) are considered combinedly to design a new objective function for segmentation. To asses the efficiency of proposed technique, experiments are done with Indian Pine dataset which captured by AVIRIS sensor and University of Pavia dataset obtained from ROSIS sensor. Three indices are used to assess the classification results: overall accuracy (OA), average accuracy (AA), and kappa coefficient (KC). The proposed method's strength is demonstrated by a comparison with two other approaches.

Keywords Hyperspectral images segmentation · Cuckoo search · Tsallis entropy · Rényi entropy

1 Inroduction

Recent developments in imaging techniques provide an opportunity to explores HSI deeply. The Hyperspectral sensors can acquire spectral information within hundreds small and contentious bands, encompassing wide variety of wavelengths in spectrum. In the study of remote sensing, increased availability of hyperspectral images has been a great success. HSIs are three-dimensional image cubes where the third dimension signifies spectral band that contain a large quantity of spectral, spatial

R. Krishna Bar (✉) · S. Mukhopadhyay
Department of Computer Science and Engineering, Assam University, Silchar, India
e-mail: rdhk_bar@yahoo.co.in

D. Chakraborty
RRSC-East, Indian Space Research Organization, Kolkata, India

© The Author(s), under exclusive license to Springer Nature Singapore Pte Ltd. 2023
J. K. Mandal and D. De (eds.), *Frontiers of ICT in Healthcare*, Lecture Notes in Networks and Systems 519, https://doi.org/10.1007/978-981-19-5191-6_49

information that may be utilized to distinguish and classify spectrally unique objects [1]. Because of the presence of huge spectral-signatures and spatial information in HSI, they are potential for mapping of land-cover and detection [2, 3]. The purpose of image segmentation is to split the image into several homogeneous-region in such a way that no two adjacent regions are similar when integrated. Hyperspectral image segmentation is challenging because of confusing regions, weak local co-relation amongst pixels and smaller abundant regions of interest. In their work, the researchers observed challenges identifying agricultural areas from satellite images due to bad resolution, bad illumination, as well as severe environmental conditions that occurred when acquiring the images [4]. Optimization algorithms were introduced with the goal of solving the difficult issues like these with limited time and minimal resources. Hyperspectral image segmentation algorithms can be categorized into two approaches: Deep Learning-based Approach and Nature Inspired Approach.

1.1 Deep Learning Based Approach

Many recent studies [5–7] have attempted to use deep learning for HSI classification. Deep learning orinted algorithms may be divided into two types based on whether pixels in the immediate vicinity are investigated in deep networks: spectral-spatial-based methods and spectral-based methods. For HSI classification, spectral-based approaches look at the spectral characteristics of a single pixel [8]. However, the spatial information of the hyperspectral image is neglected in the spectral-based method [9]. Typically spectral-spatial methods use adjacent utilized hyperspectral pixels for HSI classification [10, 11]. Each pixel in an HSI may have the similar land-cover category like its neighbours [12, 13]. These neighbouring pixels can help to categorize the hyperspectral pixel by providing important spatial information.The traditional neural network is the mostly used deep network for spectral-spatial-based approaches [14]. The HSI cube is formed by cropping adjacent pixels inside a square region from original images to look into the spatial information of a hyperspectral pixel. Although CNN-based approaches have demonstrated to perform better in recent studies [15], CNN-based techniques still have limited generalization ability on complex layouts of land-cover [16]. Recent CNN-based algorithms [16] typically assume that neighbouring pixels belong to same land-cover category. According to this concept, HSI are intently cropped into a large number of hyperspectral cubes for classification in CNN-based algorithms [17]. A cropped HSI cube's land-cover label is first defined for training by its centre pixel. For starts, a cropped HSI cube's land-cover label is approximately specified for training by its centre pixel.

1.2 Nature Inspired Approach

Inspired from nature of swarm towards food finding tendency was introduced an evolutionary algorithm Particle Swarm algorithm (PSO). For hyperspectral and multispectral image segmentation, Martins et al. [19] employed Particle swarm optimization (FODPSO) based on fractional order. Population-based optimization method that emulates attraction of a firefly to flashing light was introduce by Brajevic and Tuba [20]. Wang et al. [21] introduced an enhanced form of the firefly algorithm (FA) that improved convergence rate for several global numerical optimizations. When the algorithm was evaluated on images, the results were not satisfactory. Based on histogram, a multilevel thresholding technique driven by the firefly algorithm approach using Brownian distribution is suggested by Raja et al. [22]. By maximizing between-class variance, the algorithm arrived at the best threshold values. In terms of segmentation quality, the test results demonstrated that the proposed technique outperformed the classic firefly algorithm.

Chen et al. [23] suggested a customized firefly algorithm that featured a diversity improved global exploration approach and a neighbourhood search method for improved local solution space exploitation. It beat DPSO, FA, Differential Evolution algorithms for normal experimental images, but it is is not so efficient for segmentation of satellite image at greater thresholding settings [23]. Akay designed the ABC and PSO methods for multilevel thresholding in [24] by improving Kapur's entropy function. However,the technique is susceptible to a condition known as earlier convergence, that prohibited it to reach global optima. Alihodzic and Tuba [25] suggested a strategy for multilayer image thresholding by combining the Bat algorithm with parts from the DE and ABC algorithms. Dimensionality reduction followed by clustering can be beneficial in some cases [26].

From the literature survey it is found that Tsallis Entropy is already employed to form the objective function of hyperspectral image segmentation. Tsallis entropic functions is efficient in some particular aspect. But that was not a generalized solution. Researchers were unable to determine whether a specific entropic function is more efficient than others in general. From this we are motivated to propose a general objective function. That's why we consider both Renyi's entropy as well as Tsallis Entropy to formulate the objective function for segment the HSI. In this research work, firstly we deal with the high dimensionality of HSI by reducing the number of bands by cuckoo search algorithm. Then the reduced banded image is segmented by multilevel thresholding method using the same approach. For band reduction we considered band correlation as objective function. To design objective function of segmentation we considered Tsallis Entropy and Rényi Entropy.

Related works are described in next section. The proposed approach is discussed in Sect. 3. In Sect. 4 we have compared the results of the proposed techniques with two other existing approaches CPSO [27] and ELM [28].

2 Related Work

2.1 Cuckoo Search Algorithm

Yang and Deb [26] introduced CS, a population-based bio-inspired metaheuristic algorithm, as a solution to global optimization challenges. The breeding behaviour of several cuckoo species helped pave the way for Cuckoo Search. Cuckoo birds lay their eggs in other birds' nests. If a cuckoo egg is found by the host bird, the foreign eggs are either thrown away or the nest is abandoned and a new nest is made. In the normal Cuckoo Search approach, every egg of the host species in a nest denotes a solution, but an egg represents a new solution. When a new solution proves to be superior to the one in the nest, it will be implemented. So, the following three main rules guide the development of the CS algorithm: (1) Each cuckoo lays one egg in a nest chosen at random. (2) The best nest with the best eggs is passed down to the next generation. (3) There is a set number of available host's nests. The new solutions are generated by the LÉvy Flight function.

2.2 *LÉvy Flight Function*

The cuckoo egg is determined by the host bird using a probability of $P_a \in [0, 1]$. When an animal detects a cuckoo egg, the nest may be abandoned or the egg discarded, and a new nest constructed. Initially, the random nest position represents a potential solutions, X_i for a cuckoo i are created. By using Lévy flight random walk, a new solution $X_{i+1}$is created from Eq. 1

$$X_{i+1} = X_i + \alpha \otimes levy(\lambda) \tag{1}$$

where α denotes scalling factor for step size having a positive value. $\otimes$ denotes the entry wise multiplication.The random walks having random size of steps that is simulated from LÉvy distribution is denoted by $levy$ and expressed as Eq. 2

$$levy(\lambda) = \frac{x}{|y|^{\frac{1}{\beta}}} \tag{2}$$

x, y are stochastic variables which are distributed normally. ($x \simeq N(0, \sigma_x^2)$) and ($y \simeq N(0, \sigma_y^2)$). The random matrix of standard deviation is as Eq. 3

$$\sigma_x(\beta) = \left[\frac{\Gamma(1+\beta)\sin(\frac{\pi\beta}{2})}{\Gamma\left(\frac{1+\beta}{2}\right)\beta 2^{\frac{(\beta-1)}{2}}} \right] \tag{3}$$

and $\sigma_y = 1$. Γ is a standard gamma function.

2.3 Tsallis Entropy

Constantino Tsallis introduced the Tsallis entropy measure, which is a variation of the Boltzmann-Gibbs entropy. A non-extensive system driven by the entropy formula described in Eq. 4 is a generalization of Tsallis' entropy measure using the multi-fractal theory.

$$S_q = \frac{1 - \sum_{n=1}^{k} p_n^q}{q - 1} \tag{4}$$

The system's probability to be in state n denoted by p_i which distributed between 0 and 1. It denotes number of unique intensity levels in grayscale photographs. Tsallis parameter is used to describe the measurement of non-extensivity of the system and denoted by q. Pseudo additivity entropy rule is described as Eq. 5.

$$S_q(f_g^c + b_g^c) = S_q(f_g^c) + S_q(b_g^c) + (1 - q).S_q(f_g^c).S_q(b_g^c) \tag{5}$$

b_g, f_g represent the back ground and fore ground of an image. For multilevel thresholding Tsallis entropy is expressed as following equations.

$$S_q^{c_0}(t) = \frac{1 - \sum_{n=0}^{t_1-1}\left(\frac{p_n^c}{\sum_{n=0}^{t_1-1} p_n^c}\right)}{q - 1} \tag{6}$$

$$S_q^{c_1}(t) = \frac{1 - \sum_{n=t_1}^{t_2-1}\left(\frac{p_n^c}{\sum_{n=t_1}^{t_2-1} p_n^c}\right)}{q - 1} \tag{7}$$

$$S_q^{c_j}(t) = \frac{1 - \sum_{n=t_j}^{t_{j+1}-1}\left(\frac{p_n^c}{\sum_{n=t_j}^{t_{j+1}-1} p_n^c}\right)}{q - 1} \tag{8}$$

$$S_q^{c_m}(t) = \frac{1 - \sum_{n=t_m}^{N-1}\left(\frac{p_n^c}{\sum_{n=t_m}^{L-1} p_n^c}\right)}{q - 1} \tag{9}$$

2.4 Renyi's Entropy

Renyi's entropy is a generalized version of Shannon's entropy that includes an adjustable parameter α. The metric of informational coolness is very generic and adaptable, and when $x = 1$ Renyi's entropy become Shannon's entropy. it is represented as

$$R_E = \sum_{n=0}^{m} R_\alpha(A_n) \tag{10}$$

α denotes a control parameter having positive value. A_i represents the Shanon entropy's elicitation. Following Eq. 11 is used to calculate it.

$$R_\alpha = \frac{1}{1-\alpha} \ln \sum_{n=1}^{L} P_n^\alpha \tag{11}$$

A probability distribution of the $n^t h$ state is represented by P_ni. The total number of thresholds is denoted by the letter L. R_E is a maximizing function as well.

3 Proposed Methodology

To deal with the huge number of bands in HSI, firstly the band reduction is done. Then the reduced banded image is segmented. For both the purpose cuckoo search optimization approach is employed. For band reduction we use Band Correlation as objective function. Researchers were unable to establish particular entropic function

Algorithm 1 Method for Band Selection

Require: Hyperspectral image.
Ensure: Reduced banded Hyperspectral image

```
Start
Generate an initial-population having n host nests X_i (Where, i = 1, 2, ..., n)
while t < Max_Generation do
    Randomly take a cuckoo by Lévy flights using Eq. 1.
    Evaluation Fitness F_i by using Band Correlation (BC) function 12
    Randomly select one nest j among n .
    if F_j < F_i then
        j should be replaced with the new solution.
    end if
    Current nests are left and new nests are made for a fraction (pa) of worse nests.
    The best solutions, i.e. nests having quality solutions are kept.
    Solutions are arranged rankwise and take the current best (C_best)
end while
Select the fittest C_best amongst all iterations and generate the band reduced image by using it.
```

to deduce the objective function for HSI segmentation. This motivates us to formulate a new objective function for HSI segmentation. In proposed objective function we have given equal importance to both Renyi's entropy as well as Tsallis Entropy. The algorithm for band reduction is describes in Algorithm 1.

Objective Function for band reduction: The bands of a hyperspectral image are continuous and having strong spectral correlations amongst neighbouring bands. That's why, we employ an approach that prevents selecting bands which are highly related. The spectral correlation between two bands a_α and a_β is given by Eq. 12.

Algorithm 2 Proposed Method for Hyperspectral Image Segmentation

Require: Hyperspectral Image with reduced bands.
Ensure: Segmented Image
  Start
  Generate an initial-population havig n host nests X_i $(Where, i = 1, 2, \ldots, n)$
  while $t < Max_{Generation}$ **do**
    Randomly get a cuckoo by Lévy flights using Eq. 1.
    Evaluation Fitness F_i by using Reyni's and Tsallis Entropic functions 13.
    Randomly select one nest j among n
    if $F_j < F_i$ **then**
      j should be replaced with the new solution.
    end if
    Current nests are left and new nests are made for a fraction (pa) of worse nests.
    The best solutions, i.e. or nests having quality solutions are kept.
    Solutions are arranged rankwise and take the current best (C_{best})
  end while
  Fittest C_{best} solution amongst all iterations are selected and generate the segmented image

---

$$\rho(a_\alpha, a_\beta) = \frac{cov(a_\alpha, a_\beta)}{a_\alpha . \sigma a_\beta} \tag{12}$$

Here, $cov()$ is the covariance and the standard deviation is represented by σ.

Objective Function for segmentation: Both the Reyni's Entropy (RE) and Tsallis Entropy (TE) are used to design the objective function of segmentation. To make the objective function balanced and more generalized, equal importance is given to both of the entropies. The fitness of each slution is calculate by Eq. 13.

$$F_i = \frac{\left(\frac{\sum_{i=1}^{b} TE}{b}\right) + \left(\frac{\sum_{i=1}^{b} RE}{b}\right)}{2} \tag{13}$$

where b is the number of bands in reduced banded image. RE is Reyni's Entropy and TE is Tsallis Entropy.

4 Results and Discussions

Figure 2 shows the ground truth and the segmented images that are obtained from said two competing methods along with our proposed for Indian Pine hyperspectral image. Whereas the ground truth and the segmented images that are obtained from said two methods and the proposed for Pavia University hyperspectral image shown in Fig. 1.

In this section, we have shown all the experimental results in detail. All the experiments are performed in a system with the following configurations—Editor: Python-3.7, CPU: Intel(R)-Core(TM)-i7, RAM: 16 GB. The proposed method is quantitatively and qualitatively validated with respect to other 6 cutting edge algorithms.

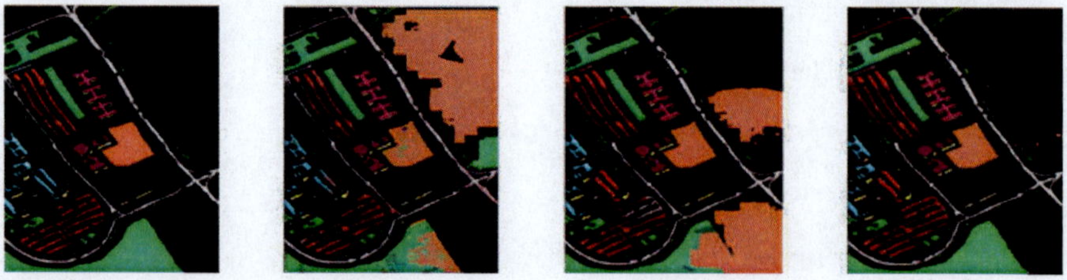

(a) Ground Truth (b) CPSO [27] (c) ELM [28] (d) Proposed Method

Fig. 1 Pavia University dataset obtained from ROSIS satellite sensor: **a** ground truth; segmented images obtained by using: **b** CPSO [27], **c** ELM [28], and **d** proposed method

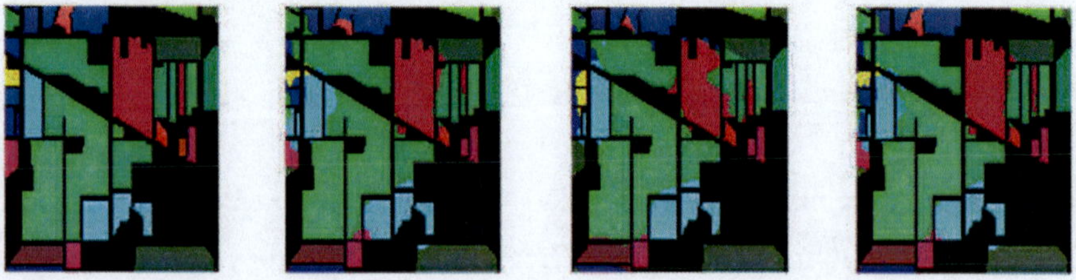

(a) Ground Truth (b) CPSO [27] (c) ELM [28] (d) Proposed Method

Fig. 2 Indiana Pine dataset obtained from AVIRIS satellite sensor: **a** ground truth; segmented images obtained by using: **b** CPSO [27], **c** ELM [28], and **d** proposed method

4.1 Dataset Description

1. Indian Pines (AVIRIS): The image of Indian Pines was acquired with the Infrared Airborne Imaging Spectrometer sensor (AVIRIS) flying above the Indian Pines location in the north-western region of Indiana. The sensor has 200 useable bands and 145 × 145 pixels per band. This hyperspectral image has a spatial resolution of 20 m. It has 16 traits for six different types of vegetation at that location, the majority of which are crop varieties. Because the spectral reflectance of many crops is so similar, identifying the different types of crops can be difficult.
2. Pavia University (ROSIS): While flying above Pavia University in Italy, the ROSIS sensor captured this image of the university. ROSIS sensor picture with a spatial resolution of 1.3 m per pixel, 610,340 pixels, and 115 bands. This HSI dataset has 9 distinct urban class regions.

4.2 Performance Analysis

For validating the performance of our proposed method, a variety of experiments are carried out. For this analysis, the reduced banded image is classified using SVM classification algorithm. That classification results are compared to that of two similar existing methods Continuous Particle Swarm Optimization method (CPSO) proposed by Liu et al. [27] (b) AdaBoost weighted composite kernel extreme learning-based method (ELM) proposed by Li et al. [28]. The performances are compared using three mostly used prominent indices: Average Accuracy (AA), Overall Accuracy (OA), and Kappa Coefficient (KC).

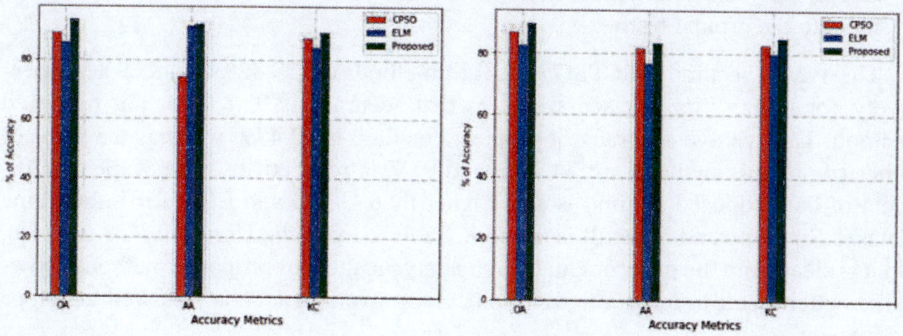

(a) Experiement with Indian Pine Dataset. (b) Experiement with Pavia University Dataset.

Fig. 3 Comparison of accuracy of the proposed pethod to other methods when experiment done with Indiana Pine data set

Table 1 Accuracy comparison with Indiana Pines data

Class	CPSO [27]	ELM [28]	Proposed method
1. Grass-trees	86.62	99.14	99.25
2. Alfalfa	38.32	97.6	98.6
3. Haywind-rowed	96.35	67.44	68.44
4. Corn notill	89.95	97.42	98.42
5. Cornmintill	67.46	80.57	81.57
6. Corn	68.27	99.78	99.8
7. Grass pasture mowed	73.84	99.44	99.54
8. Grasspasture	38.63	98.24	99.24
9. Wheat	82.83	98.23	99.23
10. Oats	21.92	98.6	99.6
11. Soybean mintill	94.36	92.72	93.72
12. Soybean clean	73.05	99.69	99.81
13. Soybean notill	94.87	89.47	90.47
14. Woods	95.49	91.89	92.89
15. Stone-steel towers	70.34	92.15	93.15
16. Building-grass trees	68.42	64.8	65.8
OA (%)	89.32	85.9	93.8
AA (%)	74.25	91.7	92.47
KC (%)	87.58	84.34	89.71

1. ***Overall Accuracy (OA)***: The percentage of pixels that are correctly identified to the total test number of tests carried out.
2. ***Average Accuracy (AA)***: The mean value of accuracy of all classification of all classes (Fig. 3 and Table 1).
3. ***Kappa Coefficient (KC)***: A statistical measure of the final classification's agreement to the ground truth.

The overall accuracy of CPSO and ELM methods are 89.32% and 85.9%, respectively, for Indian Pine dataset, where as that accuracy is 93.8% for our proposed method. The average accuracy of proposed method is 92.47% whereas the same of other competing methods are 74.25% and 91.7%, respectively. The Kappa coefficient of our proposed method is also higher than CPSO and ELM for Indian Pine dataset. Similar trend of result is found in Table 2 for Pavia University dataset also. So it is clear from the experimental result analysis, that our proposed methods shows quite better result in terms of overall accuracy, average accuracy as well as kappa coefficient.

Table 2 Accuracy comparison with Pavia University data

Class	CPSO [27]	ELM [28]	Proposed method
1. Meadows	95.7	90.93	96.7
2. Asphalt	94.14	78.02	95.14
3. Trees	89.37	86.73	91.37
4. Gravel	50.63	55.8	51.63
5. Bare soil	67.31	64.9	69.31
6. Bitumen	65.8	79.2	67.8
7. Painted metal sheets	97.34	84.7	98.34
8. Shadows	97.51	99.57	99.51
9. Self-blocking bricks	80.07	81.96	82.07
OA (%)	87.13	82.71	89.9
AA (%)	81.98	77.06	83.54
KC (%)	82.92	80.2	85.2

5 Conclusion

HSI contains a large range of spectral signature that allows for a detailed description of the objects in the scene. Segmentation of hyperspectral image is a very crucial operation for analysing the HSI data as well. But due to the high number of bands in hyperspectral images, the segmentation task become challenging. In this work we first reduce the dimension of HSI and then segment that image by Cuckoo Search algorithm. We design a new objective function by combining Renyi's Entropy and Tsallis entropy which makes our method more general and efficient to segment a hyperspectral image. We found a better accuracy than other two existing approaches.

References

1. Sawant SS, Prabukumar M (2020) A review on graph-based semi-supervised learning methods for hyperspectral image classification. Egyptian J Rem Sensing Space Sci 23(2):243–248. ISSN 1110-9823, https://doi.org/10.1016/j.ejrs.2018.11.001
2. Zhang M, Li W, Du Q (2018) Diverse region-based CNN for hyperspectral image classification. IEEE Trans Image Process 27(6):2623–2634
3. Liu W, Shen X, Du B, Tsang IW, Zhang W, Lin X (2019) Hyperspectral imagery classification via stochastic HHSVMs. IEEE Trans Image Process 28(2):577–588
4. Romshoo SA, Rashid I (2014) In: Assessing the impacts of changing land cover and climate on Hokersar Wetland in Indian Himalayas. Arab J Geo-sci 7(1):143–160
5. Mou L, Zhu XX (2020) Learning to pay attention on spectral domain: a spectral attention module-based convolutional network for hyperspectral image classification. IEEE Trans Geosci Rem Sens 58(1):110–122
6. Feng J et al (2019) CNN-based multilayer spatial-spectral feature fusion and sample augmentation with local and nonlocal constraints for hyperspectral image classification. IEEE J Sel Topics Appl Earth Observ Rem Sens 12(4):1299–1313

7. Paoletti ME, Haut JM, Fernandez-Beltran R, Plaza J, Plaza AJ, Pla F (2019) Deep pyramidal residual networks for spectral-spatial hyperspectral image classification. IEEE Trans Geosci Rem Sens 57(2):740–754
8. Hu W, Huang Y, Wei L, Zhang F, Li H (2015) Deep convolutional neural networks for hyperspectral image classification. J Sens 2015:1–12
9. Sun H, Zheng X, Lu X, Wu S (2020) Spectral-spatial attention network for hyperspectral image classification. IEEE Trans Geosci Rem Sens 58(5):3232–3245
10. Fang L, Liu G, Li S, Ghamisi P, Benediktsson JA (2019) Hyperspectral image classification with squeeze multibias network. IEEE Trans Geosci Rem Sens 57(3):1291–1301
11. Zhong Z, Li J, Luo Z, Chapman M (2018) Spectral-spatial residual network for hyperspectral image classification: a 3D deep learning framework. IEEE Trans Geosci Rem Sens 56(2):847–858
12. He L, Li J, Liu C, Li S (2018) Recent advances on spectral-spatial hyperspectral image classification: an overview and new guidelines. IEEE Trans Geosci Rem Sens 56(3):1579–1597
13. Luo F, Zhang L, Zhou X, Guo T, Cheng Y, Yin T (2020) Sparseadaptive hypergraph discriminant analysis for hyperspectral image classification. IEEE Geosci Rem Sens Lett 17(6):1082–1086
14. Yu C et al (2019) Hyperspectral image classification method based on CNN architecture embedding with hashing semantic feature. IEEE J Sel Topics Appl Earth Observ Rem Sens 12(6):1866–1881
15. Li S, Song W, Fang L, Chen Y, Ghamisi P, Benediktsson JA (2019) Deep learning for hyperspectral image classification: an overview. IEEE Trans Geosci Rem Sens 57(9):6690–6709
16. Audebert N, Le Saux B, Lefevre S (2019) Deep learning for classification of hyperspectral data: a comparative review. IEEE Geosci Rem Sens Mag 7(2):159–173
17. Liu B, Yu X, Zhang P, Yu A, Fu Q, Wei X (2018) Supervised deep feature extraction for hyperspectral image classification. IEEE Trans Geosci Rem Sens 56(4):1909–1921
18. Han J, Zhang D, Cheng G, Guo L, Ren J (2015) Object detection in optical remote sensing images based on weakly supervised learning and high-level feature learning. IEEE Trans Geosci Rem Sens 53(6):3325–3337
19. Ghamisi P, Couceiro MS, Martins FM, Atli Benediktsson J (2014) Multilevel image segmentation based on fractional-order Darwinian particle swarm optimization. IEEE Trans Geosci Rem Sens 52(5):2382–2394
20. Brajevic I, Tuba M (2014) Cuckoo search and firefly algorithm applied to multilevel image thresholding. In: Cuckoo search and firefly algorithm. Springer, pp 115-139
21. Wang G-G, Guo L, Duan H, Wang H (2014) A new improved firefly algorithm for global numerical optimization. J Comput Theor Nanosci 11(2):477–485
22. Raja N, Rajinikanth V, Latha K (2014) Otsu based optimal multilevel image thresholding using firefly algorithm. Model Simul Eng 2014:37
23. Chen K, Zhou Y, Zhang Z, Dai M, Chao Y, Shi J (2016) Multilevel image segmentation based on an improved firefly algorithm. Math Prob Eng
24. Akay B (2013) A study on particle swarm optimization and artificial bee colony algorithms for multilevel thresholding. Applied Soft Comput 13(6):3066–3091
25. Alihodzic A, Tuba M (2014) Improved bat algorithm applied to multilevel image thresholding. Sci World J
26. Schclar A, Averbuch A (2019) A diffusion approach to unsupervised segmentation of hyperspectral images. In: Sabourin C, Merelo JJ, Madani K, Warwick K (eds) Proceedings of 9th international joint conference computational intelligence (IJCCI). Springer, Cham, Switzerland, pp 163–178. https://doi.org/10.1007/978-3-030-16469-0
27. Liu X, Zhang C, Cai Z, Yang J, Zhou Z, Gong X (2021) Continuous particle swarm optimization-based deep learning architecture search for hyperspectral image classification. Rem Sens 13(6):1082
28. Li L, Wang C, Li W, Chen J (2018) Hyperspectral image classification by AdaBoost weighted composite kernel extreme learning machines. Neurocomputing 275:1725–1733

Deep SqueezeNet-Based Diagnosis of the Breast Cancer Using Ultrasound (US) Images

Mithun Karmakar and Amitava Nag

Abstract Breast cancer affects millions of women. It is the most common cause of death in the world. Therefore, the detection and diagnosis of breast cancer is very necessary. The conventional method for diagnosis of breast cancer relies on manual analysis and interpretation by radiologists. However, this process is slow and the success of the diagnosis is proportional to the radiologist's capabilities and experiences. Thus there is a need for a system that can perform a successful automatic diagnosis. Over the last few years, extensive research has been done on deep learning (DL)-based diagnostic processes of breast cancer. In this work, we fine tune a pre-trained deep convolutional neural network (SqueezeNet) for breast cancer detection from ultrasound (US) images. The experimental results reveal that the proposed work achieves more than 98% accuracy.

Keywords Breast cancer diseases · Convolutional neural network · Deep learning · SqueezeNet

1 Introduction

Breast cancer is the most common type of cancer in women of all cancers. In 2020, the World Health Organization (WHO) reported 2.3 million women diagnosed with breast cancer with 685,000 deaths. The main reason for the high death rate is the lack of mechanism for early detection and diagnosis of breast cancer tumours. Timely and accurate detection of it may increase survival rate [1]. To improve the accuracy of diagnosis, various radiological-based diagnosis approaches are now being used. Mammography, Ultrasound imaging, and magnetic resonance imaging (MRI) are the traditional approaches [2]. Among all other, Ultrasound imaging is mostly preferred as a diagnostic tool because it is inexpensive, easily accessible, reproducible and it prevents radiation exposure of the breast [3]. Breast cancer diagnosis using US

M. Karmakar (✉) · A. Nag
Department of Computer Science and Engineering, CITK, Kokrajhar, Assam, India
e-mail: m.karmakar@cit.ac.in

© The Author(s), under exclusive license to Springer Nature Singapore Pte Ltd. 2023

J. K. Mandal and D. De (eds.), *Frontiers of ICT in Healthcare*, Lecture Notes in Networks and Systems 519, https://doi.org/10.1007/978-981-19-5191-6_50

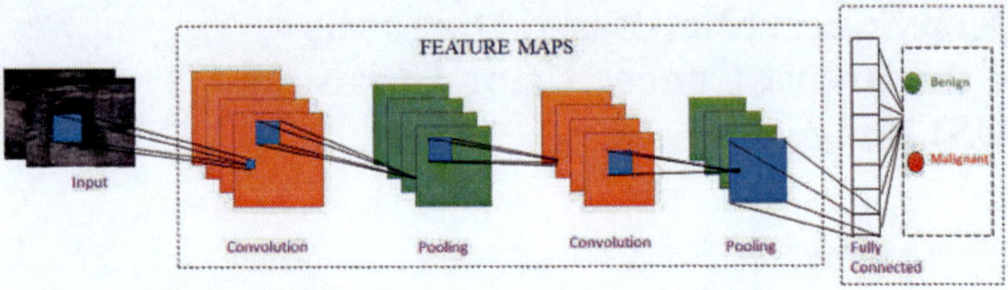

Fig. 1 An architecture of Convolution Neural Network (CNN)

imaging is dependent on manual analysis and interpretation by radiologists, which can lead to inaccurate analyses due to shortage of expert radiologists and human mistakes. This reason is enough to justify the need for automated computer-aided diagnosis (CAD) systems for detection of breast cancer. The use of CAD systems aims to reduce the efforts of radiologists and prevent observational oversights.

The recent technological development in artificial intelligence (AI) has made it simple and effective to build intelligent CAD systems for breast cancer diagnosis. The ability of machines to replicate human intellect is referred to as AI. Machine learning (ML), a subset of AI, is used to execute tasks by learning from available data [4]. Many researchers have developed CAD tools for detecting breast cancer [5]. However, the traditional machine learning techniques are time-consuming and challenging to design [6]. Deep learning (DL) is currently applied to develop CAD systems for breast cancer. Deep learning, a type of machine learning, is a set of multi-layer "artificial neural networks (ANN)" based automatic learning methods. The most common DL method for analysing the US image is convolutional neural networks (CNN). The primary goal of this study is to use a deep CNN model for detecting breast cancer from Ultrasound images.

Deep Convolutional Neural Network models are used in this study to find patterns in ultrasound pictures that are undetected to the naked eye. The convolutional neural network is a class of deep learning techniques that is used to identify useful and distinctive representations of images. A typical CNN is depicted in Fig. 1. However, the fundamental issue that a deep CNN model encountered during training was a large volume of image data. This problem has been addressed using a technique known as transfer learning (TL) which is designed for the CNNs. Several pre-trained models with transfer learning that have already trained on a huge annotated image library have been designed.

Recently, a number of CNN Architectures such as VGG16 [7], ResNet50 [8], DenseNet201 [9], InceptionV3 [10] and Exception [11] etc. have been proposed for diagnosis of breast cancer.

The following is how the rest of this article is organized: Sect. 2 summarizes the numerous relevant works that have been completed in this area. The methods used is shown in Sect. 3. The experimental results are presented in Sect. 4. The last section concludes the overall work.

2 Related Work

In recent years deep learning is being extensively used for image classification. Many researchers reported that the DL technique achieves high accuracy in breast cancer detection. Rakhlin et al. [12] adopted three pre-trained models (VGG16, InceptionV3, and ResNet50) for feature extraction. Then they merged the extracted features to a single feature vector using the 3-norm pooling approach. Finally, breast US images are classified as normal or malignant using the LightGBM classifier. They achieved an average of 87.2% accuracy on their experimental analysis. Kwok [13] developed a method to detect breast cancer on histological images using four established, state-of-the-art CNNs (VGG-19, InceptionV3, InceptionV4, and ResNet50) with an accuracy of 91%.

Instead of training a CNN from scratch with randomly initialized parameters, Byra et al. [14] used the transfer learning (TL) approach on a pre-trained model Visual Geometry Group (VGG)-19 for breast mass analysis. Similarly, Tanaka et al. [15] in their work applied an ensemble TL model that combined VGG-19 and ResNet-152 in order to develop a diagnosis system for breast cancer classification applied on US images. Fujioka et al. [16] presented CNN models to discriminate between benign and malignant breast masses on ultrasound shear wave elastography images. Zhang et al. [17] integrated deep learning-based radiomics signatures derived into the B-mode US (BUS) and Shear-wave elastography (SWE) images. The authors also determine their diagnostic performances in classifying breast masses. Another approach using automatic intra-operative ultrasound image processing through the transfer learning method using Inception V3 was presented by Cepeda et al. [18]. Another diagnosis system was developed by Wang et al. [19] which used Inception V3 for classification of breast cancer. The method obtained an average of 87.2% accuracy on their experiments.

3 Materials and Methods

The goal of this research is to use a lightweight deep CNN model in terms of model size. SqueezeNet has been chosen for this purpose.

3.1 US Image DataSet

We used Rodrigues's [20] publicly available breast US images dataset which contains 250 images. Among the 250 images, 40% images (100) corresponded to benign and 60% malignant (150). The images are different sizes. The images' minimum and maximum sizes, in grey and RGB colours, are 57×75 and 61×199 pixels,

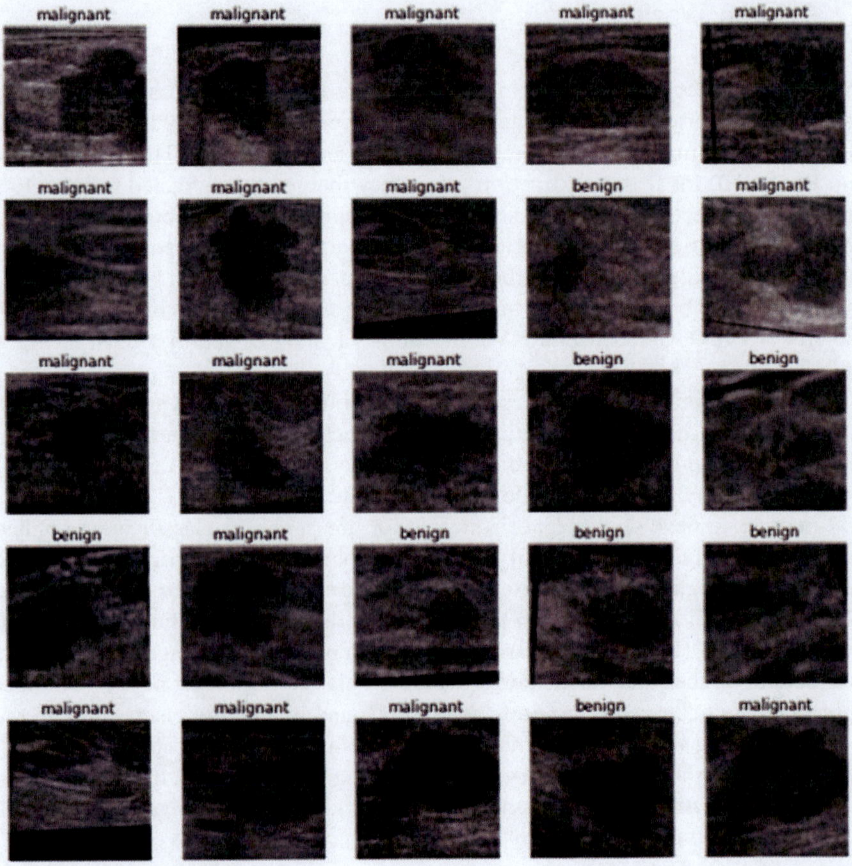

Fig. 2 Sample of Ultrasound images from dataset

respectively. As a result, all of the images are resized to 224 × 224 in order to fit within the model. The sample of Ultrasound images are shown in Fig. 2.

We used two different classes in this work (i.e. Benign and Malignant). The whole mechanism for detecting breast cancer is depicted in Fig. 3. In this work, first US images are collected from public datasets [20]. Then, image preprocessing was done. The only preprocessing used in this work was a simple resizing of the US images. Finally, the pre-trained CNN (SqueezeNet) model with weights from ImageNet and with the proper fine-tuning are used for classification.

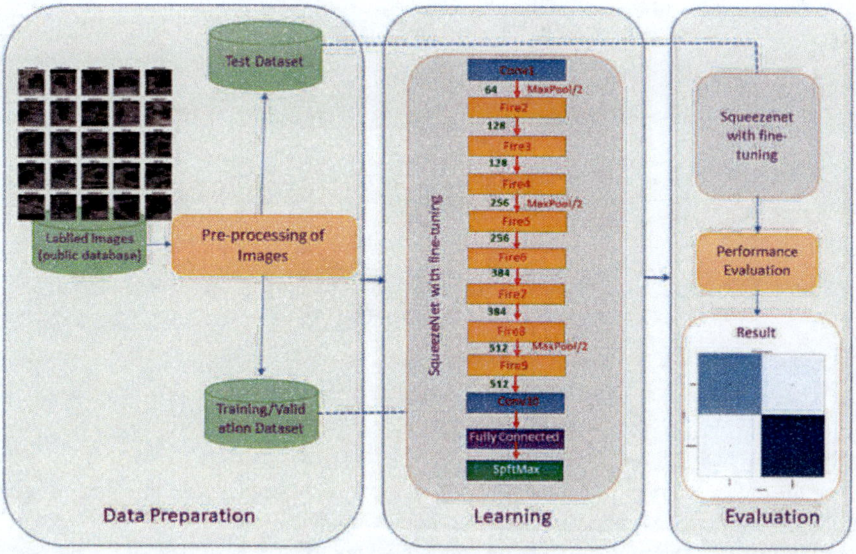

Fig. 3 Architecture of deep learning (SqueezeNet)-based breast cancer diagnosis system

3.2 *The Pre-trained SqueezeNet Architecture and Fine-Tuning Procedure*

The overall architecture of the proposed deep SqueezeNet-based system is presented in Fig. 3. SqueezeNet is proposed by Iandola et al. [21]. SqueezeNet is a CNN model that starts with convolutional layer, followed by eight fire layers and another convolutional layer. The structure of fire layer which uses squeeze and expansion phases is illustrated in Fig. 4. Squeeze as well as expansion both phases are connected to the ReLU units. The fire layer with the help of squeeze and expansion layers make the SqueezeNet smaller and more effective CNN model.

Training deep CNN models from scratch is complex as well as demand large amount of data in order to converge the model. Fine-tuning on a pre-trained CNN model can be an alternate solution. In this work, fine-tuning was performed on pre-trained CNN (SqueezeNet) model with US image dataset [20]. The models were pre-trained with weights from ImageNet. Furthermore, the top layer of SqueezeNet was truncated by adding a new fully-connected softmax layer to the top layer.

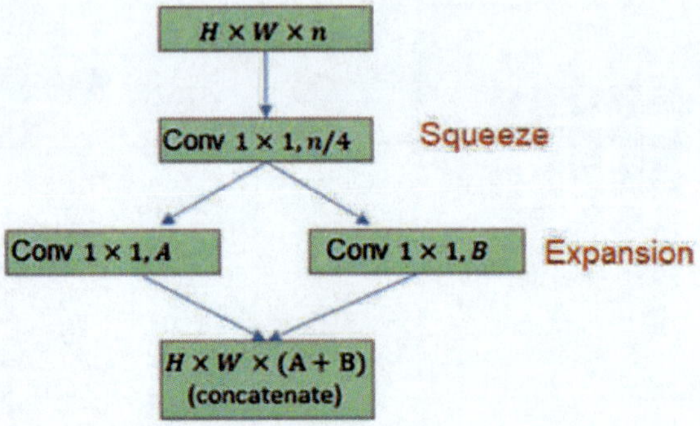

Fig. 4 Structure of the fire layer

4 Results

Using the datasets given in Sect. 3.1, the classification of breast cancer is performed. The CNN models described in Sect. 3.2 was evaluated for breast cancer detection from US images. Training and testing are carried out on 80% and 20% of the dataset, respectively, in the experiment.

4.1 Tools Used

We used Fast.ai wrapper on top of PyTorch deep learning framework in python 3.8.5 by Google Colab GPU (Tesla K80 12GB GDDR5 VRAM).

4.2 Performance Evaluation

The performance has been evaluated using measured in terms of classification accuracy (CA) which is defined as follows:

The performance has been evaluated using five metrics which are defined as follows:
Classification accuracy (CA): CA is the ratio of correct predictions of the proposed scheme to the total number of predictions performed on a given set of data which is given as:

$$\text{Classification Accuracy (CA)} = \frac{\text{TP} + \text{TN}}{\text{TP} + \text{TN} + \text{FP} + \text{FN}}$$

Precision: It is the ratio of positive data points that are correctly predicted as positive to the number of data points predicted as positive by the classifier, which is represented by the formula:

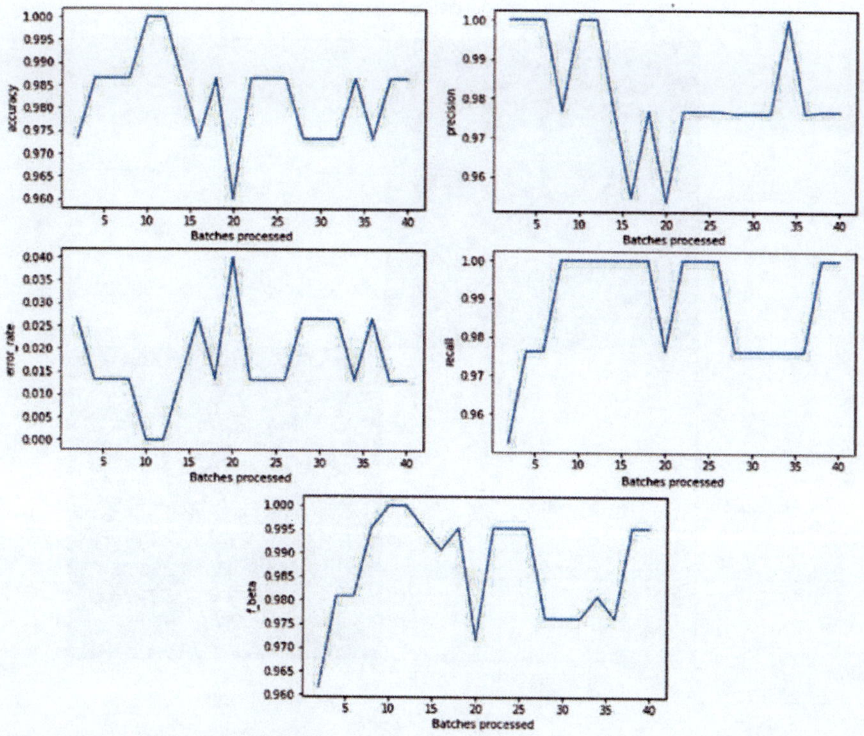

Fig. 5 Model accuracy and loss curve

Table 1 Performance of SqueezeNet on the US image dataset

No. of epoch	Accuracy	Error rate	Precision	Recall	Tim
20	0.9867	0.0133	0.9767	1.0000	0.02

$$\text{Classification Accuracy (CA)} = \frac{\text{TP}}{\text{TP} + \text{FP}}$$

Sensitivity: It is defined as the ratio of positive data points that are correctly predicted as positive to the total number of positive data points.

$$\text{Sensitivity} = \frac{\text{TP}}{\text{TP} + \text{FN}}$$

F1-score: It is used to determine the accuracy of a test dataset. The harmonic mean of precision and sensitivity is the F1-score.

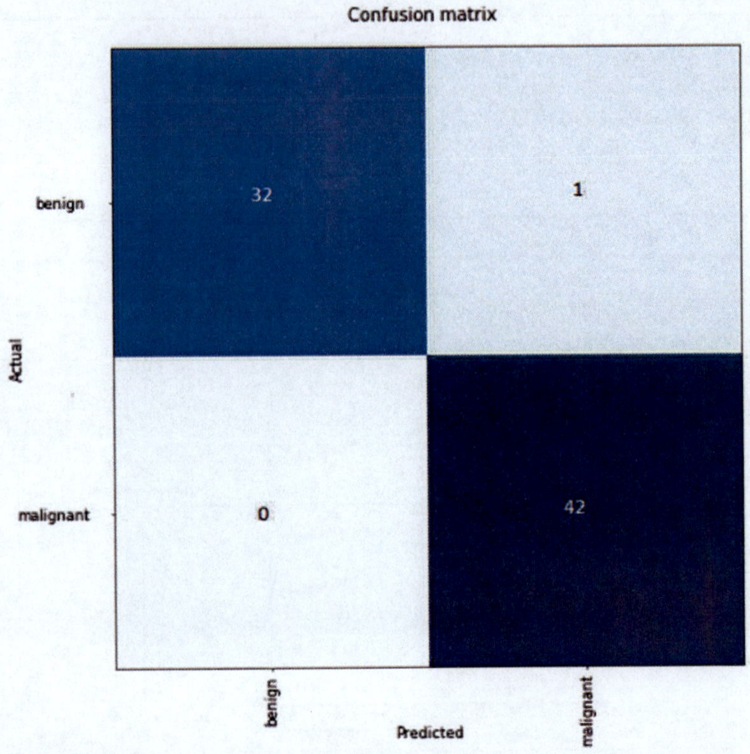

Fig. 6 Confusion matrix of the proposed CNN model in testing phase

$$\text{F1-Score} = 2 * \frac{1}{\frac{1}{\text{precision}} + \frac{1}{\text{sensitivity}}}$$

Here, True Positive, True Negative, False Positive, and False Negative are represented by TP, TN, FP, and FN, respectively.

4.3 Result Analysis

The results for the performance of the used model are illustrated in Fig. 5 and given in Table 1. From curve plot in Fig. 6, it can be seen that the model performed very well with accuracy over 98%. The confusion matrix of SqueezeNet model on test dataset is shown in Fig. 6.

5 Conclusions

This work presents an approach for the classification of Breast cancer using deep CNN architecture. The work fine tuned SqueezeNet model on US images for breast cancer detection instead of designing a new model as SqueezeNet is a state-of-the-art deep learning model with lightweight model size. Experimental results show that our method gives an overall accuracy over 98%. As a result, this work can be successfully applied for deep learning-based mobile-aided diagnostic tools for breast cancer detection.

References

1. Mao N, Yin P, Wang Q, Liu M, Dong J, Zhang X, Xie H, Hong N (2019) Added value of radiomics on mammography for breast cancer diagnosis: a feasibility study. J Am College Radiol 16(4):485–491
2. Masud M, Hossain MS, Alhumyani H, Alshamrani SS, Cheikhrouhou O, Ibrahim S, Muhammad G, Eldin Rashed AE, Gupta BB (2021) Pre-trained convolutional neural networks for breast cancer detection using ultrasound images. ACM Trans Internet Technol 21(4):1–17
3. Eroglu Y, Yildirim M, Çinar A (2021) Convolutional Neural Networks based classification of breast ultrasonography images by hybrid method with respect to benign, malignant, and normal using mRMR. Comput Biol Med 133:104407
4. Senapati A, Nag A, Mondal A, Maji S (2021) A novel framework for COVID-19 case prediction through piecewise regression in India. Int J Inform Technol 13(1):41–48
5. Cai L, Wang X, Wang Y, Guo Y, Yu J, Wang Y (2015) Robust phasebased texture descriptor for classification of breast ultrasound images. Biomed Eng OnLine 14(1):26
6. Misra S, Jeon S, Managuli R, Lee S, Kim G, Yoon C, Lee S, Barr RG, Kim C (2021) Bi-modal transfer learning for classifying breast cancers via combined B-mode and ultrasound strain imaging. IEEE Trans Ultrasonics Ferroelectr Frequency Control
7. Iandola F, Moskewicz M, Karayev S, Girshick R, Darrell T, Keutzer K (2014) Densenet: implementing efficient convent descriptor pyramids. arXiv preprint arXiv:1404.1869
8. He K, Zhang X, Ren S, Sun J (2016) Deep residual learning for image recognition. In: Proceedings of the IEEE conference on computer vision and pattern recognition, pp 770–778
9. Zhang X, Zou J, He K, Sun J (2015) Accelerating very deep convolutional networks for classification and detection. IEEE Trans Pattern Anal Mach Intell 38(10):1943–1955
10. Szegedy C, Vanhoucke V, Ioffe S, Shlens J, Wojna Z (2016) Rethinking the inception architecture for computer vision. In: Proceedings of IEEE conference on computer vision and pattern recognition, June 2016, pp 2818–2826
11. Chollet F (2017) Xception: deep learning with depthwise separable convolutions. In: Proceedings of the IEEE conference on computer vision and pattern recognition, pp 1251–1258
12. Rakhlin A, Shvets A, Iglovikov V, Kalinin AA (2018) Deep convolutional neural networks for breast cancer histology image analysis. In: International conference image analysis and recognition. Springer, Cham, pp 737–744
13. Kwok S (2018) Multiclass classification of breast cancer in whole-slide images. In: Proceedings of the 15th international conference on image analysis and recognition (ICIAR'18). IEEE, Los Alamitos, CA, pp 931–940
14. Byra M, Galperin M, Ojeda-Fournier H, Olson L, O'Boyle M, Comstock C, Andre M (2019) Breast mass classification in sonography with transfer learning using a deep convolutional neural network and color conversion. Med Phys 46(2):746–755

15. Tanaka H, Chiu S-W, Watanabe T, Kaoku S, Yamaguchi T (2019) Computer-aided diagnosis system for breast ultrasound images using deep learning. Phys Med Biol 64(23):235013
16. Fujioka T, Katsuta L, Kubota K, Mori M, Kikuchi Y, Kato A, Oda G, Nakagawa T, Kitazume Y, Tateishi U (2020) Classification of breast masses on ultrasound shear wave elastography using convolutional neural networks. Ultrasonic Imaging 42(4–5):213–220
17. Zhang X, Liang M, Yang Z, Zheng C, Wu J, Ou B, Li H, Wu X, Luo B, Shen J (2020) Deep learning-based radiomics of B-mode ultrasonography and shear-wave elastography: improved performance in breast mass classification. Frontiers Oncol 10:1621
18. Cepeda S, García-García S, Arrese I, Fernández-Pérez G, Velasco-Casares M, Fajardo-Puentes M, Zamora T, Sarabia R (2021) Comparison of intraoperative ultrasound B-mode and strain elastography for the differentiation of glioblastomas from solitary brain metastases. An automated deep learning approach for image analysis. Frontiers Oncol 10:3322
19. Wang Y, Choi EJ, Choi Y, Zhang H, Jin GY, Ko S-B (2020) Breast cancer classification in automated breast ultrasound using multiview convolutional neural network with transfer learning. Ultrasound Medi Biol 46(5):1119–1132
20. Rodrigues PS (2017) Breast ultrasound image. Mendeley Data. Retrieved 10 Apr. 2020 from http://dx.doi.org/10.17632/wmy84gzngw.1
21. Iandola FN, Han S, Moskewicz MW, Ashraf K, Dally WJ, Keutzer K (2016) SqueezeNet: AlexNet-level accuracy with 50x fewer parameters and <0.5 MB model size. arXiv preprint arXiv:1602.07360

Automated Brain Tumor Segmentation Using GAN Augmentation and Optimized U-Net

Swathi Jamjala Narayanan, Adithya Sreemandiram Anil, Chinmay Ashtikar, Sasank Chunduri, and Sangeetha Saman

Abstract Children and adults with brain tumors are among the top causes of death in the world. Deep learning-based approaches have seen considerable success in brain tumor segmentation in recent years. Medical image tasks like tumor segmentation are severely limited by the time and effort necessary to collect paired medical imaging datasets. When gathering multi-modal image data, the problem becomes more complicated. However, this problem can be overcome by leveraging generative adversarial networks (GAN), which can generate synthesized images. The proposed automated brain tumor segmentation is made up of two modules. The first is a DCGAN network, which produces a binary tumor mask that is to be overlayed on a healthy brain image. Then, the overlayed brain image is used as an input for the pix2pix GAN network that applies for style transfer and generates realistic output that is indistinguishable from a real input. Thus, we are able to generate synthetic paired data to augment our dataset. The next module is the segmentation model that comprises a U-Net architecture that is optimized with residual blocks, the addition of residual blocks improves training time, training accuracy, and validation accuracy. The experimental results show that the synthesized dataset created by our proposed method and optimized U-Net model significantly improve the tumor segmentation performance and achieves the dice and IOU scores of 0.93 and 0.87, respectively.

Keywords Dataset augmentation · Generative adversarial network · ResNet · U-Net · Convolution neural networks · Tumor segmentation

1 Introduction

Gliomas are brain tumors that arise from glial cells. They are the leading types of brain tumors on which current brain tumor segmentation research is largely focused. Gliomas are graded into low grade gliomas (LGG) and high-grade gliomas (HGG),

S. J. Narayanan (✉) · A. S. Anil · C. Ashtikar · S. Chunduri · S. Saman
School of Computer Science and Engineering, Vellore Institute of Technology, Vellore 632014, Tamil Nadu, India
e-mail: swathi.jns@gmail.com

© The Author(s), under exclusive license to Springer Nature Singapore Pte Ltd. 2023
J. K. Mandal and D. De (eds.), *Frontiers of ICT in Healthcare*, Lecture Notes in Networks and Systems 519, https://doi.org/10.1007/978-981-19-5191-6_51

with HGG being the more aggressive. In clinical processes, tumors are often segmented manually. Manual segmentation is tedious, laborious, and prone to intra and inter observer variations [1]. Convolutional neural networks [2] require a large amount of data to be trained successfully. Networks generalize poorly with small datasets. Data augmentation approaches enhance the generalizability of neural networks by making better use of existing training data. To create new data and improve the performance of CNNs, generative adversarial networks (GANs) have been used.

A review by Nalepa et al. [3] covers a variety of data augmentation methods specific to brain tumor segmentation, such as image transformation (affine, elastic, and pixel-level) and synthetic transformation techniques. Bowles et al. [1] demonstrate the feasibility of using GAN networks to augment datasets, and notes the performance increase in segmentation task by using GAN networks to augment data. Sandfort et al. [4] use TumorGAN to generate image segmentation pairs, this approach states that adding a regional perceptual loss to the discriminator increases the efficiency of the network. Mok et al. [5] propose a novel GANs to synthesize high resolution data from coarse noise. The system uses two generators to synthesize data. Shin et al. [4] implement a pix2pix network for synthesis of brain tumor datasets in which the original tumor is transformed and added back, then used as input for the pix2pix network in order to generate new paired data. Han et al. [6] propose PG-GAN network for a multistage GAN method, in which the data is synthesized from latent space (noise). Ghaffari et al. [7] presented the review for automated brain tumor segmentation in the BRATS challenge from 2012 to 2018. This review states that the best performing algorithm for the data segmentation tasks is the U-Net. McKinley et al. [8] propose an architecture for brain tumor segmentation through the use of dense unit in the DEEPSCAN network. The goal of which is to build an architecture using skip connections, which assists the training of very profound networks. Khan et al. [9] propose a pipeline in which three features are extracted in a spatial neighborhood and were passed to SVM resulting in the generation of confidence surface modality (CSM) which served as the foregoing knowledge and fed to novel three pathways CNN model along with the given MRIs. Zhang et al. [10] study adopted a post-processing strategy in which small ET was relabeled as non-enhancing tumors to correct some false positive ET segmentations. Syed et al. [11] propose an extension of 3D U-Net architecture called E1D3.

Summary of gaps identified in the survey: The existing GAN networks for data augmentation employ standalone GAN networks that synthesize paired data. However, these are computationally expensive, and thus, we propose a multistage data augmentation pipeline that uses two separate GAN networks, one that creates a tumor mask and another that combines it with a healthy brain MRI slice. Thus, we are able to produce anatomically correct paired data that can be used as input in our segmentation network. Batch normalization and dropout layers are used to improve accuracy of the CNN-based segmentation networks, so we also chose to opt to use these layers to improve the original U-Net model. Residual blocks used in ResNet and DenseNet can also be added to the original U-Net model to improve performance of the network.

The architecture proposed consists of two phases. The first phase deals with dataset augmentation, second phase deals with identifying and segmenting tumor cells from healthy tumor cells in the given input data. Three neural networks are used in our application workflow. The first is a DCGAN network, which generates a binary tumor mask to be overlaid on a healthy brain image. The overlaid brain image is then used as input for the second network, a pix2pix GAN network that uses style transfer to generate realistic output that is indistinguishable from a real input. As a result, we can generate synthetic paired data to augment our dataset. The segmentation model is the next phase, and it consists of a U-Net network that has been improved with residual blocks. The addition of residual blocks improves training time, training accuracy, and validation accuracy. The segmentation model is fed an MRI brain slice (T2-Flair) as input and separates the tumor from the healthy brain cells. We have used various metrics to assess the performance of our network such as IOU, dice, precision, and recall.

2 Proposed System for Brain Tumor Segmentation

2.1 Module 1: Data Augmentation

An architecture of the GAN model has two sub-models: a generator model for generating examples from the domain and a discriminator model for determining whether examples generated by the generator model are real or not. DCGAN [12] network proposes the synthesis of images from the latent space, which is initially randomized. In this work, we employ DCGAN to produce a randomized binary tumor mask that is based on real tumor masks which is obtained from the training dataset. DCGAN network comprises of a generator and a discriminator networks that is interconnected. For our use case, we have modified the original DCGAN network to synthesize 128×128 sized images. The generator shown in Fig. 1 consists of a dense layer that accepts the latent space as input, immediately after which is reshaped into a $512 \times 8 \times 8$ layer. The reshaped input layer is then passed through four deconvolution layers (or transposed convolution layer) or filter sizes 512, 256, 128, and 64, which uses LeakyReLU activation. Finally, passed through an output convolution layer with sigmoid activation that produces an 128×128 image, which is then fed into the discriminator as input.

The output received from convolution layer is then compressed and passed through a dense layer with sigmoid activation, after which the final output is fed into the discriminator network. Binary cross-entropy (Eq. 1) is used to calculate the loss in both the generator and discriminator models (Fig. 2).

Where y is the label for all the true values and $p(y)$ is the predicted probability of the point being true for all N points. Adam optimizer is used as an optimization function with a learning rate of 0.0001. The network is then trained for 25 epochs with a dataset size of 4000.

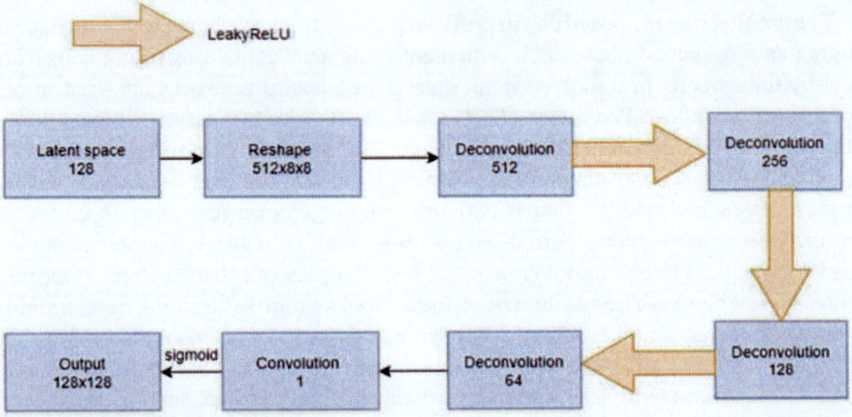

Fig. 1 Generator network of DCGAN

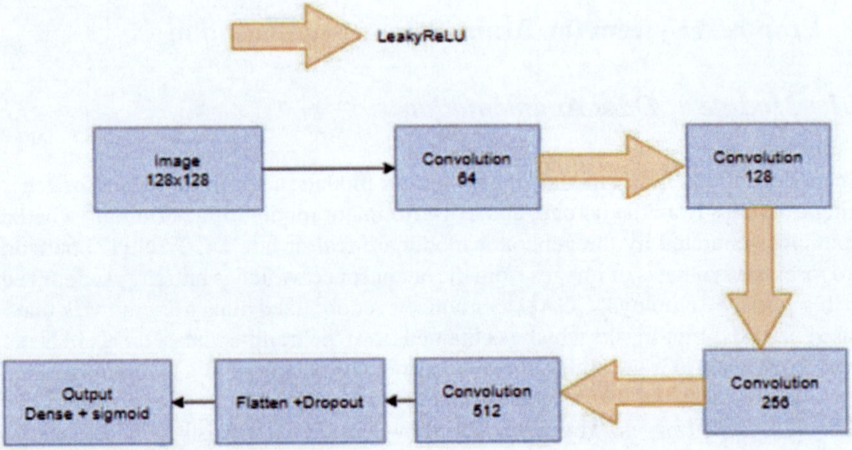

Fig. 2 Discriminator network of DCGAN

$$L = \left(\frac{-1}{\text{Output Size}}\right) \sum_{i=1}^{\text{Output Size}} y_i \cdot \log(\check{y}_i) + (1 - y_i) \cdot \log(1 - \check{y}_i) \tag{1}$$

Pix2Pix GAN network perform image-to-image translation [13], pix2pix is a generic and covers a wide range of translations such as B&W to color, edge to photo, label to scene and style transfer. In the proposed system, we use a pix2pix network to produce realistic MRI slices. This is done through overlaying the binary tumor mask produced by the DCGAN network onto a healthy brain image, and then feeding it into a pix2pix network to transform it into a realistic MRI slice. Thus, we are able to augment our dataset through the successful addition of paired data. The pix2pix

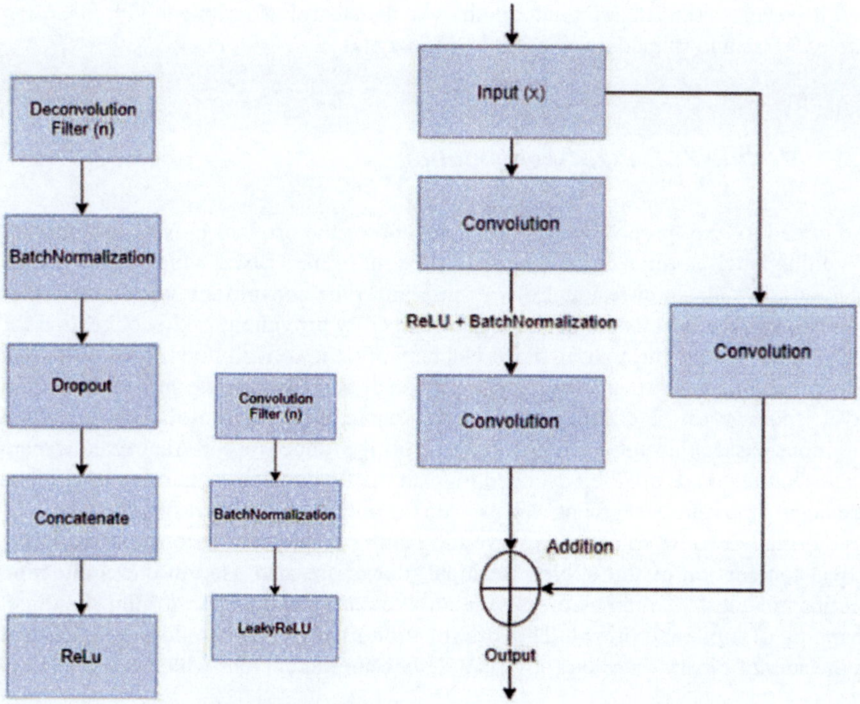

Fig. 3 Decoder, encoder, and ResBlock

consists of two interconnected networks namely the generator and discriminator. The generator is a U-Net network, consisting of six encoder blocks, one bottleneck layer and six decoder blocks, the output of corresponding encoder and decoder blocks (by filter size) is then concatenated (Fig. 3).

This is done so as to preserve the features learned during encoding, is also used during decoding, greatly improving performance. The working illustration of decoder and encoder blocks is shown in Fig. 4. The encoder blocks use LeakyReLU activation, while the decoders use ReLU activation layers. The discriminator network of pix2pix consists of two input layers, one for the real image (source) and one for the fake image (generated). These two inputs are merged and used as input for the convolution layers. The convolution layers consist of six layers with increasing filter size of 32, 64, 128, 256, and 256, with LeakyReLU activation function and batch normalization performed between each convolution layers. The final output Layer consists of a convolution 1 layer with a sigmoid activation function. The loss function for the discriminator is binary cross-entropy (Eq. 3), and L1 loss for the generator, which is defined as follows:

$$\text{Smooth } L1(x) = \begin{cases} 0.5x^2, & \text{if } |x| < 1. \\ |x| - 0.5, & \text{otherwise.} \end{cases} \quad (2)$$

The generator and discriminator both use Adam learning optimizer with a learning rate of 0.001 and trained using 8000 input images.

2.2 Module 2: Image Segmentation

We intend to have proposed a modified version of the original U-Net algorithm by including batch normalization layer and dropout to the U-Net, which improves the accuracy. We also add residual blocks instead to the convolution layers, to further preserve the gradient as the network gets deeper by providing a skip connection for the gradient to pass through. In the U-Net network, the convolution layers are known as the encoding layers in the contraction section of the U-Net, while the deconvolution layer is known as the decoder layers in the expansion section of the U-Net. When the input passes through each encoding layer, it produces a different feature map, these features maps are then decoded to form the final image output, in our case the predicted brain tumor segment. We also add the outputs of the corresponding encoder layer to the decoder so as to preserve the feature map, while reconstructing in the expansion section of the U-Net. Residual blocks are also used in the contraction sections of the U-Net so as to provide an alternative connection to find the direct mapping of input and output. The loss function used is a custom loss function that is the sum of binary cross-entropy (1) and dice coefficient loss which is defined as

$$L_{(\text{true},\text{pred})} = \text{Binary Crossentropy}(\text{true}, \text{pred}) + (1 - \text{Dice}(\text{true}, \text{pred})) \quad (3)$$

The optimizer used is SGD optimizer with an initial learning rate of 0.1, hyper-parameter optimizer such as EarlyStopping, and ReduceLROnPlateau as used to automatically stop at plateau and reduce learning rate (minimum of 0.00001).

2.3 Module 3: All Modules Integrated

We integrate the above module to complete our brain segmentation pipeline as shown in Fig. 4. In our pipeline, first the dataset is pre-processed, pre-processing includes N4 bias field correction and intensity normalized using Z-score normalization. The pre-processed input is then passed through the DCGAN network to produce randomized binary tumor masks. The tumor mask is then overlaid on a healthy brain slice and passed into the pix2pix network, which produces a realistic paired data that is then added into the working dataset. The augmented dataset is then used to train the segmentation network, i.e., optimized U-Net algorithm to obtain the predicted output for the input.

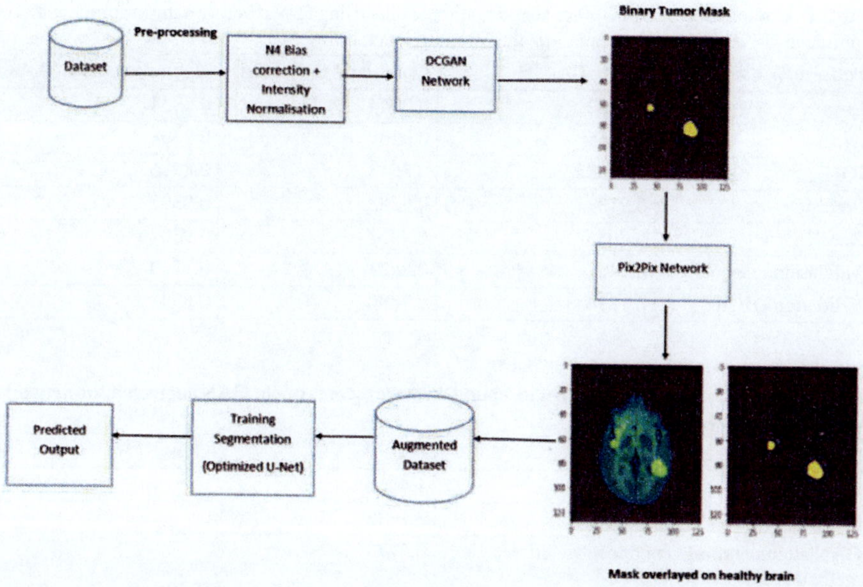

Fig. 4 ResBlock diagram

3 Experimental Result

The MICCAI BRATS-2017 dataset has been used to evaluate our proposed method. The input consists of total 10000 images, which is broken down into: 6000 real images used for training, 2000 images which are synthesized, and 2000 images, which are used for validation metrics. For implementation of proposed method, SimpleITK, Keras libraries are used. We used dice similarity coefficient, intersection over union (IOU), precision, and recall metrics for measuring the accuracy of our proposed segmentation method. The more value of the dice and Jaccard coefficient close to 1, the higher the accuracy of segmentation. The proposed optimized U-Net after dataset segmentation achieves the dice score of 0.9308 and Jaccard score of 0.8716, which is higher than conventional U-Net-based segmentation methods (Table 1).

If we compare Fréchet inception distance (FID) [14] scores of our GAN augmentation network with existing networks it is evident there is no loss in quality of the GAN network. Here a lower FID score indicated more similarity to the training data (Table 2).

Before augmentation, we first explore the performance of our residual block optimized U-Net and regular U-Net (with batch normalization and dropout). Figures 5 shows a noticeable improvement in training accuracy and all other performance metrics. This is visible in Fig. 9 as the predicted output of the from an input from the validation set, where it is noted that the optimized U-Net prediction has more detail compared to the regular U-Net prediction. Fig. 6 shows the difference in validation

Table 1 Comparison of brain tumor segmentation results using U-Net before dataset augmentation, optimized U-Net before augmentation and after augmentation

Performance measure	U-Net BA	Optimized U-Net BA	Optimized U-Net AA
Loss	0.1122	0.0944	0.0834
Dice	0.9055	0.9207	0.9308
IOU	0.8288	0.8543	0.8716
Precision	0.9187	0.9283	0.9397
Recall	0.9056	0.9231	0.9307
Validation loss	0.2481	0.2421	0.1750
Validation DICE	0.7814	0.7880	0.8548

Table 2 Comparison of FID (Fréchet inception distance) scores of our GAN augmentation network with existing networks

Method	FID
CBGAN	1.4406
Pix2pix	3.1472
GAN augmentation via concentric circles method [15]	0.5273
Our method	0.4117

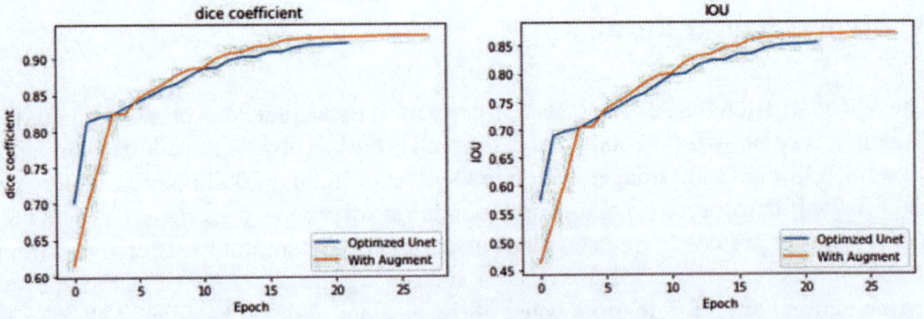

Fig. 5 Comparison of dice and IOU before and after dataset augmentation

accuracy (dice coefficient), since we use early stopping when the validation loss plateaus it is clear that the ResBlock optimized U- Net learns faster, as it plateaus are a much lower epoch number than the regular U-Net, the higher validation accuracy is also proof that the optimized U-Net also has better generalization ability than the regular U-Net. In Fig. 10, we observe that there is a discrepancy between the training loss and validation loss in the optimized U-Net algorithm. This indicates that overfitting occurs. Thus, we opt to perform data augmentation on our dataset to overcome this (Figs. 7 and 8).

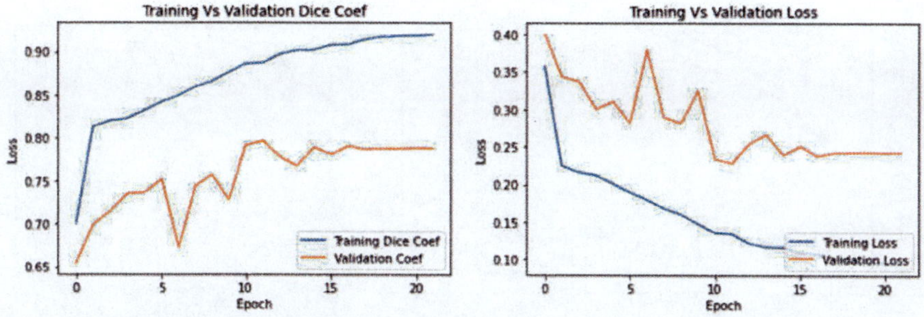

Fig. 6 Left: training versus validation dice coefficient of optimized U-Net. Right: training versus validation loss of optimized U-Net

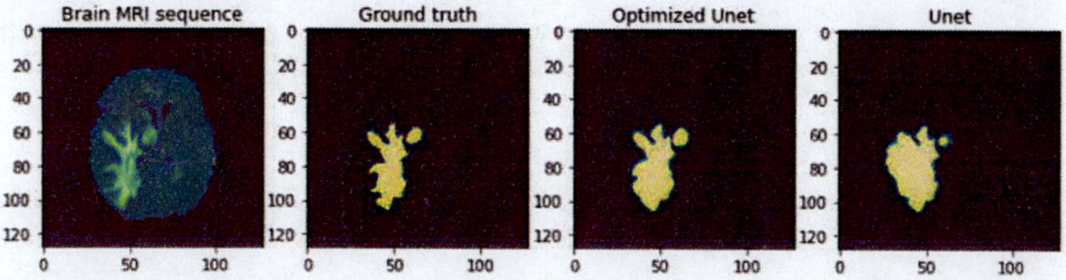

Fig. 7 Output before augmentation

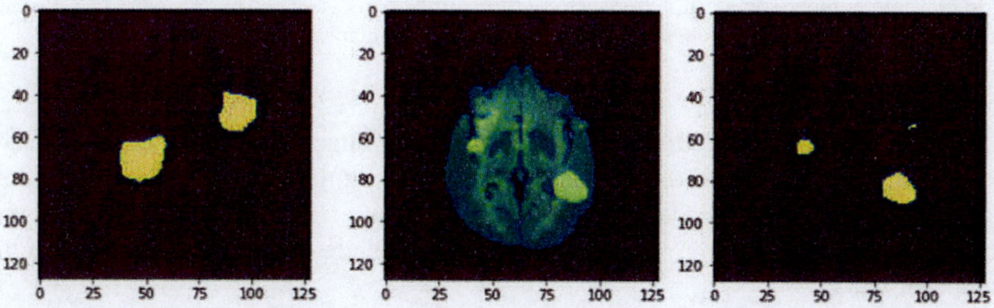

Fig. 8 Generated binary tumor mask (DCGAN), overlaying tumor mask with healthy brain (pix2pix output)

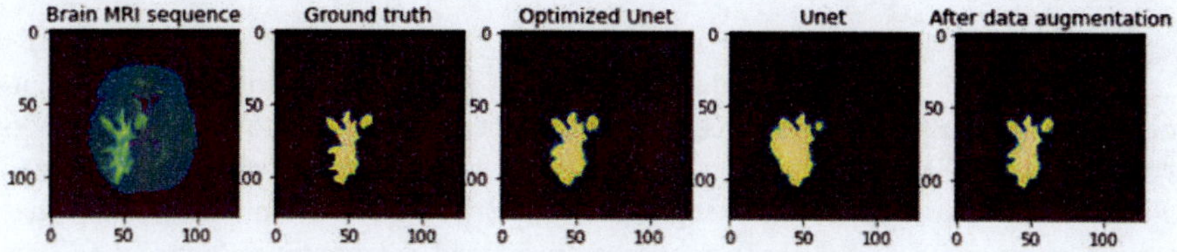

Fig. 9 Output after dataset augmentation with GAN

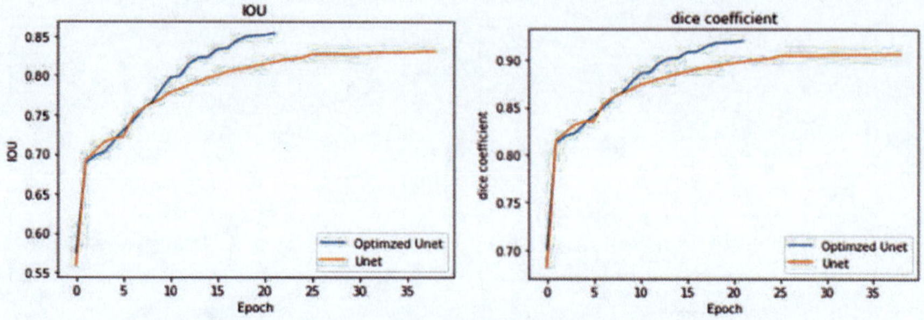

Fig. 10 Comparison of IOU and dice between U-Net and optimized U-Net

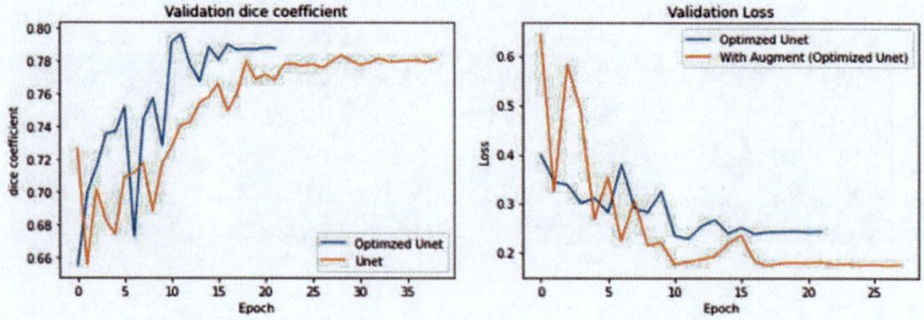

Fig. 11 Left: comparison of validation dice coefficient between U-Net and optimized U-Net. Right: comparison of validation loss before and after dataset augmentation

Figure 11 shows the reduction in loss after data augmentation. The increase in validation accuracy of 5% shows that overfitting is significantly decreased, and the ability of the network to generalize outside of the dataset is improved. This is evident in Fig. 9, as after data augmentation the predictions are closer to the ground truth than ever before.

4 Conclusion

Early detection of gliomas in brain MR images is important for enhancing the treatment options. In this paper, the need for large dataset for training of deep neural networks is accomplished by use of an efficient GAN-based augmentation and optimized U-Net for automatic brain tumor segmentation. BraTS 2017 brain tumor dataset has been used to evaluate the performance of proposed segmentation approach. Dice coefficient, Jaccard similarity, precision, and recall measures are used as performance metric in the proposed system which demonstrates the better performance compared to traditional U-Net-based deep learning model. In the future, we plan to combine the multi-task learning technique with the proposed architecture to improve accuracy and increase the number of classes, perhaps providing more information on the grades of glioma tumors.

References

1. Bowles C, Chen L, Guerrero R, Bentley P, Gunn R, Hammers A, Dickie DA, Hernández MV, Wardlaw J, Rueckert D (2018) Gan augmentation: augmenting training data using generative adversarial networks. arXiv preprint arXiv:1810.10863
2. Iqbal S, Ghani MU, Saba T, Rehman A (2018) Brain tumor segmentation in multi-spectral MRI using convolutional neural networks (CNN). Microsc Res Tech 81(4):419–427
3. Nalepa J, Marcinkiewicz M, Kawulok M (2019) Data augmentation for brain-tumor segmentation: a review. Front Comput Neurosci 13:83
4. Sandfort V, Yan K, Pickhardt PJ, Summers RM (2019) Data augmentation using generative adversarial networks (CycleGAN) to improve generalizability in CT segmentation tasks. Sci Rep 9(1):1–9
5. Mok TC, Chung AC (2018) Learning data augmentation for brain tumor segmentation with coarse-to-fine generative adversarial networks. In: International MICCAI brainlesion workshop. Springer, Cham, pp 70–80
6. Han C, Murao K, Noguchi T, Kawata Y, Uchiyama F, Rundo L, Nakayama H, Satoh SI (2019) Learning more with less: conditional PGGAN-based data augmentation for brain metastases detection using highly-rough annotation on MR images. In: Proceedings of the 28th ACM international conference on information and knowledge management, pp 119–127
7. Ghaffari M, Sowmya A, Oliver R (2019) Automated brain tumor segmentation using multimodal brain scans: a survey based on models submitted to the BraTS 2012–2018 challenges. IEEE Rev Biomed Eng 13:156–168
8. McKinley R, Meier R, Wiest R (2018) Ensembles of densely-connected CNNs with label-uncertainty for brain tumor segmentation. In: International MICCAI brainlesion workshop. Springer, Cham, pp 456–465
9. Khan H, Shah PM, Shah MA, ul Islam S, Rodrigues JJ (2020) Cascading handcrafted features and convolutional neural network for IoT-enabled brain tumor segmentation. Comput Commun 153:196–207
10. Zhang Y, Zhong P, Jie D, Wu J, Zeng S, Chu J, Liu Y, Wu EX, Tang X (2021) Brain tumor segmentation from multi-modal MR images via ensembling UNets. Front Radiol 11
11. Bukhari ST, Mohy-ud-Din H (2021) E1D3 U-Net for brain tumor segmentation: submission to the RSNA-ASNR-MICCAI BraTS 2021 challenge. arXiv preprint arXiv:2110.02519
12. Isola P, Zhu JY, Zhou T, Efros AA (2017) Image-to-image translation with conditional adversarial networks. In: Proceedings of the IEEE conference on computer vision and pattern recognition, pp 1125–1134
13. Ronneberger O, Fischer P, Brox T (2015) U-net: convolutional networks for biomedical image segmentation. In: International conference on medical image computing and computer-assisted intervention. Springer, Cham, pp 234–241
14. Heusel M, Ramsauer H, Unterthiner T, Nessler B, Hochreiter S (2017) Gans trained by a two time-scale update rule converge to a local nash equilibrium. Adv Neural Inf Proc Syst 30
15. Kim S, Kim B, Park H (2021) Synthesis of brain tumor multicontrast MR images for improved data augmentation. Med Phys 48(5):2185–2198. https://doi.org/10.1002/mp.14701
16. Li Q, Yu Z, Wang Y, Zheng H (2020) TumorGAN: a multi-modal data augmentation framework for brain tumor segmentation. Sensors 20(15):4203
17. Madani A, Moradi M, Karargyris A, Syeda-Mahmood T (2018) Chest x-ray generation and data augmentation for cardiovascular abnormality classification. In: Medical imaging 2018: image processing, vol 10574. International Society for Optics and Photonics, p 105741M

18. Radford A, Metz L, Chintala S (2015) Unsupervised representation learning with deep convolutional generative adversarial networks. arXiv preprint arXiv:1511.06434
19. Shin HC, Tenenholtz NA, Rogers JK, Schwarz CG, Senjem ML, Gunter JL, Andriole KP, Michalski M (2018) Medical image synthesis for data augmentation and anonymization using generative adversarial networks. In: International workshop on simulation and synthesis in medical imaging. Springer, Cham, pp 1–11

Estimation of Different Transformation Parameters Based on Optimised Scale Invariant Feature Transform for Image Registration

Joydev Hazra, Aditi Roy Chowdhury, Kousik Dasgupta, and Paramartha Dutta

Abstract Image registration uses attributes or similarity measures to align images taken at various times or from different points of view. In this work, we provide an image registration parameter estimation approach based on structural features. The scale invariant feature transform (SIFT) retrieves structural features such as edge, corner, and so on. To choose the most intrinsic element from the retrieved feature vector, the arithmetic optimisation algorithm (AOA) is applied. On image databases that are publicly accessible such as standard benchmark images, synthetic aperture radar (SAR) and medical images, the proposed technique's effectiveness is compared to different earlier state-of-the-art methodologies. According to the results of this experiment, this strategy can reduce the mean square error of inaccurate image registration parameter predictions.

Keywords Image registration · SIFT · AOA · Parameter estimation

1 Introduction

For the last few decays, image registration and matching has been the most challenging interest of researchers. Two or more images, captured from different perspectives, times, or modalities, are aligned to form a single 2D/3D scene [1]. Image registration is used in a range of applications, such as fusing two or more images, compressing inter- or intra-patient MRI, CT, or SPET images, the construction of a 3D image from

J. Hazra (✉)
Heritage Institute of Technology, Kolkata, India
e-mail: joydevhazra@gmail.com

A. R. Chowdhury
Women's Polytechnic, Kolkata, India

K. Dasgupta
Kalyani Government Engineering College, Kalyani, India

P. Dutta
Visvabharati University, Santiniketan, India

© The Author(s), under exclusive license to Springer Nature Singapore Pte Ltd. 2023

J. K. Mandal and D. De (eds.), *Frontiers of ICT in Healthcare*, Lecture Notes in Networks and Systems 519, https://doi.org/10.1007/978-981-19-5191-6_52

numerous 2D images, remote sensing, and so on. The goal of image registration is to anticipate the transformation parameters between the input and target images, such as rotation, translation, and scale.

Two crucial processes in image registration are feature extraction and matching. Various feature extraction algorithms extract features such as points, edges, curves, and corners from images. The most effective feature-based matching algorithms include scale invariant feature transform (SIFT) [2], speed up robust feature (SURF) [3], histogram of oriented gradients (HOG) [4], Kanade Lucas Tomasi (KLT) [5, 6], and geometric invariants using local features [7]. For deriving structural features, the histogram of oriented gradients (HOG) [4] method is well-known. The final feature vector is separated into cells, which are overlapping blocks that are utilised to compute the HOG descriptor. Its efficiency against image rotation, on the other hand, is insufficient [8]. The feature tracking and extraction approach Kanade Lucas Tomasi (KLT) is utilised in image registration [5, 6]. It uses spatial information from the pixels to find the best match point. In the year 2004 [2], Lowe proposed the SIFT algorithm. SIFT is a highly effective feature-based image registration approach, however, it is computationally demanding. A number of analysts have created SIFT modifications such as SAR-SIFT [9], DSP Filter [10], and PCA-SIFT [11], to minimise computational unpredictability. In [12], the SURF feature was combined with the maximum submatrix. The SURF algorithm is a faster version of the SIFT method, but it is not rotationally stable. The authors offer an image registration technique based on the NSCT, mutual information (MI), and particle swarm optimisation (PSO) [13, 14]. An optimisation search strategy known as a genetic algorithm (GA) [15] is used to find exact or approximate target solutions. Equilibrium optimisation (EO) [16], a recently developed optimisation technique, has been combined with the feature extraction algorithm (SIFT) to determine different affine transformation parameters for image registration [17]. The main problem of EO is that it tends to become trapped in local minima. The newly developed arithmetic optimisation algorithm (AOA) [18] is employed as a feature selection strategy in this paper to overcome this challenge. The mathematical presentation of AOA is straightforward and transparent. Due to the random and adaptive parameters, the AOA's search solutions diverged and converged quickly.

2 Proposed Methodology

The suggested approach for image registration is clearly illustrated in this section. To create the keypoint description in the first phase, SIFT is performed. Then, using an arithmetic optimisation approach (AOA), the best features are selected.

2.1 Feature Extraction by SIFT

SIFT is a method of recognising important, steady feature points in an image ($I(x, y)$). It is comprised of the following steps:

(a) Determine the approximate location and scale of prominent feature points, i.e. keypoints: Gaussian kernels (G) are used to produce scale space in the initial phase of scale-space extrema identification.

$$R(x, y, \sigma) = G(x, y, \sigma) * I(x, y) \tag{1}$$

The difference of Gaussian (DoG) is often used to detect local maxima and minima in scale space.

$$D(x, y, \sigma) = R(x, y, k\sigma) - R(x, y, \sigma) \tag{2}$$

(b) Refine the location and scale of salient keypoints: The low-contrast points and weak feature points on the edges of images are filtered out by keypoint localization. The position of the extremum, F, is determined using Eq. 3.
If the value of F is less than a threshold value, this point is excluded. This removes low-contrast extrema.

$$F = -\frac{\partial^2 D^{-1}}{\partial x^2} \frac{\partial D}{\partial x} \tag{3}$$

(c) Decide the orientation and magnitude (s) of each keypoint using Eqs. (4) and (5).

$$m(x, y) = \sqrt{(R(x+1, y) - R(x-1, y))^2 + (R(x, y+1) - R(x, y-1))^2} \tag{4}$$

$$\theta(x, y) = tan^{-1}(R(x, y+1) - R(x, y-1))/(R(x+1, y) - R(x-1, y)) \tag{5}$$

(d) For each keypoint, emerge appropriate descriptors.

2.2 Feature Selection by AOA

The usage of arithmetic operators in solving arithmetic issues is the main source of inspiration for the proposed AOA. The optimisation process in AOA starts with a randomly selected list of potential solutions. It is divided into two phases: exploration and exploitation. The exploring parts use the following position updating formulae as given in following equations.

$$A(r) = \min + r * (\max - \min)/\max_r \tag{6}$$

where $A(r)$ denotes the acceleration function value at the rth iteration, r lies between 1 and $\max_r$. max and min denote the minimum and maximum values of the accelerated function, respectively.

AOA's exploration operators search the search area at random. For the condition of $r_1 > A$, AOA performs exploration phase, otherwise, the algorithm performs exploitation phase. In exploration phase, $r_2 < 0.5$ is used to condition the first operator (division) as given equation (8). Otherwise, the present work will be performed by the second operator (multiplication) instead of the D, where r_1, r_2 are random numbers.

$$P(r) = 1 - \frac{r^{1/\alpha}}{\max_r^{1/\alpha}} \tag{7}$$

$$x_{i,j}(r+1) = \begin{cases} \text{best}(x_j) \div (P + \epsilon) * ((U_j - L_j) * \mu + L_j), r_2 < 0.5 \\ \text{best}(x_j) * P * ((U_j - L_j) * \mu + L_j), \text{otherwise} \end{cases} \tag{8}$$

AOA's exploitation operators scour the search area for a better solution by focusing on numerous dense regions. Here, $r_3 < 0.5$ conditions the first operator (subtraction) in this phase as given in equation (9). Otherwise, the second operator (addition) will be performed. Here, again r_3 is the random number.

$$x_{i,j}(r+1) = \begin{cases} \text{best}(x_j) - P * ((U_j - L_j) * \mu + L_j), r_3 < 0.5 \\ \text{best}(x_j) + P * ((U_j - L_j) * \mu + L_j), \text{otherwise} \end{cases} \tag{9}$$

Algorithm 1 SIFT-AOA algorithm

1: Compute the Gaussian scale-space of the input image and compute the Difference of Gaussians (DoG) using Eq. (2) and find the candidate keypoints.
2: Refine candidate keypoints location with sub-pixel precision using Eq. (3).
3: Assign a reference magnitude to each keypoint by Eq. (4).
4: Build the keypoint descriptor.
5: Randomly choose keypoint descriptor to make initial solution sets.
6: Initialize parameter a, m.
7: **while** (**do** not termination condition)
8: Calculate objective functions of the solution sets.
9: Choose the best solution based objective function.
10: Update $A(r)$ and $P(r)$ using Eqs. (6) and (7).
11: Generate three random values in the range 0 and 1 i.e R_1, R_2, R_3.
12: **if** $R_1 > A$ **then**
13: compute exploration phase and update solution sets using division operation or multiplication operation as given in (8).
14: **else**
15: Compute exploitation phase and update solution sets using subtraction operation or addition operation as given in Eq. (9).
16: **end if**
17: **end while**
18: Return the best keypoint descriptor.

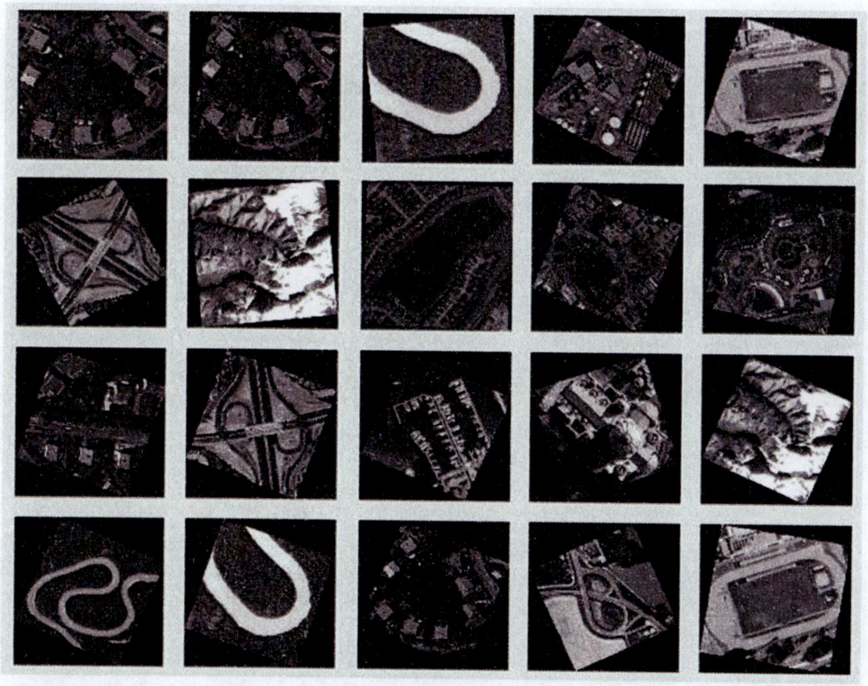

Fig. 1 Sample SAR images

3 Result Analysis

This article presents the estimated results of transformation parameters for image registration using three different types of datasets. Different types of benchmark images are included in the datasets, including typical images used in various image processing applications, medical images [19, 20], and synthetic aperture radar (SAR) [21]. In Figs. 1, 2 and 3, a sample set of images is shown. The transformational parameters were bound within a certain range for the experiments, i.e. the rotational angle is between 30° and 30° degrees, the scaling along the X and Y axes is between 0 and 3, and the translation along the X and Y axes is between 1 and 10.

The proposed methodology is compared with the original SIFT [2], KLT [5] , HOG [4], and SIFT-EO [17] algorithms in terms of parameter prediction. As a predictor, we used BPNN to estimate various transformation parameters. To compare the outcomes, we use ten repetitions to calculate the average MSE in terms of rotation (R_{MSE}), scaling (S_{MSE}), and translation (T_{MSE}). Table 1 compares the proposed method to numerous structural feature-based algorithms on the SAR dataset, medical dataset, and standard image sets. The suggested method clearly outperforms other well-known methods, as evidenced by these observations.

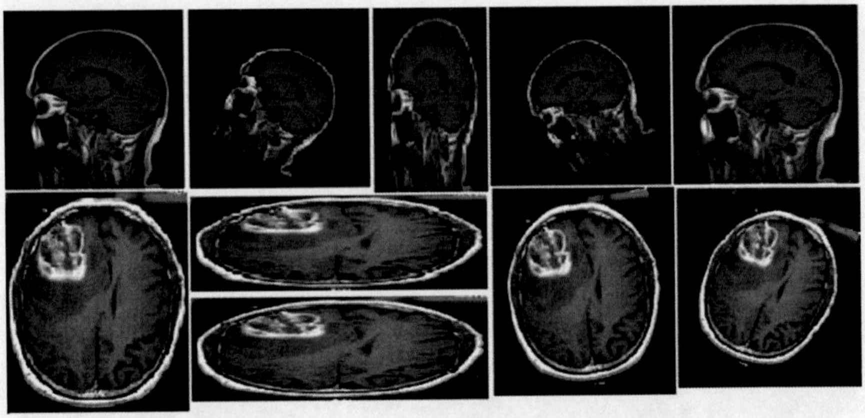

Fig. 2 Sample standard images

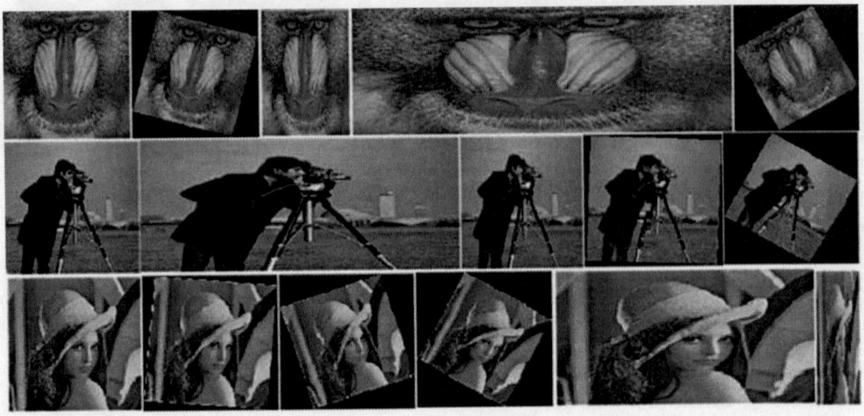

Fig. 3 Sample medical images

Table 1 MSE calculation on standard image dataset

Image datasets	SAR dataset			Medical dataset			Standard images		
Methods	R_{MSE}	S_{MSE}	T_{MSE}	R_{MSE}	S_{MSE}	T_{MSE}	R_{MSE}	S_{MSE}	T_{MSE}
SIFT	0.1202	0.1052	0.0217	0.1760	0.1845	0.0349	0.2742	0.1751	0.0289
KLT	0.146	0.2419	0.2127	0.3214	0.4142	0.1211	0.8933	0.4468	0.0311
HOG	0.066	0.1106	0.1174	0.4118	0.3343	0.0355	0.9843	0.2483	0.0359
SIFT-EO	0.0346	0.0902	0.0194	0.2185	0.2863	0.0182	0.2298	0.1448	0.0194
SIFT-AOA	0.0724	0.0747	0.0607	0.0967	0.0905	0.0738	0.0788	0.0847	0.0764

4 Conclusion

For image registration, this paper provides a structural feature-based transformational parameter estimation technique. We use SIFT to extract structural features and AOA to choose the best feature set. The backpropagation-based neural network is trained using this reduced feature vector. To estimate affine transformation parameters for image registration, the trained BPNN is used as a predictor. The efficiency of the proposed method is demonstrated by different experimental findings on various types of image datasets. In most cases, it outperforms other state-of-the-art works by a significant margin. In future, we try to improve it so that it can more reliably detect the various transformation parameters.

References

1. Zitova JFB (2003) Image registration methods: a survey. Image Vis Comput 21(1):977–1000
2. Lowe DG (2004) Distinctive image features from scale-invariant keypoints. Int J Comput Vis 5(2):91–110
3. Bay H, Tuytelaars T, LVG (2006) Surf: speeded up robust features. In: European conference on computer vision, pp 404–417
4. Navneet Dalal BT (2005) Histograms of oriented gradients for human detection, pp 886–893
5. Carlo Tomasi TK (1994) Detection and tracking of point features. Tech Rep CMU, pp 91–132
6. Nalina S, Mal A, SKVKS (2014) Image based velocity estimation by feature extraction and sub-pixel image matching. Int J Eng Res Technol 3
7. Lu Y, Gao K, TZTX (2018) A novel image registration approach via combining local features and geometric invariants. PLoS ONE 13(1)
8. Luo Z, Chen J, Takiguchi T, Ariki Y (2018) Rotation-invariant histograms of oriented gradients for local patch robust representation, pp 196–199
9. Gousseau J, Michel Y, JDFD (2015) Sift: A sift-like algorithm for sar images. IEEE Trans Geosci Remote Sens 53:453–466
10. Dong J, Soatto S (2015) Domain-size pooling in local descriptors: Dsp-sift. In: 2015 IEEE conference on computer vision and pattern recognition (CVPR). Boston, MA
11. Ke Y, RS (2004) PCA-sift: a more distinctive representation for local image descriptors. In: IEEE conference on computer vision and pattern recognition (CVPR)
12. Aljutaili DS, Almutlaq RA, Alharbi SA, Ibrahim DM (2018) A speeded up robust scale-invariant feature transform currency recognition algorithm. Int J Comput Inf Eng 12(6):365–370
13. Al-Azzawi N, Abdullah WAKW (2012) Mri monomodal feature based registration based on the efficiency of multiresolution representation and mutual information. Am J Biomed Eng
14. Malika A, Kumar M (2021) Autofer: PCA and PSO based automatic facial emotion recognition, pp 3039–3049
15. Goldberg D (1989) Genetic algorithm in search, optimization and machine learning. Addison-Wesley Professional
16. Faramarzi A, Heidarinejad M, BSSM (2020) Equilibrium optimizer: a novel optimization algorithm. Knowl.-Based Syst. 191
17. Hazra J, Chowdhury A, Dasgupta K, Dutta P (2022) Robust optimized structural feature-based transformation parameter estimation for image registration, pp 531–540
18. Abualigah L, Diabat A, Mirjalili S, Abd Elaziz M, Gandomi A (2021) The arithmetic optimization algorithm. Comput Meth Appl Mech Eng 376

19. http://www.med.wayne.edu/diagRadiology/Anatomy_Modules/brain/brain.html
20. http://www.med.harvard.edu/aanlib/home.html
21. Xia GS, Hu J, Hu F, Shi B, Bai X, Zhong Y, Zhang L, Lu X (2017) Aid: a benchmark data set for performance evaluation of aerial scene classification. IEEE Trans Geosci Remote Sens 55(7):3965–3981. http://dx.doi.org/10.1109/TGRS.2017.2685945

Designing an Iterative Adaptive Arithmetic Coding-Based Lossless Bio-signal Compression for Online Patient Monitoring System (IAALBC)

Uttam Kr. Mondal, Asish Debnath, N. Tabassum, and J. K. Mandal

Abstract Various new generation research works on real-time healthcare monitoring system are performing on to fulfill the demands of medical signal compression. In this paper, we proposed a state-of-the-art technique to compress and transmit large number of bio-signals like EEG, ECG, etc., of multiple patients over a network. The proposed bio-signal lossless compression system formed on iterative adaptive arithmetic coding technique. In an online patient monitoring system, using the proposed technique, multiple signals from large number of patients are compressed and sent over the network to the control room by saving bandwidth. The technique is comprised of restructuring frequency and magnitude and phase components followed by adaptive arithmetic coding. Therefore, the proposed mechanism reduces the complexities and at the same time increase the compression performance compared to the existing encoders. Assessing the performance of the methodology and the quality of the signal, several parameters such as compression ratio, SNR, PSNR, and entropy are used to analyze the experimental data.

Keywords Lossless compression · Bio-signal · Discrete Fourier transforms · Inverse Fourier transforms · Adaptive arithmetic coding

1 Introduction

Nowadays, high quality signal recording demand for mobile products and portable health monitoring systems needs a lossless compressor [2] for handling electrocardiogram (ECG), electroencephalogram (EEG), electromyogram (EMG), electrooculogram (EOG), electroretinogram (ERG), electrogastrogram (EGG), electrodermal activity (EDA), etc., bio-signals with reduced storage need [26, 27]. Bio-signals are bioelectrical signals in living beings that can be monitored and measured.

U. Kr. Mondal (✉) · A. Debnath · N. Tabassum
Department of Computer Science, Vidyasagar University, Midnapore, West Bengal, India
e-mail: uttam_ku_82@yahoo.co.in

J. K. Mandal
Department of CSE, Kalyani University, Kalyani, West Bengal, India

© The Author(s), under exclusive license to Springer Nature Singapore Pte Ltd. 2023

J. K. Mandal and D. De (eds.), *Frontiers of ICT in Healthcare*, Lecture Notes in Networks and Systems 519, https://doi.org/10.1007/978-981-19-5191-6_53

In current Internet and streaming era, communicating multiple signals in reduced compacted form [1] are becoming more prevalent [10]. Lossless compression [14] technique reconstructs the original data from the compressed data without compromising the data quality [21, 25]. Nowadays, various research with new emerging technologies is going on to improve the performance of the lossless compression [24, 25]. The fast Fourier transform [6, 7] method is a mathematical operation which is applicable in many fields like signal processing, image processing, signal analysis [30], etc. Arithmetic coding [9, 23] is a type of entropy [16] encoding which is used in lossless data compression. The latest method applied in data compression technique is arithmetic coding [5, 22]. Arithmetic coding [19] provides higher compression and is faster for adaptive models. The fast Fourier transform (FFT) [3, 4] is generally used to reconstructing the signals into frequency domain and analyzes its properties.

In an online patient monitoring system, various captured bio-signals like ECG, EEG, EMG, EOG, etc., are sent over the network to the control room for monitoring purpose. In this paper, a low complexity and high compression capable method for bio-signal compression technique is introduced. This lossless encoder will receive the signals and encoded into compressed format and transmit over the network to the control room. The lossless compression technique is fabricated using two steps. In the initial step, the transformation of bio-signals into frequency domain using the fast Fourier transform (FFT) [8] occurred. The extraction of frequency, magnitude, and phase components is occurred in frequency domain. The total number of (frequency/magnitude) components is being divided into a set of equal size blocks, and each of the blocks is divided into equal size sub-blocks successively. In the subsequence phase, adaptive arithmetic coding is applied over each sub-block of the frequencies and magnitudes separately. Repeatedly, applying the same process over the entire frequency and magnitude components in sub-blocks of each block produces a compressed representation of signal without losing any signal information or audible quality.

2 The Technique

The compression algorithm namely encoding of frequency and magnitude components (IAALBC-EFMC) depicts how the bio-signal is transformed into the frequency domain and components (frequency, magnitude, and phase) are segregated. Adaptive arithmetic coding is applied to constituted components to generate compressed data stream. The decoding algorithm namely decoding of frequency and magnitude components (IAALBC-DFMC) performs as the inverse process of the (IAALBC-EFMC) algorithm and regenerates input bio-signal. The compression technique is depicted in Fig. 1.

The encoding technique works in three steps.

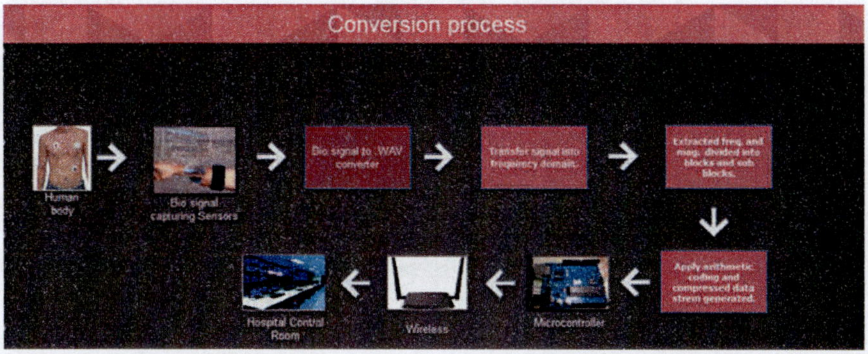

Fig. 1 Conversion process

Step 1: MATLAB programming artifacts convert the bio-signals to waveform audio file format. We have used audiowrite function to develop the programming stuff.
Step 2: The bio-signal transformation in frequency domain is performed by applying fast Fourier transform (FFT). Magnitude, frequency, and phase components are computed from the transformed signal.
Step 3: The total number of frequency and magnitude components is divided into equal size block and sub-block subsequently. Then, process each block and applies arithmetic encoding separately on each sub-block belongs to the corresponding block.

2.1 Encoding Frequency and Magnitude Components (IAALBC-EFMC)

The encoding technique is outlined in Algorithm 1.

Algorithm 1 The IAALBC-EFMC compression algorithm

Require: A strip of bio-signal

1: Convert the slice of a bio-signal input signal into waveform format.

2: Transfer the bio-signal into frequency domain. With the help of fast Fourier transformations (FFT), a time domain bio-signal is transformed in frequency domain. $Y = \text{FFT}(x)$ enumerates the discrete Fourier transform (DFT) of X using FFT algorithm. The bio-sampled values in spatial domain are denoted as x.

3: Segregation of the magnitude, frequency, and phase components of the corresponding signal. Magnitude, frequency, and phase information are extracted from transformed signal using Eq. (1).

$$x_{p(t)} = \sum_{n=-\infty}^{\infty} x_n e^{j2\pi n f_0 t} \quad (1)$$

Equation 1 states that $x_{p(t)}$ normally is constructed by the frequency components at DC, fundamental, and corresponding higher harmonics. The $|x_p|$ versus n (or nf_0) plot is called the magnitude spectrum, and φ_n versus n (or nf_0) is termed as the phase spectrum. $|x_p|$ denotes the magnitude of the component in $x_{p(t)}$ at nf_0 (frequency) and φ_n (its phase). The spectrum of the periodic signal available at discrete frequencies only, which is at nf_0, where $n = 0, \pm 1, \pm 2, \ldots$, etc. The values of $(n, f_0, \emptyset)$, $\emptyset =$ initial angle of phase signal and $n = 0, \pm 1, \pm 2, \ldots$, etc., represent the phase component of bio-signal.

4: Distribute the extracted frequency and magnitude into blocks. The total number of frequency and magnitude components is divided into sets of equal size blocks and blocks are divided into equal size sub-block subsequently. The size of the block and sub-block is considered as 125 and 5 (due to machine limitations but it can be varied), respectively. The arithmetic coding technique is applied to each sub-block. Let, N represents the total number of frequency/magnitude components.

$R =$ size of block (i.e., 125)

$S_b =$ Sub-block size (i.e., 5)

$$\text{Total number of blocks} = \frac{N}{R} \quad (2)$$

5: While (Range blocks exist that do not covered yet), do.

5.1: Calculate number of sub-blocks in each block. In each block, total range of entries (frequency/magnitudes) is divided into number of sub-blocks.

$$\text{Total number of sub blocks} = \frac{R}{Sb} \quad (3)$$

5.1.1: while (Range sub-blocks exist that do not covered yet), do.

Arithmetic coding is applied separately on each of the sub-blocks. The arithmetic encoding technique [27] is represented by intervals in the form $\theta_k(H) = (\gamma_k, \delta_k), k = 0, 1, 2, \ldots, N$, where H is the input data sequence,

γ_k and δ_k are denoted as real numbers such that $0 \leq \gamma_k \leq \gamma_{k+1}$ and $\delta_{k+1} \leq \delta_k \leq 1$.

For simple representation of the above intervals

$$|s, t\rangle = [\gamma, \delta) \text{ if } s = \gamma \text{ and } t = \delta - \gamma \tag{4}$$

In this new notation, set of recursive equations [25, 26]

$$\theta_0(H) = |s_0, t_0\rangle = |0, 1\rangle, \tag{5}$$

$$\theta_k(H) = |s_k, t_k\rangle = |s_{k-1} + c(h_k)t_{k-1}, p(h_k)t_{k-1}\rangle, k = 1, 2, \ldots, N \tag{6}$$

The characteristics of the intervals ensures that $0 \leq s_k \ll s_{t+1} < 1$, and $0 \leq t_{k+1} < t_k \leq 1$. A code value in the final interval, which is $\hat{v} \in \theta_N(H)$.

End While;

5.2: Single arithmetic compressed form of bio-data which is the combination of frequency and magnitude components generated at the end of processing of each block.

End While;

6: A stream of arithmetic encoded frequency and magnitude combined entity generated, which is equal to the number of block.

7. Stop.

2.2 *Decoding Frequency and Magnitude Components (IAALBC-DFMC)*

The decoding algorithm process the encoded streams generated from the encoding algorithm (IAALBC-EFMC). The decoding algorithm regenerates the input bio-signal in spatial domain from encoded compressed values in the frequency domain. The decoding method is outlined in Algorithm 2.

Algorithm 2 The IAALBC-DFMC decompression algorithm

Require: A IAALBC-EFMC encoded datastream.

1: Apply Arithmetic decoding techniques on the encoded input streams. In the arithmetic decoding technique [27], the decoded sequence is purely dependent on the compressed sequence code value $\hat{v}$. Therefore, the decoded sequence is represented as below

$$\widehat{H}(\hat{v}) = \left\{\widehat{h_1}(\hat{v}), \widehat{h_2}(\hat{v}), \ldots, \widehat{h_N}(\hat{v})\right\} \tag{7}$$

So, with the help of decoding technique, any code value $\hat{v} \in \theta_N(H)$ can be used to decode the correct sequence, i.e., $\widehat{H}(\hat{v}) = H$.

2: Complex format entity with magnitude and phase component generated. Apply the Eq. (8) on the magnitude and phase value (getting from step 1 of Algorithm 2) to convert into complex value format of the magnitude as magnitude m and phase phi (in radians) can be written in phase form using Eq. (8)

$$F(x) = m * e^{j*\emptyset} \tag{8}$$

where $j =$ square root of -1 (i.e., $\sqrt{-1}$).

3: Apply inverse fast Fourier transform (IFFT). Applying the inverse fast Fourier transform (IFFT) over produced values of step 2 (Algorithm 2). At the end of the step 3, bio-signal sampled values will be generated in the spatial domain.

4: Stop.

3 Results and Analysis

To evaluate the performance of our state-of-the-art technique for bio-signal lossless compression, we used three bio-signals like ECG, EEG, and EMG. We have used ECG dataset [19] sampled at 360 Hz, EEG dataset [28] sampled at 200 Hz, and EMG dataset [29] sampled at 4 kHz from PhysioNet for experimental purpose. We have developed a programming artifact to convert above mentioned three bio-signals to waveform using MATLAB. Here, for experimental purpose, the ECG signals were acquired from the "MIT-BIH Arrhythmia" [31] database. The MATLAB code converts the files belongs to the ECG, EEG, and EMG signals to waveform audio file format. Three existing lossless audio compression techniques considered for the performance evaluation of the present technique are Monkey's Audio [11], WavPack lossless [12] and FLAC [13]. The compression efficiency of the present technique is evaluated by using the statistical parameter metric compression ratio and it is

Table 1 Average compression ratio (%) for WavPack lossless [12], Monkey's audio [11], and FLAC [13] and IAALBC for three different types of signals

Metrics	Signal category	Monkey's audio	WavPack	FLAC	IAALBC
Compression ratio (%)	ECG	46.78	48.7	68.63	91.91
	EEG				
	EMG				

computed by Eqs. (9) and (10), respectively [17].

$$\text{Compression ratio} = \frac{\text{Uncompressed data file size}}{\text{Compressed data file size}} \tag{9}$$

$$\text{Space saving(\%)} = \frac{(\text{Uncompressed data file size} - \text{Compressed data file size})}{\text{Uncompressed data file size}} * 100 \tag{10}$$

Considering the results set of Table 1, IAALBC demonstrates higher compression performance compared to other existing lossless audio signal compression techniques, i.e., Monkey's audio, wave pack, and FLAC. Table 1 and Fig. 2 clearly established that the compression ratio (%) of the present system is better than that of WavPack lossless [12], Monkey's Audio [11], and FLAC [13]. Overall average SNR values of the present technique and referenced techniques are represented in Table 2. Evaluated PSNR values over the dataset are represented in Table 3. PSNR and SNR values are calculated between the compressed signals and the original [15]. Lower SNR and higher PSNR values represent good signal quality. Table 4 is showing the entropy value of the present technique concerning WavPack lossless [12], Monkey's Audio [11], and FLAC [13] lossless technique.

SNR [18] is the measurement of the strength of the signal comparing to the noise. The SNR value calculation is performed using the Eq. 11.

$$\text{SNR} = \sum_{i,j} X_{i,j}^2 / \sum_{i,j} \left(X_{i,j} - \overline{X}_{i,j}\right)^2 \tag{11}$$

Here, $X_{i,j}$ is the input sampled value and $\overline{X}_{i,j}$ is the regenerated sampled value for ith sampled value in jth channel.

PSNR [18] is used to measure the quality between original and reconstructed bio-signal. PSNR calculation is performed using the Eq. 12.

$$\text{PSNR} = I\,J \max_{i,j} X_{i,j}^2 / \sum_{i,j} \left(X_{i,j} - \overline{X}_{i,j}\right)^2 \tag{12}$$

Entropy [16] is used to measure the randomness. It denotes the average information of a symbol. Entropy is calculated using the below Eq. 13

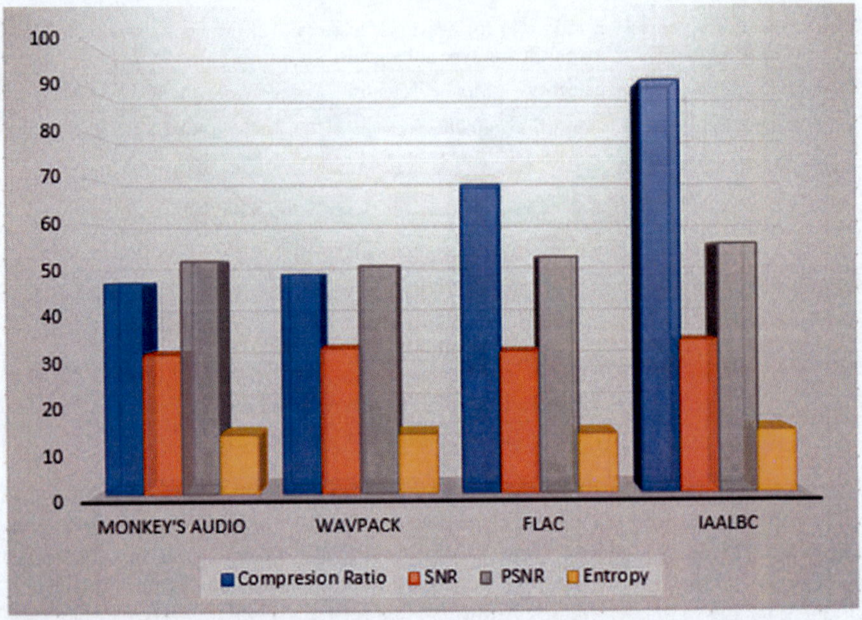

Fig. 2 Graphical representation of performance comparisons

Table 2 Average SNR for three different types of signals for WavPack lossless [12], Monkey's audio [11], FLAC [13], and IAALBC

Metrics	Signal category	Monkey's audio	WavPack	FLAC	IAALBC
SNR	ECG	30.99	32.27	31.43	33.89
	EEG				
	EMG				

Table 3 Average PSNR for three different types of signals for WavPack lossless [12], Monkey's audio [11], FLAC [13], and IAALBC

Metrics	Signal category	Monkey's audio	WavPack	FLAC	IAALBC
PSNR	ECG	51.79	50.59	52.47	55.46
	EEG				
	EMG				

Table 4 Average Entropy for three different types of signals for WavPack lossless [12], Monkey's audio [11], FLAC [13], and IAALBC

Metrics	Signal category	Monkey's audio	WavPack	FLAC	IAALBC
Entropy	ECG	13.1	13.08	13.06	13.78
	EEG				
	EMG				

$$H(X) = -\sum_{k=1}^{m} P(x_k)\log_2 P(x_k) \tag{13}$$

where X represents the discrete random variable with possible values in the signal sampled value set $\{x_1, x_2, \ldots, x_m\}$ with corresponding probabilities $p_1, p_2, \ldots, p_m$, where $\sum_{j=1} p_j = 1$. $H(X)$, the entropy value of X denotes the average information hold in X.

Figure 2 graphically compares the performance of IAALBC with other referenced encoders. Therefore, from experimental outcome, it is evident that the proposed technique (IAALBC) is more efficient.

4 Conclusions

The current compression algorithm is designed in the frequency domain. Extracting individual components, i.e., frequency, magnitude, and phase, and reprocessing their values adaptively using a standard arithmetic coding accomplished greater than 90% audio signal compression without information loss. The robustness characteristics of current proposed algorithm was evaluated using various quality parameters like SNR, PSNR, and entropy. The efficiency of the proposed algorithm may be further improved by searching for more efficient coding techniques along with improvise effective representation of individual components. Experiment with a greater number of different bio-signal is the scope of future work.

References

1. Tejedor J et al (2019) Search on speech from spoken queries: the Multi-domain International ALBAYZIN 2018 Query-by-Example Spoken Term Detection Evaluation. EURASIP J Audio Speech Music Process 2019. Article number: 13
2. Uthayakumar J et al A survey on data compression techniques: from the perspective of data quality, coding schemes, data type and applications. J King Saud Univ Comput Inform Sci. https://doi.org/10.1016/j.jksuci.2018.05.006
3. Cooley JW, Lewis PAW, Welch PD (1969) The fast Fourier transform and its applications. IEEE Trans Educ 12(1):27–34. https://doi.org/10.1109/TE.1969.4320436
4. Serov V Formulation of Fourier series. In: Fourier series, Fourier transform and their applications to mathematical physics, vol 197. ISSN 0066-5452. Springer International Publishing. https://doi.org/10.1007/978-3-319-65262-7
5. Wong MW Discrete Fourier analysis. Birkhäuser Basel. eBook ISBN 978-3-0348-0116-4, https://doi.org/10.1007/978-3-0348-0116-4
6. Brigham EO, Morrow RE (1967) The fast Fourier transform. IEEE Spectr 4(12):63–70. https://doi.org/10.1109/MSPEC.1967.5217220
7. Bergland GD (1969) A guided tour of the fast Fourier transform. IEEE Spectr 6(7):41–52. https://doi.org/10.1109/MSPEC.1969.5213896
8. Loan CV Computational frameworks for the fast Fourier transform. ISBN 978-0-89871-285-8, https://doi.org/10.1137/1.9781611970999

9. Howard PG, Vitter JS (1994) Arithmetic coding for data compression. Proc IEEE 82(6):857–865. https://doi.org/10.1109/5.286189
10. Howard PG, Vitter JS (1992) Practical implementations of arithmetic coding. In: Storer JA (ed) Image and text compression. The Kluwer international series in engineering and computer science (Communication and information theory), vol 176. Springer, Boston, MA. https://doi.org/10.1007/978-1-4615-3596-6_4
11. http://www.monkeysaudio.com/. Accessed on 15.08.2021 at 11 AM
12. http://www.wavpack.com/. Accessed on 14.08.2021 at 9 AM
13. https://xiph.org/flac/. Accessed: 19-09-2021
14. Chou CH, Wu TL (2003) Embedding color watermarks in color images. EURASIP J Adv Sig Process 2003:548941. https://doi.org/10.1155/S1110865703211227
15. Manju M, Abarna P, Akila U, Yamini S (2018) Peak signal to noise ratio and mean square error calculation for various images using the lossless image compression in CCSDS algorithm. Int J Pure Appl Math 119(12):14471–14477
16. Shannon CE (1948) A mathematical theory of communication. Bell Syst Tech J 27(3):379–423. https://doi.org/10.1002/j.1538-7305.1948.tb01338.x
17. Li ZN, Drew MS, Liu J (2014) Internet multimedia content distribution. In: Fundamentals of multimedia. Texts in computer science. Springer, Cham. https://doi.org/10.1007/978-3-319-05290-8_16
18. Kutter M, Petitcolas F (1999) A fair benchmark for image watermarking systems. Proc SPIE Int Soc Opt Eng 3657. https://doi.org/10.1117/12.344672
19. https://data.mendeley.com/datasets/7dybx7wyfn/3. Accessed: 19-09-2021
20. Arnold M (200) Audio watermarking: features, applications and algorithms. In: 2000 IEEE international conference on multimedia and expo. ICME2000. Proceedings. Latest advances in the fast-changing world of multimedia (Cat. No.00TH8532), vol 2, pp 1013–1016. https://doi.org/10.1109/ICME.2000.871531
21. Kim H, Wen J, Villasenor JD (2007) Secure arithmetic coding. IEEE Trans Sig Process 55(5):2263–2272. https://doi.org/10.1109/TSP.2007.892710
22. Huang S-J, Jou M-J (2004) Application of arithmetic coding for electric power disturbance data compression with wavelet packet enhancement. IEEE Trans Power Syst 19(3):1334–1341. https://doi.org/10.1109/TPWRS.2004.825899
23. Rubin F (1979) Arithmetic stream coding using fixed precision registers. IEEE Trans Inf Theor 25(6):672–675. https://doi.org/10.1109/TIT.1979.1056107
24. Mondal U, Debnath A (2021) Developing a dynamic cluster quantization based lossless audio compression (DCQLAC). Multimedia Tools Appl 80:1–24. https://doi.org/10.1007/s11042-020-09886-3
25. Mondal U, Debnath A, Mandal J (2020) Deep learning-based lossless audio encoder (DLLAE). https://doi.org/10.1007/978-981-15-4288-6_6
26. Chua E, Fang WC (2011) Mixed bio-signal lossless data compressor for portable brain-heart monitoring systems. IEEE Trans Consum Electron 57:267–273
27. Sriraam N, Eswaran C (2008) An adaptive error modeling scheme for the lossless compression of EEG signals. IEEE Trans Inf Tech Biomed 12:587–594
28. https://physionet.org/content/auditory-eeg/1.0.0/. Accessed: 19-09-2021
29. https://physionet.org/content/emgdb/1.0.0/. Accessed: 19-09-2021
30. Debnath A, Mondal U, Roy B, Panja N (2020) Achieving lossless audio encoder through integrated approaches of wavelet transform, quantization and Huffman encoding (LAEIWQH), pp 1–5. https://doi.org/10.1109/ICCSEA49143.2020.9132865
31. https://physionet.org/content/mitdb/1.0.0/. Accessed: 19-09-2021

Healthcare Security of Patient's Medical Images by PEE-Based RIW Without Location Mapping

Soumen Bhowmick, Debashis De, and Sudip Ghosh

Abstract Here, we propose a new effective technique for prediction error expansion-based digital reversible watermarking of a color image where embedding the location map (mapping the data of overflow/underflow pixel) into a watermarked image is not required at all. So this technique gives the extra space to embed more secret bits or increase the payload. Basically, we have done a prepossessing of the cover image so that no location map is required but it degrades the quality of the cover image a little bit which is negligible. But it does not affect the embedded 3 bpp color secret/watermarking image. We have done it on MATLAB, and the results are quite good.

Keywords Reversible watermarking · Prediction error expansion (PEE) · Color image watermarking · Location map

1 Introduction

In today's world, digital watermarking of the image is very much essential due to some factors like copyright protection, source tracing, annotations, etc.

Reversible watermarking is a lossless data embedding technique. Where secret image/information is being embedded into a cover image and as a result a watermarked image will be generated. But the quality degradation of the cover image must be as much as low so that distinction between cover image and watermarked image by human eyes is impossible. And the reversibility feature helps us to restore the original secret image and cover image from the watermarked image.

Prediction error expansion (PEE) is a spatial domain algorithm for data hiding. PEE algorithm actually consists of two algorithm which are histogram shifting (HS) and differential expansion (DE). The important features of the PEE algorithm are

S. Bhowmick · S. Ghosh (✉)
Indian Institute of Engineering Science and Technology (IIEST), Shibpur, India
e-mail: soumenbhowmick22@gmail.com

D. De
Maulana Abul Kalam Azad University of Technology, Kolkata, West Bengal, India

© The Author(s), under exclusive license to Springer Nature Singapore Pte Ltd. 2023

J. K. Mandal and D. De (eds.), *Frontiers of ICT in Healthcare*, Lecture Notes in Networks and Systems 519, https://doi.org/10.1007/978-981-19-5191-6_54

large payloads and low distortion, which make this algorithm superior to the other available algorithms in the spatial domain for reversible watermarking. Early PEE-based reversible watermarking is used to embed the problematic pixels location where secret bit cannot be embedded or this location data use as a secret key. But the proposed technique is fully free from the above hindrance that's why this method blindly decodes the secret image as well as cover image and also increases the payload.

Please note that PEE-based reversible watermarking is a very sensitive technique. That is mean if watermarked image is being manipulated or compressed, then restoration of the secret image will be impossible. That is give a huge security to the secret image. So, we use this feature where authentication of the cover image image is important concern and also we can use in covert communication where secret image carry some very sensitive information. For example, we can use this in military field image processing, image sharing in medical field [1], some remote sensing application, and also to archive the multimedia management, etc.

2 Proposed Algorithm

2.1 *Embedding Process*

A digital color image is made by three different color planes that are the RED plane, GREEN plane, and BLUE plane. These three individual planes are like a 2D matrix. Here, each pixel of each plane of the cover image is 8 bpp and the secret image is 1 bpp. This is represented by Fig. 1.

For illustration purposes, we have taken a single plane of cover image as well as a secret image in Fig. 2, which are 2D matrices. Here, the cover image size is (6×6)

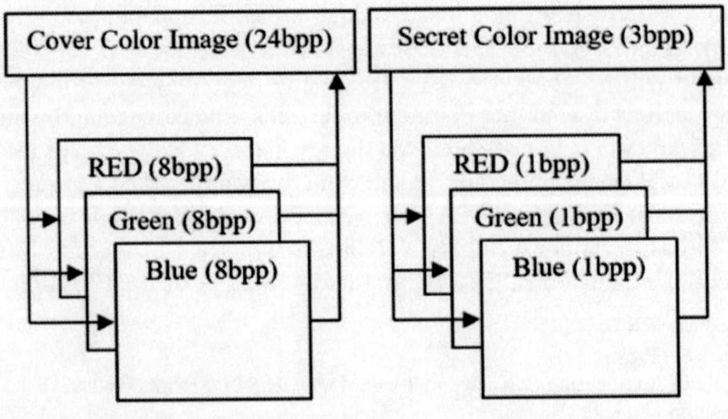

Fig. 1 Here used cover and secret color image format

(a)

154	156	153	153	155	155
154	156	150	148	150	154
154	157	157	157	154	154
151	158	157	155	155	155
255	158	158	159	0	156
154	156	150	148	150	154

Cover Image (6x6)

(b)

1	1
0	1

Secret Image (2x2)

Fig. 2 Example 1: **a** Cover image (6 × 6). **b** Secret image (2 × 2)

and each pixel depth is 8bit so the value will be in the range of [0, 255]. The secret image size is (2 × 2), and pixel depth is 1 so the value will be in the range of [0, 1]. Then, we have to scan cover image pixels in Fig. 2a from left to right first and then top to bottom up to (5 × 5) and for each pixel of a single plane of the cover image, we have to do the next three steps, i.e., pre-processing, prediction algorithm [2], encoding [2, 3].

- **Pre-processing:**

Here, this is the major step for which embedding the location map is not required. So that payload of watermarked image is increased and complexity of this PEE-based reversible watermarking is reduced.

Here, $T(> 0)$ is called capacity parameter [3] by which we may also increase the payload. Capacity parameter actually shifts the pixel intensity value, so it has a significant role in the embedding performance.

Case 1: If pixel intensity value (x) is within the range [$(255 - T)$, 255], then we decrease the pixel value as,

$$x = 255 - T$$

Case 2: If pixel intensity value (x) is within the range [0, T], then we increase the pixel value as,

$$x = T$$

Here, in the Example 1, we have taken $T = 1$. So, pixel value 255 will be 254, and 0 will be 1. They are shown as bold in Fig. 4a.

$$P_x = \begin{cases} \max(a, b) & \text{if } c \le \min(a, b) \\ \min(a, b) & \text{if } c \ge \max(a, b) \\ a + b - c & \text{otherwise} \end{cases}$$

x	b
a	c

Fig. 3 Used prediction algorithm

(a)

154	156	153	153	155	
154	156	150	148	150	
154	157	157	157	154	
151	158	157	155	155	
254	158	158	159	1	

Pre-Processed Cover Image (5x5)

(b)

0	0	0	0	4	
0	6	2	-5	-4	
3	-1	0	3	0	
-103	1	2	-4	154	
98	0	-1	158	-151	

Prediction Error matrix (5x5)

Fig. 4 Example 1: **a** Pre-processing cover image (5 × 5). **b** Prediction error matrix (5 × 5)

- **Prediction Algorithm:**

Here, We have used a low complexity prediction algorithm with an inherent primitive edge detector [2]. The predictor operates on a three neighbor pixels. The prediction algorithm and the contexts pixels are in Fig. 3. Where x is the current pixel and a, b, c are the context of x, and P_x is the predicted value. The pixels in the last row and last column have only one pixel in their context, so this pixels are not considered for embedding.

After computing the prediction value(P_x), then we compute the prediction error P_e as follows and prediction error matrix for example 1 is represented by Fig. 4b.

$$P_e = x - P_x$$

- **Encoding:**

Here, we first check the prediction error (P_e) and according to this P_e, we do the following operation.

Expansion embedding: If the prediction error $P_e \in [-T, T)$, then P_e is expanded and the watermarked pixel intensity value is computed by

$$x^w = x + P_e + S_b\,, \quad \text{if } P_e \in [-T, T)$$

Here, $S_b \in [0, 1]$ is the secret bit, which is the information of secret image bit and secret image row and column binary array followed by a end of secret bit (EOS), that

(a)

155	**157**	**153**	**154**	156	
154	157	151	147	149	
155	**157**	**157**	158	**155**	
150	159	158	154	156	
255	**159**	**157**	160	0	

Encoded matrix up to (5x5)

(b)

155	**157**	**153**	**154**	156	155
154	157	151	147	149	154
155	**157**	**157**	158	**155**	154
150	159	158	154	156	155
255	**159**	**157**	160	0	156
154	156	150	148	150	154

Watermarked Image Matrix (6x6)

Fig. 5 Example 1: **a** Encoded matrix up to (5×5). **b** Watermarked image matrix (6×6)

is 1. After the embedding of EOS, then only we embed the bit 0, which will help us to find the EOS at the time of decoding.

Histogram Shifting: If the prediction error $P_e \in (-\infty, -T) \cup [T, \infty)$, then the pixel does not carry any information and the prediction error is shifted simply by T. The watermarked pixel intensity value is computed by

$$x^w = \begin{cases} x + T, \text{ if } P_e \geq T \\ x - T, \text{ if } P_e < -T \end{cases}$$

Finally, when we complete all the previous three steps for each pixel of the cover image except the last row and last column, then we have to just copy the last row and last column to the watermarked image as it is as in the cover image.

Here, in the example 1, we have done the previous three steps for pixel up to (5×5) in Fig. 5a, then we copy the sixth column and sixth row from the cover image to watermarked image. In this way, we have successfully completed the embedding process and we have got the watermarked image which is in Fig. 5b.

The bolded number in Fig. 5b represents where the secret data has been embedded. Which secret bit has embedded in which location of the watermarked image that is given in Table 1 (Fig. 6).

2.2 *Extraction and Image Restoration Process*

In this process, the input is the watermarked image that is generated in the embedding process. By this process, we cannot restore the cover image instead of getting the cover image we get the pre-process cover image at Fig. 7b. For this, we get a negligible error and we will discuss it in the result and analysis section. But in this process, we are able to restore the secret image without any distortion.

Table 1 Information of embedded bit location on the watermarked image

(Row, column)	Secret bit	Embedded information
(1, 1)	1	This are the secret Image bit (2 × 2) which is shown in Fig. 2b
(1, 2)	1	
(1, 3)	0	
(1, 4)	1	
(2, 1)	0	This is secret image column as binary array
(3, 2)	1	
(3, 3)	0	This is secret image row as binary array
(3, 5)	1	
(5, 2)	1	EOS bit
(5, 3)	0	After EOS, all bit 0

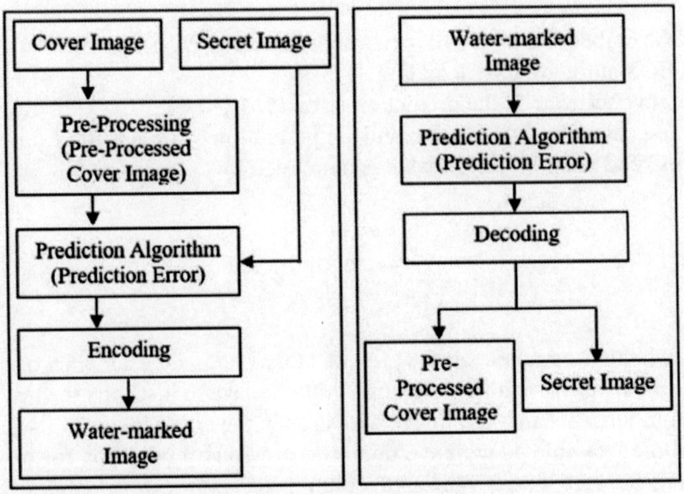

Fig. 6 Left: embedding process || right: extraction and restoration process

To get the original cover image as well as the secret image, we have to process each pixel from downward but leaving the last row and last column of the watermarked image. So in the example, the first selected pixel position in Fig. 5b is (5, 5), whose value is 0. Then, we go in the left and upward direction.

- **Prediction Algorithm:**

The prediction algorithm [2] of the extraction process is exactly the same as described in the embedding process section at Fig. 3. After getting the prediction value($\overline{P_x}$) of the selected pixel, we compute the prediction error($\overline{P_e}$) using the following formula

$$\overline{P_e} = x^w - \overline{P_x}$$

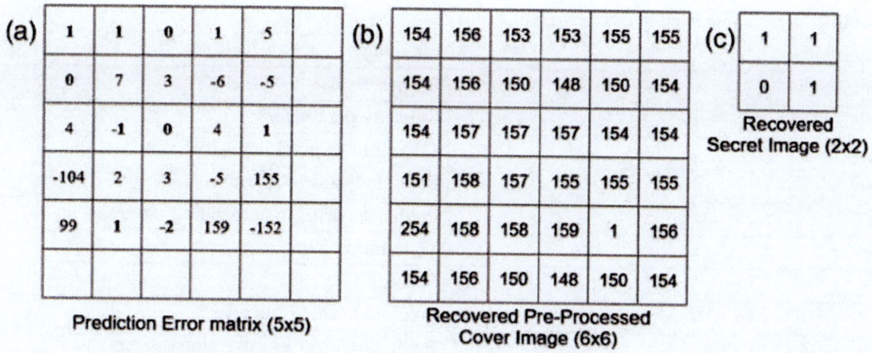

Fig. 7 Example 1: **a** prediction error matrix ($\overline{P_e}$). **b** Pre-process cover image. **c** Secret image

- **Decoding Algorithm:**

Secret image and the cover image can be extracted and be restored according to the $\overline{P_e}$, as follows:

Case 1: If the prediction error($\overline{P_e}$) $\in [-2T, 2T)$

$$S_b = \overline{P_e} - 2\lfloor \overline{P_e}/2 \rfloor$$

$$x = x^w - \lfloor \overline{P_e}/2 \rfloor - S_b$$

Case 2: If the prediction error(P_e) $\in (-\infty, -2T) \cup [2T, \infty)$

$$x = \begin{cases} x^w - T, & \text{if } \overline{P_e} \geq 2T \\ x^w + T, & \text{if } \overline{P_e} < -2T \end{cases}$$

In the example, after completing the decoding process from position (5, 5) to (1, 1) of the watermarked image, then we have copied the last row and column from watermarked image to pre-process cover image. At the time of the decoding process, whenever we will get the first 1 as a S_b, then we skip it and then we will get the row binary array followed by the column binary array of the secret image. Then, we will get the actual secret image data (Table 2).

3 Software Implementation of Proposed Algorithm

We have implemented this proposed algorithm in MATLAB [4] to check the functionality. We take a cover image (Lena) of 24 bpp and whose dimensions is (256 × 256) and a 3 bpp secret image (also Lena) of dimensions (128 × 128) and do

Table 2 Here some used symbols meaning

Symbols	Meaning
bpp	Bit per pixel
T	Capacity parameter
x	Cover image pixel intensity value
P_x	Predicted value of pixel x
P_e	Prediction error in embedding process
x^w	Watermarked image pixel intensity value
S_b	Secret bit
$\overline{P_x}$	Predicted value of pixel x^w
$\overline{P_e}$	Prediction error in extraction process

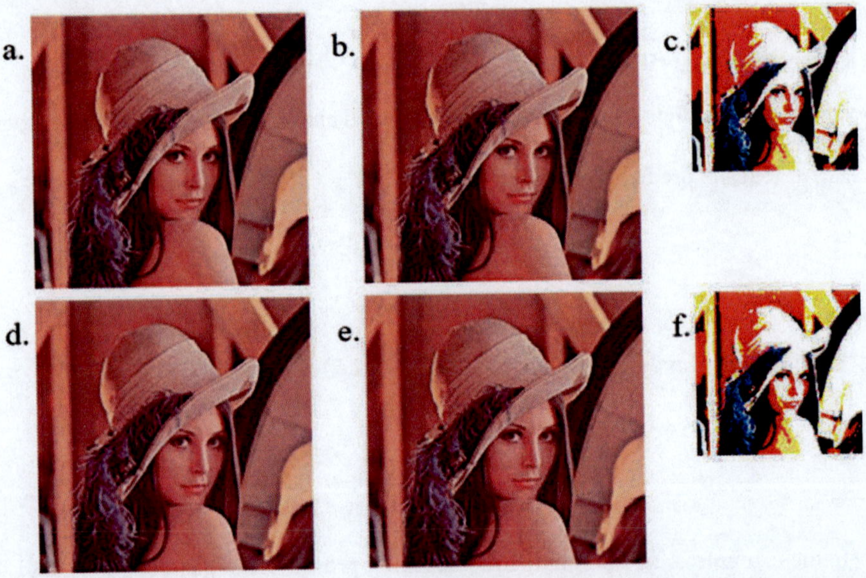

Fig. 8 Example 2: **a** Cover image [Lena (256 × 256)]. **b** Pre-process cover image [Lena (256 × 256)]. **c** Secret image [Lena (128 × 128)]. **d** Watermarked image [Lena (256 × 256)]. **e** Restored pre-process cover image [Lena (256 × 256)]. **f** Restored secret image [Lena (128 × 128)]

the experiment for T equal to 1. Then, we have embedded the three planes of secret image into three planes of cover image by selecting one plane at a time. As a result of this process, we get the watermarked image. After getting the watermarked image, we run the extraction process on it and get the pre-process cover image and the secret image. This is represented by Fig. 8.

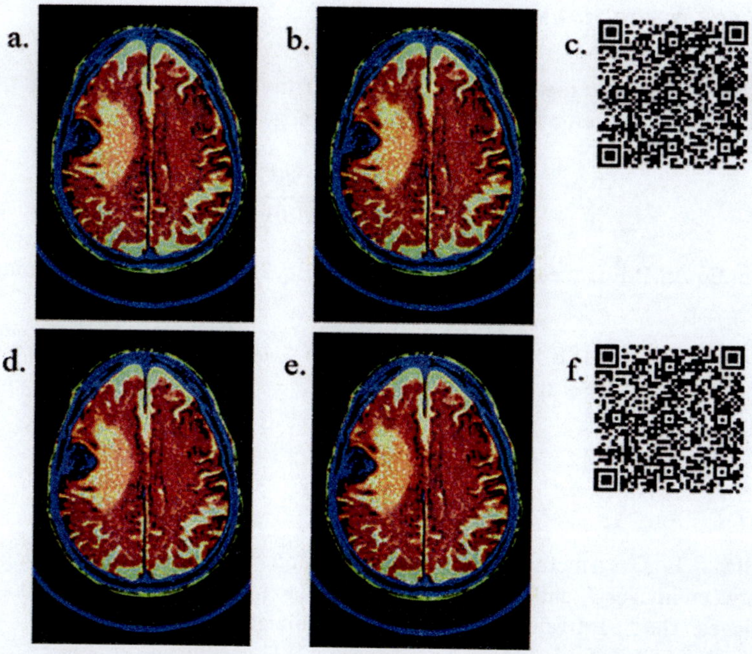

Fig. 9 Example 3: **a** Cover image [CT scan (800 × 545)]. **b** Pre-process cover image (800 × 545). **c** Secret image [QR Code (200 × 200)]. **d** Watermarked image (800 × 545). **e** Restored pre-process cover image (800 × 545). **f** Restored secret image [QR code (200 × 200)]

Then in the other example in Fig. 9 we have taken a color 24 bpp CT scan of brain (800 × 545) which is got from www.sciencephoto.com (https://www.sciencephoto.com/media/254798/view/coloured-ct-scan-of-metastatic-brain-cancer) and a QR code as 3 bpp secret image (200 × 200) into which we embed the arbitrary name and age of a patient and the web address of the cover image. Here, QR code has been embedded into the CT scan and successfully again that QR code has been restored from the watermarked image with no distortion. But in the recovered CT scan image, there was some negligible distortion for $T = 1$.

4 Results and Analysis

Here, we have focused only on two performance parameters. They are PSNR and SSIM [5, 6].

4.1 Peak Signal-to-Noise Ratio (PSNR)

The PSNR in Eq. 1 is a method to measure the quality between image I_1 and image I_2 in dB. The PSNR value for exactly the same images is ∞.

$$\text{PSNR} = 10 \log_{10} \left(\frac{255^2}{\text{MSE}} \right) \tag{1}$$

where in Eq. 1 MSE is mean square error and in Eq. 2 (r x c) is the size of image I_1 and I_2.

$$\text{MSE} = \frac{1}{rc} \sum_{m=1}^{r} \sum_{n=1}^{c} [I_1(m,n) - I_2(m,n)]^2 \tag{2}$$

4.2 Structural Similarity (SSIM) Index

The SSIM in Eq. 3 is a method for predicting the perceived change in quality degradation between images I_1 and I_2. It is generally used to measure the similarity between two images. The SSIM value for the exact same image is 1.

$$\text{SSIM}(I_1, I_2) = \frac{(2\mu_{I_1}\mu_{I_2} + p_1)(2\sigma_{I_1 I_2} + p_2)}{(\mu_{I_1}^2 + \mu_{I_2}^2 + p_1)(\sigma_{I_1}^2 \sigma_{I_2}^2 + p_2)} \tag{3}$$

where μ_{I_1} and μ_{I_2} are the average of image I_1 and I_2, $\sigma_{I_1}^2$ and $\sigma_{I_2}^2$ are the variance of I_1 and I_2, $\sigma_{I_1 I_2}$ is the covariance between I_1 and I_2 and p_1, p_2 are two regularization constants.

Now, we have done some experiments on the cover image by changing the capacity parameter (T) and computed the PSNR (dB) and SSIM. We have shown the result in Tables 3 and 4.

We have taken Lena as cover image and also as secret image in Fig. 8, and the experimental results is shown in Table 3.

After that, we have plotted the percentage SSIM error between embedded Lena as cover image and restored Lena as pre-process cover image for the various capacity parameter (T) in Fig. 10. But, there is no error for T around 8 and a negligible percentage error for T more than 8 and up to 20.

In the next example, we have taken CT scan of brain as cover image and QR code as secret image in Fig. 9 and the experimental results are shown in Table 4.

Now, also we have plotted the percentage SSIM error between embedded CT scan of brain as cover image and restored CT scan of brain as pre-process cover image for a various capacity parameter (T) in Fig. 11. So, there is a negligible percentage error for T around 2. Here, error is increasing as T increases due to more number of pixels intensity values are around 0 and 255.

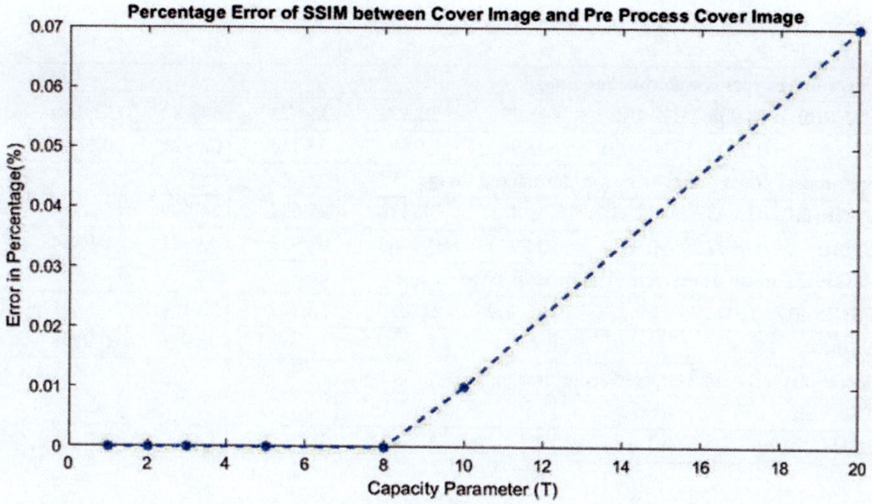

Fig. 10 Percentage SSIM error between cover and pre-process cover image of Lena

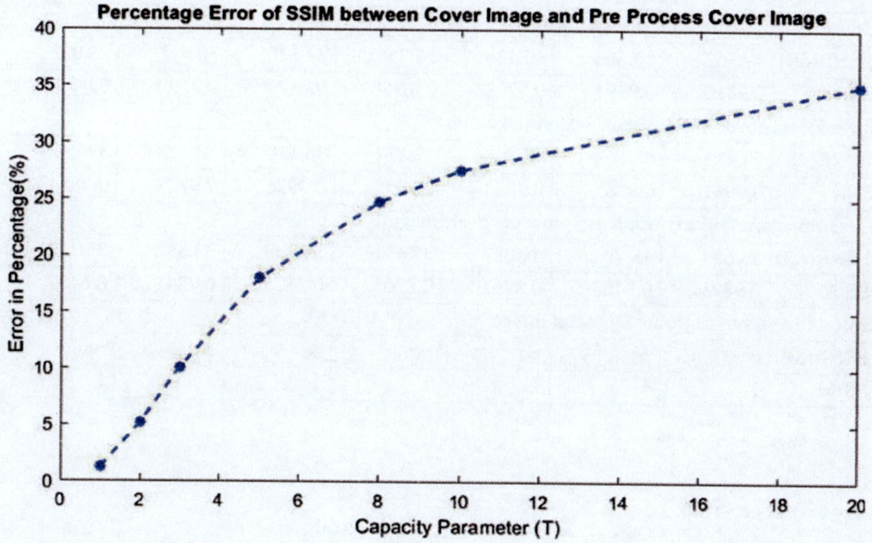

Fig. 11 Percentage SSIM error between cover and pre-process cover image of CT scan

Table 3 Effect of *T* on quality of Lena image (Fig. 8)

T	1	2	3	5	8	10	20
Cover image versus watermarked image							
PSNR(dB)	48.938	44.12	41.493	38.357	35.672	34.482	31.150
SSIM	0.9997	0.9991	0.9983	0.9965	0.9938	0.9921	0.9850
Pre-process cover image versus watermarked image							
PSNR(dB)	48.933	44.116	41.491	38.358	35.682	34.499	31.314
SSIM	0.9997	0.9991	0.9983	0.9965	0.9938	0.9921	0.9854
Cover image versus extracted pre-process cover image							
PSNR(dB)	76.043	69.793	65.969	60.879	55.782	53.154	43.421
SSIM	1	1	1	1	1	0.9999	0.9993
Secret image versus extracted secret image							
PSNR(dB)	∞	∞	∞	∞	∞	∞	∞
SSIM	1	1	1	1	1	1	1

Table 4 Effect of *T* on quality of CT scan image (Fig. 9)

T	1	2	3	5	8	10	20
Cover image versus watermarked image							
PSNR(dB)	49.152	43.668	40.424	36.355	32.610	30.812	25.023
SSIM	0.9810	0.9391	0.8908	0.8144	0.7473	0.7192	0.6440
Pre-process cover image versus watermarked image							
PSNR(dB)	50.133	45.668	42.361	39.114	36.510	35.422	32.892
SSIM	0.9961	0.9965	0.9964	0.9955	0.9936	0.9923	0.9884
Cover image versus extracted pre-process cover image							
PSNR(dB)	55.617	48.79	44.627	39.431	34.739	32.537	25.742
SSIM	0.9873	0.9483	0.8991	0.8205	0.7525	0.7245	0.6497
Secret image versus extracted secret image							
PSNR(dB)	∞	∞	∞	∞	∞	∞	∞
SSIM	1	1	1	1	1	1	1

5 Conclusion

By this algorithm, we have evaluated the performance metrics for various test images. And we have seen that if the cover image pixel intensity value is within a certain range, then we recover the exact cover image from watermarked image. Otherwise, we get a negligible distortion in the cover image. But there is no error in the recovered secret image. So in the application, where a little bit of distortion in the cover image is allowable there, we can use this algorithm.

References

1. Ghosh S, Bhateja Y, Palathinkal JR, Rahaman H (2021) Hardware design with real-time implementation for security of medical images and EPMR. Circ Syst Sig Proc. https://doi.org/10.1007/s00034-021-01807-5
2. Thodi DM, Rodriguez JJ (2004) Prediction-error based reversible watermarking. In: 2004 international conference on image processing, 2004. ICIP '04., vol 3, pp 1549–1552. https://doi.org/10.1109/ICIP.2004.1421361
3. Li X, Yang B, Zeng T (2011) Efficient reversible watermarking based on adaptive prediction-error expansion and pixel selection. IEEE Trans Image Proc 20(12):3524–3533. https://doi.org/10.1109/TIP.2011.2150233
4. MATLAB (2021) version 9.10.0.1739362 (R2021a) Update 5. Natick, Massachusetts, The MathWorks Inc
5. Ahmad Shaik V, Thanikaiselvan, Amitharajan R (2017) Data security through data hiding in images: a review. J Artific Intell 10:1–21. https://doi.org/10.3923/jai.2017.1.21
6. Ghosh SS, Rahaman H (2020) A new digital color image watermarking algorithm with its FPGA and ASIC implementation. In: International symposium on devices. Circuits and systems (ISDCS), pp 1–6. https://doi.org/10.1109/ISDCS49393.2020.9263003

Deep Cervix Model Development from Heterogeneous and Partially Labeled Image Datasets

Anabik Pal, Zhiyun Xue, and Sameer Antani

Abstract Cervical cancer is a significant disease affecting women worldwide. Regular cervical examination with gynecologists is important for early detection and treatment planning for women with precancers. Precancer is the direct precursor to cervical cancer. However, there is a scarcity of experts and the experts' assessments are subject to variations in interpretation. In this scenario, the development of a robust automated cervical image classification system is important to augment the experts' limitations. Ideally, for such a system the class label prediction will vary according to the cervical inspection objectives. Hence, the labeling criteria may not be the same in the cervical image datasets. Moreover, due to the lack of confirmatory test results and inter-rater labeling variation, many images are left unlabeled. Motivated by these challenges, we propose to develop a pretrained cervix model from heterogeneous and partially labeled cervical image datasets. Self-supervised learning (SSL) is employed to build the cervical model. Further, considering data-sharing restrictions, we show how federated self-supervised learning (FSSL) can be employed to develop a cervix model without sharing the cervical images. The task-specific classification models are developed by fine-tuning the cervix model. Two partially labeled cervical image datasets labeled with different classification criteria are used in this study. According to our experimental study, the cervix model prepared with dataset-specific SSL boosts classification accuracy by 2.5% than ImageNet pretrained model. The classification accuracy is further boosted by 1.5%↑ when images from both datasets are combined for SSL. We see that in comparison with the dataset-specific cervix model developed with SSL, the FSSL is performing better.

Keywords Deep Learning · Self-supervised Learning · Federated Learning · Cervical image classification

A. Pal (✉)
SRM University, Amaravati, Guntur District 522502, Andhra Pradesh, India
e-mail: anabik.p@srmap.edu.in

A. Pal · Z. Xue · S. Antani
National Library of Medicine, National Institutes of Health, Bethesda, MD 20894, USA
e-mail: zhiyun.xue@nih.gov

S. Antani
e-mail: sameer.antani@nih.gov

© The Author(s), under exclusive license to Springer Nature Singapore Pte Ltd. 2023

J. K. Mandal and D. De (eds.), *Frontiers of ICT in Healthcare*, Lecture Notes in Networks and Systems 519, https://doi.org/10.1007/978-981-19-5191-6_55

1 Introduction

In the global scenario, cervical cancer is the fourth most common cancer in women. Early detection of pre-cancerous cervical lesions can reduce the premature death of the woman. Hence, it is important to screen the cervix on a regular basis. Among all cervical screening techniques, visual inspection with acetic acid (VIA) is commonly used as it is cheap and available easily. The key limitation of this technique is that it is suffering from inter-and intra-expert variability. Recently growing artificial intelligence and machine learning-based automated image analysis system could address this limitation [6, 10]. Note that hand-crafted feature-based classifiers are known to under performing [5, 7, 12] than the deep learning approaches [8, 9]. Therefore, the researchers prefer to employ deep learning to solve cervical image analysis problems. However, by nature deep learning is data-hungry and needs experts' involvement for annotating the data [3]. From the current image analysis challenge perspective, cervical image labeling is costly, needs multiple experts' agreements, and requires multiple diagnostic information. Therefore, to overcome the limitations in developing a robust deep model with limited data, transfer learning [15], i.e., transferring knowledge from natural images becomes a commonly used method. However, the development of domain-specific deep models is the current research focus as it will be providing better image representation.

The conventional approach to overcome data scarcity is uniting data from multiple institutions or organizations. However, conducting such collaboration for centralized learning (CL) has several limitations. First, there might be variations in the visual quality of the images contributed by different organizations. This variation comes from the use of different imaging devices for image acquisition. Moreover, images may not be allowed to share among the collaborated institutions for which federated learning (FL) is an effective solution [14]. However, for federated supervised learning, a special research effort is required to deal with the different class distribution among the institutions [13]. Finally, and most importantly, the cervical image labeling criteria vary and depend on: the availability of other diagnostic results, population under study, treatment planning, severity grading strategy, etc. The variety in the image labeling criteria across datasets makes the task more challenging as it restricts researchers in performing any kind of supervised collaborative (CL or FL) learning.

This paper develops a pretrained cervix model (or cervix model) with self-supervised learning (SSL) using two cervical image datasets that are partially labeled (a part of the dataset is labeled) and labeled with different classification criteria (heterogeneous). Both centralized SSL and federated SSL are experimented. The self-supervised learning is used as the images do not need any expert annotation. Hence, it allows uniting all images from both datasets for cervix model development. There is no way to evaluate the effectiveness of the developed pretrained models. Therefore, a downstream task having labeled data is considered and the pretrained model is fine-tuned to build a deep model which can be evaluated. In this paper, as a downstream task, we choose to develop two cervical image classification models: (i) classify an image based on the presence of cervical infection and (ii) classify a cervical image based on whether the cervical infection is a precursor of pre-malignancy. Two different datasets are used for these two downstream tasks. Note that, to the best of our knowledge, no cervical image dataset is available in the public domain which can be utilized for automating the visual assessment of acetic acid-applied cervix.

In summary, the research presented in Zhou et al. [16] and Chen et al. [2] motivate us to do this work. Model genesis presented in Zhou et al. [16] proposed to train an encoder-decoder-based deep model to reconstruct original images from synthetically distorted images for obtaining a pretrained model for medical image representation. In Chen et al. [2], visual contrastive learning was employed to learn the natural image representation. In this paper, we hire the concept of contrastive learning from Chen et al. [2] and utilize it for developing pretrained cervical model development. We experiment on both centralized and federated self-supervised learning. Our work is novel in the following two perspectives: (a) it is the first research attempt that focuses on the development of a pretrained cervix model with zero annotation cost; (b) believe to be the first medical image representation research work which consider Federated Self-Supervised Learning (FSSL).

The rest of the paper is organized as follows: Sect. 2 discusses the background of self-supervised learning, and federated learning and ends with describing how federated self-supervised learning is used for pretrained cervix model development. The experimental protocol is available in Sect. 3. The analysis of experimental results is presented in Sect. 4. Finally, Sect. 5 concludes the paper and mentions the future scope of this work.

2 Methods

2.1 *Self-supervised Learning*

Self-supervised learning (SSL) is a visual representation learning approach that releases the requirement of expert annotation. Machine learners design a discriminative task directly from the raw images without any expert supervision. The designed task is called the pretext task. The deep model is trained to learn the pretext task which can capture the image semantics (i.e., good initialization weights for related domain's downstream tasks).

This paper considers contrastive feature learning as the pretext task—i.e., embedding of the images will be well separated and the image and an augmented version will have closer embedding [2]. The SSL model can be trained with the mini-batch of size $2N$ constructed with N random images and an augmented version of every image. The training loss ($L_{i,j}$) between an image i and its augmented version j is given as:

$$L_{i,j} = -\log \frac{\exp(f_i^T f_j/\tau)}{\sum_{i=1}^{2N} 1_{[k \neq i]} \exp(f_i^T f_k/\tau)} \tag{1}$$

where f_i is the feature vector of i-th image; $1_{[k \neq i]} \in \{0, 1\}$ is an indicator function evaluating to 1 iff $k \neq i$; ^{T} representation transpose operation and τ is a constant. The loss in a mini-batch is computed across all pairs constructed with an image and its augmented version.

2.2 *Federated Self-supervised Learning (FSSL)*

Unauthorized access to sensitive data is harmful and is a social threat. Hence, several laws and regulations (GDPR 2018 by the EU, CCPA 2020 in the US, etc) are formed to stop sensitive information sharing (especially medical/banking domain). Therefore due to these legal issues related to data protection collaborated institutions may not be allowed to share raw data among them. In this regard, federated learning (FL) is an effective approach for robust inter-institutional collaborated deep model development from the data distributed in multiple institutions (clients) without sharing the raw data [14].

In this paper, two cervical image datasets are used for developing the cervix model. We assume that two datasets are residing in two different clients and clients are not allowed to share raw data. All images (both labeled and unlabeled) from both datasets are utilized for Federated Self-supervised Learning (FSSL). Two naive federated learning approaches namely, Client-server federated self-supervised learning (CSFSSL) and Peer-to-Peer federated self-supervised learning (PPFSSL) are considered in this research. In the client-server approach (CSFSSL) there is no direct communication channel among the clients and a central server controls the learning. In this approach, first, the server broadcast a model to both clients, and then independently, at every client, the model is updated based on the loss computed with its images. This weight updating is performed for E-epochs. After that, the clients send the updated models to the server which aggregates the model weights received from both clients. Note that the value of E may vary among the clients. The whole communication round is repeated until the model is fully trained. For simplicity, this paper adopts federated averaging for aggregating the client models. On the other hand, in the Peer-to-Peer approach, no server is present- clients can directly communicate with each other. In this approach, first, a random client is chosen which initialize a model and update weights with SSL by using the available images. The updated model is then sent to another client where SSL is performed and weights are updated further. Thus the communication among the clients takes place circularly. Like CSFSSL, the weight updating in a client is performed for E-epochs and the value of E can be varied among clients. The whole communication round is repeated until the model is fully trained. It is worth mentioning that in both cases clients are not sharing the images however the potential of all images available in both clients are utilized for cervix model building.

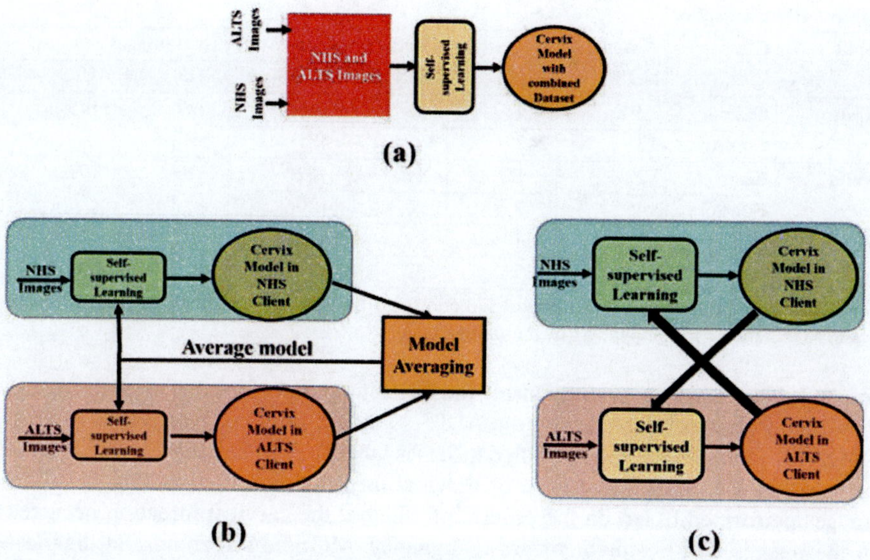

Fig. 1 Block diagram of the SSL training system. **a** Centralized SSL (CSSL), **b** Client-Server FSSL (CSFSSL) and **c** Peer-to-Peer FSSL (PPFSSL)

2.3 Proposed Approach: Cervical Model Development

This paper considers two different FSSL approaches presented in Sect. 2.2 for cervix model development. Finally, the performance of the FSSL model is compared with centralized SSL (CSSL). As a downstream task, client-specific classification model building is considered. The pictorial representation of the learning frameworks for the CSSL, CSFSSL, and PPFSSL are shown in Fig. 1a–c, respectively. The SSL algorithm discussed in Sect. 2.1 is used for model building. The augmented version of an image is obtained with rotation, horizontal and vertical flipping, random shift, random zoom, gamma changing, and brightness changing.

3 Experimental Protocol

3.1 Dataset Description

The datasets used in this research come from two distinct cohort studies for cervical examination (NHS [1] and ALTS [11]). These studies are conducted by the researchers at the National Cancer Institute (NCI) of the US National Institutes of Health (NIH). NCI shared a subset of acetic acid-applied cervix images for our

Table 1 Data set splits

Split	Class	Patients		Labeled images		Total images	
		NHS	ALTS	NHS	ALTS	NHS	ALTS
Train	Case	91	124	182	248	2029	3145
	Control	181	242	361	481		
Valid	Case	22	31	44	62	520	791
	Control	45	60	90	120		
Test	Case	25	34	49	68		
	Control	50	65	99	130		

For NHS case refers presence of cervical infection and for ALTS case refers cervical infection occurred in a image is a precursors of pre-malignancy

research. The images generated during the NHS study are referred to as NHS dataset and the images generated during the ALTS study are referred to as ALTS dataset. Only a subset of the images for both datasets is labeled. The labeling of NHS images performed based on the presence of cervical infection and the labeling of ALTS images performed based on the criteria of whether the cervical infection occurred in the images is a precursor of pre-malignancy. Multiple screening and diagnostic information like visual assessment, HPV, cytology, histopathology, colposcopy, etc. are analyzed for labeling the images. For experimental evaluation, both datasets are splitted at the women's level into three disjoint subsets - train, validation, and test. Table 1 represents the subset-wise number of patients, labeled images, and total available images for the datasets.

3.2 *Network Architecture*

In this paper, ResNet-50 a widely used state-of-the-art deep model is used as the backbone. During SSL, the final classification layer is replaced with a dense layer with a ReLU activation. The number of neurons in the dense layer is varied among [64, 128, 256] and our experimental outcome shows that performances are very closer. Hence, to reduce the computational burden we set the number of the neuron to 64. For the downstream classification task, this dense layer (along with the activation layer) is replaced with a single output neuron with sigmoid activation. The predicted case probability is obtained from the sigmoid layer. Note that full fine-tuning is employed for the dataset-specific downstream classification tasks.

3.3 *Competing Methods*

This paper compares the performance of cervical image classification for the following six different varying initialization approaches: (i) **Random**: Random network weights initialization, (ii) **ImageNet**: Network initialization with pretrained ImageNet model, (iii) **Self-supervised Learning (SSL)**: Network initialization with

SSL with the available images in a client. (iv) **Centralized Self-supervised Learning (CSSL)**: Network initialization with SSL with the available images in both clients, (v) **Client-Server Federated Self-supervised Learning (CSFSSL)**: Network initialization with the Client-Server Federated Self-supervised Learning, and (vi) **Peer-to-Peer Federated Self-supervised Learning (PPFSSL)**: Network initialization with the circular SSL. Note that in **Random** no knowledge is transferred, in **ImageNet** the knowledge is transferred from a different domain (natural image) than cervical images, and knowledge is transferred from the same domain for the rest of the approaches.

3.4 Parameter Settings

The optimal hyper-parameters for both SSL training and downstream classification model training are chosen empirically. The validation loss is analyzed for parameter selection. SSL uses $\tau = 0.1$ (see Eq. 1), learning rate 0.01, momentum = 0.9, weight decay = $1e - 5$, and trained for 50 epochs. The downstream classification models are trained with batch size = 4, learning rate 0.001, momentum = 0.09, weight decay = $1e - 6$, and trained for 50 epochs. Random shuffling of images is done for both SSL and downstream classification model training. Reverse class weighting is employed to tackle the class imbalance issue during classification model training.

3.5 Implementation

The networks are implemented with Keras [4] a popularly used deep learning toolkit. Regarding computing hardware, two (2) GeForce RTX 2080 Ti GPUs installed with an Intel(R) Xeon(R) Gold 5218 CPU (@ 2.30 GHz) is used for training. Note that the federated learning algorithms are logically implemented in the same computing resources.

3.6 Evaluation Metrics

As there is no known evaluation metric for evaluating the quality of the developed pretrained model, we evaluate only the dataset-specific downstream class label prediction performances. We constraint the learning approach for the downstream classification task and vary the network initialization (see Sect. 3.3). The following four commonly known matrices are computed for performance comparison: (1) Accuracy (ACC), (2) Recall, (3) Precision, (4) F1-Score.

4 Experimental Results and Discussion

Figure 2 contains the Receiver Operating Curves (ROC) for all downstream classification tasks developed with different model initialization approaches. The quantitative performance (used matrices are described in Sect. 3.3) for the same is shown in Table 2. Table 2 shows that for both datasets ImageNet initialization improves the accuracy than random initialization but is unable to improve the recalls. The pretrained network built with SSL is better than transferring knowledge from the ImageNet model (built with natural images). In case of cervical model development with the NHS image dataset, the NHS classification model provides the best accuracy, recall, and F1_Score when the SSL approach with $N = 16$ is used and the best precision is received when $N = 8$ is used. In case of cervical model development with the ALTS image dataset, ALTS classification model provides the best accuracy and precision when the SSL approach with $N = 16$ is used and the best recall and F1_Score is received when $N = 8$ is used. Our experimental results show that pretrained model developed with SSL makes a noticeable performance improvement over the ImageNet pretrained model which justifies the importance of SSL-based cervical model development. We find that the cervix model initialized with CSSL improves the performance than SSL-based initialization for both downstream tasks which advocates the importance of uniting images from both datasets. For CSSL-based initialization when $N = 8$, for most cases, the best classification performance are received for both datasets. Therefore, for developing the cervix model with federated self-supervised learning (FSSL) we set $N = 8$. For CSFSSL-based cervix model development, The value of E (iteration during local model updating) is varied among 1, 5, 10 and according to our experiment $E = 1$ provides best performance. The PPFSSL-based cervix model development is done with two different approaches. The approaches

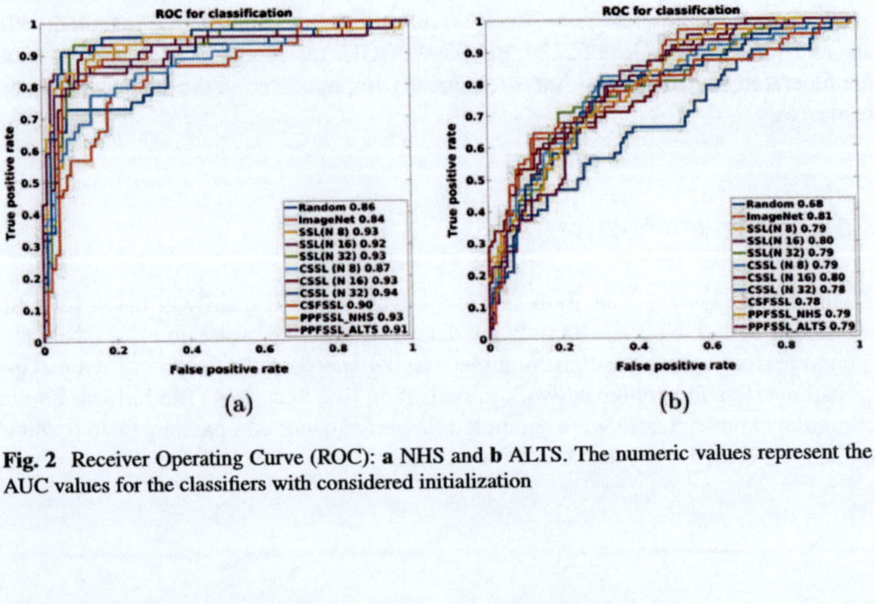

(a) (b)

Fig. 2 Receiver Operating Curve (ROC): **a** NHS and **b** ALTS. The numeric values represent the AUC values for the classifiers with considered initialization

Table 2 Performance evaluation

Initialization method	NHS				ALTS			
	ACC	Recall	Precision	F1_Score	ACC	Recall	Precision	F1_Score
Random	79.73	0.5306	0.7879	0.6341	76.77	0.5735	0.6964	0.6290
ImageNet	80.41	0.4898	**0.8571**	0.6234	77.78	0.5588	0.7308	0.6333
SSL (N 8)	83.11	0.6327	0.8158	0.7126	79.80	0.7206	0.7000	0.7101
SSL (N 16)	83.11	0.6939	0.7727	0.7312	80.30	0.6029	0.7736	0.6777
SSL (N 32)	83.11	0.6531	0.8000	0.7191	79.29	0.6176	0.7368	0.6720
CSSL (N 8)	**86.49**	0.7143	0.8537	0.7778	**81.82**	**0.7794**	0.7162	**0.7465**
CSSL (N 16)	85.81	0.7551	0.8043	0.7789	81.31	0.6324	**0.7818**	0.6992
CSSL (N 32)	85.14	**0.7959**	0.7647	**0.7800**	81.31	0.6471	0.7719	0.7040
CSFSSL	84.46	0.6735	0.8250	0.7416	79.80	0.6912	0.7121	0.7015
PPFSSL_NHS	84.46	0.7347	0.7826	0.7579	80.81	0.6618	0.7500	0.7031
PPFSSL_ALTS	84.46	0.7755	0.7600	0.7677	80.30	0.6618	0.7377	0.6977

vary based on the starting client. If the SSL learning starts with the NHS client we term this approach as PPFSSL_NHS and if the SSL learning starts with the ALTS client we term this approach PPFSSL_ALTS. For experimental similarity and comparison, we consider $E = 1$ for both PPFSSL_NHS and PPFSSL_ALTS. The experimental results show that the development of the cervix model with both PPFSSL and CSF-SSL produces comparative classification performance. From Table 2, it is evident that in general, federated SSL performs better than SSL with single client images. Hence, our experimental results support the usefulness of FSSL to overcome data-sharing constraints and utilize data from multiple clients to develop a better cervix model.

5 Conclusion and Scope of Future Work

In this paper, we highlighted the cervical image analysis challenges owing to labeling scarcity, and variability. Finally, we propose an innovative federated self-supervised learning approach to tackle this. The experimental outcome justifies that the self-supervised learning approach is efficient to cope with the label scarcity and the labeling heterogeneity. The use of federated self-supervised learning illuminates to tackle data privacy. We believe that the cervix model development presented in this paper is the inaugural attempt in light of a domain-specific task agnostic pretrained model construction.

The immediate future scope of this work will include the development of an improved cervix model combining multi-source image datasets that are unlabelled, have labeling heterogeneity, and have variation in pixel properties due to imaging devices. The experiment on federated learning is shown in a synthetic environment, however, actual deployment of the proposed federated learning algorithm for uniting multiple institutions is the next future challenge. The proposed concept is generic and can be hired by other medical image analysis tasks.

Acknowledgements This work was supported by the Intramural Research Program of the National Library of Medicine, part of the National Institutes of Health, USA. The authors of this paper want to thank Dr. Mark Schiffman of the Division of Cancer Epidemiology and Genetics, National Cancer Institute, National Institutes of Health, and his colleagues for sharing the cervical images with us.

References

1. Bratti MC, Rodríguez AC, Schiffman M, Hildesheim A, Morales J, Alfaro M, Guillén D, Hutchinson M, Sherman ME, Eklund C, Schussler J, Buckland J, Morera LA, Cárdenas F, Barrantes M, Pérez E, Cox TJ, Burk RD, Herrero R (2004) Description of a seven-year prospective study of human papillomavirus infection and cervical neoplasia among 10000 women in Guanacaste, Costa Rica. Pan Am J Public Health 2(15):75–89
2. Chen T, Kornblith S, Norouzi M, Hinton G (2020) A simple framework for contrastive learning of visual representations. In: Singh A (eds) Proceedings of the 37th international conference on machine learning. Proceedings of machine learning research, vol 119, PMLR, Virtual, 13–18 Jul 2020, pp 1597–1607
3. Ching T, Himmelstein DS, Beaulieu-Jones BK, Kalinin AA, Do BT, Way GP, Ferrero E, Agapow PM, Zietz M, Hoffman MM, Xie W, Rosen GL, Lengerich BJ, Israeli J, Lanchantin J, Woloszynek S, Carpenter AE, Shrikumar A, Xu J, Cofer EM, Lavender CA, Turaga SC, Alexandari AM, Lu Z, Harris DJ, DeCaprio D, Qi Y, Kundaje A, Peng Y, Wiley LK, Segler MHS, Boca SM, Swamidass SJ, Huang A, Gitter A, Greene CS (2018) Opportunities and obstacles for deep learning in biology and medicine. J Royal Soc Interface
4. Chollet F et al (2015) Keras. https://keras.io
5. Fernandes K, Cardoso JS, Fernandes J (2018) Automated methods for the decision support of cervical cancer screening using digital colposcopies. IEEE Access 6:33910–33927
6. Hu L, Bell D, Antani S, Xue Z, Yu K, Horning MP, Gachuhi N, Wilson B, Jaiswal MS, Befano B, Long LR, Herrero R, Einstein MH, Burk RD, Demarco M, Gage JC, Rodriguez AC, Wentzensen N, Schiffman M (2019) An observational study of deep learning and automated evaluation of cervical images for cancer screening. JNCI: J Natl Cancer Inst 111(9):923–932
7. Kim E, Huang X (2013) A data driven approach to cervigram image analysis and classification. Springer, Dordrecht, pp 1–13
8. Litjens G, Kooi T, Bejnordi BE, Setio AAA, Ciompi F, Ghafoorian M, van der Laak JA, van Ginneken B, Sánchez CI (2017) A survey on deep learning in medical image analysis. Med Image Anal 42:60–88
9. Pal A, Chaturvedi A, Chandra A, Chatterjee R, Senapati S, Frangi AF, Garain U (2022) Micaps: multi-instance capsule network for machine inspection of munro' microabscess. Comput Biol Med 140:105071
10. Pal A, Xue Z, Befano B, Rodriguez AC, Long LR, Schiffman M, Antani S (2021) Deep metric learning for cervical image classification. IEEE Access 9:53266–53275
11. Schiffman M, Adrianza ME (2000) Ascus-lsil triage study. Design, methods and characteristics of trial participants. Acta Cytol 44(5):726–742
12. Srinivasan Y, Nutter B, Mitra S, Phillips B, Sinzinger E (2006) Classification of cervix lesions using filter bank-based texture mode. In: 19th IEEE symposium on Computer-Based Medical Systems (CBMS'06), pp 832–840
13. Yang M, Wong A, Zhu H, Wang H, Qian H (2020) Federated learning with class imbalance reduction
14. Yang Q, Liu Y, Cheng Y, Kang Y, Chen T, Yu H (2019) Federated learning
15. Yang Q Zhang Y, Dai W, Pan SJ (2020) Transfer learning. Cambridge University Press, Cambridge
16. Zhou Z, Sodha V, Pang J, Gotway MB, Liang J (2021) Models genesis. Med Image Anal 67:101840

Region Separated Vessel Segmentation in Fundus Image Using Multi-scale Layer-Based Convolutional Neural Network

Supratim Ghosh, Mahantapas Kundu, and Mita Nasipuri

Abstract A region-based Multi-scale Convolutional Neural Network is used in this work to automatically segment the blood vessel pixels in Fundus images. Firstly, a region-based image partitioning method is implemented which separates each image into a set of three homogenous regions, namely Optic Disc, High Contrast and Low Contrast regions. kNN-based clustering approach is used for the image partitioning. Three Multi-scale Layer-based CNN models are then trained individually for each of the regions and tested on the DRIVE and STARE datasets. The obtained output is evaluated based on Accuracy, Sensitivity and Specificity, respectively, and the achieved results are reported in this work.

Keywords Classification · Neural network · Fundus · Retina · Vessel segmentation · Retinopathy · Clustering · K-Means

1 Introduction

Retinal vessel analysis forms a core part of the diagnosis process for the detection of Diabetic Retinopathy in pathological patients. However, the process of diagnosis requires medical expertise and human intervention for blood vessel segmentation which is not available in regions lacking medical facilities [1]. Consequently, automated systems are becoming popular in modern times in the segmentation and analysis of blood vessels present in the Fundus images to detect anomalies and retinal diseases [1, 2]. The work done by Fraz et al. [3] highlights a list of approaches which have been implemented in the past research works. The past works in the literature can be broadly classified into three major categories, namely Unsupervised Algorithms,

S. Ghosh (✉)
Techno India University, EM-4, EM Block, Sector V, Bidhannagar, Kolkata, West Bengal 700091, India
e-mail: supratimghosh2772@gmail.com

M. Kundu · M. Nasipuri
Jadavpur University, 132, Raja Subodh Chandra Mallick Rd, Jadavpur, Kolkata, West Bengal 700032, India

© The Author(s), under exclusive license to Springer Nature Singapore Pte Ltd. 2023
J. K. Mandal and D. De (eds.), *Frontiers of ICT in Healthcare*, Lecture Notes in Networks and Systems 519, https://doi.org/10.1007/978-981-19-5191-6_56

Supervised Algorithms and Deep Learning models. Unsupervised Algorithms refer to approaches which do not require labeled data for performing analysis. Line detectors [4], matched filtering [5], morphological transformations [6, 7], model-based methods [8, 9] and Multi-scale segmentation methods [10–12] are some of the common approaches used under Unsupervised Algorithms. Alternatively, methodologies have been proposed in the past which utilize annotated data for the design of learning models using Supervised Algorithms. k-Nearest Neighbor [13], Gaussian Mixture Model (GMM) [14], Support Vector Machine (SVM) [15], Neural Networks [16], Decision Trees [17], AdaBoost [18] and Conditional Random Fields [19] are some of the popular approaches which have been adopted in the past research works. Analysis of the computational complexity of the different sets of approaches highlights that Unsupervised Algorithms are unsuitable for the detection of diseases in pathological images. Conversely, traditional Supervised Learning approaches depend upon handcrafted feature sets which are extensively dependent on the training datasets and often lack robustness for translating the prediction capabilities to unseen datasets. To mitigate such issues, a third category of approaches, namely Deep Learning, had been studied in literature in the past, notably by Liskowski et al. [1] and Yan et al. [2], which had proposed Convolutional Neural Network models for learning the feature sets needed for effective classification. The Deep Learning approaches existing in past literature [1, 2, 20, 21] focus extensively on designing models using custom loss functions and different patch sizes that can be used for performing pixel-wise classification.

An earlier work in this field [20] was based on the design of a low-cost solution based on a U-Net model for learning. In the previous work, the input Fundus image was separated into three different regions based on the intensity value thresholding of the image and each of these resultant regions is segmented using a separate U-Net model for isolating the blood vessel pixels. The distribution of the segmentation task across three individual Convolutional models resulted in the design of a solution that provided the advantage of Convolutional Neural models while significantly reducing the prediction time required on a low-cost standard system. However, the solution proposed in the previous work [20] suffered due to the quality of region separation based on thresholding which impacted the performance of the approach. In this work, we propose the use of a k-Means-based clustering method for generating the three separate regions for the distribution of the segmentation task among three separate classifier models. For the purpose of classification, we have used an InceptionNet and GRU-inspired Multi-scale Layer-based Convolutional model [21] which had been proposed for use in this domain in an earlier work [21].

Our primary contributions in this work include: (a) The use of a k-Means clustering approach for region separation using pixel intensity and Neighborhood Difference. (b) The use of separate Multi-scale Layer-based Convolutional Neural Network for vessel pixel segmentation in individual regions of Fundus image.

The paper has been organized as follows. Section 2 of the paper describes in detail the proposed methodology and our contribution in this work. Section 3 highlights the experimental results obtained in this work, and the comparative analysis of our proposed solution is presented. Section 4 analyzes the results obtained and final conclusion.

2 Proposed Methodology

Our proposed approach here is an extension of the work done in [20] and is based on the need for designing an algorithm having minimal computational complexity while maintaining the quality of blood vessel pixel segmentation in the input Fundus images. The previous work in this field focused on the separation of the Fundus image into three regions, namely Optic Disc, High Contrast and Low Contrast regions, respectively. The region of the Fundus image, after removing the Optic Disc region, having the greatest difference in intensity between blood vessel pixels and non-blood vessel pixels is considered as the High Contrast region of the Fundus image. Similarly, the region of the Fundus image, after removing the Optic Disc region and the High Contrast region, comprised of blood vessel pixels having minimal intensity difference with non-blood vessel pixels is considered to be the Low Contrast region. A threshold-based segmentation approach based on the intensity of the pixels in the Fundus image had been designed in the work [20] for the separation of the regions. However, the approach for separation of the input image into regions solely on the basis of intensity of the pixels does not take into consideration any contrast information. As a result, regions obtained after separation lacked sufficient uniformity characteristics in the respective region and thus led to subsequent loss of accuracy in the final blood vessel segmented output image.

In this work, firstly, we have calculated two features for each given pixel in the input Fundus image, namely, Intensity and Neighborhood Difference. The resultant feature vector is used for clustering all the pixels in the Fundus image into three clusters using a k-Means algorithm for forming the homogenous regions. The principle for clustering the pixels into three regions is based on the definition of a Fundus image as combination of three homogenous regions, namely Optic Disc, High Contrast and Low Contrast regions. The resultant regions are each passed through a separate Convolutional Neural Network for final classification of the image pixels. In this work, we have utilized a model, Multi-scale Layer Convolutional Network model, which we had proposed in an earlier work [21], for the classification of the Fundus image pixels as blood vessel pixels. This section of the paper highlights the individual stages of our proposed methodology.

2.1 Region Separation

The first stage of the proposed solution involves the separation of the input Fundus image into a set of three non-overlapping individual regions. Two features are taken into consideration for separating the input Fundus image into individual regions, namely Pixel Intensity and Neighborhood Difference. Let the input RGB Fundus image be denoted as I. For the purpose of segmentation of blood vessel pixels, the green channel information of image I is considered for our approach. The choice of the green channel of image I for analysis is based on an observation made by

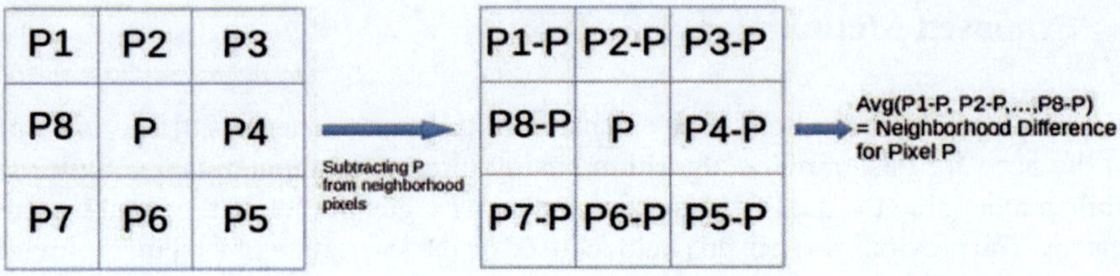

Fig. 1 Neighborhood difference calculation

Liskowski et al. [1]. The green channel of a Fundus image is found to provide the best contrast of intensities between background and blood vessel pixels. Let the green channel of image I be denoted as I_G. As the task of region segmentation is determinant on the values of background pixels rather than blood vessel pixels, the intensities of pixels corresponding to the blood vessel pixels are removed from the image I_G. The ground truth images present in the training dataset are used as a mask for removing the blood vessel pixels from the image I_G. Let the vessel removed image I_G be named as I'_G. After removal of the vessel pixels, for each pixel in the image I'_G, two features are computed. The pixel intensity value of the vessel removed image I'_G for each pixel is considered as the first feature, namely F_1.

For each pixel P in I'_G, the second feature, namely, Neighborhood Difference (F_2), is calculated based on the intensity of pixel P and the intensities of the pixels present in the 8-neighborhood of the pixel P. The intensity value of pixel P is subtracted from the 8-neighborhood pixel intensities and the average intensity of the neighborhood is considered as value of feature F_2. The neighborhood pixels, which have minimal intensity difference with the central pixel P, correspond to regions having Low Contrast in the Fundus image. Similarly, the neighborhood pixels having high intensity difference with the central pixel P correspond to regions having High contrast in the Fundus image. A representation of the process is shown in Fig. 1.

The two features, namely, F_1 and F_2, are collectively used to compute the region separation using a k-Means clustering algorithm. The k-Means clustering algorithm is used in this work with a cluster value of 3 for generating 3 separate clusters, each corresponding to one region in the image. The obtained clusters each correspond to one region, namely Optic Disc, High Contrast Region and Low Contrast Region. To identify the clusters and associate the same with the respective regions in the obtained output, we have used the feature values of F_1 and F_2 for each cluster. The cluster having the highest pixel intensity (F_1) data points corresponds to the Optic Disc region. The cluster having the highest Neighborhood Difference intensity (F_2) data points corresponds to the High Contrast Region and the remaining data cluster corresponds to the Low Contrast Region in the input image I'_G. The region separated image is shown in Fig. 2. The regions thus formed are passed individually through separate networks for obtaining the final output. In this work, we have utilized a Multi-scale Convolutional Network model, which we had proposed in an earlier work, for final region-based segmentation.

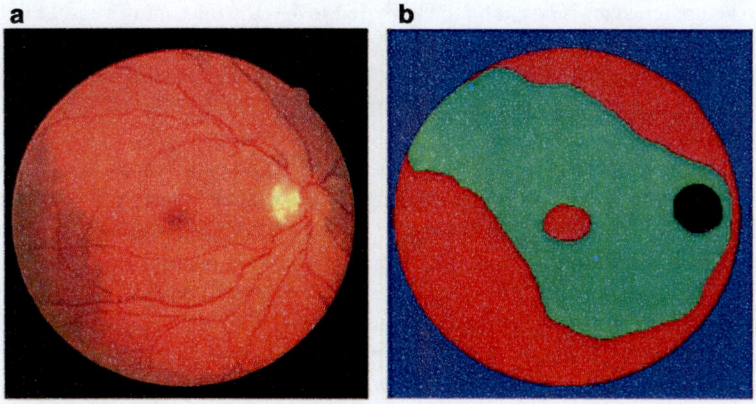

Fig. 2 **a** Original Fundus image. **b** Region separated image

2.2 *Multi-scale Layer Network*

The region separated image is used to segment the blood vessel pixels from the Fundus image. For each region formed, a separate Multi-scale Layer Network [21] is used for training and segmentation of the blood vessel pixels. The Multi-scale Layer Network is a modified Convolutional Neural Network, inspired from the designs of InceptionNet architecture and GRU Networks. The model was proposed and tested on the problem of blood vessel pixel segmentation in Fundus image in an earlier work [21] and was found to perform comparably with current state-of-the-art automated systems. The network is designed to perform classification of the pixels in the input image based on the concept of varying context sizes. The network had been designed to reduce the dependency of model performance on the selection of the patch sizes for final classification. In the previous works [20], a U-Net-based architecture had been utilized for the final segmentation of the blood vessel pixels in the Fundus images. However, the U-Net architecture provided an architecture for a multi-pixel classification approach, where, multiple pixels of a given patch were classified and segmented in a single iteration. For a light weighted model, such a task of multi-pixel classification and segmentation often leads to poor results as the network is unable to learn adequately due to lack of sufficient number of weights. In order to achieve a better output, we propose the use of the Multi-scale Layer Network which is capable of learning the features based on different context information for a single pixel in the input image. The incorporation of the context information is important as blood vessels having larger widths require larger context for accurate segmentation. Similarly, blood vessels having smaller widths require smaller context for better segmentation. In such conditions, it is not much useful to use a single context information for all vessel segmentation.

For each pixel P in a given region R, three patch sizes of dimensions $9 \times 9, 11 \times 11, 13 \times 13$ are extracted from the green channel I_G of the Fundus image I. The selection of the given patch sizes is based on the knowledge that the maximum vessel thickness usually observed in a blood vessel of input Fundus image is approximately 22 pixels. As such, the average vessel width can be considered to be approximately 11 pixels. Each individual patch is provided as an input to a separate Convolutional channel for generating the feature vector. Each patch is transformed into a 1D vector firstly by using a Convolutional Neural Network which contains an input layer followed by four consecutive Convolutional layers. A flatten layer is attached at the end of each patch channel to build a set of three 1D feature vectors which are provided as input to the Multi-scale Layer of the model for the final classification of the pixel. The Multi-scale Layer combines the 1D feature vectors from each patch to form a single 1D feature vector. The obtained 1D feature vector is finally provided as an input to a simple ANN model for obtaining the final classification of the pixel P. For each region R, a separate Multi-scale Convolutional Neural Network is used for pixel classification. A diagram of the Multi-scale Layer Convolutional Neural Network is provided in Fig. 3. The results obtained for separate regions are combined finally into a single vessel segmented output image.

3 Experimental Observation

The performance of the proposed solution in this work is evaluated using two standard benchmark datasets, namely DRIVE [22] and STARE [5]. The DRIVE dataset comprises two sets of data, training set and testing set, which are, respectively, used for training and testing of the proposed solution. The DRIVE dataset contains a total of 20 training images and 20 testing images each having a dimension of 768×584 pixels with 8-bit resolution. The STARE dataset comprises 20 images each having a dimension of 605×700 pixels. As the STARE dataset does not contain any division, so, the leave-one-out testing approach is used in this work for evaluation. The model performance is calculated using four different metrics, namely, Area Under Curve (AUC), Accuracy (ACC), Sensitivity (Se) and Specificity (Sp), and the obtained results in this work are compared with the past literature and reported in this work.

The data presented in Table 1 highlights our obtained results. For analysis of the results obtained for vessel segmentation, the value of Sensitivity plays an equally important role as Accuracy in the evaluation of a system as Sensitivity correlates with the number of vessel pixels correctly segmented by the algorithm. From the analysis of a Fundus image, it can be observed that blood vessel pixels only constitute 10–15% of the total pixels in an image. Hence, Accuracy metric is not sufficient to evaluate the classification of a model as the dataset is heavily negatively skewed. In such scenario, the metric for True Positive, namely, Sensitivity, is important for analyzing the strength of a model in this domain. In Table 1, it can be observed that most of the existing works in the literature have not performed well in Sensitivity, whereas our achieved Sensitivity for DRIVE dataset has obtained the highest sensitivity value, and for STARE dataset, it has achieved the second best performance to Liskowski et al. Additionally, the work by Liskowski et al. has achieved a poor performance

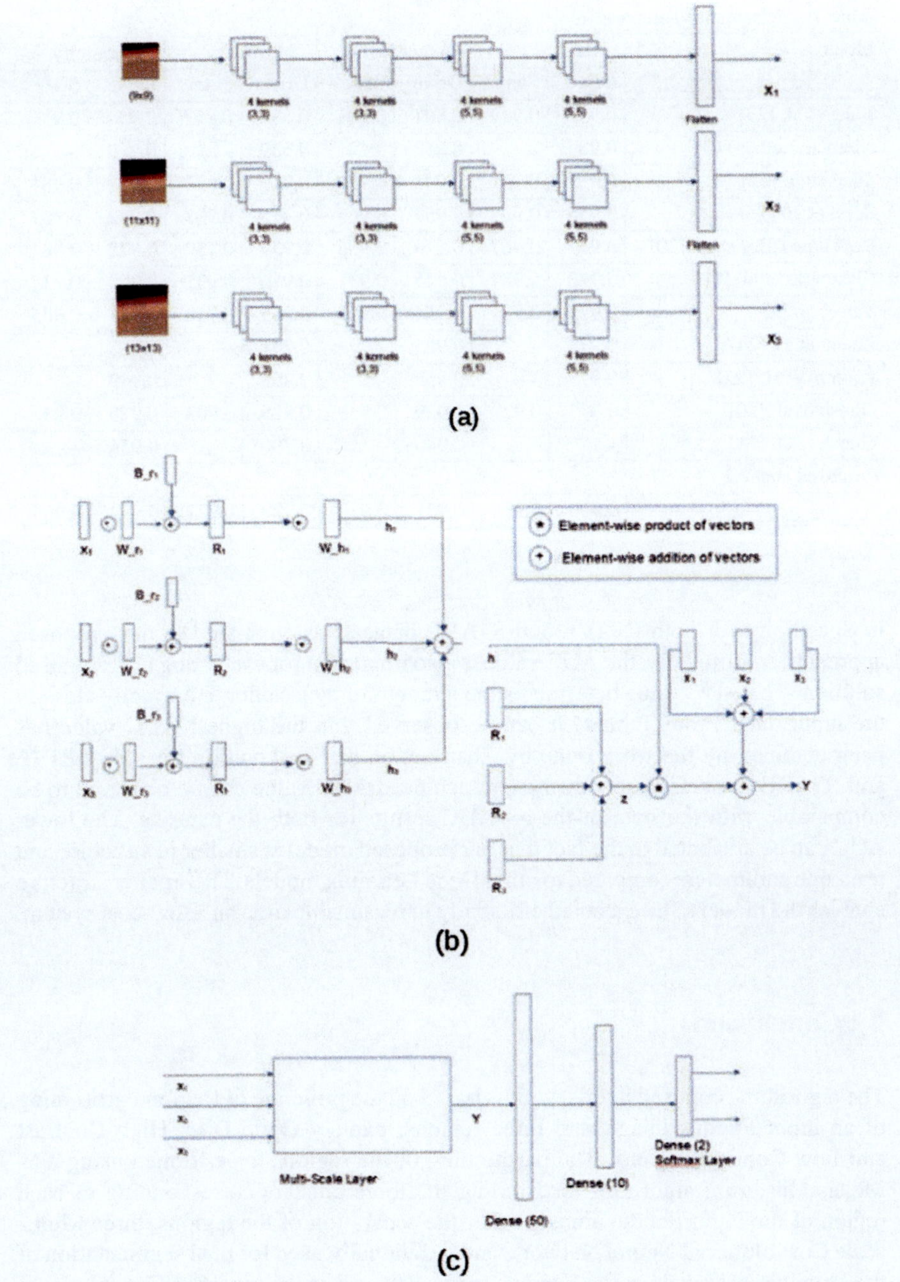

Fig. 3 **a** Convolutional Neural Network for feature extraction. **b** Multi-scale Layer. **c** ANN classifier

Table 1 Performance comparison

Methods	AUC		Accuracy		Sensitivity		Specificity	
	Drive	Stare	Drive	Stare	Drive	Stare	Drive	Stare
Jiang et al. [23]	0.932	0.929	0.891	0.901	0.83	0.857	0.9	0.9
Niemeijer et al. [13]	0.93	–	0.942	–	0.689	–	0.969	–
Staal et al. [22]	0.952	0.961	0.944	0.952	0.719	0.697	0.977	0.981
Ricci et al. [15]	0.955	0.96	0.959	0.965	0.775	0.903	0.972	0.939
Roychowdhury et al. [10]	0.967	0.967	0.949	0.956	0.739	0.732	0.978	0.984
Liskowski et al. [1]	0.973	0.982	0.925	0.931	0.916	0.931	0.924	0.93
Yan et al. [2]	0.975	0.98	0.954	0.961	0.765	0.758	0.981	0.985
Zhang et al. [24]	0.977	–	0.965	–	0.731	–	0.988	–
Kromm et al. [25]	0.975	–	0.955	–	0.765	–	0.982	–
Ghosh et al. [20]	0.93	0.92	0.929	0.928	0.925	0.903	0.929	0.93
Ghosh et al. [21]	–	–	0.940	–	0.780	–	0.956	–
Proposed method								
	0.968	0.974	0.931	0.933	0.929	0.927	0.932	0.935

in Specificity for both DRIVE and STARE datasets as compared to our proposed approach. Additionally, the AUC value is also important for evaluating any proposed solution. The AUC value determines the strength of a classifier to correctly classify the input data. From Table 1, it can be observed that the highest AUC value has been obtained by the work done by Zhang et al. and Liskowski et al. for DRIVE and STARE datasets, respectively. Our achieved AUC value can be observed to be comparable with the state-of-the-art AUC results for both the datasets. The lower AUC can be attributed to the fact that our proposed model is smaller in structure and trainable parameters compared to other Deep Learning models. The smaller structure enables the model to be executed efficiently in reasonable time on a low-cost system.

4 Conclusion

The algorithm proposed in this work is based on the principle of Region Partitioning of an input Fundus image into three regions, namely Optic Disc, High Contrast and Low Contrast regions. The partitioning of the regions is performed using a k-Means clustering algorithm for forming the three clusters corresponding to each region of the input Fundus image. After the separation of the regions, three Multi-scale Convolutional Neural Networks are individually used for final segmentation of the blood vessel pixels in the Fundus image. The use of the modified Convolutional Neural Network helps in segmenting the blood vessel pixels without the need for any handcrafted feature vectors and specific patch size. The proposed solution requires a low-cost system for deployment and execution while maintaining the performance standard with current state-of-the-art models.

References

1. Liskowski P, Krawiec K (2016) Segmenting retinal blood vessels with deep neural networks. IEEE Trans. Med. Imaging 35(11):2369–2380
2. Yan Z, Yang X, Cheng KTT (2018) Joint segment-level and pixel-wise losses for deep learning based retinal vessel segmentation. IEEE Trans Biomed Eng 65(9):1912–1923
3. Fraz MM et al (2012) Blood vessel segmentation methodologies in retinal images–a survey. Comput Methods Programs Biomed 108(1):407–433
4. Nguyen UTV, Bhuiyan A, Park LAF, Ramamohanarao K (2013) An effective retinal blood vessel segmentation method using multi-scale line detection. Pattern Recognit 46(3):703–715
5. Hoover A (2000) Locating blood vessels in retinal images by piecewise threshold probing of a matched filter response. IEEE Trans Med Imag 19(3):203–210
6. Mendonca AM, Campilho A (2006) Segmentation of retinal blood vessels by combining the detection of centerlines and morphological reconstruction. IEEE Trans Med Imag 25(9):1200–1213
7. Miri MS, Mahloojifar A (2011) Retinal image analysis using curvelet transform and multistructure elements morphology by reconstruction. IEEE Trans Biomed Eng 58(5):1183–1192
8. Vermeer KA, Vos FM, Lemij HG, Vossepoel AM (2004) A model based method for retinal blood vessel detection. Comput Biol Med 34(3):209–219
9. Lam BSY, Gao Y, Liew AW-C (2010) General retinal vessel segmentation using regularization-based multiconcavity modeling. IEEE Trans Med Imag 29(7):1369–1381
10. Roychowdhury S, Koozekanani DD, Parhi KK (2015) Iterative vessel segmentation of fundus images. IEEE Trans Biomed Eng 62(7):1738–1749
11. Budai A, Michelson G, Hornegger J (2010) Multiscale blood vessel segmentation in retinal fundus images. Bild für die Medizin 261–265
12. Palomera-Perez MA, Martinez-Perez ME, Benitez-Perez H, Ortega-Arjona JL (2010) Parallel multiscale feature extraction and region growing: application in retinal blood vessel detection. IEEE Trans Inf Technol Biomed 14(2):500–506
13. Niemeijer M, Staal J, van Ginneken B, Loog M, Abramoff MD (2004) Comparative study of retinal vessel segmentation methods on a new publicly available database, p 648
14. Soares JVB, Leandro JJG, Cesar RM, Jelinek HF, Cree MJ (2006) Retinal vessel segmentation using the 2-D Gabor wavelet and supervised classification. IEEE Trans Med Imag 25(9):1214–1222
15. Ricci E, Perfetti R (2007) Retinal blood vessel segmentation using line operators and support vector classification. IEEE Trans Med Imag 26(10):1357–1365
16. Marín D, Aquino A, Gegúndez-Arias ME, Bravo JM (2011) A new supervised method for blood vessel segmentation in retinal images by using gray-level and moment invariants-based features. IEEE Trans Med Imag 30(1):146–158
17. Fraz MM et al (2012) An ensemble classification-based approach applied to retinal blood vessel segmentation. IEEE Trans Biomed Eng 59(9):2538–2548
18. Lupascu CA, Tegolo D, Trucco E (2010) FABC: retinal vessel segmentation using AdaBoost. IEEE Trans Inf Technol Biomed 14(5):1267–1274
19. Orlando JI, Prokofyeva E, Blaschko MB (2017) A discriminatively trained fully connected conditional random field model for blood vessel segmentation in fundus images. IEEE Trans Biomed Eng 64(1):16–27

20. Ghosh S, Kundu M, Nasipuri M (2021) Retinal vessel segmentation in fundus image using low-cost multiple U-net architecture. In: 2nd international symposium on computer vision and machine intelligence in medical image analysis (ISCMM), November 2021 (Accepted and Presented)
21. Ghosh S, Kundu M, asipuri M (2021) Retinal blood vessel segmentation using a multi-scale layer in deep learning. In: 2021 IEEE 18th India council international conference (INDICON), pp 1–6. https://doi.org/10.1109/INDICON52576.2021.9691545
22. Staal J, Abrámoff MD, Niemeijer M, Viergever MA, van Ginneken B (2004) Ridge-based vessel segmentation in color images of the retina. IEEE Trans Med Imag 23(4):501–9
23. Jiang X, Mojon D (2003) Adaptive local thresholding by verification-based multithreshold probing with application to vessel detection in retinal images. IEEE Trans Pattern Anal Mach Intell 25(1):131–137
24. Zhang M, Li W, Chen D (2019) Blood vessel segmentation in fundus images based on improved loss function. In: 2019 Chinese automation congress (CAC), pp 4017–4021
25. Kromm C, Rohr K (2020) Inception capsule network for retinal blood vessel segmentation and centerline extraction. In: 2020 IEEE 17th international symposium on biomedical imaging (ISBI), pp 1223–1226
26. Martinez-Perez ME, Hughes AD, Thom SA, Bharath AA, Parker KH (2007) Segmentation of blood vessels from red-free and fluorescein retinal images. Med Image Anal 11(1):47–61
27. Zana F, Klein J-C (2001) Segmentation of vessel-like patterns using mathematical morphology and curvature evaluation. IEEE Trans Image Process 10(7):1010–1019
28. Lam BSY, Yan H (2008) A novel vessel segmentation algorithm for pathological retina images based on the divergence of vector fields. IEEE Trans Med Imag 27(2):237–246
29. Budai A, Bock R, Maier A, Hornegger J, Michelson G (2013) Robust vessel segmentation in fundus images. Int J Biomed Imaging 2013:1–11
30. Roychowdhury S, Koozekanani DD, Parhi KK (2014) DREAM: diabetic retinopathy analysis using machine learning. IEEE J Biomed Heal Inf 18(5):1717–1728
31. Ronneberger O, Fischer P, Brox T (2015) U-Net: convolutional networks for biomedical image segmentation

MsMED-Net: An Optimized Multi-scale Mirror Connected Encoder-Decoder Network for Multilingual Natural Scene Text Recognition

Kalpita Dutta, Shuvayan Ghosh Dastidar, Mahantapas Kundu, Mita Nasipuri, and Nibaran Das

Abstract End-to-end multi-script text recognition from natural scene text images is a difficult task as compared to document text recognition due to the complex background semantics, distinct font style of multilingual data, and fancy font style with low-quality images. Multilingual text recognition in the natural scene can be divided into three distinct tasks: (a) text localization, (b) script identification, and (c) text recognition. The proposed text localization part involves fine-tuning using a multi-scale mirror connection-based encoder-decoder network (MsMED-Net) by replacing the Adam optimizer with the experimentally selected diffGrad optimizer to segment each text pixel correctly. The MsMED-Net outperforms the other popular deep semantic segmentation algorithms for the same task. The detected regions contain three different languages. Local and global feature learning by InceptionNet-V3 with MISH activation function model is applied to identify the script of the detected portions. Finally, Tesseract OCR version-4 is applied to the identified scripts to recognize them. The text recognition part involves fine-tuning Tesseract 4 by applying pre-processing steps to the input data and training the Tesseract with our new camera captured data set. The proposed method is tested on a new camera captured multilingual natural scene text data set entitle JUDVLP-MNSITextdb.v1 (multilingual natural scene Indic text data set) text data set. The data set contains 700 multilingual (Bengali, English, Hindi) text images with their ground truth showing encouraging results.

Keywords Text localization · Text recognition · Diffgrad optimizer · Multilingual scene text data set · Tesseract OCR

K. Dutta (✉) · S. G. Dastidar · M. Kundu · M. Nasipuri · N. Das
CMATER Department of CSE, Jadavpur University, Kolkata, India
e-mail: dutta.kalpita@gmail.com

M. Nasipuri
e-mail: mita.nasipuri@jadavpuruniversity.in

N. Das
e-mail: nibaran@ieee.org

© The Author(s), under exclusive license to Springer Nature Singapore Pte Ltd. 2023
J. K. Mandal and D. De (eds.), *Frontiers of ICT in Healthcare*, Lecture Notes in Networks and Systems 519, https://doi.org/10.1007/978-981-19-5191-6_57

1 Introduction

In a multi-script environment, end-to-end text recognition is a difficult task. Text localization and script identification are essential prior to end-to-end multi-script recognition. In the last decade, many research studies were carried out in the domain of text localization [1], multi-script identification [2–4], and end-to-end recognition [5, 6]. Recently, many end-to-end text recognition methods have focused on the oriented and curved text [6, 7], this significantly improves the performance of those on a single script rather than a multilingual text. End-to-end recognition from multilingual natural scene text images using deep learning-based method has attracted the attention of researchers in the recent past years. Few samples of our camera captured JUDVLP-MNSITextdb.v1 are shown in Fig. 1. Apart from different writing style of the multi-script with fancy font style, natural scene text may include some haze affects illustrated in Fig. 2 with few sample images taken from camera captured multilingual natural scene Indic text data set.

1.1 Past Works

Busta et al. [5] presented scene text localization and recognition in a single end-to-end framework, which simultaneously localize and recognize text in the input image. YOLOv2 architecture is used with 18 convolution layers, 5 max pool layers based on 3 × 3 kernel, and double the number of channels after each pooling operation.

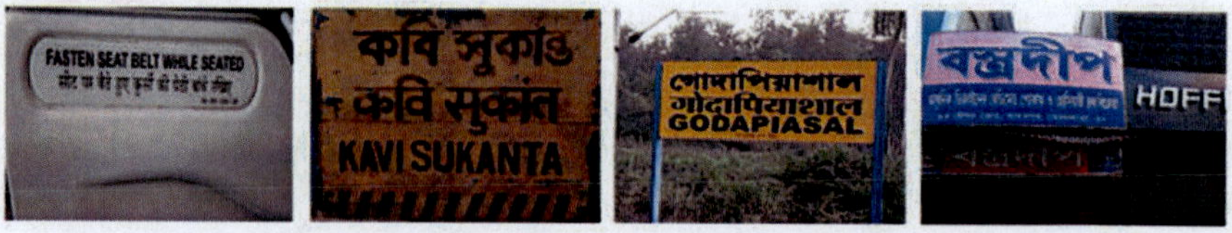

Fig. 1 Few samples of camera captured multilingual natural scene text images

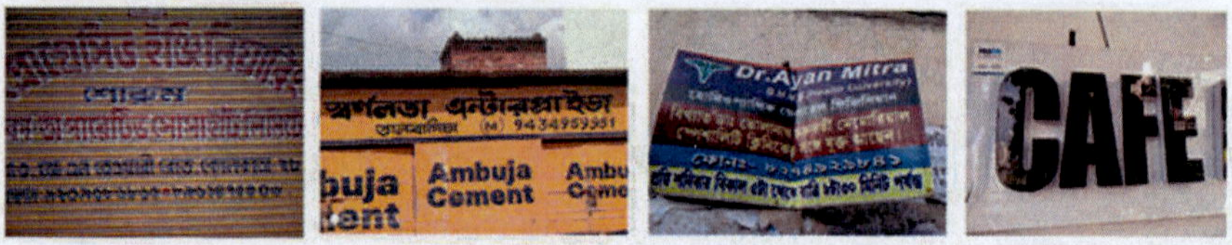

a b c d

Fig. 2 Few samples of difficult input images taken from camera captured multilingual natural scene text data set, **a** contains complex background, **b** has some shadow effects, **c** has difficult text area, and **d** has different light effects

YOLOv2 allows to process images with higher resolution and it helps to recognize the text region. Region proposal network (RPN) is used to generate regions with addition of a rotation value for accurate recognition. The detected regions with different rotated angle and different size are mapped in a fixed size by using faster R-CNN with ROI pooling approach to amp the feature vector into a canonical dimension tensor. It is useful for text recognition task. Finally, a fully convolutional neural network is trained to recognize text. Li et al. [8] proposed a deep learning-based end-to-end text recognition model using a two-stage framework. ROI pooling operation is used to joint detection and recognition task. But all the previous methods are focused on horizontal text. In the work of zhan et al. [7], an end-to-end iterative rectification model is developed to remove perspective distortion and text line curvature to improve the performance of curved scene text recognition. End-to-end scene text recognition system can rectify scene text distortions iteratively. A rectification network corrects curvature distortions of the text, and then the rectified image is fed to a recognition network for text recognition. A unique line-fitting transformation is employed by the iterative rectification network. Any extra annotation of fitting lines is not required for training the localization network because it is completely derived from the gradients which are back-propagated from the recognition network. In the work of liu et al. [6], an attempt has been made an effective and simple end-to-end framework for recognize curved scene text by using Adaptive Bezier Curve Network. Curved text is represented by parameterized Bezier curve and a feature alignment layer or BezierAlign is incorporated with the network to accurately calculate convolutional features of text line instances in a curved shape text.

1.2 Motivation

One major focus of all these recent research efforts is developing end-to-end text recognition by using different deep learning-based models. In this context, a pipeline can recognize multilingual scripts from natural scene text images by combining three tasks (text localization, script identification, and recognition). For text localization, the multi-scale mirror connection-based encoder-decoder network (MsMED-Net) [9] model with diffGrad optimizer [10] is trained to classify each image pixel as text or non-text. MsMED-Net is trained to encode the input image through several intermediate layers of transformation and then to decode it in a way that each pixel in the decoded images is represented with a '1' for the text and '0' for non-text. To boost this network performance, experimentally selected diffGrad optimizer is used to further optimize the network. Confirms the observation, diffGrad performs better than other optimizer like Adam, SGD, AdaDelta, RMSProp, AMSGrad, made by dubey et al. [10]. Different optimizer learning rate computation rules are different described in Table 1. It is a gradient descent optimization technique that considers the local gradient change information between two consecutive iterations, containing updated gradient information in a small time span. It is used to regulate the rate of

Table 1 Different optimization methods

Optimizer	Specification
SGD	1. Update all parameters with the same learning rate
SGDM	1. It is an extended version of SGD with momentum
	2. Incorporates the past gradients in each dimension
	3. In each dimension, SGDM maintains momentum
	4. Want to achieve a high velocity with a accurate gradient in any dimension
	5. It can solve the jittering problem by reducing the high velocity, and by using the past gradient, saddle point problem is reduced
AdaGrad	1. It can deal with sparse data
	2. AdaGrad performs more significant updates for infrequent parameters; as a result, the magnitude of gradients is smaller
	3. It also performs minor updates for frequent parameters; as a result, the magnitude of gradients increases
	4. The learning rate may turn slower for the monotonically increasing sum of squaring the gradient after some iteration kill the learning process
AdaDelta	1. Solve the dying learning problem of AdaGrad
	2. It collects the square of previous gradients but only includes a few recent past gradients rather than all previous gradients
RMSProp	1. Similar to AdaDelta, it corrects the diminishing learning rate of AdaGrad
	2. RMSProp uses a learning rate, but AdaDelta does not use any learning rate
Adam	1. Each parameter's learning rate computation is adaptive, and it uses both first and second moments
	2. Like other optimization tasks like SGDM by decaying the average of past gradient as the first moment, similar to AdaDelta and RMSProp. AdaDelta and RMSProp decay the average of squares of past gradients as a second moment
	3. It performs better than other adaptive optimizers
AMSGrad	1. It updates the parameter by considering the maximum of the past second moment of past gradients as "long-term memory"
	2. To avoid the overshooting of the minimum, it imposes more friction
	3. Learning rate cannot be changed based on current gradient behaviour and does not handle the saddle point issue
DiffGrad	1. It overcomes the problem of AMSGrad and Adam by controlling the learning rate based on gradient change with "short-term gradient behaviour"
	2. DiffGrad incorporates the immediate past gradient information, but Adam does not utilize it

learning based on the optimization stage for each cycle. Then, the trained model Inception net V3 with MISH [4] is used to classify the detected text image into their specific script class, Bengali, Hindi, and English. Finally, for the recognition part, the Tesseract OCR version 4 [11] is trained to classify a word image in a word class represented with ASCII values of its constituent characters.

The remaining portion of this paper is structured as follows: The proposed approach has been described in Sect. 2. The data set preparation and description,

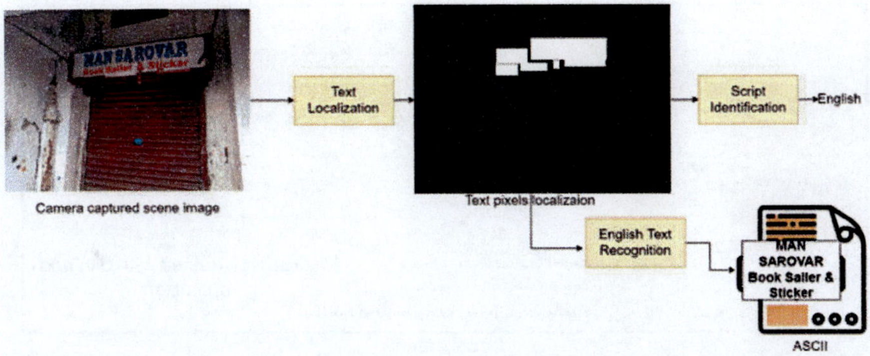

Fig. 3 Pictorial representation of the end-to-end text recognition task

experimental results, and comparative results analysis of the proposed work are presented in Sect. 3. Finally, the work is concluded, and the future scope is discussed in Sect. 4.

1.3 Contribution

- The significant contributions of this work come from making an end-to-end multi-script natural scene text recognition methodology indicated in Fig. 3 which is subdivided into three steps, localization, script identification, and recognition.
- The algorithm is applied on our camera captured multilingual natural scene text data set (JUDVLP-MNSITextdb.v1).
- The methodology to learn multi-scale features through fine-tuning MsMED-Net with diffGrad optimizer has achieved satisfactory results. And we have compared the results with other semantic segmentation models. Then, classify localized crop word using pretrained model Inception net V3 with MISH.
- Finally, Tesseract with LSTM is trained to recognize text from scene text images. Our primary focus is on localization tasks to improve recognition.

2 Proposed Methodology

The methodology demonstrates in Fig. 4. JUDVLP-MNSITextdb.v1 images are supplied as input in the MsMED-Net model optimized with diffGrad optimizer. This model classifies each pixel as a text or non-text pixel, by considering the maximum of the sums of the weighted probability values. By using mirror skip connection, find better feature re-usability and faster convergence of the learning process. Outputs

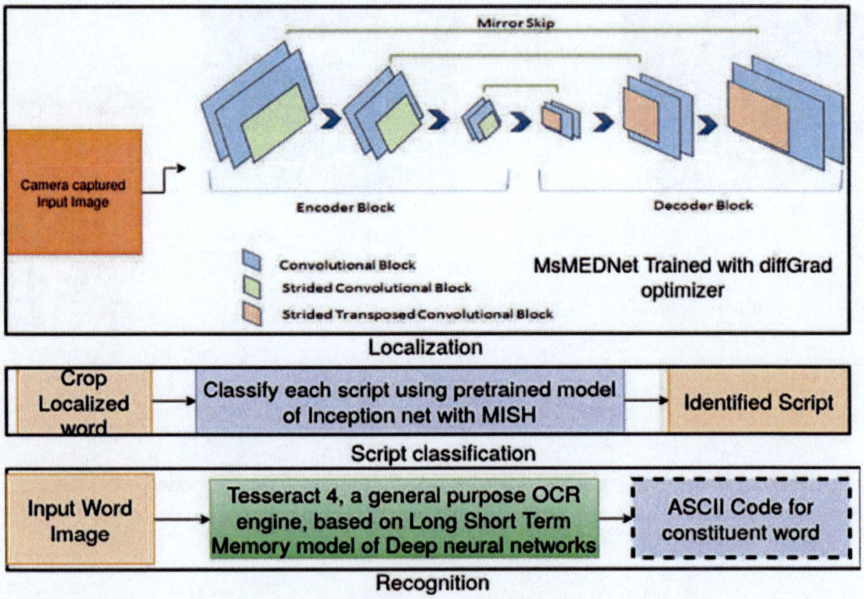

Fig. 4 Intermediate network diagram of the end-to-end text recognition

from this models (linear, parametric, and convolutional) trained on various kernel sizes ($3 \times 3, 5 \times 5, 7 \times 7$) are combined. The segmented images are generated using the localization model. Then by finding the connectivity of the segmented text region, draw rectangular bounding box over each text word. After cropping each segmented text words, the text words are classified into specific script using pretrained model of Inception net V3 with MISH activation function [4]. Finally, the identified script (Bengali, English, and Hindi) is passed as an input to the trained Tesseract OCR engine version 4 model [11]. Available Tesseract 4 is basically trained on document text data set. In this paper, we have trained the Tesseract 4 model with natural scene text word data for each script (Bengali, English, and Hindi). DiffGrad optimizer controls the learning rate by using a diffGrad friction coefficient (DFC) [10]. DFC (ξ) for jth parameter in kth iteration is defined as

$$\xi_{k,j} = \text{AbsSig}\left(\Delta g_{k,j}\right) \tag{1}$$

where a nonlinear sequence function is AbsSig and the computed gradient is $g_{k,j}$ for jth parameter in kth iteration. AbsSig maps all values between 0.5 and 1 and described as

$$\text{AbsSig}(x) = \frac{1}{1 + e^{-|x|}} \tag{2}$$

$\Delta g_{k,j}$ is gradient change between current iteration and its immediate past iteration. It is defined as

$$\Delta g_{k,j} = g_{k-1,j} - g_{k,j} \tag{3}$$

The diffGrad optimizer changes the jth parameter at the kth iteration using the given equation

$$\theta_{k+1,j} = \theta_{k,j} - \frac{\alpha_t \times \xi_{k,j} \times \hat{m}_{k,j}}{\sqrt{\hat{v}_{k,j}} + \epsilon} \tag{4}$$

where weight value is $\theta_{k+1,j}$, learning rate is α_k, a small ϵ value is added, $\xi_{k,j}$ is DFC, and saddle regions are $\hat{v}_{k,j}$ and $\hat{m}_{k,j}$. DFC allows the step size with sufficient magnitude due to high moment gained. So, the diffGrad emerges from flat saddle regions and flat local optima.

The recognition task is executed by using Tesseract, an open source OCR engine [12, 13], which was developed by HP. Now, it is maintained and developed by Google. Tesseract version 4 [11] incorporates a new neural network-based subsystem long short-term memory (LSTM), configured as a text line recognizer.

2.1 Data set Preparation

JUDVLP-MNSITextdb.v1 consists of three Indian languages, like Bengali, English, and Hindi. This data set contains 700 fully annotated data. The ground truth contains word-wise annotation of the text portion, each word is localized with a bounding box with their respective script name and recognized word. The data set images are mostly shop heading, different advertisement posters, road signs, advertisements written on the bus or car, car or bus number plate, object labels and banners, etc., different texts present in the wild presented in Fig. 1. The images are captured using an Android mobile device. At the time of image collection, maintains some image capturing protocols are

- Maintain the front view of the images.
- The image should contain at least 70% text portion.
- Most of the image has captured in the day light.

Some previously available data sets with single script (English) are ICDAR 2015 [14], ICDAR 2017 [15] or COCO text data set, Google street view data set (SVT) [16], KAIST [17]. ICDAR 2019 [18] robust reading challenge was conducted a challenge on multilingual scene text data set (Fig. 5).

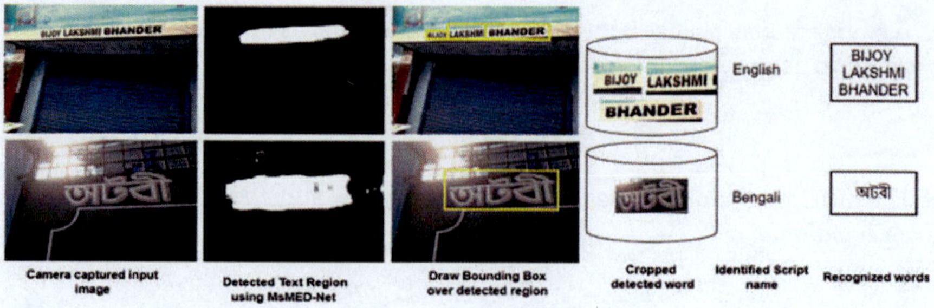

Fig. 5 Few sample results of the end-to-end text recognition task

2.2 *Experiments*

The proposed work is compiled on our camera captured multilingual scene text image mentioned above. Bengali, English, and Hindi three Indian scripts are included in this data set. The proposed method is implemented here in PyTorch and MATLAB. For the text localization part, the input images are resized with the size 512×512. Training is done for 200 epochs, with diffGrad optimizer and loss is calculated with cross entropy loss with learning rate 0.001. Optimization controls the learning rate and convergence the network performance. Performances of the model are tested on various semantic segmentation model indicated in Table 4. It can be observed from Table 4 that models optimize with diffGrad optimizer performs better than other models with Adam optimizer. The detailed performances of the MsMED-Net with diffGrad optimizer indicated in Table 2. Bounding boxes are drawn over the segmented text pixel regions and crop those text word region. To classify those script of the crop word, apply pre-trained Inception net V3 with MISH model [4]. Each script is classified and passed

Table 2 Text localization using encoder-decoder network with diffGrad optimizer applied on camera captured multilingual natural scene text data set

Model	Kernel size	Mirror skip	Precision	Recall	F-score
L3	3×3	Linear	0.6392	0.7384	0.7016
L5	5×5	Linear	0.4793	0.6141	0.3069
L7	7×7	Linear	0.4324	0.6227	0.5104
P3	3×3	Parametric	0.5771	0.6505	0.5988
P5	5×5	Parametric	0.6254	0.9782	0.4051
P7	7×7	Parametric	0.6509	0.7027	0.6744
C3	3×3	Convolutional	0.6948	0.7096	0.7011
C5	5×5	Convolutional	0.5344	0.6080	0.5688
C7	7×7	Convolutional	0.5271	0.6252	0.5720
Overall mean	–	–	59.78	61.82	69.61

Table 3 Text localization results of different models applied on camera captured multilingual natural scene text data set

Models	Accuracy	Precision	Recall	F-score	Dice score	IOU
SegNet with Adam	67.25	47.24	68.05	55.76	63.58	48.27
SegNet with diffGrad	69.58	49.30	67.49	57.53	64.94	49.81
UNet with Adam	75.49	63.50	70.04	66.61	70.32	56.68
UNet with diffGrad	78.54	68.40	66.45	67.41	72.64	60.10
PSPNet with Adam	78.92	67.47	57.66	62.18	72.55	59.60
PSPNnet with diffGrad	80.15	56.37	62.35	71.03	59.21	59.61
DeepLab with Adam	74.97	58.25	58.90	58.57	67.55	54.35
DeepLab with diffGrad	74.99	59.48	56.13	67.88	57.23	53.99
MsMED-Net with Adam	75.27	52.20	53.76	52.96	64.16	52.08
MsMED-Net with diffGrad	80.95	59.78	61.82	69.61	65.17	52.43

Table 4 Recognition results on camera captured multilingual natural scene text data set using Tesseract OCR 4

Language	English		Bengali	
Accuracy	Without training	With training	Without training	With training
	47.97	75.79	32.86	60.91

as an input image patch for the trained Tesseract OCR 4. The Tesseract 4 is trained using natural scene text word patch with 10,00,000 iterations with PSM value 7 and learning rate 0.0001. The performance of trained model of Tesseract and without trained model is indicated in Table 4. The performance of trained model outperforms without trained model of Tesseract OCR engine 4 (Table 3).

3 Conclusion and Future Scope

This paper has proposed an end-to-end multilingual script recognition approach. Text localization is performed by fine-tuning MsMED-Net using diffGrad optimizer. Experiments have been performed in our camera captured JUDVLP-MNSITextdb.v1 data set. MsMED-Net with diffGrad optimizer reports better accuracy rates in comparison with a number of other well-known semantic segmentation methods. DiffGrad is found to boost the text localization performance. The localization results contain both small and large text regions with the help of multi-scale property of MsMED-Net network. The next step of script identification by pre-trained model of learning local and global script specific features using Inception net V3 with MISH activation function improves the result of recognition step. The last recognition step recognizes each script using trained model of Tesseract OCR 4. Training the Tesseract OCR 4 with individual script increases our recognition accuracy. In future, the rate of results can be increased by incorporating other novel approaches.

Acknowledgements This work was supported by Rashtriya Uchchatar Shiksha Abhiyan (RUSA) 2.0, Government of India, Ministry of Human Resource Development project.

References

1. Zhou X, Yao C, Wen H, Wang Y, Zhou S, He W, Liang J (2017) East: an efficient and accurate scene text detector. In: Proceedings of the IEEE conference on computer vision and pattern recognition, pp 5551–5560
2. Bhunia AK, Konwer A, Bhunia AK, Bhowmick A, Roy PP, Pal U (2019) Script identification in natural scene image and video frames using an attention based convolutional-lSTM network. Pattern Recogn 85:172–184
3. Dastidar SG, Dutta K, Das N, Kundu M, Nasipuri M (2021) Exploring knowledge distillation of a deep neural network for multi-script identification. In: International conference on computational intelligence in communications and business analytics. Springer, pp 150–162
4. Dutta K, Ghosh Dastidar S, Das N, Kundu M, Nasipuri M (2021) Script identification in natural scene text images by learning local and global features on inception net. In: 6th IAPR international conference on computer vision and image processing (CVIP 2021). Spinger (Accepted and Presented)
5. Busta M, Neumann L, Matas J (2017) Deep textspotter: an end-to-end trainable scene text localization and recognition framework. In: Proceedings of the IEEE international conference on computer vision, pp 2204–2212
6. Liu Y, Chen H, Shen C, He T, Jin L, Wang L (2020) Abcnet: real-time scene text spotting with adaptive bezier-curve network. In: Proceedings of the IEEE/CVF conference on computer vision and pattern recognition, pp 9809–9818
7. Zhan F, Lu S (2019) ESIR: end-to-end scene text recognition via iterative image rectification. In: Proceedings of the IEEE/CVF conference on computer vision and pattern recognition, pp 2059–2068
8. Li H, Wang P, Shen C (2017) Towards end-to-end text spotting with convolutional recurrent neural networks. In: Proceedings of the IEEE international conference on computer vision, pp 5238–5246
9. Dutta K, Bal M, Basak A, Ghosh S, Das N, Kundu M, Nasipuri M (2020) Multi scale mirror connection based encoder decoder network for text localization. Pattern Recogn Lett 135:64–71
10. Dubey SR, Chakraborty S, Roy SK, Mukherjee S, Singh SK, Chaudhuri BB (2019) Diffgrad: an optimization method for convolutional neural networks. IEEE Trans Neural Netw Learn Syst 31(11):4500–4511
11. Tesseract(1) manual page. https://github.com/tesseract-ocr/tesseract/wiki/TrainingTesseract-4.00. Accessed on 26 Jan 2022
12. Patel C, Patel A, Patel D (2012) Optical character recognition by open source ocr tool tesseract: a case study. Int J Comput Appl 55(10):50–56
13. Smith R (2007) An overview of the tesseract ocr engine. In: Ninth international conference on document analysis and recognition (ICDAR 2007), vol 2. IEEE, pp 629–633
14. Karatzas D, Gomez-Bigorda L, Nicolaou A, Ghosh S, Bagdanov A, Iwamura M, Matas J, Neumann L, Chandrasekhar VR, Lu S, et al (2015) Icdar 2015 competition on robust reading. In: 2015 13th international conference on document analysis and recognition (ICDAR). IEEE, pp 1156–1160

15. Grüning T, Labahn R, Diem M, Kleber F, Fiel S (2018) Read-bad: a new dataset and evaluation scheme for baseline detection in archival documents. In: 2018 13th IAPR international workshop on document analysis systems (DAS). IEEE, pp 351–356
16. Wang T, Wu DJ, Coates A, Ng AY (2012) End-to-end text recognition with convolutional neural networks. In: Proceedings of the 21st international conference on pattern recognition (ICPR2012). IEEE, pp 3304–3308
17. Choi Y, Kim N, Hwang S, Park K, Yoon JS, An K, Kweon IS (2018) Kaist multi-spectral day/night data set for autonomous and assisted driving. IEEE Trans Intell Transp Syst 19(3):934–948
18. Nayef N, Patel Y, Busta M, Chowdhury PN, Karatzas D, Khlif W, Matas J, Pal U, Burie JC, Liu Cl et al (2019) Icdar2019 robust reading challenge on multi-lingual scene text detection and recognition—RRC-MLT-2019. In: 2019 international conference on document analysis and recognition (ICDAR). IEEE, pp 1582–1587

Author Index

© The Editor(s) (if applicable) and The Author(s), under exclusive license to Springer Nature Singapore Pte Ltd. 2023

J. K. Mandal and D. De (eds.), *Frontiers of ICT in Healthcare*, Lecture Notes in Networks and Systems 519, https://doi.org/10.1007/978-981-19-5191-6